HUMAN PAPILLOMAVIRUS AND RELATED DISEASES – FROM BENCH TO BEDSIDE

RESEARCH ASPECTS

Edited by **Davy Vanden Broeck**

Human Papillomavirus and Related Diseases – From Bench to Bedside – Research Aspects
Edited by Davy Vanden Broeck

Published by InTech

Janeza Trdine 9, 51000 Rijeka, Croatia

Publishing Process Manager Ivona Lovric

Technical Editor Teodora Smiljanic

Cover Designer InTech Design Team

Additional hard copies can be obtained from orders@intechopen.com

Human Papillomavirus and Related Diseases – From Bench to Bedside
– Research Aspects, Edited by Davy Vanden Broeck
p. cm.
ISBN 978-953-307-855-7

For EU product safety concerns:
IN TECH d.o.o., Prolaz Marije Krucifikse Kozulić 3, 51000 Rijeka, Croatia,
info@intechopen.com or visit our website at intechopen.com.

Meet the editor

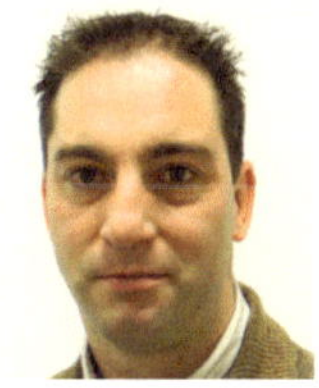

Professor Dr Davy Vanden Broeck, MSc, PhD, obtained his MSc degree in Biochemistry from Antwerp University, in Belgium, with judicium Cum Laude. Afterwards, he pursued a PhD in Biomedical Sciences at Antwerp University. Later, he joined the International Centre for Reproductive Health (ICRH) and dedicated his research efforts on the focus of sexually transmitted viruses. Finally, he obtained two consecutive post-doc grants at Ghent University in Ghent, Belgium, with a specific focus on papilloma virus research. Currently, Dr Vanden Broeck holds the position of professor of Molecular Virology and heads the ICRH HPV/cervical cancer research team. Within this team, multi-disciplinary research is performed on the prevention of cervical cancer (vaccine, screening), as well as clinical/translational aspects of cervical cancer research, with equally fundamental research forming a part of the research agenda.

Contents

Preface

Cervical cancer is the second most prevalent cancer among women worldwide, mainly affecting young women. Infection with Human Papilloma Virus (HPV) has been identified as the causal agent for this condition. The natural history of cervical cancer is characterized by slow disease progression, generally taking over 10 years, from the initial infection with HPV, to the diagnosis of cancer. In essence, cervical cancer is a preventable disease, and treatable if diagnosed in early stage. Historically, the introduction of the Pap smear has markedly reduced the number of new cases in countries with an effective prevention program. The burden of disease is highest in developing countries, with peak incidence in Eastern Africa. Recently, prophylactic vaccines became available, equally contributing to a better disease prevention. Unfortunately, the global burden of disease is still very high.

Cervical cancer research is a multidisciplinary matter, combining efforts of clinicians (gynaecologists, pathologists, clinical chemists), epidemiologists, fundamental scientists, and sociologists. In this book, focus has been put on research and fundamental aspects of HPV related research. Section 1 is titled: Epidemiology of Human Papillomavirus and Cervical Lesions. In this section, epidemiological data per age group are presented, and data that has been collected in asymptomatic women are equally included. In the second section, translation of fundamental findings into novel HPV diagnostic and treatment options are summarized. Molecular biology has found its way into this field and created many new possibilities, comprising molecular biomarkers, and allowing more accurate diagnosis and targeted treatment. The final section outlines recent advances in fundamental HPV research. New insights on the role of ion channels and the cytoskeleton are presented. Furthermore, signal pathways in carcinogenesis are dissected, as well as immunological implications in the carcinogenic transformation. Among the novelties in fundamental research, Dr. Maramis and co-workers have developed software allowing automation of HPV genotyping assays. In addition, new molecular biological tools in the diagnosis and treatment of cervical cancer are included, next to the development of a research tool to investigate the cellular uptake of the HPV virus.

This book will be a useful tool for both researchers and clinicians dealing with cervical cancer, and will provide them with the latest information in this field.

Prof. Dr. Davy Vanden Broeck, MSc, PhD.
Team leader HPV/Cervical Cancer Research
International Centre for Reproductive Health
Ghent University
Belgium

Acknowledgements

The editor of this book would like to express sincere thanks to all authors for their high quality contributions. The editor expresses the gratefulness to Ms. Bojana Zelenika and Ms. Ivona Lovric, process managers, for their continued cooperation.

Part 1

Epidemiology of Human Papillomavirus and Cervical Lesions

1

Epidemiology of Mucosal Human Papillomavirus (HPV) Infections Among Adult and Children

Helen Trottier
Sainte-Justine University Hospital Research Center
Department of Social and Preventive Medicine, University of Montreal
Canada

1. Introduction

Human papillomavirus (HPV) infection is recognized today as the main causal factor for ~100% of cervical cancer cases in the world and of a substantial proportion of many other anogenital neoplasms (anal, vaginal, vulvar, and penile cancer). HPV is also implicated in the genesis of several other cancers, such as head and neck (oral cavity, pharynx, and larynx) cancer and non-melanoma skin cancer and is suspected also to play a causal role in the genesis of a few other neoplasms (Trottier et al, 2009). The epidemiology of mucosal human papillomavirus (HPV) as been well studied today, especially cervicovaginal HPV infection among young women and there are also more available epidemiologic data for older women, men and as well as for children. HPV infection is the most common sexually transmitted infections in the world. The predominant route of transmission is via sexual contact, although vertical and horizontal transmissions also occur. This chapter will review the epidemiology of mucosal HPV infections affecting genital, oral and conjunctival mucosa in adults and children. This chapter will detail the epidemiology of HPV in adult considering young versus older population rather than focussing on adolescent and adult populations separately because there is no universal cut-off age group to define high risk population as HPV is highly dependant on the onset of sexual activity.

2. Classification and carcinogenicity of HPVs

More than 100 HPV genotypes have been catalogued so far and can be classified according to the phylogenetics in genera and species (De Villiers et al, 2004) (table 1). The L1 protein is highly conserved among all HPV genotypes and is thus used for taxonomical purposes. Different genera of the Papillomaviridae (Alpha, Beta, etc.) share less than 60% nucleotide sequence identity in the L1 protein whereas species within a genus share between 60% and 70% nucleotide identity. A new HPV isolate is recognized as a new genotype when the nucleotide sequence of the L1 gene differs by more than 10% from the genotype with which it has greatest homology in DNA sequence.

Papillomaviruses can also be classified according to their tissue tropism (mucosal or cutaneous) and oncogenic potential (table 2) (De Villiers et al, 2004). Although it is possible

Genus	Species	Genotypes of HPV
Alpha-papillomavirus	Alpha-1	42
	Alpha-2	3, 10, 28,29, 77, 78, 94
	Alpha-3	61, c62, 72, 81, 83, c87, c86, c89, 84,
	Alpha-4	2, 27, 57
	Alpha-5	26, 51, 69, 82
	Alpha-6	30, 53, 56, 66
	Alpha-7	18, 45, 59, c85, 39, 68, 70
	Alpha-8	7, 40, 43, c91
	Alpha-9	16, 31, 33, 35, 52, 58, 67
	Alpha-10	6, 11, 13, 44, 55, 74
	Alpha-11	34, 73
	Alpha-12	RhPV1
	Alpha-13	54
	Alpha-14	c90
	Alpha-15	71
Beta-papillomavirus	Beta-1	5, 8, 12, 14, 19, 20, 21, 24, 25, 36, 47, 93
	Beta-2	9, 15, 17, 22, 23, 37, 80,
	Beta-3	38, 49, 75, 76
	Beta-4	92
	Beta-5	96
Gamma-papillomavirus	Gamma-1	4, 65, 95
	Gamma-2	50
	Gamma-3	48
	Gamma-4	60
	Gamma-5	88
Mu-papillomavirus	Mu-1	1
	Mu-2	63
Nu-papillomavirus	Nu	41

Adapted from De Villiers et al, 2004.

Table 1. Phylogenetics of Papillomaviridae affecting humans

to find all these genotypes in both mucosal and cutaneous tissue, they are classified according to their tissue tropism as shown in table 2. This chapter will focus on the genotypes of HPV that infect the epithelial lining of the anogenital tract and other mucosal areas of the body (mucosal HPV). There are over than 40 genotypes of HPV that infect human mucosal from which 13–25 genotypes have been identified as probable or definite high-oncogenic risk (HR-HPV) according to their frequency of association with cervical cancer and other anogenital cancers (review in Trottier et al, 2006; IARC 2007; IARC 2011). Although, the vast majority of infected people will clear mucosal HPV infections without any clinical consequences, its role in the pathogenesis of malignant tumours has been well described. HR-HPV is recognized unequivocally as the main causal factor for (~100%) cervical cancer, is responsible for a substantial proportion of many other (60-90 %) anogenital neoplasms (anal, vaginal, vulvar and penile cancers), and a non negligible portion (~30%) of head and neck cancers (oral cavity, pharynx, and larynx), and is suspected to play a causal role in many other neoplasms, such as conjunctiva carcinoma and lung cancer (Trottier et al, 2009). The latest classification published by the World Health Organization's International Agency for Research on Cancer (IARC) referred HPV-16, 18, 31, 33, 35, 39, 45, 51, 52, 56, 58, 59 as HR-HPVs (IARC, 2011). This classification included also many other genotypes as probably carcinogenic such as HPV genotypes 26, 30, 34, 53, 66, 67, 68, 69, 70, 73, 82, 85, 97. Infection with low-oncogenic risk HPVs (LR-HPV), such as HPV-6 and 11, can cause benign lesions of the anogenital areas known as *Condylomata acuminate* (genital warts), a large proportion of low-grade squamous intraepithelial lesions (LSIL) of the cervix, oral papillomas as well as conjunctival papillomas. HPV-6 or 11 may also cause in rare instance recurrent respiratory papillomatosis, which in infants and young children can be very morbid and usually perinatally transmitted (Armstrong et al. 2000) whereas in adult it is usually sexually transmitted and less severe than in children (Kashima et al, 1992).

Tissue tropism	Genotypes of HPV
Mucosal	High-risk: 16, 18, 31, 33, 35, 39, 45, 51, 52, 56, 58, 59 Low-risk (or probably carcinogenic): 6, 11, 13, 26, 30, 32, 34, 42, 44, 53, 54, 61, 62, 66, 67, 68, 69, 70, 71, 72, 73, 74, 81, 82, 83, 84, 85, 86, 87, 89, 90
Cutaneous	1, 2, 4, 5, 8, 9, 12 ,1 4, 15 ,17, 19, 20, 21, 22, 23, 25, 27, 36, 37, 38, 41, 47, 48, 49, 50, 57, 60, 63, 65, 75, 76, 80, 88, 92, 93, 95, 96
Both (mixte)	3, 7, 10, 28, 29, 40, 43, 78, 91, 94

Adapted from De Villiers et al, 2004. Carcinogenic potential classification based on IARC monograph, Vol 100B, 2009.

Table 2. Classifications of HPVs according to their tissue tropism and oncogenic potential

3. Mode of transmission of mucosal HPV

3.1 Predominant route of transmission is via sexual contact

There is a strong and consistent association between sexual activity and mucosal HPV infections (Winer et al 2008). The number of lifetime and recent partners is one of the strongest risk factors for prevalent infection as well as acquisition in adult (Trottier et al, 2006). Further data supporting sexual intercourse as the primary route of genital HPV infection include documented transmission of genital warts between sex partners, concordance in sex partners for genotype-specific HPV infection, the rarity of genital HPV infection in virgin women, and increased risk of HPV acquisition following new and recent sex partners (Winer et al, 2008; Winer et al, 2008b; Burchell et al, 2006). The practice of anal intercourse is also associated with HPV detection in the anal canal in men who have sex with men and to a lesser degree for women (Dunne et al, 2006; Moscicki et al, 1999). Transmission may also occur via other sexual practices, such as oral sex, digital-vaginal sex and use of insertive sex toys (Edwards et al, 1998; Sonnex et al, 1999; Gervaz et al, 2003). For example, oral sex may explain why husband of women with cervical cancer are at higher risk of upper aerodigestive track cancer (Hemminki et al, 2000). Studies on genital HPV infection between women who have sex with women also suggest the possibility of transmission between female sex partners (Marrazzo et al 2000). More studies are also available on the transmissibility of HPV; the evidence is that HPV is highly transmissible (Barnabas et al, 2006; Burchell et al, 2010). For example, Barnabas et al. (2006) estimated the per-partner male-to-female transmission probability as much as 60% for HPV-16.

3.2 Vertical transmission

Non-sexual routes of transmission are believed to be far less common, but possible. Transmission of HPV from mother to child (perinatal infection) was first reported in 1956 (Hajek, 1956) in a case of juvenile laryngeal papillomatosis (JLP). Confirmation of the perinatal transmission of HPV in different mucosa (genital, oral) was subsequently supported by several studies although the route of transmission is not well understood (Syrjänen et al, 2000). Direct maternal transmission during vaginal delivery or at caesarean section following early membrane rupture is possible as well as in utero through semen or ascending infection from mother's genital tract (Syrjänen et al, 2000; Favre et al, 1998). Transplancental transmission is also possible since HPV DNA has been detected by PCR in amniotic fluid of HPV positive pregnant women. HPV 16 DNA has also been found in cord blood cells. See section on children for an estimate of the probability of transmission of HPV at birth.

3.3 Horizontal transmission and other route

Horizontal transmission had also been reported; possible routes of infection are the fingers and mouth, fomites and skin contact outside sexual contact. For example, transmission from the anogenital region to hands is possible via self-inoculation (Hernandez et al, 2008). Although possible, this non-sexual route of transmission is also believed to be far less common than sexual contact route, especially in adult. Obviously, the horizontal route is more important in children (excluding sexually abused children) than the sexual route although vertical transmission do occurs. For example, the presence of oral HPV DNA is detected in buccal cavities of 19–35% of healthy children aged 6–11 years (Puranen et al, 1997; Summersgill et al, 2001; Kojima et al, 2003). Blood transmission of HPV as well as transmission via breast milk is implausible since HPV infection does not produce viremia (Cason et al, 2005).

4. Epidemiology of HPV infection in adult

4.1 Anogenital HPV infection in women

4.1.1 Prevalence, incidence, duration, co-infection and re-infection

There are many studies that have reported on cervical HPV epidemiology. Studies on the prevalence of HPV around the world show that the prevalence of cervical HPV infection ranges from 2 to 44%. This wide variation in the prevalence estimates is largely explained by the age and the region of the populations studied. Typically, HPV prevalence increases rapidly following the onset of sexual activity (highest prevalence occurs among young women / adolescent). In fact, cervicovaginal HPV infection is rarely observed among virgins, even among those who engage in sexual activity other than intercourse (Kjaer et al, 2001). The peak after sexual debut is usually followed by an age-related decline in prevalence, and occasionally a second but more modest peak in prevalence among older women.(~› 45 years) (Trottier et al, 2006). The prevalence of cervical HPV infection is estimated at 5.2%, 8.7%, 12.9%, 14.3% and 25.6% in Europe, Asia, North America, South America and Sub-Saharan Africa, respectively (Clifford et al., Lancet 2005, Burchell et al. 2006). HPV-16 is the most common genotype in all regions of the world except in Eastern Africa, Japan and Taiwan, where HPV 52 is the most frequent genotype but overall, the top ranked genotypes are HPVs 16, 18, 31, 58, and 52 (de Sanjosé et al, 2007). Coinfection with multiple HPV genotypes is also a very common finding of many epidemiologic studies. For example, among the cohort of Brazilian women, between 1.9% to 3.2% were co-infected with multiples genotypes at a same visit (concurrently infected) whereas when considering cumulatively (period prevalence) during the first year and the first 4 years of follow-up, 12.3% and 22.3% were infected with multiple genotypes, respectively (Trottier et al, 2006b). We also have to take into account that positivity for HPV is typically higher in cervicovaginal than in exclusively cervical specimens (Bauer et al; 1991).

The incidence of cervical HPV infections has also been well studied in many cohorts of young or college-aged women. These cohort studies have shown that the cumulative incidence of cervical HPV infection exceeded 40% after 3 years among women who were initially HPV negative at enrolment (Trottier et al, 2006). These studies also had shown that the cumulative incidence is higher for high risk genotypes than for low-risk genotypes. As with prevalence, incidence rates of HPV in women tend to decline with age, although second peaks are sometimes observed in older women. In fact, over 75% of sexually active women will contract HPV in their lifetime and its detection is strongly and consistently associated with the number of sexual partners. In most cases, HPV infection is transient or intermittent; only a very small proportion of cervical HPV infection will persist and progress toward cervical cancer (Schiffman et al, 2003). The median duration of cervical infection for any HPV genotype appears to range between 4 and 20 months (Trottier et al, 2006).

Recent evidence shown that re-infection with HPV (with a different or either a same genotype) is a common occurrence (Trottier et al, 2010). Prior infection with HPV does not provide women with adequate immunity against subsequent infections. In fact, serum antibody levels after natural HPV infection when detectable are low and 40-50% of women do not develop measurable antibody response after HPV natural infection (Viscidi et al, 2004; Nonnenmacher et al, 1995; Park et al, 1998; Heim et al, 2002; Skjeldestad et al, 2008). Moreover, it has been shown that an infection with a specific genotype does not decrease the probability of being infected by a phylogenetically-related genotype (Thomas et al, 2000). Recent studies have shown that re-infection with a same genotype, as well as incident infection in older women who had multiple lifetime sexual partners, are associated with new sexual partners suggesting that infection in adult women may results not only from reactivation (infections acquired at a young age that never completely cleared but become undetectable and appeared later in life) but also from new exposure via sexual activity (Trottier et al, 2010; Munoz et al, 2004).

Relatively little is known about the epidemiology of anal HPV infection in women compare to cervical infection. However the few studies that reported on anal HPV infection shown that it is very common (Goodman et al, 2008; 2010; Shvetsov et al, 2009). When both cervical and anal HPV testing is done, anal HPV is more common than cervical HPV (Williams et al, 1994; Palefsky et al, 2001). More recently, Goodman et al. (2010) reported that cervical and anal HPV infections do occur consecutively and that the risk of one increases the risk of the other and vice versa. They also reported on prevalence, incidence and clearance rates of genotype-specific anal HPV infection in women. The period prevalence of anal HPV was as much as 70% for a follow-up period that averaged 1.3 years (Goodman et al, 2008). The incidence of anal HPV infection was 50% through a follow-up period of average duration of 1.2 years whereas the median duration of anal HPV infection was 150 days (Shvetsov et al, 2009). In sum, data suggest that women's risk of anal HPV infection is at least as common (if not more common) as their risk of cervical HPV infection.

4.2 Anogenital HPV infection in men

4.2.1 Prevalence, incidence, duration

Compared to women, far fewer studies have been conducted among men but evidence suggests that the prevalence may even be more important in male. Depending of the anatomic sites (specifically the glans, corona, prepuce/foreskin and shaft, with improved HPV detection if a scrotal, perianal and/or anal canal sample is also obtained), the prevalence of anogenital HPV-DNA positivity among men ranges from 0 to 73% and is usually more than 20% (Giuliano et al, 2007; 2008; Dunne et al, 2006; Weaver et al, 2004). Also, HR-HPV appears to occur in a higher proportion of male than female infections (Giuliano et al, 2008b) and such as for women, penile HPV prevalence typically increases with the number of sex partners (Giuliano et al, 2007; Dunne et al, 2006; Weaver et al, 2004). Importantly and unlike for women, the available data do not indicate marked differences in HPV prevalence across age groups in men (Giuliano et al, 2008c). In fact, after the onset of sexual activity, HPV prevalence in men is relatively stable across age group.

Some cohort studies revealed that anogenital HPV incidence is at least as high among men as it is in women, with cumulative incidences ranging from 14 to 62% within 3 to 24 months (Dunn et al, 2006; Giuliano et al, 2008, Partridge et al, 2006; 2007). Although far fewer data are available for men, infection seems to be of short duration compare to women with a median duration of 5.9 months and no evidence for a difference in duration between oncogenic and non-oncogenic infections (Giuliano et al, 2008; Kjaer et al, 2005; Lajous et al, 2005). Only one study has reported on the risk of infection with multiple types in male and found that coinfection with multiple HPV genotypes was very common; the cumulative incidence of multiple genotypes after 24 months of follow-up of heterosexually active male university students 18–20 years was 35.6% (Partridge et al, 2007). There is no available study concerning the probability of re-infection with a same or a different genotype in men.

4.2.2 Special case for men who have sex with men

Men who have sex with men (MSM) have been observed to have a particularly high prevalence of HPV infections (Chin-Hong et al, 2004; Palefsky et al, 1998) and especially HIV positive MSM (de Pokomandy et al, 2009). Cohort studies of HIV-positive MSM revealed that the prevalence of anal HPV is more than 95% in these men, with high rates of multiple HPV genotype infections and lower genotype-specific HPV clearance rates (de Pokomandy et al, 2009; Kiviat et al, 1990; Palefsky et al 2005).

4.3 Oral HPV infection in adults

It is clear that oral mucosa act as a reservoir for HPV. A systematic review (Kreimer et al, 2010) of studies on oral HPV infection among 4070 healthy and cancer free individuals estimated the prevalence of oral HPV infection (any genotypes) of 4.5%. More specifically, 1.3% had oral HPV-16 and 3.5% had carcinogenic HPV. In this systematic review oral HPV-16 accounted for 28% of all HPV detected in the oral region and there was no difference in the oral prevalence between men and women. Other recent studies had shown nearly the same prevalence. A study among 1,688 healthy men aged 18 to 74 (median = 31 years) in United States, Mexico, and Brazil shown that the prevalence of oral HPV infection was 4% (Kreimer et al, 2011) whereas the study of Matsushita et al (2011) estimate oral HPV prevalence at 6.1%. Genotypes mostly detected included HPVs -16 and -18 and the tonsil appears to be the site with the highest prevalence.

4.4 Conjunctival HPV infection in adult

It is also clear that conjunctival mucosa act as a reservoir for HPV. LR-HPV such as HPVs -6 and -11 as well as HR-HPV, such as genotypes 16 and 33 are associated with the occurrence of conjunctival papilloma (Sjö et al, 2007). Ateenyi-Agaba et al. (2010) have tested conjunctival biopsy samples from healthy individuals to estimate the prevalence of HPV. The prevalence of mucosal HPVs was 3.5%, the prevalence of cutaneous HPVs was 10.5% whereas the prevalence multiple-genotype infections was present in 13.3% (Ateenyi-Agaba et al, 2010). It is possible that conjunctival tissues are more likely to be infected with cutaneous genotypes because of horizontal transmission.

5. Epidemiology of HPV infection in infant and children

The few studies available on genital and oral HPV infection in children have shown clear evidence of HR-HPV infections in healthy children (Kojima et al, 2003; Summersgill et al, 2001; Smith et al, 2007; Rice et al, 2000; Syrjänen et al, 2000). Sexual abuse and vertical and horizontal transmission may explain the positivity in children. This chapter focuses on the evidence about the epidemiology of HPV in children and not on the possible route of transmission since it is impossible to distinguish between both routes based simply on the clinical/epidemiological data. What is well known is that both routes (sexual and non-sexual) are possible. For example, perinatal HPV transmission has been unequivocally identified as a possible cause for the rare disease called Juvenile-Onset Recurrent Respiratory papillomatosis (JORRP) (Wiatrak et al, 2004).

Confirmation of the perinatal transmission of HPV in different mucosa (genital, oral) is supported by several studies. These studies have reported widely varying probability of infection in newborns, with estimates from the first couple of days of life ranging from 4 to 79% among infants born to mothers testing positive for HPV DNA during pregnancy (Table 3). Although perinatal transmission may be observed in baby born by caesarean, it is usually admitted that caesarean decreases the risk of perinatal infection. For example, a significantly higher rate of HPV 16/18 infection was found at birth when infants were delivered vaginally than when infants were delivered by cesarean (51.4% versus 27.3%) (Tseng et al, 1998). A systematic review (Medeiros et al, 2005) reported a higher risk of HPV infection after vaginal delivery than after cesarean section (RR: 1.8; 95%CI: 1.3-2.4). The risk of transmission has also been identified as increasing with the rupture of membranes; the longer time rupture of membranes occurred before delivery, higher risk of transmission (Tenti et al, 1999).

Study, year; country	Genotype of HPV	Sample (number of HPV+ pregnant mother)	Transmission rate at birth	Follow-up
Tseng et al, 1998; Taiwan	16, 18	68	40 % (buccal and genital)	delivery
Puranen et al, 1997; Finland	6, 11, 16, 18	42	79% (nasopharyngeal)	delivery
Chatterjee et al, 1998; India	6, 11, 16, 18	12	42% (buccal)	delivery
Tenti et al, 1999; Italy	6, 11, 16, 18, 31, 33, 35, 39, 51, 54, 56, 58, 59, 66, 68, 69, 70, 83, 84	37	30% (oropharyngeal)	18 mths
Bandyopadhyay et al, 2003; India	6, 11, 16, 18, 31, 33	38	18% (buccal)	12 mths
Smith et al, 2004; United States	6, 11, 16, 18, 31, 33, 53, 66	172	4% (buccal, genital)	6 mths
Rintala et al, 2005; Finland	16, 18, 31, 33, 35, 39, 45, 51, 52, 54, 56, 58	Include 77 newborns	(15% and 9% of newborns had genital or oral HPV infection, at birth, respectively	2 yrs
Rombaldi et al, 2009; Brazil	6/11, 16, 18, 31, 33, 42, 52, 58	49	20% (buccal, axillary and inguinal regions)	1 yr
Castellsagué et al, 2009; Spain	6, 11, 16, 18, 31, 33, 39	66	19.7% (mouth and anogenital exfoliated cells)	2 yrs

Table 3: Cohort studies on HPV perinatal transmission

Only a few studies have analysed the probability of persistence among babies born to HPV-infected mothers such as Rombaldi et al (2009) and Watts et al. (1998) who have reported a very low proportion of persistent infection in infants (reported 0% in a 1 and 3-year follow-up study, respectively) whereas some reported very high proportions ranging from 27 to

56% (Fredericks et al, 1993; Kaye et al, 1994; Pakarian et al, 1994; Cason et al, 1995, 2005; Syrjänen et al, 2000). These studies have shown that perinatally acquired HPV can persist for at least 2 years and that HPV is mostly prevalent during the first year of infancy reaching a peak at 6 months of age.

Anogenital warts may also be transmitted perinatally (Jayasingue et al, 2006; Sinal et al, 2005; Marcoux et al, 2006; Sinclair et al, 2005; Jones et al, 2007). Boyd (1990) has shown that at least 20% of anogenital warts occur because of perinatal transmission. Although the incubation period for children is not known, a period of several months typically elapses between viral infection at delivery and clinical manifestations (Monk et al, 2007). A review of studies of the HPV genotype distribution in anogenital warts in children has shown that 75% are caused by genotypes 6 and 11, 11% by HPV-2, 6% by HPV-16 and -18 and 3% by HPV-27 and -57 (Syrjänen et al, 2000; Sinal et al, 2005; Marcoux et al, 2006; Aguilera-Barrantes et al, 2007). Since the 1990s, the incidence of anogenital warts has dramatically increased in adults as well as in children (Syrjänen et al, 2000). To summarize, it is clear that perinatal transmission of HPV occurred although the frequency at which it occurred and persist remains controversial.

It is also clear that infants and children might acquire oral and genital HPV infection postnatally from a variety of sources such as direct transmission (person-to-person or auto-inoculation), indirect transmission (via contaminated objects) and sexual abuse (Syrjänen et al, 2000). For example, in their longitudinal study of the prevalence of HR-HPV in oral and genital mucosa of infants during their first 3 years of life, Rintala et al. (2005b) found that 42% of infants (negative at birth) had acquired an oral HR-HPV infection (from which 10% had persistent infection) and 36% had acquired a genital HR-HPV infection (from which 1.5% had persisted). Some cross-sectional studies have estimated the prevalence of HPV among children of different age-groups. The estimates of prevalence of HPV (detected by PCR) in oral swabs from children aged 0-13 years range from 32 to 52% (Rice et al, 2000; Syrjänen et al, 2000). In their review of studies that analyzed PCR-detected HR-HPV during infancy and childhood, Cason et al. (2005) reported HPV prevalences ranging from 9 to 55%. However, oral HPV infection is likely to decrease with age. The study of Marais et al. (2006) had compared oral HPV prevalence among children, adolescent and adult. They found that oral HPV infection was highest in children (7.9%), followed by adolescents (5.1%), and lowest in normal adults (3.5%). Mamas et al. (2011) also shown the presence of HPV in the lower respiratory tract of healthy children; 8% of bronchoalveolar lavage of children (2-12 years old) they tested were positive for HPV. Finally, there are no available studies on the prevalence of conjunctival HPV in children although papilloma represents 7-10% of conjunctival benign tumors in childhood where HPV-6 and -11 are the major genotypes responsible for conjunctival lesions (Okan et al, 2010).

There are some studies that reported cases of squamous cell carcinoma (SCC) involving the larynx/lung in childhood which transformed from the recurrent respiratory papillomatosis with HPV (Lin et al, 2010; Katsenos et al, 2011) but cancers associated with HPV in childhood are not frequent. However, although rare, cancers related to HPV are increasing in recent years in children and this increasing correlates with increased prevalence of HPV in the community (Chow et al, 2007). Moreover and importantly, they are no longitudinal studies available to clarify whether children exposed to HPV (oral, anogenital or conjunctival) are at risk of developing carcinoma in adulthood. A better understanding the natural history of HPV infection in children is clearly needed.

6. Conclusion

Anogenital HPV infection is very common with high prevalences found in both females and males. Typically, anogenital HPV prevalence increases rapidly in adolescents/young adults following sexual debut, and the highest prevalence occurs among this population (Kjaer et al, 2001). The probability of finding a cervicovaginal HPV infections in women decrease after that according to age with a possible peak at older age whereas it is relatively stable according to age for men. The predominant route of HPV transmission is through sexual contact although vertical and horizontal transmissions are possible. Most sexually-active individuals are likely to be exposed to anogenital HPV infection during their lifetimes and most infections will be cleared spontaneously within a year. A small fraction of people will have persistent infection with HR-HPVs, which is unequivocally established as a necessary cause of cervical cancer and is likely to be responsible for a substantial proportion of other anogenital neoplasms and non negligible number of head and neck cancers. Persistent infection result in substantial morbidity and invoke high costs associated with the treatment of clinically relevant lesions. Oral and conjunctival infections may also exist in adults although the epidemiology of these infections has been less studied. Children are also exposed to HPV as anogenital and oral samples of healthy children have often been found positive. The incidence of HPV-associated diseases, such as squamous cell carcinomas, has increased in children in recent years which may be, in part, related to an increase in HPV prevalence (Syrjänen et al, 2000; Chow et al, 2007). HPV vaccination, one of the most remarkable discoveries of the past decade, is currently implanted all around the world and is expected to prevent a substantial proportion of cervical and other HPV-related cancers in the future.

7. References

Aguilera-Barrantes I, Magro C, Nuovo GJ. Verruca vulgaris of the vulva in children and adults: a nonvenereal type of vulvar wart. Am J Surg Pathol 2007; 31(4):529-35.

Ateenyi-Agaba C, Franceschi S, Wabwire-Mangen F, Arslan A, Othieno E, Binta-Kahwa J, van Doorn LJ, Kleter B, Quint W, Weiderpass E. Human papillomavirus infection and squamous cell carcinoma of the conjunctiva. Br J Cancer 2010; 102(2):262-7.

Armstrong LR, Preston EJ, Reichert M, Phillips DL, Nisenbaum R, Todd NW, Jacobs IN, Inglis AF, Manning SC, Reeves WC. Incidence and prevalence of recurrent respiratory papillomatosis among children in Atlanta and Seattle. Clin Infect Dis. 2000; 31(1):107-9.

Bandyopadhyay S, Sen S, Majumdar L, Chatterjee R. Human papillomavirus infection among Indian mothers and their infants. Asian Pac J Cancer Prev 2003; 4(3):179-84.

Barnabas R, Laukkanen P, Koskela P, Kontula O, Lehtinen M, Garnett G: Epidemiologyof HPV 16 and cervical cancer in Finland and the potential impact of vaccination: mathematical modelling analyses. PLoS Med 2006; 3:e138.

Bauer HM, Ting Y, Greer CE, Chambers JC, Tashiro CJ, Chimera J, Reingold A, Manos MM. Genital human papillomavirus infection in female university students as determined by a PCR-based method. JAMA 1991; 265:472-7.

Boyd AS. Condylomata acuminata in the pediatric population. Am J Dis Child 1990; 144(7):817-24.

Burchell AN, Winer RL, de Sanjosé S, Franco EL: Epidemiology and transmission dynamics of genital human papillomavirus infection. Vaccine 2006; 24:S52–S61.

Burchell AN, Tellier PP, Hanley J, Coutlée F, Franco EL. Human papillomavirus infections among couples in new sexual relationships. Epidemiology 2010; 21(1):31-7.

Cason J, Kaye J, Pakarian F, Raju KS, Best JM. HPV-16 transmission. Lancet 1995; 345: 197-8.

Cason J, Mant CA. High-risk mucosal human papillomavirus infections during infancy & childhood. J Clin Virol 2005; 32 Suppl 1:S52-8.

Castellsagué X, Drudis T, Cañadas MP, Goncé A, Ros R, Pérez JM, Quintana MJ, Muñoz J, Albero G, de Sanjosé S, Bosch FX. Human Papillomavirus (HPV) infection in pregnant women and mother-to-child transmission of genital HPV genotypes: a prospective study in Spain. BMC Infect Dis 2009; 9:74.

Chaterjee R, Mukhopadhyay D, Murmu N, Mitra PK. Correlation between human papillomavirus DNA detection in maternal cervical smears and buccal swabs of infants. Indian J Exp Biol 1998; 36(2):199-202.

Chin-Hong PV, Vittinghoff E, Cranston RD, Buchbinder S, Cohen D, Colfax G, Da Costa M, Darragh T, Hess E, Judson F, Koblin B, Madison M, Palefsky JM. Age-specific prevalence of anal human papillomavirus infection in HIV-negative sexually active men who have sex with men: the EXPLORE study. J Infect Dis 2004; 190:2070–76.

Chow CW, Tabrizi SN, Tiedemann K, Waters KD. Squamous cell carcinomas in children and young adults: a new wave of a very rare tumor? J Pediatr Surg. 2007; 42(12):2035-9.

Clifford GM, Gallus S, Herrero R, Muñoz N, Snijders PJ, Vaccarella S, Anh PT, Ferreccio C, Hieu NT, Matos E, Molano M, Rajkumar R, Ronco G, de Sanjosé S, Shin HR, Sukvirach S, Thomas JO, Tunsakul S, Meijer CJ, Franceschi S. Worldwide distribution of human papillomavirus genotypes in cytologically normal women in the International Agency for Research on Cancer HPV prevalence surveys: a pooled analysis. Lancet 2005; 366(9490):991-8.

de Pokomandy A, Rouleau D, Ghattas G, Vézina S, Côté P, Macleod J, Allaire G, Franco EL, Coutlée F. Prevalence, clearance, and incidence of anal human papillomavirus infection in HIV-infected men. J Infect Dis 2009;199:965-73.

de Sanjosé S, Diaz M, Castellsagué X, Clifford G, Bruni L, Muñoz N, Bosch FX. Worldwide prevalence and genotype distribution of cervical human papillomavirus DNA in women with normal cytology: a meta-analysis. Lancet Infect Dis 2007; 7(7):453-9.

de Villiers EM, Fauquet C, Broker TR, Bernard HU, zur Hausen H. Classification of papillomaviruses. Virology 2004; 324:17–27.

Dunne EF, Nielson CM, Stone KM, Markowitz LE, Giuliano AR. Prevalence of HPV infection among men: a systematic review of the literature. J Infect Dis 2006; 194:1044–57.

Edwards S, Carne C. Oral sex and the transmission of viral STIs. Sex Transm Infect 1998; 74:6–10.

Favre M, Majewski S, De Jesus N, Malejczyk M, Orth G, Jablonska S. A possible vertical transmission of human papillomavirus genotypes associated with epidermodysplasia verruciformis. J Invest Dermatol 1998; 111(2):333-6.

Fredericks BD, Balkin A, Daniel HW, Schonrock J, Ward B, Frazer IH. Transmission of human papillomavirus from mother to child. Aust NZ.J Obstet Gynaecol 1993; 33:30–2.

Gervaz P, Allal AS, Villiger P, Buhler L, Morel P. Squamous cell carcinoma of the anus: another sexually transmitted disease. Swiss Med Wkly 2003; 133:353–9.

(c) Giuliano AR, Lazcano-Ponce E, Villa LL, Flores R, Salmeron J, Lee JH, Papenfuss MR, Abrahamsen M, Jolles E, Nielson CM, Baggio ML, Silva R, Quiterio M. HPV prevalence and type-distribution among men residing in Brazil, Mexico and the US. Cancer Epidemiol Biomarkers Prev 2008; 17: 2036–43.

(b) Giuliano AR, Tortolero-Luna G, Ferrer E, Burchell AN, de Sanjosé S, Kjaer SK, Muñoz. N, Schiffman M, Bosch FX. Epidemiology of human papillomavirus infection in men, cancers other than cervical and benign conditions. Vaccine 2008; 26(S10):K17-K28.

Giuliano AR, Lu B, Nielson CM, Flores R, Papenfuss MR, Lee JH, Abrahamsen M, Harris RB. Age-specific prevalence, incidence, and duration of human papillomavirus infections in a cohort of 290 US men. J Infect Dis 2008; 198: 827–35.

Giuliano AR, Nielson CM, Flores R, Dunne EF, Abrahamsen M, Papenfuss MR, Markowitz LE, Smith D, Harris RB. The optimal anatomic sites for sampling heterosexual men for human papillomavirus (HPV) detection: the HPV Detection in Men Study. J Infect Dis 2007; 196: 1146–52.

Goodman MT, Shvetsov YB, McDuffie K, Wilkens LR, Zhu X, Thompson PJ, Ning L, Killeen J, Kamemoto L, Hernandez BY. Sequential acquisition of human papillomavirus (HPV) infection of the anus and cervix: the Hawaii HPV Cohort Study. J Infect Dis 2010; 201:1331-9.

Goodman MT, Shvetsov YB, McDuffie K, Wilkens LR, Zhu X, Ning L, Killeen J, Kamemoto L, Hernandez BY. Acquisition of anal human papillomavirus (HPV) infection in women: the Hawaii HPV Cohort study. J Infect Dis 2008; 197:957-66.

Hajek EF. Contribution to the etiology of laryngeal papilloma in children. J Laryngol Otol. 1956; 70(3):166-8.

Heim K, Widschwendter A, Pirschner G, Wieland U, Awerkiew S, Christensen ND, Bergant A, Marth C, Höpfl R. Antibodies to human papillomavirus 16 L1 virus-like particles as an independent prognostic marker in cervical cancer. Am J Obstet Gynecol 2002; 186(4):705-11.

Hemminki K, Dong C. Cancer in Husbands of Cervical Cancer Patients. Epidemiology 2000; 11(3): 347-9.

Hernandez BY, Wilkens LR, Zhu X, Thompson P, McDuffie K, Shvetsov YB, Kamemoto LE, Killeen J, Ning L, Goodman MT. Transmission of human papillomavirus in heterosexual couples. Emerg Infect Dis 2008; 14: 888–94.

International Agency for Research on Cancer (IARC). Monographs on the evaluation of carcinogenic risks to humans. Human papillomaviruses, vol. 90. Lyon, France; 2007.

International Agency for Research on Cancer (IARC). Monographs on the Evaluation of Carcinogenic Risks to Humans, vol. 100B, Lyon, France; 2011.

Jayasinghe Y, Garland SM. Genital warts in children: what do they mean? Arch Dis Child 2006; 91(8):696-700.

Jones V, Smith SJ, Omar HA. Nonsexual transmission of anogenital warts in children: a retrospective analysis. ScientificWorld Journal 2007; 7:1896-9.

Kashima HK, Shah F, Lyles A, Glackin R, Muhammad N, Turner L, Van Zandt S, Whitt S, Shah K. A comparison of risk factors in juvenile-onset and adult-onset recurrent respiratory papillomatosis. Laryngoscope 1992; 102(1):9-13.

Katsenos S, Becker HD. Recurrent respiratory papillomatosis: a rare chronic disease, difficult to treat, with potential to lung cancer transformation: apropos of two cases and a brief literature review. Case Rep Oncol. 2011; 4(1):162-71.

Kaye JN, Cason J, Pakarian FB, Jewers RJ, Kell B, Bible J, Raju KS, Best JM. Viral load as a determinant for transmission of human papillomavirus type 16 from mother to child. J Med Virol 1994; 44(4):415-21.

Kiviat N, Rompalo A, Bowden R, Galloway D, Holmes KK, Corey L, Roberts PL, Stamm WE. Anal human papillomavirus infection among human immunodeficiency virus-seropositive and -seronegative men. J Infect Dis 1990; 162:358-61.

Kjaer SK, Chackerian B, van den Brule AJ, Svare EI, Paull G, Walbomers JM, Schiller JT, Bock JE, Sherman ME, Lowy DR, Meijer CL. High-risk human papillomavirus is sexually transmitted: evidence from a follow up study of virgins starting sexual activity (intercourse). Cancer Epidemiol Biomarkers Prev 2001; 10: 101–6.

Kjaer SK, Munk C, Winther JF, Jorgensen HO, Meijer CJLM, van den Brule AJC. Acquisition and persistence of human papillomavirus infection in younger men: a prospective follow-up study among Danish soldiers. Cancer Epidemiol Biomarkers Prev 2005; 14: 1528–33.

Kojima A, Maeda H, Kurahashi N, Sakagami G, Kubo K, Yoshimoto H, Kameyama Y. Human papillomaviruses in the normal oral cavity of children in Japan. Oral Oncol 2003; 39(8):821–8.

Kreimer AR, Bhatia RK, Messeguer AL, González P, Herrero R, Giuliano AR. Oral human papillomavirus in healthy individuals: a systematic review of the literature. Sex Transm Dis 2010; 37(6):386-91.

Kreimer AR, Villa A, Nyitray AG, Abrahamsen M, Papenfuss M, Smith D, Hildesheim A, Villa LL, Lazcano-Ponce E, Giuliano AR. The epidemiology of oral HPV infection among a multinational sample of healthy men. Cancer Epidemiol Biomarkers Prev 2011; 20(1):172-82.

Lajous M, Mueller N, Cruz-Valdez A, Aguilar LV, Franceschi S, Hernandez-Avila M, Lazcano-Ponce E. Determinants of prevalence, acquisition, and persistence of human papillomavirus in health Mexican military men. Cancer Epidemiol Biomarkers Prev 2005; 14: 1710–16.

Lin HW, Richmon JD, Emerick KS, de Venecia RK, Zeitels SM, Faquin WC, Lin DT. Malignant transformation of a highly aggressive human papillomavirus type 11-associated recurrent respiratory papillomatosis. Am J Otolaryngol 2010; 31:291-6.

Mammas IN, Zaravinos A, Sourvinos G, Spandidos DA. Detection of human papillomavirus in bronchoalveolar lavage samples in immunocompetent children. Pediatr Infect Dis J. 2011; 30(5):384-6.

Marais DJ, Sampson C, Jeftha A, Dhaya D, Passmore JA, Denny L, Rybicki EP, Van Der Walt E, Stephen LX, Williamson AL. More men than women make mucosal IgA antibodies to Human papillomavirus type 16 (HPV-16) and HPV-18: a study of oral HPV and oral HPV antibodies in a normal healthy population. BMC Infect Dis 2006; 6:95.

Marcoux D, Nadeau K, McCuaig C, Powell J, Oligny LL. Pediatric anogenital warts: a 7-year review of children referred to a tertiary-care hospital in Montreal, Canada. Pediatr Dermatol 2006; 23(3):199-207.

Marrazzo JM, Stine K, Koutsky LA. Genital human papillomavirus infection in women who have sex with women: a review. Am J Obstet Gynecol 2000; 183: 770–4.

Matsushita K, Sasagawa T, Miyashita M, Ishizaki A, Morishita A, Hosaka N, Saikawa K, Hoshina S, Bi X, Ichimura H. Oral and cervical human papillomavirus infection among female sex workers in Japan. Jpn J Infect Dis 2011; 64(1):34-9.

Medeiros LR, Ethur AB, Hilgert JB, Zanini RR, Berwanger O, Bozzetti MC, Mylius LC. Vertical transmission of the human papillomavirus: a systematic quantitative review. Cad Saude Publica. 2005;21(4):1006-15.

Monk BJ, Tewari KS. The spectrum and clinical sequelae of human papillomavirus infection. Gynecol Oncol 2007; 107(2 Suppl 1):S6-13.

Moscicki AB, Hills NK, Shiboski S, Darragh TM, Jay N, Powell K, Hanson E, Miller SB, Farhat S, Palefsky J. Risk factors for abnormal anal cytology in young heterosexual women. Cancer Epidemiol Biomarkers Prev 1999; 8: 173–8.

Muñoz N, Méndez F, Posso H, Molano M, van den Brule AJ, Ronderos M, Meijer C, Muñoz A; Instituto Nacional de Cancerologia HPV Study Group. Incidence, duration, and determinants of cervical human papillomavirus infection in a cohort of Colombian women with normal cytological results. J Infect Dis 2004; 190:2077–87.

Nonnenmacher B, Hubbert NL, Kirnbauer R, Shah KV, Muñoz N, Bosch FX, de Sanjosé S, Viscidi R, Lowy DR, Schiller JT. Serologic response to human papillomavirus type 16 (HPV-16) virus-like particles in HPV-16 DNA-positive invasive cervical cancer and cervical intraepithelial neoplasia grade III patients and controls from Colombia and Spain. J Infect Dis 1995; 172(1):19-24.

Okan G, Ayan I, Karslioğlu S, Altiok E, Yenmiş G, Vural G. Conjunctival papilloma caused by human papillomavirus type 11 treated with systemic interferon in a five-year-old boy. Turk J Pediatr 2010; 52(1):97-100.

Pakarian F, Kaye J, Cason J, Kell B, Jewers R, Derias NW, Raju KS, Best JM. Cancer associated human papillomaviruses: perinatal transmission and persistence. Br J Obstet Gynaecol 1994; 101(6):514-7.

Palefsky JM, Holly EA, Efirdc JT, Da Costa M, Jay N, Berry JM, Darragh TM. Anal intraepithelial neoplasia in the highly active antiretroviral therapy era among HIV-positive men who have sex with men. AIDS 2005; 19:1407-14.

Palefsky JM, Holly EA, Ralston ML, Da Costa M, Greenblatt RM. Prevalence and risk factors for anal human papillomavirus infection in human immunodeficiency virus (HIV)-positive and high-risk HIV-negative women. J Infect Dis 2001; 183:383-91

Palefsky JM, Holly EA, Ralston ML, Jay N. Prevalence and risk factors for human papillomavirus infection of the anal canal in human immunodeficiency virus (HIV)-positive and HIV-negative homosexual men. J Infect Dis 1998; 177: 361–7.

Park J, Sun D, Genest DR, Trivijitsilp P, Suh I, Crum CP. Coexistence of low and high grade squamous intraepithelial lesions of the cervix: morphologic progression or multiple papillomaviruses? Gynecol Oncol 1998; 70(3):386-91.

Partridge J, Koutsky L: Genital human papillomavirus infection in men. Lancet Infect Dis 2006; 6: 21–31.

Partridge JM, Hughes JP, Feng Q, Winer RL, Weaver BA, Xi LF, Stern ME, Lee SK, O'Reilly SF, Hawes SE, Kiviat NB, Koutsky LA. Genital human papillomavirus infection in men: incidence and risk factors in a cohort of university students. J Infect Dis 2007; 196: 1128–36.

Puranen MH, Yliskoski MH, Saarikoski SV, Syrjänen KJ, Syrjänen SM. Exposure of an infant to cervical human papillomavirus infection of the mother is common. Am J Obstet Gynecol 1997; 176(5):1039–45.

Rice PS, Mant C, Cason J, Bible JM, Muir P, Kell B, Best JM. High prevalence of human papillomavirus type 16 infection among children. J Med Virol 2000; 61(1):70-5.

Rintala MA, Grénman SE, Puranen MH, Isolauri E, Ekblad U, Kero PO, Syrjänen SM. Transmission of high-risk human papillomavirus (HPV) between parents and infant: a prospective study of HPV in families in Finland. J Clin Microbiol 2005; 43(1):376-81.

(b) Rintala MA, Grénman SE, Järvenkylä ME, Syrjänen KJ, Syrjänen SM. High-risk types of human papillomavirus (HPV) DNA in oral and genital mucosa of infants during their first 3 years of life: experience from the Finnish HPV Family Study. Clin Infect Dis 2005; 15;41(12):1728-33.

Rombaldi RL, Serafini EP, Mandelli J, Zimmermann E, Losquiavo KP. Perinatal transmission of human papilomavirus DNA. Virol J. 2009 Jun 21;6:83.

Schiffman M, Castle PE. Human papillomavirus: epidemiology and public health. Arch Pathol Lab Med 2003; 127: 930–4.

Shvetsov YB, Hernandez BY, McDuffie K, Wilkens LR, Zhu X, Ning L, Killeen J, Kamemoto L, Goodman MT. Duration and clearance of anal human papillomavirus (HPV) infection among women: the Hawaii HPV cohort study. Clin Infect Dis 2009; 48:536-46.

Sinal SH, Woods CR. Human papillomavirus infections of the genital and respiratory tracts in young children. Semin Pediatr Infect Dis 2005; 16(4):306-16.

Sinclair KA, Woods CR, Kirse DJ, Sinal SH. Anogenital and respiratory tract human papillomavirus infections among children: age, gender, and potential transmission through sexual abuse. Pediatrics 2005; 116(4):815-25.

Sjö NC, von Buchwald C, Cassonnet P, Norrild B, Prause JU, Vinding T, Heegaard S. Human papillomavirus in normal conjunctival tissue and in conjunctival papilloma: types and frequencies in a large series. Br J Ophthalmol 2007; 91: 1014–15.

Skjeldestad FE, Mehta V, Sings HL, Øvreness T, Turpin J, Su L, Boerckel P, Roberts C, Bryan J, Jansen KU, Esser MT, Liaw KL. Seroprevalence and genital DNA prevalence of HPV types 6, 11, 16 and 18 in a cohort of young Norwegian women: study design and cohort characteristics. Acta Obstet Gynecol Scand 2008; 87(1):81-8.

Smith EM, Swarnavel S, Ritchie JM, Wang D, Haugen TH, Turek LP. Prevalence of human papillomavirus in the oral cavity/oropharynx in a large population of children and adolescents. Pediatr Infect Dis J 2007; 26(9):836-40.

Smith EM, Ritchie JM, Yankowitz J, Swarnavel S, Wang D, Haugen TH, Turek LP. Human papillomavirus prevalence and types in newborns and parents: concordance and modes of transmission. Sex Transm Dis. 2004;31(1):57-62.

Sonnex C, Strauss S, Gray JJ. Detection of human papillomavirus DNA on the fingers of patients with genital warts. Sex Transm Infect 1999; 75: 317–9.

Summersgill KF, Smith EM, Levy BT, Allen JM, Haugen TH, Turek LP. Human papillomavirus in the oral cavities of children and adolescents. Oral Surg Oral Med Oral Pathol Oral Radiol Endod 2001; 91(1):62-9.

Syrjänen S, Puranen M. Human papillomavirus infections in children: the potential role of maternal transmission. Crit Rev Oral Biol Med 2000; 11(2):259-74.

Tenti P, Zappatore R, Migliora P, Spinillo A, Belloni C, Carnevali L. Perinatal transmission of human papillomavirus from gravidas with latent infections. Obstet Gynecol 1999; 93(4):475-9.

Thomas KK, Hughes JP, Kuypers JM, Kiviat NB, Lee SK, Adam DE, Koutsky LA. Concurrent and sequential acquisition of different genital human papillomavirus types. J Infect Dis 2000; 182: 1097–102.

Trottier H, Franco EL: The epidemiology of genital human papillomavirus infection. Vaccine 2006; 24(suppl 1):S1–S15.

(b) Trottier H, Mahmud S, Costa MC, Sobrinho JP, Duarte-Franco E, Rohan TE, Ferenczy A, Villa LL, Franco EL. Human papillomavirus infections with multiple types and risk of cervical neoplasia. Cancer Epidemiol Biomarkers Prev 2006; 15(7):1274-80.

Trottier H, Burchell AN. Epidemiology of mucosal human papillomavirus infection and associated diseases. Public Health Genomics 2009; 12(5-6):291-307.

Trottier H, Ferreira S, Thomann P, Costa MC, Sobrinho JS, Prado JC, Rohan TE, Villa LL, Franco EL. Human papillomavirus infection and reinfection in adult women: the role of sexual activity and natural immunity. Cancer Res 2010; 70(21):8569-77.

Tseng CJ, Liang CC, Soong YK, Pao CC. Perinatal transmission of human papillomavirus in infants: Relationship between infection rate and mode of delivery. Obstet. Gynecol 1998; 91:92–6.

Viscidi RP, Schiffman M, Hildesheim A, Herrero R, Castle PE, Bratti MC, Rodriguez AC, Sherman ME, Wang S, Clayman B, Burk RD. Seroreactivity to human papillomavirus (HPV) types 16, 18, or 31 and risk of subsequent HPV infection: results from a population-based study in Costa Rica. Cancer Epidemiol Biomarkers Prev 2004; 13(2):324-7.

Watts DH, Koutsky LA, Holmes KK, Goldman D, Kuypers J, Kiviat NB, Galloway DA. Low risk of perinatal transmission of human papillomavirus: results from a prospective cohort study. Am J Obstet Gynecol 1998; 178(2):365-73.

Weaver BA, Feng Q, Holmes KK, Kiviat N, Lee SK, Meyer C, Stern M, Koutsky LA. Evaluation of genital sites and sampling techniques for detection of human papillomavirus DNA in men. J Infect Dis 2004; 189: 677–85.

Wiatrak BJ, Wiatrak DW, Broker TR, Lewis L. Recurrent respiratory papillomatosis: a longitudinal study comparing severity associated with human papilloma viral types 6 and 11 and other risk factors in a large pediatric population. Laryngoscope 2004; 114(11 Pt 2 Suppl 104):1-23.

Williams AB, Darragh TM, Vranizan K, Ochia C, Moss AR, Palefsky JM. Anal and cervical human papillomavirus infection and risk of anal and cervical epithelial abnormalities in human immunodeficiency virus-infected women. Obstet Gynecol 1994; 83:205-11.

Winer RL, Koutsky LA: Genital human papillomaviruses; in Holmes KK, et al (eds): Sexually Transmitted Diseases, ed 4. New York, McGraw Hill Medical 2008, pp 489–508.

b) Winer RL, Feng Q, Hughes JP, O'Reilly S, Kiviat SB, Koutsky LA. Risk of female human papillomavirus acquisition associated with first male sex partner. J Infect Dis 2008; 197: 279–82.

2

Human Papillomavirus Type Distribution in Southern China and Taiwan

Chung-Yung Chen[1] and Chin-Hung Wang[2]
[1]*Department of Bioscience Technology, Chung Yuan Christian University, Chung-Li, 320,*
[2]*Genelite Life Science Centre, Taipei, 105,*
Taiwan

1. Introduction

In 2007, a worldwide analysis was published that assessed the types of HPV infection found in women without cervical disease (1). Of the 291 million women suffered with cervical diseases around the world, it was found that 32% are infected with either HPV16 or HPV18, or both. Data regarding the HPV burden and incidence rates are available on the WHO/ICO Information Centre on HPV and Cervical Cancer Web site (http://www.who.int/hpvcentre). However, HPV prevalence in different regions of Southern China is not mentioned in this website. Hence the diversity of HPV prevalence and distribution in Taiwan, Hong Kong, and various regions of China is the major focus in this chapter.

In Hong Kong, HPV DNA has been detected in 4% of women in 1996 and in 11% in 2002 by utilizing polymerase chain reaction methods on cervical samples, the most common high-risk (HR) HPV types identified being, in decreasing order, HPV 16, 58, 53, 18, 33, 45, and 52. Moreover, HPV 6 and 11, two types responsible for about 90% of genital warts, are among the most frequent HPV types found in Hong Kong population. In Taiwan, the five most common HPV types, also listed in decreasing order of frequency, are: HPV 16, 18, 58, 33, and 52 for women with cervical cancer, and HPV 16, 52, 58, 18, and 51 for women with normal cytology (2, 3). According to literature, there are, to date, fifty cities and provinces including Hong Kong and Taiwan whose predominant HPV types are already known. Table 1 shows the prevalence of HR-HPV in different regions in China such as, Zhejiang Province, Tianjin City, Shanxi Province, Hong Kong (HK), Guangzhou, Shandong Province, Shenzhen, Fujian, Liaoning Province, Beijing, Gansu province, Shanghai, Sichuan province, Guangdong province, Shenyang City, and in Taiwan. HPV type 16 exhibits the highest incidence in majority of these regions except Zhejiang province, Guangzhou, Fujian province, and in Taiwan (3), where HPV 52 has the highest prevalence. However, an investigation by Jin *et al.* (2010) in the Tibet Autonomous Region (TAR) which included both Tibetan and non-Tibetan populations pointed out that the frequency of HPV 33 may be higher than HPV 16 for non-Tibetan people, with the order of frequency of HPV genotypes being 16, 58, 31, 33, and 52 for Tibetan people. Incidentally, HPV 58 is also the second most common HPV type found in Taiwan (2), Chengdu, Liaoning, Beijing, Shenzhen, Shenyang, Shanxi, and Hong Kong (Table 1).

The three major HR-HPV types which can be deduced from Table 1 infect over 50% of patients in every city/region included in the list. In Taiwan (2), the TAR, Liaoning,

Shenzhen, and Shanxi, the order of frequency of HPV type is 16, 58 and 52, while the order that can be found in Shandong, Hong Kong, and Shenyan is 16, 52 and 58. Another combination of frequency order, namely, HPV 52, 16, and 58, has also been discovered in Taiwan (3), Guangzhou, and Zhejiang, whereas the order 16, 58, and 33 is inherent to Beijing, Shanxi, and Shenzhen (4). Both Chengdu and Shenyang (cancer cases) are represented by the order HPV 16, 58, and 18. Only cancer cases in Shanxi consist of the order 16, 58, and 56. To summarize, HPV 16, 52, and 58 are the three major types affecting 87% of the geography that includes these selected areas.

The relationship between geography and HPV types is demonstrated in Figure 1, with A~D corresponding to the distribution of HPV 16, 18, 52, and 58, respectively. Coastal areas in the southeast such as Taiwan and Hong Kong display a higher prevalence than inland cities. HPV prevalence may vary among different regions due to geographical separation, an example of which is Taiwan and Hong Kong. The political separation of Taiwan and Hong Kong most likely caused the HPV types diverse than mainland China. Moreover, the TAR is isolated by mountains from mainland China while Taiwan and Hong Kong are separated by sea. Thus, the lower number of HPV patients in the TAR compared with other regions can

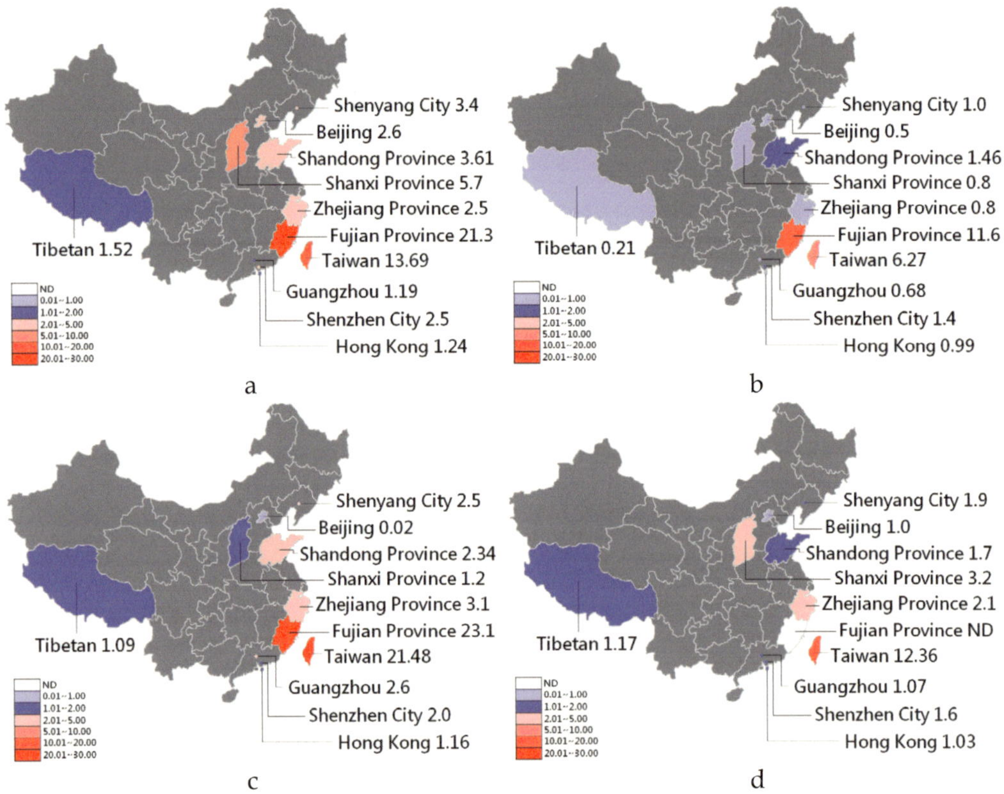

Fig. 1. The prevalence of major HPV types in some of China areas, Hong Kong and Taiwan. Four different HPV types show as (A) HPV16 (B) HPV18 (C) HPV52 (D) HPV58

be attributed to population conservation. In Taiwan, from 52 HPV types screening, HPV type 52 has the highest frequency (21.48% flowing HPV type 16, 58, 56, 39, 51, 18, 68, 31, 33, 59, 45, and 35(3) among HR-HPV types that is distinguish HPV combination compared to other regions. This also demonstrates the effect of geography despite Taiwan and China essentially being of the same ethnicity only partitioned over 60 years to affect two generations of people including marriage. The more independent, younger generation and their sexual culture are two major factors that cause the variations in HPV types distribution.

Since the prevalence of HPV types in each age group can be linked to sexual behavior, it is reasonable to investigate the multiple HPV infection types that can be found in patients (Table 2). In Taiwan, the multiple HPV infection rate is over 19%, only slightly lower than Hong Kong's (22.8%) but distinctly higher compared to others. For instance, most of the cities/regions that belong to mainland China, specifically inland cities like Beijng, Shangdong, Shanxi, Shengyang, Shenzhen, and Zhejiang, possess only 4~5% multiple HPV infection rates. Only Guangdong province has 11.1% between inland and island; however, Guangdong province is closest to Hong Kong and is more well-developed than inland cities. In contrast to Hong Kong and Taiwan, the TAR is isolated from immigration and might have conservative social behaviors, resulting to the lowest fraction of multiple HPV types (1.3%).

Regions\ HPV types (%)	16	18	31	33	35	39	45	51	52	56	58	59	68	References
Beijing	2.6	0.5	0.4	0.8	0.6	0.1	0.1	0.2	0.02	0.7	1.0	0.3	0.5	(Zhao et al., 2009)
Chengdu, western China (Cancer)	68.1	4.9	ND	0.7	ND	ND	0.7	ND	2.8	ND	8.3	ND	ND	(Li et al., 2011)
Fujian province	21.3	11.6	ND	11.2	ND	ND	ND	ND	23.1	ND	ND	ND	ND	(Wu et al., 2010)
Gansu Province (Cancer)	80.4	3.6	1.8	1.8	ND	ND	ND	ND	3.6	ND	3.6	3.6	ND	(Wu et al., 2009)
Guangdong province (Cancer)	25.0	20.8	ND	ND	ND	ND	ND	ND	20.8	ND	ND	ND	ND	(Lin et al., 2008b)
Guangzhou	1.19	0.68	1.16	0.59	0.07	0.32	0.24	0.14	2.6	0.27	1.07	0.15	0.39	(Liu et al., 2011)
Hong Kong	1.24	0.99	0	0.25	0	0.04	0.15	0	1.16	0	1.03	0.09	0.23	(Liu et al., 2011)
Hong Kong (Cancer)	18.3	9.1	ND	ND	ND	ND	ND	8	18.3	ND	17.7	ND	ND	(Chan et al., 2009a)
Hong Kong (Cancer)	43.2	4.8	3.2	3.2	0.8	0.8	1.1	0.5	9.1	0	5.9	0.8	0.8	(Chan et al., 2009b)
Liaoning province (Cancer)	19.64	1.8	3.03	4.6	1.03	1.59	0.29	0.77	6.4	0.61	8.39	ND	ND	(Sun et al., 2010)
Taiwan (Cancer)	18.4	1.7	0.3	3.6	0.6	1.5	0.6	2.9	9.4	0.6	7.6	1.5	0.6	(Chen et al., 2006)

Regions\ HPV types (%)	16	18	31	33	35	39	45	51	52	56	58	59	68	References
Taiwan	13.4	4.6	3.2	5.8	1.6	3.7	1.8	6.0	10.4	3.7	7.6	1.2	1.4	(Lin et al., 2008a)
Taiwan	13.69	6.27	3.52	3.42	0.95	8.46	2.38	8.17	21.48	9.03	12.36	2.66	4.66	(Wang et al., 2010)
Tibetan	1.52	0.21	1.17	1.17	0.04	0.21	0.17	0.21	1.09	0.21	1.17	0.08	0.5	(Jin et al., 2010)
Shandong Province	3.61	1.46	0.85	1.46	0.21	0.42	0.21	0.21	2.34	1.27	1.7	0	2.76	(Yuan et al., 2011)
Sichuan province (Cancer)	41.6	3.2	1.1	ND	ND	ND	1.1	ND	2.1	2.6	1.1	ND	ND	(Wu et al., 2008)
Shanxi Province	5.7	0.8	0.5	1.2	ND	0.6	0.6	0.6	1.2	0.8	3.2	0.3	0.2	(Dai et al., 2006)
Shenyang City	3.4	1	1	0.9	0.3	0.9	0.6	0.6	2.5	0.9	1.9	0.6	0.3	(Li et al., 2006)
Shenzhen City	2.5	1.4	1.5	0.3	0.4	1.5	0.7	0.6	2	1	1.6	0.9	0.5	(Wu et al., 2007)
Shenzhen City (Cancer)	29.7	18.9	5.4	9	6.3	ND	1.8	ND	1.8	3.6	18.9	9	ND	(Shi et al., 2006)
Zhejiang Province	2.5	0.8	0.8	0.8	0.2	0.3	0.3	0.9	3.1	0.4	2.1	0.7	1.0	(Ye et al., 2010)

Table 1. The HR-HPV types distribution in China, Hong Kong and Taiwan

Numerous investigations focused on HR-HPV due to its higher relationship to cervical cancer and high-grade squamous intraepithelial lesion. To survey high-risk and low-risk HPV, HR-HPV frequently found in women with ASCUS and CIN3/cervical cancer, and might be at least double frequencies than LR-HPV cases (Table 2). The average incidence of HR-HPV in population is over 10%, but an extremely high incidence has been found in CIN3/cervical cancer cases (Taiwan reports, Table 2). However, the LR-HPV prevalence might not be estimated correctly due to less LR-HPV types screening. A survey of 52 HPV types reported in Taiwan suggests that the prevalence of LR-HPV (37 types) and HR-HPV (15 types) is 10% and 5%, respectively (3). Other HPV reports listed less than 37 LR-HPV types and focused only on HR-HPV. The same HPV screening type but few LR-HPV screening types caused underestimation for the incidence of LR-HPV that showed in Table 2. For example, incidences of LR-HPV in Beijing, Hong Kong, the TAR, Shandong, Shanxi, Shenyang, Shenzhen, and Zhejiang are 2.0, 2.4, 2.1, 1.7, 3.8, 6.4, 6.6, and 3.5, respectively, and 5.8, 74.8, 7.1, 11.0, 12.2, 11.7, 12.2, and 10.2 for HR-HPV.

To compare HPV infections in different geographies around the world, the data from IARC and Table1 combined into Appendix 1. For overall HPV infection rate, Kenya has the highest HPV prevalence (38.8%) region and Span has the lowest HPV infection (1.5%). The Asia region including, China, Hong Kong, Japan, Korea, Taiwan and Thailand, are around 10~15% of overall infection rate except Thailand (4.8%). The most of developed countries, such as, Italy, Japan, Span, Sweden, UK, and USA are less HPV prevalence than most of the developing countries and under-developed countries, such as Argentina, Honduras, Kenya and Nigeria. For East-Asia, like, China, Japan, Hong Kong and Taiwan, HPV type 52 is higher HPV incidence than HPV 16. Other regions, HPV type 16 is the major incidence. HPV type 51 is another typical case for geographic : HPV 51 is higher incidence than HPV 52 in Brazil, Costa Rica, Republic of Korea, Scotland, and USA. In China and Hong Kong, HPV 51 is not significant prevalence in population. For top five prevalence of HR-HPV, HPV 16, 18, 31, 52, 58 are found in most of the countries/regions but different orders. However, the geography separated populations to cause the diverse of HPV infection types can be deduced from Appendix 1.

Regions\HPV types (%)	Multiple HPV %	LR	HR	References
Beijing	2.6	2.0	5.8	(Zhao et al., 2009)
Guangdong province (Cancer)	11.1	ND	7.4	(Lin et al., 2008)
Hong Kong (Cancer)	22.8	2.4	74.8	(Chan et al., 2009)
Taiwan	4.9	4.4	52.3	(Chen et al., 2006)
Taiwan (Cancer)	19.9	70.4	29.6	(Chao et al., 2008)
Taiwan (Cancer)	19.4	68.9	31.1	(Lai et al., 2008)
Taiwan	4.5	10.0	5.0	(Wang et al., 2010)
Tibetan	1.32	2.14	7.05	(Jin et al., 2010)
Shandong Province	4.2	1.70	11.04	(Yuan et al., 2011)
Shanxi Province	4.5	3.8	12.2	(Dai et al., 2006)
Shenyang City	5.3	6.4	11.7	(Li et al., 2006)
Shenzhen City	4.4	6.6	12.2	(Wu et al., 2007)
Zhejiang Province	3.5	2.7	10.2	(Ye et al., 2010)

Table 2. A list of Multiple HPV infection rate in individual region.

2. Age related to HPV genotypes

Based on our previous study of Taiwan cases, the prevalence of LR-HPV is diverse among different age groups. For instance, HPV 84 is found most frequently in the 20–29 age group, HPV 54 in the 30–39 age group, HPV 53 in the 40–49 age group, and HPV 72 in the over-50 age group. When the range of HPV genotypes that could be identified among cases of multiple infections was examined, 38 HPV genotypes were found in the over-50 age group and 40 genotypes in the 40–49 age group. In addition, 41 HPV genotypes were identified in the 30–39 age group, while 42 genotypes were discovered in the 20–29 age group (3). HR-HPV genotypes in Taiwan have the highest peak in the younger population (<20 years old, 28.1%), subsequently decreasing as it moved from the 20-29 age group (26.7%), 30-39 age group (15.5%), and 40-49 (12.1%) age group, to the over-50 age group (10.4%). This pattern, however, is different from those found in other regions (Table 3).

Based on the epidemiological distribution of HPV in Beijing city, the 30-34 age group has the highest HPV frequency, while the 25-29 and 50-54 age groups have the lowest (5). By contrast, according to Guangdong province cervical cancer cases, older women tended to have higher HPV infection rates, as evidenced by the 11.7%, 8.2%, 8.1%, and 3.4% rates representing the 51-60, 41-50, 31-40, and 21-30 age groups, respectively (6). For people in Guangzhou, a high HPV rate (15.1%) is evident in the 20-29 age group and lower HPV rates

(11.7% and 11.8%) can be observed in the 40-49 and over-60 age groups (7). However, there is no significant difference in HPV rates among age groups in Guangzhou. In Hong Kong, the 20-29 age group has the highest peak in both cancer report and population screening; however, the 40-49 age group had less HPV frequency (7, 8) which remains without clear explanation. In other south coast cities, namely, Shanghai and Shenzhen, the 20-29 age group also exhibited the highest HPV infection rate but in Shanghai only; an opposite trend was found in Shenzhen city, where a high infection rate manifested in older people (45-59 age group). Two recent reports related to Shenzhen city have pointed out the discrepancy about HPV prevalence. One demonstrated an increased HPV infection along with elder people and another report mentioned the 25-29 age group is the lowest. However, Shenzhen city has many plants with numerous temporary residents and tertiary sector workers from other counties that might cause residential status being significantly associated with HPV positivity.

Regions\Age Groups (%)	A	B	C	D	E	F	G	H	References
Beijing	25-29 4.9%	30-34 8.2%	35-39 7.1%	40-44 7.5%	45-49 6.4%	50-54 4.9%			(Zhao et al., 2009)
Guangdong province (Cancer)	21-30 3.4%	31-40 8.1%	41-50 8.2%	51-60 11.7%					(Lin et al., 2008)
Guangzhou	20-29 15.1%	30-39 14.2%	40-49 11.7%	50-59 14.0%	≧60 11.8%				(Liu et al., 2011)
Hong Kong	20-29 13.0%	30-39 4.9%	40-49 4.6%	50-59 7.1%	≧60 9.6%				(Liu et al., 2011)
Hong Kong (Cancer)	<26 10.0%	26-30 14.0%	31-35 9.5%	36-40 6.0%	41-45 5.6%	46-50 7.5%	51-55 6.5%	>55 3.5%	(Chan et al., 2009)
Taiwan	<20 28.1%	20-29 26.7%	30-39 15.5%	40-49 12.1%	≧50 10.4%				(Wang et al., 2010)
Tibetan	19-29 9.2%	30-39 9.2%	40-49 9.1%	≧50 9.1%					(Jin et al., 2010)
Shanxi Province	15-24 13.3%	25-34 7.5%	35-44 20.5%	45-54 17.0%	55-59 14.3%				(Dai et al., 2006)
Shanghai	18-20 54.4%	21-30 26.4%	31-40 30%	41-50 32.0%	51-60 31.0%	61-78 31.5%			(Zhang et al., 2008)
Shenyang City	<25 2.7%	25-34 11.8%	35-44 12.5%	45-54 13.0%	55-59 6.3%				(Li et al., 2006)
Shenzhen City	<25 14.3%	25-34 16.2%	35-44 15.2%	45-59 24.4%					(Wu et al., 2007)
Shenzhen City	15-24 15.5%	25-29 17.7%	30-34 12.6%	35-39 8.8%	40-44 10.2%	45-49 15.3%	50-59 21.0%		(Wu et al., 2010)
Zhejiang Province	20-24 14.5%	25-29 9.3%	30-34 8.4%	35-39 10.7%	40-44 10.7%	45-49 9.2%	50-54 14.4%	55-79 8.6%	(Ye et al., 2010)

Table 3. A list of HPV infection rates among different age groups

Zhejiang province provided more interesting data (9) showing a similar low HPV frequency in each age group (Table 3). Although both the 20-24 and 50-54 age groups have slightly higher rates, the highest (14.4%) and lowest (8.4%) frequencies indicated a less diverse range of HPV prevalence than in other cities/regions. For the north coast city of Shenyang, HPV infection rate initially increases with respect to age, starting from 2.7% for women <25 years old to 13% for women 45-54 years old, but then drops to 6.3% for the 55-59 age group. This pattern is unique among coastal cities and is compatible with the flat age-curves that have been described in other countries such as India and Africa (10). A flat age-curve indicates that young women are not infected with new HPV types more frequently than older women (11). The number of sexual partners as well as the husband's extramarital sexual relationships are believed to be explanatory of this flat age-curve. For inland cities, the TAR has consisted of HPV prevalence around 9% in every age group. For Shanxi province, the 35-44 age group has the highest peak of infection distribution (20.5%), followed by age groups 45-54 with 17.0%, 55-59 with 14.3%, 15-24 with 13.3%, and 25-34 with 7.5%. Finally, for Guangzhou, Hong Kong, Shenzhen, and Zhejiang, the age distribution of cervical HPV infection shows a bimodal curve in half of the regions, with a first peak at younger women, a lower prevalence plateau at middle-aged women, and a variable rebound at older ages (≧45 years). One explanation for this is sexual behavior, which is considered an important risk factor for HPV infection. On the other hand, HPV incidence associated with unmarried status along with a high peak of HPV infection suggests that younger, single women may have an increased possibility of encountering complicated sexual relationships (11). However, the lower prevalence plateau at middle-aged women may be caused by less sexual frequency and single sex partners for married Chinese women.

3. HPV type distribution in invasive cervical cancer and high-grade squamous intraepithelial lesion

Overall HPV prevalence in invasive cervical cancer (ICC) is 87%, ranging from 86% to 94% by region, according to literature. In Jiashan, data for the incidence of invasive cervical cancer (ICC) from 1998 to 2002 has been reported. Incidence rates of cervical cancer ranged from 2.4 per 100,000 women to 4.6 per 100,000 women in Guangzhou (12). Some areas have notably high cervical cancer incidence rates, such as in Yangcheng and Shanxi, where there is an estimated rate of about 81 per 100,000 women between 1998–2002 (12). Incidentally, the incidence rates for cervical cancer in Hong Kong, Singapore, and Taiwan are 9.6, 10.6, and 18.6 per 100,000 women, respectively (13). Between these three regions, the incidence of cervical cancer is highest in Taiwan and is nearly double than Hong Kong's. However, it has declined since 1993 to 2003.

Tay *et al.* (2008) has reported the five most common HPV types in Taiwan to be, in decreasing frequency order: HPV 16, 18, 58, 33, and 52 for women with cervical cancer, and HPV 16, 52, 58, 18, and 51 for women with normal cytology (13). Due to a high HPV prevalence, the Taiwanese National Health Insurance launched a screening program in 1995 for women aged 30 years old and above. This program included quality control monitoring and a training system for medical doctors, public health nurses, cytologists, and medical technicians. By 2001, the screening program has been estimated to reduce cervical cancer incidence by 29% and mortality by 50%, and has been shown to be cost-effective for Taiwanese public health (14). Upon analysis of HPV genotypes present in ICC, HPV 16 was found to be the most common type, rating 52% in Asia and 58% in Europe, while HPV18 was the second most common type which rated from 13% in South/Central America to 22%

Regions\Abnormal (HPV%)	ASCUS	ICC	HSIL	LSIL	CIN1	CIN2	CIN3	References
Beijing	56.0	Unknown	93.3	Unknown	Unknown	Unknown	85.7	(Zhao et al., 2009)
Chengdu, western China	Unknown	80.6	61.9	Unknown	Unknown	Unknown	Unknown	(Li et al., 2011)
Fujian province	Unknown	94.3	Unknown	Unknown	70.5	90.2	Unknown	(Wu et al., 2010a)
Gansu Province	Unknown	Unknown	Unknown	Unknown	70.5	Unknown	Unknown	(Wu et al., 2009)
Guangdong province	12.4	1	Unknown	2.1	Unknown	Unknown	Unknown	(Lin et al., 2008)
Guangdong and Jiangxi	Unknown	89.9	Unknown	Unknown	68.8	80.3	90.2	(Wu et al., 2006)
Liaoning province	54.6	83.1	Unknown	Unknown	64.1	Unknown	Unknown	(Sun et al., 2010)
Taiwan	13.4	Unknown	89.4	84.7	Unknown	Unknown	Unknown	(Chen et al., 2006)
Taiwan	41.2	66.7	87.5	Unknown	Unknown	5.7	Unknown	(Chao et al., 2008)
Taiwan	Unknown	Unknown	Unknown	Unknown	81	84	90	(Tsai et al., 2005)
Tibetan	7.41	Unknown	56.8	24.3	Unknown	Unknown	Unknown	(Jin et al., 2010)
Shandong Province	Unknown	81.3	Unknown	Unknown	34.8	59.8	74.5	(Yuan et al., 2011)
Shanghai	Unknown	52.9	Unknown	Unknown	34.4	31.7	47.1	(Zhang et al., 2008)
Shanxi Province	Unknown	Unknown	Unknown	Unknown	46.2	68.8	92.5	(Dai et al., 2006)
Shanxi Province	7.3	Unknown	25.8	2.7	13.1	5.7	Unknown	(Shi et al., 2009)
Shenzhen City	Unknown	Unknown	Unknown	Unknown	16.6	11.9	68.2	(Wu et al., 2007)
Shenzhen City	47.8	Unknown	Unknown	Unknown	77.8	100	100	(Wu et al., 2010b)

Table 4. Incidence of HPV infection related to ICC, HSIL and LSIL in China, Hong Kong and Taiwan

in North America (13). Other HPV types most commonly related to ICC were HPV 31, 33, 35, 45, and 52. However, the prevalence of both HPV 58 and 52 were notably higher in ICC cases in Asia. For example, the prevalence of HPV 58 and 52 was found to be as important as the prevalence of HPV 16 and 18 in early cervical cancer patients as well as patients with advanced cervical cancer in Taiwan (15). As shown in Table 4, the frequency of HPV in HSIL, ICC, and CIN3 samples is higher than in ASCUS, LSIL, CIN1, and CIN2.

In Beijing, 85.7% of CIN3 patients have been diagnosed with HPV infections similar to 93.3% of HSIL patients (Table 4). In ASCUS cases, only 56.0% involve HPV infection (5). In all of these cases, HPV 16 was found to be the most common type (2.6% overall; 39.1% of HPV-positive women), followed by HPV 58 (1.0% overall) and HPV 33 (0.8% overall). For inland regions like Shandong and Shanxi province, CIN3/ICC patients have the highest HPV infection rate. HPV types 16, 52, 58, and 31 are the most prevalent HPV genotypes found in Shandong, whereas HPV 16, 58, 52, 33, and 18 are the predominant genotypes in Shanxi province (16, 17). In the TAR, HPV prevalence in HSIL cases is twice that of LSIL patients (Table 4). The descending order of HPV incidence among Tibetan women is HPV 16, 33, 58, 31, 52, and 68 (18).

For coastal areas like Fujian, Guangdong, Jiangxi, Liaoning, Shanghai, Shenzhen, and Taiwan, a similar prevalence of HPV types in ICC/CIN3 cases is observable (Table1 and Table 4). In Fujian province, HPV 16 (24.5%), HPV 33 (21.6%), and HPV 52 (19.6%) are the major genotypes present in CIN2/3 patients. In addition, HPV 16 (42.7%), HPV 18 (20.8%), and HPV 33 (12.5%) are also frequently found in squamous cell carcinoma (SCC) and adenocarcinoma (ADCA) (19). For Guangdong and Jiangxi, there is a significantly increased risk of elevating the CIN stage with high viral load. Thus, 68.8% of CIN1, 80.3% of CIN2, 90.2%of CIN3 and 90.0% of CIS contain HR-HPV genotypes like HPV 16 (79.6%), HPV 58 (5.92%), HPV 33 (3.29%), HPV 18 (1.97%), HPV 6 (1.97%), HPV 31 (1.31%), HPV 39 (1.31%), and HPV 68 (1.31%) (20). In Liaoning province, the most common HPV genotypes are HPV 16, HPV 58, HPV 52, HPV 33, HPV 53, and HPV 31, occurring in 54.6% of ASCUS patients, 64.1% of CIN, and 83.1% of ICC (21). For the island of Taiwan, the HPV prevalence for ASCUS, LSIL, HSIL, and squamous cell carcinoma are 41.2%, 76.9%, 87.5%, and 66.7%, respectively. The five high-incidence HPV genotypes are HPV 52, 18, 58, 53, and 70 in Taiwanese CIN2 patients (22). For Shanghai city, HPV viral load values in women with CINs and cervical cancer were calculated to be 68.8% in CIN1, 66.7% in CIN2, 76.5% in CIN3, and 94.1% in cervical cancer (23). For Shenzhen city, the incidence of HR-HPV genotypes increased with increasing severity of cervical lesions, such as 50.0% of CIN1, and 74.0% of CIN2 /CIN3. However, the most common types were HPV52, 16, and 18 in CIN samples that are different with population screening which the most common genotypes are HPV 16, 52, 58, 31 and 39 (24).

4. HPV vaccination in Southern China, Hong Kong, and Taiwan

Based on statistical calculations to determine the link between HPV and cervical cancer, many strategies for the prevention of cervical cancer have been proposed, including vaccination in younger women and improved HPV screening in older women (25). Two HPV vaccines have been generated from the recombinant L1 protein into non-infectious capsids (virus-like particles, VLPs). Gardasil™ (Merck and Co, USA) already has approval for vaccination against HPV6/11/16/18 in several countries including Singapore and Hong Kong. The bivalent vaccine, Cervarix™ (GlaxoSmithKline, Belgium), has also been approved in both countries. Both vaccines were developed for HPV16 and HPV18, which cause approximately 70% of all reported cervical cancer cases worldwide (26). Thus, the quadrivalent vaccine can be expected to prevent CIN-2 and CIN-3 (CIN-2,3), cervical cancer, as well as genital warts. However, HPV 18 is less common than HPV 52 and 58 in places like China, Hong Kong, and Taiwan (Table 1) where there is no publicly funded vaccination program. Hence vaccination is voluntary and paid by individuals.

HPV vaccination does not increase the clearance of established infections; therefore, young females are ideally targeted before the development of sexual behavior. Initiation of HPV vaccination in younger cohorts combined with HPV screening in older women is a good strategy for HPV prevention. In China and Taiwan, evaluation of HPV vaccination as primary care HPV and assessment of the threshold cost per vaccinated girl (CVG) became potential feasible strategies in public health. Singapore's policy regarding the management of HPV can be a reference for China and Taiwan. In a cervical cancer awareness survey for Singaporean women aged 30-55 years in 2006, 80% have had at least one Pap smear although 25% did not fully understand the significance behind it (13). Furthermore, 80% were unaware of HPV. In Hong Kong, most women have never heard of HPV or its infection by sexual transmission (27). Thus, participants had no knowledge or means of understanding the link between cervical cancer and HPV infection. However, participants agreed to HPV vaccination for both themselves and their teenage daughters if a health department endorsement was provided. Another study demonstrated that 32% of participants accepted HPV vaccination prior to receiving an educational booklet, and that this number increased to 52% after reading the pamphlet (28). About 48% of women remained undecided or disagreed with vaccination after education; 84% were worried about the side effects of vaccination, and 63% of women augmented fear of earlier sexual activity and unsafe sex. In China, a population-based survey related to knowledge concerning HPV vaccination reported that 15.8% of women between the ages of 15–54 have never heard of HPV, of which 49% bewared that HPV was related to cervical cancer. Around 87% of women agreed to be vaccinated with the prophylactic HPV vaccine and, in addition, 88% of women expressed that they would like to have their daughters vaccinated (29). In rural Shanxi, 67% of surveyed women did not believe that they were at risk of HPV infection and cervical cancer, while 65% of women thought there would be no difference whether or not they were vaccinated. However, 98% of the surveyed women preferred to receive information about the HPV vaccine from doctors, nurses, and hospital staff rather than from family members or friends.

To improve the coverage of vaccination programs, a low vaccine price is one important issue to consider, and 83% of the women hoped that health insurance or the government can cover all or part of vaccine-related costs (30). When asked about the vaccine cost, 42% of women said they are willing to pay USD 2.50 or less and 50% agreed to pay USD 2.50–14.00, while only 8% can afford to pay more than USD 15.00 (31). However, according to investigation conducted by Canfell *et al.* (2011), vaccination combined with once- or twice-in-a-lifetime screening is sufficiently cost-effective with a CVG of USD 52. But the maximum vaccine unit cost per dose is USD 9.00-14.00 that is also implied by maximum CVG of $50–54. Therefore, HPV vaccination is potentially feasible for Chinese women at a reasonable price. However, in order to sustain a wide vaccine coverage, vaccine price would be one of the largest barriers for promotion (31).

In terms of HPV vaccine safety, data from pharmaceutical companies responsible for bivalent and quadrivalent vaccines suggest that some patients could be expected to experience mild, transient vaccine-related side effects upon receiving the HPV vaccine (32, 33). From reports, pain is the most frequently reported adverse effect, with a prevalence ranging from 83% to 93% in tested vaccine group (34). With the exception of pain, no differences in serious vaccine-related events were prominent between vaccine and placebo groups. Data regarding the long-term safety of these vaccines are not yet available. HPV vaccination tests also did not include pregnant women. Although incidence of spontaneous abortion occurred in 10% of the vaccine group, it also occured in 7% of the placebo group, hence there is no significant difference between the two groups (35). Similarly, results from the quadrivalent vaccine Phase III studies indicated no observable differences in relation to the incidence of spontaneous abortions, late fetal death, or congenital abnormal infants between both groups. Even women who became pregnant more than 30 days after vaccine administration did not contribute any statistical difference whatsoever (35).

Currently, available vaccines contain HPV 16 and 18; however, HPV types 52 and 58 are more prevalent in Southeast Asia, especially in Hong Kong and Taiwan. Although, HPV16 and 18 are major genotypes found in CIN3 and cervical cancer patients, HPV types 52 and 58 also have high prevalence rate in cancer cases. For example, HPV types 52 and 58 have 25% and 12.5% infection rate in Taiwan (15), As shown in Table 1, the prevalence of HPV 52 and HPV 58 in Chengdu, Fujian, Gansu, Guangzhou, Hong Kong, Liaoning, Taiwan, Shandong, Shanxi, Shenyang, Shenzhen, and Zhejiang is higher than HPV 18, 6, and 11. This indicates that bivalent and quadrivalent vaccines are only capable of covering a small part of prospective patients infected with HPV. The emerging question then is, *Should women pay for HPV vaccines without understanding their HPV infection types or not*? It is safe to say at the present time that a vaccination program, combined with HPV Pap smear screening, is necessary to avoid useless vaccine treatment. The prevalence of HPV 52 and HPV 58 is nearly equal to the frequency of HPV 16 in China, Hong Kong, and Taiwan whether in cervical cancer-related or population-based surveys (Table 1). Moreover, a 1997–2007 report in Hong Kong showed that aside from 68.0% of all histological groups combined, 62.6% of squamous cell carcinoma and 93.8% of adenocarcinoma and adenosquamous cell carcinoma were covered by HPV 16 and HPV 18. Hence if vaccines included HPV 52 and HPV 58, it could increase the coverage by 15.9% for cervical cancers overall, 18.4% for squamous cell carcinoma, and 4.1% for adenocarcinoma and adenosquamous cell carcinoma (8). To summarize, pharmaceutical companies should make an effort to include more high prevalence HPV types in the next generation of vaccines they develop.

The limitations of vaccine programs must also be recognized, because HPV 16 and 18 account for approximately 70% of all invasive cervical cancers in nine countries (36), excluding Chinese people. Thus, women should be advised that the HPV vaccine does not confer full protection against cervical cancer. To reduce the risk of HPV infection and cervical cancer, safe sexual practices, which include the use of condoms and routine Pap smear testing, are necessary. Another important issue is the HPV genotypes screening. There are over 100 different HPV types, but only 13 HR-HPVs were routine in Pap smear screening. In our previous data, 52 HPV genotypes were adopted to screen 10,543 cases, of which 1,021 involve HR-HPVs and 556 involve non-HR-HPVs. Our investigation supported more HPV genotypes prevalence than other literatures. Majority of existing reports focus on HR-HPV due to a high risk of cervical cancer associated with it. However, other LR-HPV types may be valuable, especially when indicating the risk in women's sexual behavior which could bring about a high chance of incurring HR-HPV infection in the future. Any HR-HPV/LR-HPV infection is worth to notice the cervical cancer possibility in women even HR-HPV is significant in ICC/CIN3 samples. Although there are little evidences to prove the relationship between LR-HPV and cervical cancer, we would like to point out the importance of LR-HPV screening, which could be useful to get rid of HPV attack, if the cost is reasonable for both HR-HPV and LR-HPV tests.

5. Conclusion

HPV 16, 52, and 58 are the most predominant types of HPV in China, Hong Kong, and Taiwan. HPV 18, on the other hand, may have lower prevalence than types 39, 51, and 56 in some regions, such as Taiwan. Single/multiple HPV infection types do not distinguish between different age groups. The incidence of HPV types reflect women's sexual behavior in different ages. However, HPV 16 is clearly the most common type of HPV in the world. Because HPV 16, 52, and 58 are more common than HPV 18 in China, Hong Kong, and Taiwan, the protective effect of an HPV16/18 vaccine against HR-HPV infection in these regions should be a major consideration because both subtypes are not powerful enough to reduce the prevalence of cervical cancer. Geographic variation with regard to distribution of HPV genotypes should also be an important consideration, especially in the tailoring of vaccines in different regions. The prevalence of HPV genotypes may be caused by the complex interplay among different HPV genotypes, safety of sexual practices, and host immunogenetic factors.

6. Appendix: The HPV prevalence around the world

Area	Overall HPV (%)	HPV Genotypes (%)																	Reference
		6	11	16	18	31	33	35	39	45	51	52	56	58	59	68	73	82	
Argentina	16.7	0.1	0.3	4.0	1.9	1.8	1.4	1.9	1.0	1.1	0.4	1.2	0.9	1.3	0.8	0.8	0.2	0.1	(Matos et al., 2003)
Brazil	13.8	0.5	0.5	2.7	0.8	1.1	0.4	0.2	0.1	0.5	0.7	0.6	0.6	2.1	0.1	0.4	0.2	0.1	(Franco et al., 1999)
Chile	11.2	0.2	0.4	2.2	0.4	0.5	0.1	0.3	0.7	0.7	0.7	0.8	1.3	1.0	0.9	0.0	0.2	0.0	(Ferreccio et al., 2004)
China (Beijing)	7.9	ND	ND	2.6	0.5	0.4	0.8	0.6	0.1	0.1	0.2	0.0	0.7	1.0	0.3	0.5	0.1	ND	(Zhao et al., 2009)
China (Guangzho)	8.9	ND	ND	1.2	0.7	1.2	0.6	0.1	0.3	0.2	0.1	2.6	0.3	1.1	0.2	0.4	ND	ND	(Liu et al., 2011)
China (HK)	5.2	ND	ND	1.2	1.0	0.0	0.3	0.0	0.1	0.2	0.0	1.2	0.0	1.0	0.1	0.2	ND	ND	(Liu et al., 2011)
China (Shandong)	16.5	ND	ND	3.6	1.5	0.9	1.5	0.2	0.4	0.2	0.2	2.3	1.3	1.7	0.0	2.8	ND	ND	(Yuan et al., 2011)
China (Shanxi)	15.9	ND	ND	5.7	0.8	0.5	1.2	ND	0.6	0.6	0.6	1.2	0.8	3.2	0.3	0.2	ND	0.2	(Dai et al., 2006)
China (Shenyang)	14.8	ND	ND	3.4	1.0	1.0	0.9	0.3	0.9	0.6	0.6	2.5	0.9	1.9	0.6	0.3	ND	0.2	(Li et al., 2006)

China (Shenzhen)	15.2	ND	ND	2.5	1.4	1.5	0.3	0.4	1.5	0.7	0.6	2.0	1.0	1.6	0.9	0.5	0.1	0.2	(Wu et al., 2007)
China (Zhejiang)	13.9	ND	ND	2.5	0.8	0.8	0.8	0.2	0.3	0.3	0.9	3.1	0.4	2.1	0.7	1.0	0.0	ND	(Ye et al., 2010)
China (Tibetan)	7.8	ND	ND	1.5	0.2	1.2	1.2	0.0	0.2	0.2	0.2	1.1	0.2	1.2	0.1	0.5	ND	ND	(Jin et al., 2010)
Costa Rica	22.4	0.4	0.2	2.2	1.1	1.1	0.5	0.2	0.4	0.5	1.5	1.1	0.5	1.3	0.3	0.2	0.3	0.3	(Herrero et al., 2005)
Ho Chi Minh.	10.9	0.0	0.0	3.3	1.2	0.8	1.1	0.3	0.9	0.7	0.8	1.1	1.1	1.5	0.0	0.7	0.1	0.0	(Ahn et al., 2003)
Honduras	39.0	0.2	1.8	10.9	4.1	3.4	0.7	0.2	0.0	0.0	0.0	0.2	0.0	1.8	0.0	0.0	0.0	0.0	(Ferrera et al., 1999)
Italy	7.8	0.1	0.2	2.7	0.1	0.3	0.1	0.1	0.3	0.6	0.1	0.3	0.4	0.4	0.1	0.2	0.0	0.0	(Ronco et al., 2005)
Japan	10.2	0.1	0.0	0.5	0.2	0.3	0.4	0.8	0.1	0.0	0.9	1.2	0.6	0.2	0.2	0.5	0.0	0.0	(Asato et al., 2004)
Kenya	38.8	0.5	0.5	3.5	2.2	3.3	1.9	2.7	1.4	1.6	1.1	6.2	1.4	2.7	0.3	1.6	ND	ND	(De Vuyst et al., 2003)
Mexico	13.5	0.5	1.0	1.8	1.1	1.5	1.0	0.3	1.0	0.6	0.8	0.8	0.3	1.0	0.2	0.3	0.1	0.3	(Lazcano-Ponce et al. 2001)
Nigeria	24.8	0.4	0.4	3.0	1.7	2.6	0.6	3.0	0.4	2.1	1.1	1.5	2.1	2.5	0.6	0.2	0.5	0.4	(Thomas et al., 2004)
Republic of Korea	15.2	0.7	0.3	1.3	1.2	0.7	0.4	0.3	0.9	0.1	1.8	1.3	1.5	0.7	0.4	0.5	0.5	0.0	(Shin et al., 2004)
Scotland	12.7	ND	ND	3.4	1.4	0.7	0.5	0.3	0.4	0.9	0.9	0.8	0.6	0.7	0.7	0.2	0.8	0.1	(Cuschieri et al., 2004)
Senegal	12.5	0.2	0.0	1.0	0.9	0.4	0.7	0.0	0.1	0.2	0.3	0.5	0.3	0.7	0.4	0.1	0.3	0.1	(Xi et al., 2003)
South India	14.0	0.2	0.0	2.8	0.8	0.8	0.8	0.8	0.6	0.3	0.4	0.7	1.1	0.2	0.7	0.0	0.2	0.2	(Franceschi et al., 2005)
Spain Hanoi, Vietnam	1.5	0.1	0.0	1.0	0.0	0.4	0.0	0.5	0.1	0.0	0.4	0.0	0.2	0.1	0.2	0.2	0.0	0.0	(de Sanjose et al., 2003)
Sweden	6.8	ND	ND	2.1	0.6	1.1	0.4	0.3	0.2	0.8.	0.4	0.3	0.5	0.3	0.1	ND	ND	ND	(Forslund et al., 2002)
Taiwan	15.0	0.5	0.1	1.4	0.6	0.3	0.3	0.1	0.8	0.2	0.8	2.1	0.9	1.2	0.3	0.1	0.2	1.6	(Wang et al., 2010)
Thailand	4.8	0.0	0.0	0.7	0.3	0.3	0.5	0.2	0.3	0.1	0.2	0.3	0.2	0.4	0.1	0.2	0.0	0.0	(Sukvirach et al., 2003)
UK	3.5	ND	ND	1.3	0.7	0.9	0.7	ND	ND	ND	ND	ND	ND	ND	ND	ND	ND	ND	(Cuzick et al., 1995)
USA	15.8	0.6	0.6	2.5	0.8	0.9	0.6	0.3	0.7	0.9	1.8	0.8	0.5	0.9	0.7	0.2	0.0	0.0	(Liaw et al., 1999)

Appendix 1. Data summarized from IARC and this article.

7. References

[1] de Sanjose, S., Diaz, M., Castellsague, X., Clifford, G., Bruni, L., Munoz, N. and Bosch, F.X. (2007) Worldwide prevalence and genotype distribution of cervical human papillomavirus DNA in women with normal cytology: a meta-analysis. *Lancet Infect Dis*, 7, 453-459.

[2] Chen, C.A., Liu, C.Y., Chou, H.H., Chou, C.Y., Ho, C.M., Twu, N.F., Kan, Y.Y., Chuang, M.H., Chu, T.Y. and Hsieh, C.Y. (2006) The distribution and differential risks of human papillomavirus genotypes in cervical preinvasive lesions: A Taiwan Cooperative Oncologic Group Study. *Int J Gynecol Cancer*, 16, 1801-1808.

[3] Wang, C.H., Garvilles, R.G. and Chen, C.Y. (2010) Characterization of human papillomavirus infection in north Taiwan. *J Med Virol*, 82, 1416-1423.

[4] Shi, J.F., Wu, R.F., Liu, Z.H., Zhou, Q.Z., Li, N., Wu-Lan, N., Li, Q., Wang, Q., Liu, B., Li, R.Z. *et al.* (2006) (Distribution of human papillomavirus types in Shenzhen women). *Zhongguo Yi Xue Ke Xue Yuan Xue Bao*, 28, 832-836.

[5] Zhao, R., Zhang, W.Y., Wu, M.H., Zhang, S.W., Pan, J., Zhu, L., Zhang, Y.P., Li, H., Gu, Y.S. and Liu, X.Z. (2009) Human papillomavirus infection in Beijing, People's Republic of China: a population-based study. *Br J Cancer*, 101, 1635-1640.

[6] Lin, M., Yang, L.Y., Li, L.J., Wu, J.R., Peng, Y.P. and Luo, Z.Y. (2008) Genital human papillomavirus screening by gene chip in Chinese women of Guangdong province. *Aust N Z J Obstet Gynaecol*, 48, 189-194.

[7] Liu, S.S., Chan, K.Y., Leung, R.C., Chan, K.K., Tam, K.F., Luk, M.H., Lo, S.S., Fong, D.Y., Cheung, A.N., Lin, Z.Q. *et al.* (2011) Prevalence and risk factors of Human Papillomavirus (HPV) infection in southern Chinese women - a population-based study. *PLoS ONE*, 6, e19244.

[8] Chan, P.K., Ho, W.C., Yu, M.Y., Pong, W.M., Chan, A.C., Chan, A.K., Cheung, T.H., Wong, M.C., To, K.F. and Ng, H.K. (2009) Distribution of human papillomavirus types in cervical cancers in Hong Kong: current situation and changes over the last decades. *Int J Cancer*, 125, 1671-1677.

[9] Ye, J., Cheng, X., Chen, X., Ye, F., Lu, W. and Xie, X. (2010) Prevalence and risk profile of cervical Human papillomavirus infection in Zhejiang Province, southeast China: a population-based study. *Virol J*, 7, 66.

[10] Li, L.K., Dai, M., Clifford, G.M., Yao, W.Q., Arslan, A., Li, N., Shi, J.F., Snijders, P.J., Meijer, C.J., Qiao, Y.L. *et al.* (2006) Human papillomavirus infection in Shenyang City, People's Republic of China: A population-based study. *Br J Cancer*, 95, 1593-1597.

[11] Vaccarella, S., Franceschi, S., Herrero, R., Munoz, N., Snijders, P.J., Clifford, G.M., Smith, J.S., Lazcano-Ponce, E., Sukvirach, S., Shin, H.R. *et al.* (2006) Sexual behavior, condom use, and human papillomavirus: pooled analysis of the IARC human papillomavirus prevalence surveys. *Cancer Epidemiol Biomarkers Prev*, 15, 326-333.

[12] Shi, J.F., Qiao, Y.L., Smith, J.S., Dondog, B., Bao, Y.P., Dai, M., Clifford, G.M. and Franceschi, S. (2008) Epidemiology and prevention of human papillomavirus and cervical cancer in China and Mongolia. *Vaccine*, 26 Suppl 12, M53-59.

[13] Tay, S.K., Ngan, H.Y., Chu, T.Y., Cheung, A.N. and Tay, E.H. (2008) Epidemiology of human papillomavirus infection and cervical cancer and future perspectives in Hong Kong, Singapore and Taiwan. *Vaccine*, 26 Suppl 12, M60-70.

[14] Koong, S.L., Yen, A.M. and Chen, T.H. (2006) Efficacy and cost-effectiveness of nationwide cervical cancer screening in Taiwan. *J Med Screen*, 13 Suppl 1, S44-47.

[15] Ho, C.M., Chien, T.Y., Huang, S.H., Lee, B.H. and Chang, S.F. (2006) Integrated human papillomavirus types 52 and 58 are infrequently found in cervical cancer, and high viral loads predict risk of cervical cancer. *Gynecol Oncol*, 102, 54-60.

[16] Dai, M., Bao, Y.P., Li, N., Clifford, G.M., Vaccarella, S., Snijders, P.J., Huang, R.D., Sun, L.X., Meijer, C.J., Qiao, Y.L. *et al.* (2006) Human papillomavirus infection in Shanxi Province, People's Republic of China: a population-based study. *Br J Cancer*, 95, 96-101.

[17] Yuan, X., Yang, Y., Gu, D., Liu, H., Yang, H. and Wang, M. (2011) Prevalence of human papillomavirus infection among women with and without normal cervical histology in Shandong Province, China. *Arch Gynecol Obstet*, 283, 1385-1389.

[18] Jin, Q., Shen, K., Li, H., Zhou, X.R., Huang, H.F. and Leng, J.H. (2010) Age-specific prevalence of human papillomavirus by grade of cervical cytology in Tibetan women. *Chin Med J (Engl)*, 123, 2004-2011.

[19] Wu, D., Cai, L., Huang, M., Zheng, Y. and Yu, J. (2010) Prevalence of genital human papillomavirus infection and genotypes among women from Fujian province, PR China. *Eur J Obstet Gynecol Reprod Biol*, 151, 86-90.

[20] Wu, Y., Chen, Y., Li, L., Yu, G., Zhang, Y. and He, Y. (2006) Associations of high-risk HPV types and viral load with cervical cancer in China. *J Clin Virol*, 35, 264-269.

[21] Sun, Z.R., Ji, Y.H., Zhou, W.Q., Zhang, S.L., Jiang, W.G. and Ruan, Q. (2010) Characteristics of HPV prevalence among women in Liaoning province, China. *Int J Gynaecol Obstet*, 109, 105-109.

[22] Chao, A., Hsu, K.H., Lai, C.H., Huang, H.J., Hsueh, S., Lin, S.R., Jung, S.M., Chao, F.Y., Huang, S.L., Huang, C.C. *et al.* (2008) Cervical cancer screening program integrating Pap smear and HPV DNA testing: a population-based study. *Int J Cancer*, 122, 2835-2841.

[23] Zhang, W.Y., Xue, Y.Z., Chen, M., Han, L. and Luo, M. (2008) Prevalence of high-risk human papillomavirus infection in different cervical lesion among organized health-examination women in Shanghai, China. *Chin Med J (Engl)*, 121, 1578-1582.

[24] Wu, R.F., Dai, M., Qiao, Y.L., Clifford, G.M., Liu, Z.H., Arslan, A., Li, N., Shi, J.F., Snijders, P.J., Meijer, C.J. *et al.* (2007) Human papillomavirus infection in women in Shenzhen City, People's Republic of China, a population typical of recent Chinese urbanisation. *Int J Cancer*, 121, 1306-1311.

[25] Schiffman, M., Castle, P.E., Jeronimo, J., Rodriguez, A.C. and Wacholder, S. (2007) Human papillomavirus and cervical cancer. *Lancet*, 370, 890-907.

[26] Smith, J.S., Lindsay, L., Hoots, B., Keys, J., Franceschi, S., Winer, R. and Clifford, G.M. (2007) Human papillomavirus type distribution in invasive cervical cancer and high-grade cervical lesions: a meta-analysis update. *Int J Cancer*, 121, 621-632.

[27] Kwan, T.T., Chan, K.K., Yip, A.M., Tam, K.F., Cheung, A.N., Young, P.M., Lee, P.W. and Ngan, H.Y. (2008) Barriers and facilitators to human papillomavirus vaccination among Chinese adolescent girls in Hong Kong: a qualitative-quantitative study. *Sex Transm Infect*, 84, 227-232.

[28] Chan, S.S., Cheung, T.H., Lo, W.K. and Chung, T.K. (2007) Women's attitudes on human papillomavirus vaccination to their daughters. *J Adolesc Health*, 41, 204-207.

[29] Lai, H.C., Lin, W.Y., Lin, Y.W., Chang, C.C., Yu, M.H., Chen, C.C. and Chu, T.Y. (2005) Genetic polymorphisms of FAS and FASL (CD95/CD95L) genes in cervical carcinogenesis: An analysis of haplotype and gene-gene interaction. *Gynecol Oncol*, 99, 113-118.

[30] McIntosh, J., Sturpe, D.A. and Khanna, N. (2008) Human papillomavirus vaccine and cervical cancer prevention: practice and policy implications for pharmacists. *J Am Pharm Assoc (2003)*, 48, e1-13; quiz e14-17.

[31] Canfell, K., Shi, J.F., Lew, J.B., Walker, R., Zhao, F.H., Simonella, L., Chen, J.F., Legood, R., Smith, M.A., Nickson, C. *et al.* (2011) Prevention of cervical cancer in rural China: evaluation of HPV vaccination and primary HPV screening strategies. *Vaccine*, 29, 2487-2494.

[32] Villa, L.L., Costa, R.L., Petta, C.A., Andrade, R.P., Ault, K.A., Giuliano, A.R., Wheeler, C.M., Koutsky, L.A., Malm, C., Lehtinen, M. *et al.* (2005) Prophylactic quadrivalent human papillomavirus (types 6, 11, 16, and 18) L1 virus-like particle vaccine in young women: a randomised double-blind placebo-controlled multicentre phase II efficacy trial. *Lancet Oncol*, 6, 271-278.

[33] Villa, L.L., Costa, R.L., Petta, C.A., Andrade, R.P., Paavonen, J., Iversen, O.E., Olsson, S.E., Hoye, J., Steinwall, M., Riis-Johannessen, G. *et al.* (2006) High sustained efficacy of a prophylactic quadrivalent human papillomavirus types 6/11/16/18 L1 virus-like particle vaccine through 5 years of follow-up. *Br J Cancer*, 95, 1459-1466.

[34] Garland, S.M., Hernandez-Avila, M., Wheeler, C.M., Perez, G., Harper, D.M., Leodolter, S., Tang, G.W., Ferris, D.G., Steben, M., Bryan, J. *et al.* (2007) Quadrivalent vaccine against human papillomavirus to prevent anogenital diseases. *N Engl J Med*, 356, 1928-1943.

[35] (2007) Quadrivalent vaccine against human papillomavirus to prevent high-grade cervical lesions. *N Engl J Med*, 356, 1915-1927.

[36] Munoz, N., Bosch, F.X., de Sanjose, S., Herrero, R., Castellsague, X., Shah, K.V., Snijders, P.J. and Meijer, C.J. (2003) Epidemiologic classification of human papillomavirus types associated with cervical cancer. *N Engl J Med*, 348, 518-527.

[37] Matos, E., Loria, D., Amestoy, G.M., Herrera, L., Prince, M.A., Moreno, J., Krunfly, C., van den Brule, A.J., Meijer, C.J., Munoz, N. *et al.* (2003) Prevalence of human papillomavirus infection among women in Concordia, Argentina: a population-based study. *Sex Transm Dis*, 30, 593-599.

[38] Franco, E.L., Villa, L.L., Sobrinho, J.P., Prado, J.M., Rousseau, M.C., Desy, M. and Rohan, T.E. (1999) Epidemiology of acquisition and clearance of cervical human papillomavirus infection in women from a high-risk area for cervical cancer. *J Infect Dis*, 180, 1415-1423.

[39] Ferreccio, C., Prado, R.B., Luzoro, A.V., Ampuero, S.L., Snijders, P.J., Meijer, C.J., Vaccarella, S.V., Jara, A.T., Puschel, K.I., Robles, S.C. *et al.* (2004) Population-based prevalence and age distribution of human papillomavirus among women in Santiago, Chile. *Cancer Epidemiol Biomarkers Prev*, 13, 2271-2276.

[40] Herrero, R., Castle, P.E., Schiffman, M., Bratti, M.C., Hildesheim, A., Morales, J., Alfaro, M., Sherman, M.E., Wacholder, S., Chen, S. *et al.* (2005) Epidemiologic profile of type-specific human papillomavirus infection and cervical neoplasia in Guanacaste, Costa Rica. *J Infect Dis*, 191, 1796-1807.

[41] Ahn, W.S., Bae, S.M., Chung, J.E., Lee, H.K., Kim, B.K., Lee, J.M., Namkoong, S.E., Kim, C.K. and Sin, J. (2003) Evaluation of adenoassociated virus 2 and human papilloma virus 16 and 18 infection in cervical cancer biopsies. *Gynecol Oncol*, 89, 105-111.

[42] Ferrera, A., Velema, J.P., Figueroa, M., Bulnes, R., Toro, L.A., Claros, J.M., De Barahona, O. and Melchers, W.J. (1999) Human papillomavirus infection, cervical dysplasia and invasive cervical cancer in Honduras: a case-control study. *Int J Cancer*, 82, 799-803.

[43] Ronco, G., Ghisetti, V., Segnan, N., Snijders, P.J., Gillio-Tos, A., Meijer, C.J., Merletti, F. and Franceschi, S. (2005) Prevalence of human papillomavirus infection in women in Turin, Italy. *Eur J Cancer*, 41, 297-305.

[44] Asato, T., Maehama, T., Nagai, Y., Kanazawa, K., Uezato, H. and Kariya, K. (2004) A large case-control study of cervical cancer risk associated with human papillomavirus infection in Japan, by nucleotide sequencing-based genotyping. *J Infect Dis*, 189, 1829-1832.

[45] De Vuyst, H., Steyaert, S., Van Renterghem, L., Claeys, P., Muchiri, L., Sitati, S., Vansteelandt, S., Quint, W., Kleter, B., Van Marck, E. *et al.* (2003) Distribution of human papillomavirus in a family planning population in nairobi, kenya. *Sex Transm Dis*, 30, 137-142.

[46] Lazcano-Ponce, E., Herrero, R., Munoz, N., Cruz, A., Shah, K.V., Alonso, P., Hernandez, P., Salmeron, J. and Hernandez, M. (2001) Epidemiology of HPV infection among Mexican women with normal cervical cytology. *Int J Cancer*, 91, 412-420.

[47] Thomas, J.O., Herrero, R., Omigbodun, A.A., Ojemakinde, K., Ajayi, I.O., Fawole, A., Oladepo, O., Smith, J.S., Arslan, A., Munoz, N. *et al.* (2004) Prevalence of papillomavirus infection in women in Ibadan, Nigeria: a population-based study. *Br J Cancer*, 90, 638-645.

[48] Shin, H.R., Franceschi, S., Vaccarella, S., Roh, J.W., Ju, Y.H., Oh, J.K., Kong, H.J., Rha, S.H., Jung, S.I., Kim, J.I. *et al.* (2004) Prevalence and determinants of genital infection with papillomavirus, in female and male university students in Busan, South Korea. *J Infect Dis*, 190, 468-476.

[49] Cuschieri, K.S., Cubie, H.A., Whitley, M.W., Seagar, A.L., Arends, M.J., Moore, C., Gilkisson, G. and McGoogan, E. (2004) Multiple high risk HPV infections are common in cervical neoplasia and young women in a cervical screening population. *J Clin Pathol*, 57, 68-72.

[50] Xi, L.F., Toure, P., Critchlow, C.W., Hawes, S.E., Dembele, B., Sow, P.S. and Kiviat, N.B. (2003) Prevalence of specific types of human papillomavirus and cervical squamous intraepithelial lesions in consecutive, previously unscreened, West-African women over 35 years of age. *Int J Cancer*, 103, 803-809.

[51] Franceschi, S., Rajkumar, R., Snijders, P.J., Arslan, A., Mahe, C., Plummer, M., Sankaranarayanan, R., Cherian, J., Meijer, C.J. and Weiderpass, E. (2005) Papillomavirus infection in rural women in southern India. *Br J Cancer*, 92, 601-606.

[52] de Sanjose, S., Almirall, R., Lloveras, B., Font, R., Diaz, M., Munoz, N., Catala, I., Meijer, C.J., Snijders, P.J., Herrero, R. *et al.* (2003) Cervical human papillomavirus infection in the female population in Barcelona, Spain. *Sex Transm Dis*, 30, 788-793.

[53] Forslund, O., Antonsson, A., Edlund, K., van den Brule, A.J., Hansson, B.G., Meijer, C.J., Ryd, W., Rylander, E., Strand, A., Wadell, G. *et al.* (2002) Population-based type-specific prevalence of high-risk human papillomavirus infection in middle-aged Swedish women. *J Med Virol*, 66, 535-541.

[54] Sukvirach, S., Smith, J.S., Tunsakul, S., Munoz, N., Kesararat, V., Opasatian, O., Chichareon, S., Kaenploy, V., Ashley, R., Meijer, C.J. *et al.* (2003) Population-based human papillomavirus prevalence in Lampang and Songkla, Thailand. *J Infect Dis*, 187, 1246-1256.

[55] Cuzick, J., Szarewski, A., Terry, G., Ho, L., Hanby, A., Maddox, P., Anderson, M., Kocjan, G., Steele, S.T. and Guillebaud, J. (1995) Human papillomavirus testing in primary cervical screening. *Lancet*, 345, 1533-1536.

[56] Liaw, K.L., Glass, A.G., Manos, M.M., Greer, C.E., Scott, D.R., Sherman, M., Burk, R.D., Kurman, R.J., Wacholder, S., Rush, B.B. *et al.* (1999) Detection of human papillomavirus DNA in cytologically normal women and subsequent cervical squamous intraepithelial lesions. *J Natl Cancer Inst*, 91, 954-960.

3

Human Papillomavirus Worldwide Distribution in Women Without Cervical Cancer

I. Dutra[1,2], I. Foroni[1,2], A.R. Couto[1,2], M. Lima[2,3] and J. Bruges-Armas[1,2]
[1] *Serviço Especializado de Epidemiologia e Biologia Molecular, Hospital de Santo Espírito de Angra do Heroísmo*
[2] *Genetic and Arthritis Research Group (GARG), Institute for Molecular and Cell Biology (IBMC), University of Porto*
[3] *Grupo de Epidemiologia e Genética Humana do Departamento de Biologia da Universidade dos Açores*
Portugal

1. Introduction

Infection by certain types of Human Papillomavirus (HPV) is closely related to the corresponding risk of cervical cancer (Trottier and Franco, 2006). Cervical cancer represents the third most common malignancy in women, and the seventh overall, with an estimate 529.000 new cases in 2008 (Ferlay et al., 2010). More than 85% of the global burden occurs in developing countries, where it accounts for 13% of all female cancer (Ferlay et al., 2010).

HPV subtypes have been associated with the development of cervical, vulvar, anal, penile and oropharyngeal cancer in 2002 (Parkin, 2006), representing 5.2% of all cancers worldwide. It has also been estimated, on basis of cross-sectional observations (Clifford et al., 2005, de Sanjose et al., 2007) that approximately 10% of women worldwide with normal cytological findings carry a detectable cervical HPV infection. Therefore, HPV can be considered as the most common known sexually transmitted agent worldwide (de Sanjose et al., 2007).

HPV vaccines hold great promise to reduce the global burden of HPV infection as well as cervical cancer development. In June 2006, the quadrivalent HPV vaccine types 6, 11, 16, and 18 (GARDASIL™, manufactured by Merck and Co., Inc., Whitehouse Station, New Jersey) was licensed for use among females aged 9-26 years for prevention of vaccine HPV-type-related cervical cancer (Markowitz et al., 2007). On October 2009, the Food and Drug Administration (FDA) licensed bivalent HPV vaccine (Cervarix, GlaxoSmithKline) for use in females aged 10 through 25 years. Cervarix is the second HPV vaccine licensed for use in females in the United States (F.D.A., 2010). Both vaccines might provide protection against some other HPV-related cancers in addition to cervical cancer, although there are currently only data sufficient to recommend Gardasil™ for protection against vulvar and vaginal cancers and precancers. Gardsil™ is also recommended for prevention of genital warts.

The well established knowledge for HPV type distribution worldwide is a key feature for the rational design of future vaccination, that would include a broadest spectrum, and for the development of new HPV screening tests (Clifford et al., 2005). To contribute for this effort, we hereby present a worldwide description of HPV type distribution in women without cervical abnormalities.

2. Population data

To describe HPV type distribution, the geographical definition of the regions was based on Globocan, a project of the International Agency for Research on Cancer, that presents incidence, prevalence and mortality estimates of 27 major cancer for all countries in the world (Ferlay et al., 2010). The geographical areas include four regions in Africa (Northern, Southern, Eastern and Western), three regions in the Americas (central, south and northern), four regions in Europe (Northern, Southern, Eastern and Western), and four regions in Asia (Eastern, Southeastern, Southern and Western).

3. Worldwide HPV type distribution in women with normal cytology

3.1 Africa

Africa has a population of 274.49 millions women ages 15 years and older who are at risk of developing cervical cancer (WHO/ICO, 2007a). Current estimates indicate that every year 80419 women are diagnosed with cervical cancer and 53334 die from the disease (WHO/ICO, 2007a). Cervical cancer ranks as the second most frequent cancer among women between 15 and 44 years of age (WHO/ICO, 2007a). The prevalence of HPV is higher in African women with normal cytology than in women from other world regions and about 24.9% of women in the general population are estimated to harbor cervical HPV infection at a given time. Furthermore, HPV16 infections are found most commonly than infections caused by other HR types in regions of the world apart from Sub-Saharan Africa, where infections by other oncogenic HPV types, most significantly, HPV35, may dominate.

3.1.1 Northern Africa

In the Northern Africa, there are available studies from Tunisia, Morocco, Egypt and Algeria that describe the HPV distribution in women with normal cytological findings.

Tunisia has a population of 3.68 millions women and every year, 314 of them are diagnosed with cervical cancer, the third most common cancer in female, and 148 die from the disease (WHO/ICO, 2007a). About 14.6% of women in the general population are estimated to harbor cervical HPV infection at a given time (WHO/ICO, 2007a). A pilot study was carried out in 2006 by De Marco et al to identify the HPV prevalence in the country (De Marco et al., 2006). HPV prevalence among healthy women was 45% and HPV16 and HPV58 were the most common high risk (HR) types with a prevalence rate of 38% and 27% respectively (Table 1). HPV82 ranked third with 15% prevalence and types 31, 33 and 35 had 4% prevalence while there were no cases of HPV18. HPV72 and HPV83 were the only low risk (LR) types with 4% each. Overall prevalence appear to be within the expected range and well in agreement with the 39% already reported in Hassen et al cohort (Hassen et al., 2003).

Region	Total tested	HPV positive n	(%)	Spectrum[a]	Common type	Single HPV[b] (%)	Multiple HPV[c] (%)	HR HPV[d] (%)	LR HPV[e] (%)	Age[f]	Method[g]
Asia											
China	1701	205	8.7	High / low	16 / 52	9.4	2.6	8.6	3.9	15 - 59	GP5+/6+PCR, DNA chip
India	3061	367	12	High / low	16 / 18	9.7	2.4	8.5	0.8	-	GP5+/6+PCR, MY09/11
Iran	400	22	5.5	High	16 / 18	-	-	5.5	-	20 - 72	GP5+/6+ PCR
Japan	1328	288	21.7	High / low	52 / 16	20.7	13.5	18	7	17 - 73	Reverse ibridization, Hybrid capture
South Korea	821	70	8.5	High / low	70 / 33	6.9	1.6	4.4	4.1	15 - 69	GP5+/6+ PCR
Thailand	1673	80	4.7	High / low	72 / 16	3.6	1.2	2.9	1.8	15 - 65	GP5+/6+ PCR
Vietnam	1878	98	5.2	High / low	16 / 52	3.2	2.0	-	-	15 - 69	GP5+/6+ PCR
America											
Brazil	2512	532	21.1	High / low	16 / 72	-	6.3	5.3	0.5	>10 - 84	GP5+/6+PCR, MY09/11PCR
Chile	921	103	11.2	High / low	16 / 56	75	28	7.7	3.5	15 - 65	GP5+/6+ PCR
Columbia	1845	275	14.9	High / low	16 / 58	10	4.4	11.4	3.2	<20 - >55	GP5+/6+ PCR
Argentina	839	130	15.4	High / low	16 / 6	8.9	3.3	56	22	17 - 69	GP5+/6+ PCR
Mexico	1340	194	14.5	High / low	16 / 53	80.4	19.6	11	19	<25 - >65	Reverse ibridization
Costa Rica	7459	1670	22.4	High / low	71 / 16	16.6	5.8	9.9	12.5	<25 - >65	MY09/11 PCR
Unites States	2356	603	25.6	High / low	16 / 52	-	-	20.9	7.4	14 - 60	MY09/11 PCR
Canada	489	124	25.4	High / low	16 / 31	16	5.9	17	14.3	15 - 69	MY09/11 PCR
Africa											
Tunisia	64	28	45	High / low	16 / 58	-	-	-	-	≤25 - ≥35	PCR
Morocco	785	124	15.9	High	16 / 18	-	-	-	-	17 - 80	MY09/11 PCR
Algeria	732	33	5.3	High / low	31 / 16	4.5	0.82	2.9	2.7	15 - 65	GP5+/6+ PCR
South Africa	848	173	20.4	High / low	83 / 53	16.3	8.8	9.7	4.9	21 - 59	Reverse line blot assay
Zimbabwe	1987	487	24.5	High / low	58 / 16	-	-	-	-	-	MY09/11 PCR
Mozambique	195	148	75.9	High / low	51 / 35	38	38	-	-	-	Reverse ibridization
Kenya	454	183	40.3	High / low	58 / 16	20.9	32.5	27.3	26.2	<25 - ≥35	GP60/GP124

Nigeria	844	209	24.8	High / low	42 / 16	16.7	8.1	18.3	6.5	<25 - >65	GP5+/6+ PCR
Guinea	831	360	47.9	High / low	16 / 45	29	37.9	29.3	29.1	18 - 64	GP5+/6+ PCR
Senegal	1639	178	13	High / low	16 / 54	6.2	1.2	6	2.9	≤35 - ≥55	Reverse ibridization
Cote d'Ivoire	120	37	31.1	High	16 / 18	-	-	31.1	-	23 - 69	MY09/11 PCR
Europe											
United Kingdom	23775	2226	11.3	High	16 / 18	-	-	11.3	-	20 - 64	HC2, Roche Linear Array
Denmark	11918	2501	22.9	High / low	16 / 31	9.3	12.1	19.2	7.4	15 - >65	Line probe assay
Sweden	282	70	24.8	High / low	16 / 18 / 42	8.8	6	23.4	3.2	24 - 88	GP5+/6+ PCR, Bioplex 200 Luminex
Ireland	886	101	11.4	High / low	16 / 18	-	-	-	-	16 - 72	MY09/11 PCR
Norway	736	78	10.6	High / low	-	-	-	-	-	≥30	Sequencing, Amplicor HPV test
Spain	-	298	-	High	16 / 31	-	-	-	-	-	HC2
Italy	3151	307	9.7	High / low	16 / 31	9.8	2.1	6.2	2.7	25 - 64	HC2, Consensus, Genotyping
Greece	1029	185	18	High / low	33 / 6	7.7	0.5	-	-	≤21 - ≥65	HC2, GP5+/6+ PCR
Croatia	205	73	35.6	High	16 / 31	32.6	2.9	35.6	-	21 - 37	HC2, PCR
Portugal	275	30	10.9	High / low	31 / 16	9.4	1.4	6.1	1.8	16 - 81	Genomica
France	980	128	13	High / low	16 / 53	-	3	8.2	3.5	≤20 - ≥50	MY09/11 PCR, sequencing
Belgium	581	155	26.7	High	-	-	-	17.9	8.8	17 - 85	HC2, MY09/11 PCR
Germany	7833	341	4.4	High / low	16 / 31	3.1	1.2	3.7	1.3	30 - ≥60	Reverse Line Blot
Netherlands	1437	75	5.2	High / low	-	-	-	3.7	1.5	40 - 60	GP5+/6+ PCR
Switzerland	680	117	17.2	High / low	16 / 31	10.9	6.3	8.1	2.7	≤20 - ≥60	Linear Array HPV
Poland	42	9	21.4	High / low	51 / 52	9.5	9.5	21.4	4.7	20 - 75	SPF10, Reverse hybridization
Hungary	1018	60	5.9	High	-	-	-	-	-	-	Digene Hybrid Capture
Russia	309	90	29	High / low	16 / 31	25	1.6	53	26	20 - 45	MY09/11 PCR
Belarus	3187	929	27.5	High	16 / 31	15.1	24.9	31.2	-	≤20 - 80	RT-PCR
Latvia	3187	929	26.2	High	16 / 31	15.1	24.9	31.2	-	≤20 - 80	RT-PCR
Romania	285	123	43.5	High / low	16 / 18	-	-	22.8	5.6	≤25 - ≥45	Reverse hybridization, line probe assay

[a] Spectrum of HPV types tested for: [b] Single infection; [c] Multiple infection; [d] High risk HPV types; [e] Low risk HPV types; [f] Age of enrolled women; [g] Main HPV testing method

Table 1. HPV prevalence in women without cervical cancer by world region.

In Morocco, statistical data showed that cervical cancer represents a serious health problem, with 500 new cases annually registered in the National Institute of Oncology, Rabat (Amrani et al., 2003). A study conducted by Alhamany et al determined the prevalence of the most oncogenic HPV in the Moroccan population (Alhamany et al., 2010). The cervix samples were collected from healthy women between 17 and 80 years of age. HPV DNA detection/typing was acquired by PCR with MY09/MY11 primers with specific probes for HPV16, 18, 31, 33, 35 and 45. HPV DNA was identified in 15.9% of women: 13.7% had HPV16, 8.9%had HPV18, 3.2% cases had HPV31, 0.8% had HPV33, 2.4% case had HPV35, 1.6% of HPV45 and 69.4% had an unknown HPV type infection (Table 1). The HPV prevalence in Moroccan women was in concordance with the overall world distribution of HPV in asymptomatic women. HPV16 was the predominant infectious type and, once again in concordance with the worldwide tendency (Figure 1).

A population-based study identified the HPV type distribution and prevalence in Algerian women (Hammouda et al., 2011), where cervical cancer is the second most common cancer. From the 11.51 millions women at risk of developing the disease, 1398 will be diagnosed per year and 797 will die (WHO/ICO, 2007a). HPV prevalence among women with normal cytology was 5.3% with 33 single infections and 6 multiple infections (Table 1). Prevalence of HR and LR types was 2.9% and 2.7% respectively, and HPV31 was the most common type (1.1%) followed by HPV16 (0.5%). Regarding LR types, HPV6 and HPV66 were the most common - 0.5%. This study is the first population-based HPV survey carried out in Northern Africa, and revealed a rather low burden of HPV infection. In addition, the prevalence of HR HPV in Algeria can be directly compared with women attending cervical screening in Europe and Canada (Figure 1).

3.1.2 Southern Africa (Sub-Saharan Africa)

In South Africa, despite the high prevalence of cervical cancer, few studies have been performed to describe the HPV type distribution in the country. A study enrolling 848 women with normal cytological findings was reported by Allan et al in 2008. The median age of the women was 44 years, ranging from 21 to 59 years. The specimens were HPV typed by a reverse line blot assay (Roche). The most prevalent types were LR HPV83 (2.6%), followed by HR HPV53 (2.2%) and HPV16 (2.0%). The prevalence of HPV16 and HPV18 was 3.3% while the HPV prevalence (20.4%) was high when compared with that reported in studies of populations elsewhere in the world (Table 1, Figure 1).

3.1.3 Eastern Africa (Sub-Saharan Africa)

A study carried out during the second phase of a cervical cancer screening project in Zimbabwe analyzed 1579 women classified as normal cytology (Womack et al., 2000). 35% of women had an HPV infection detected by HCII. Fukuchi et al performed serial HPV testing in a cohort of human immunodeficiency virus (HIV)-negative women to assess the HPV incidence and prevalence (Fukuchi et al., 2009). Testing was performed using MY09/MY11 consensus HPV L1 primers and specimens that tested positive were further studied to determine the specific HPV type. HPV prevalence at enrollment was based on a total of 1987 healthy women. The overall HPV prevalence was 24.5% and the HR HPV infection rate corresponded to 16.1% (Table 1).

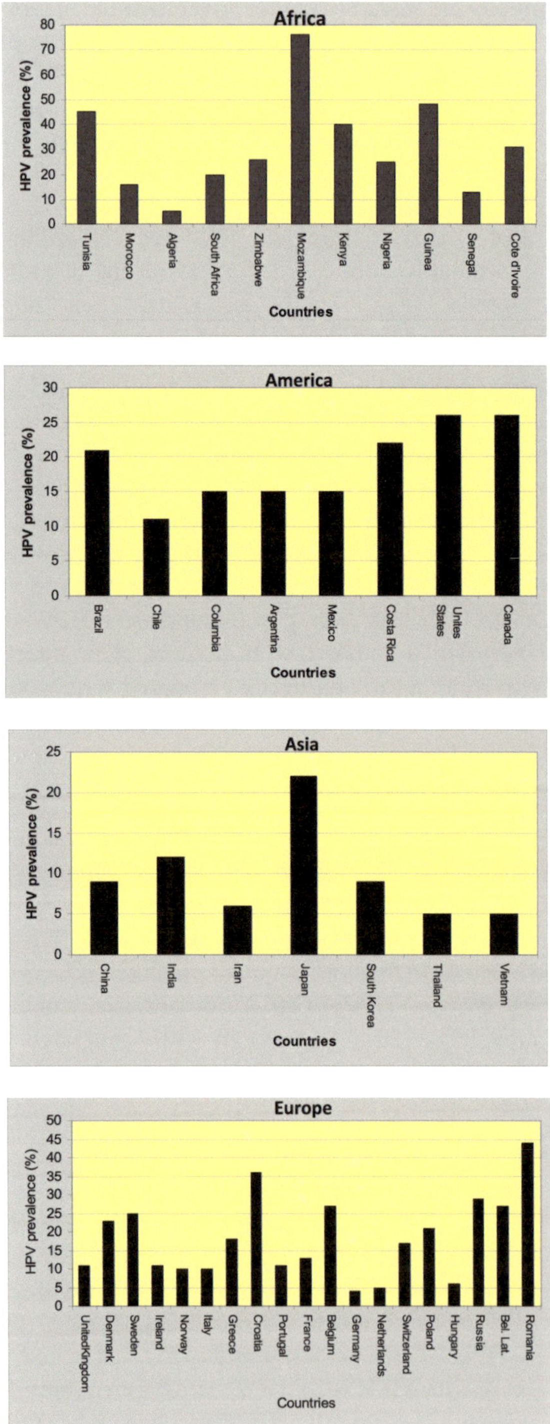

Fig. 1. HPV prevalence in women without cervical cancer

Among the prevalent infections, HPV58 was the most common HR type with 5% of women testing positive, followed by HPV16 and HPV18 with 4.7% and 2.3%, respectively. HPV70 was the most common LR type with 2,4%. HPV6 and HPV11 were rare in this cohort with 0,7% and 0,2% of women testing positive, respectively. The most common HPV types found in multiple infections were HPV types 58, 16, 70, 18, 53 and 33. The frequency of HPV58 is relatively high when compared with North America and Europe and it is associated with 3.3% of cervical cancer globally and 1.5% of cancer in Africa (WHO/ICO, 2007b).

In Mozambique, Castellsagué et al evaluated the HPV distribution in 196 women with normal Papanicolaou (Pap) smears. They used PGMY09/PGMY11 primer system in a reverse line-blot strip-based assay (Castellsague et al., 2001). The overall HPV DNA prevalence was 32%. In addition to the high prevalence of HPV infections, the most striking features in the epidemiology of HPV infection in this population were the high frequency of multiple simultaneous infections and the unexpected singularity of the type-specific HPV distribution. In 2008 Castellsagué et al reported a second study on HPV genotypes distribution in Mozambique. They collected cervical samples from 195 women without cervical abnormalities and tested them for HPV genotyping by SPF_{10}-$LIPA_{25}$ PCR system (Castellsague et al., 2008). HPV prevalence was 75.9%, the highest reported in the present work (Table 1, Figure 1). In descending order of frequency, the most frequent types were: HPV51 (23.6%), HPV35 (19.6%), HPV18 (14.2%), HPV31 (13.5%) and HPV52 (12.8%).

In Kenya, there are 10.32 million women in the general population, 2454 will be diagnosed with cervical cancer and 1676 will die from the disease (WHO/ICO, 2007a). In 1992, HPV prevalence was 19.5% among women with normal cytology (Czegledy et al., 1992). HPV16 was the most common type, followed by HPV18. To improve the epidemiological knowledge in Kenya, another HPV prevalence survey was developed in 2010 (De Vuyst et al., 2010). Among 454 women with normal cytological findings, 40.3% had a HPV DNA positive result (Table 1). The most common types were HPV58 with 9.9% prevalence, followed by HPV16 (7.5%) and HPV53 (6.6%). This study shows a high prevalence of HPV, similar to that found in other Sub-Saharan African populations. Not surprisingly for sub-Saharan Africa, half of HPV-positive women were infected with multiple types (Figure 1).

3.1.4 Western Africa (Sub-Saharan Africa)

Nigeria is the most populous country in Sub-Saharan Africa, with approximately 117 million inhabitants and an incidence of cervical cancer in Ibadan (1998-1999) of 19.9 per 100 000 (Cancer, 2003). To investigate the prevalence of cervical infection with HPV in the country, women with a sexually active life were tested (Thomas et al., 2004). HPV positivity was assessed by general primer-mediated GP5+/6+ PCR and by hybridization with an enzyme immunoassay (EIA). Among 844 women with normal cytology findings, the HPV prevalence was 24.8% with 18.3% of HR infections and 6.5% of LR infections (Table 1). The most commonly found HPV types, in either single or multiple infections, were HPV42 (4,4%), HPV16 and HPV35 (3%), HPV81 (2.7%), and HPV31 (2.6%). Other study on HPV infection in women without cervical cancer in Nigeria evaluated 844 women with normal cervical findings (Okolo et al., 2010). About 26.3% women were HPV positive. The prevalence of HPV16 and HPV35 were equally frequent (12.2%) followed by HPV 31 (11%).

Low risk and multiple HPV infections were also common with 44.9% and 27.8% respectively. The prevalence of HPV of 24.8% to 26.3% found in Nigeria studies is consistent with previous reports of the elevated prevalence of HPV in women of Sub-Saharan Africa.

To investigate HPV infection in Guinea, 831 healthy women aged 18-64 years from the general population were investigated (Keita et al., 2009). The overall presence of HPV DNA was determined by performing a general primer GP5+/6+ mediated PCR and HPV positivity was assessed by hybridization of PCR products in an EIA. HPV prevalence was 47.9% (Table 1). Prevalence of HR and LR types (29.3%, 29.1%, respectively) was similar. The commonest HR HPV types were HPV16 (6.7%), HPV45 (4.7%), HPV52 (4.0%), and HPV18, HPV35 and HPV58 (3.2% each). HPV66, HPV42 and HPV81 were the most commonly detected LR types. Totally, 29% of women had single type infection and 37.9% had multiple type infections.

In Senegal, Xi et al (2003) conducted a study among previously unscreened women to determine the prevalence of specific HPV types. HPV detection and typing analyses were carried out using a PCR-based reverse-line blot strip test (Xi et al., 2003). HPV DNA was detected in 13% women with normal cytology results, where 6.2% had a single type infection and 1.2% had a multiple type infection (Table 1). The most commonly detected types were HPV16 (1.0%), HPV54 (1.0%) and HPV18 (0.9%).

In a case-control study in the Cote d'Ivoire, the relationship between HIV infection and invasive cervical cancer was tested in 120 women with normal cytology. HPV DNA was detected by means of L1 consensus PCR assay (PGMY09/PGMY11 primer system), followed by typing in the Roche linear probe assay (Adjorlolo-Johnson et al., 2010). The prevalence of HPV infection was 31.1% and the most common types were HPV16, HPV18, HPV45, HPV35 and HPV31 (Table 1).

3.2 America

America has 336 millions of women older than 15 years which are at risk of developing cervical cancer (WHO/ICO, 2010a). Annually, 81000 of cervical cancer cases were diagnosed and 36000 of women died with the disease (WHO/ICO, 2010a). Cervical cancer ranks as the fourth most frequent cancer in women in America and the second most frequent among women between 15 and 44 years of age.

3.2.1 South and Central America

Latin America continues to be an important burden of cervical cancer (Murillo et al., 2008). South and Central America, along with Sub-Saharan Africa and Southeast Asia, exhibited some of the highest incidence rates worldwide (Gage et al., 2003). The incidence of cervical cancer is highest among poor women with few years of schooling, who tend to be diagnosed at advanced stages of the disease (Murillo et al., 2008). Even when these women are screened or diagnosed, less than one fourth of them receive adequate follow-up and care (Gage et al., 2003). Numerous countries in the region have attempted to implement cytology-based screening programs but without success, even in countries where cytology has been available for many years and where organized health care systems exist. While the lack of impact is frequently attributed to problems associated with program performance, new screening technology and prophylactic HPV vaccines emerge as promising alternatives for cervical cancer control (Murillo et al., 2008). Nevertheless, to ensure success of these technological advances, public health programs will still need to be organized and structured to maximize the benefits that could be obtained with the adoption and implementation of novel methods to control cervical cancer (Murillo et al., 2008). Latin America has a high HPV prevalence among women with normal cytology (Table 1) but the incidence of this disease varies between rich and poor countries, even between regions within a country (Figure 1). Age-specific prevalence ranges from 30% among women younger than 25 to 11% among women aged 45-54 (Figure 2). It is very high among teen-agers and then it slowly declined until 45-54 years of age to increase again significantly among women more than 55 years (20%). HPV16 was the most prevalent type among women with normal cervical histology but other common HPV genotypes are HPV18, HPV52, HPV31, and HPV6.

In Mexico cervical cancer is the most common cancer among women and its incidence rate is the highest world-wide. Mexico has a population of 37.45 million women aged 15 years and older who are at risk of developing cervical cancer (WHO/ICO, 2010k). Annually 10000 women are diagnosed with cervical cancer and 5000 die from the disease (WHO/ICO, 2010k). In countries like Mexico, cervical cancer early detection programs have had a minimal impact on the incidence and death rates (Lazcano-Ponce et al., 1999, Lazcano-Ponce et al., 2003, Ogedegbe et al., 2005). In addition, in poor regions, Pap smears have generally proven to be ineffective (Chu et al., 2007), frequently due to inadequate sampling of the specimen (Raab et al., 2008), poor fixation, and lack of competencies (Tworek et al., 2007). The consequence is a very high number of false-negative results (DeMay, 1996). The HPV prevalence among women with normal cervical cytology in Mexico was 14.5% (Table 1). As in Chile, Columbia, and Costa Rica, the age standardized–HPV prevalence among healthy women follows a bimodal distribution. HPV DNA was detected in 16.7% among women less than 25 years, with the prevalence declining rapidly to 3.7% between 45 and 54 years (12.3%), and increasing again to a maximum of 23% among women with 65 years of age. The HR HPV types were predominant in the first peak while LR HPV types were more frequent among women over 65 years of age. The most common genotype was HPV16, followed by HPV53 and HPV31.

Cervical cancer and breast cancer are leading causes of cancer-related morbidity and mortality in Costa Rica. In a population where every year 1.5 million of teenagers are at risk for cervical cancer, 403000 cervical cancer cases were diagnosed and 158000 women older than 15 years died with the disease (WHO/ICO, 2010h). HPV prevalence among women with normal cervical histology was high (22.4) (Table 1). Infection with a single type occurred in 16.6%, and 5.8% of women were infected with at least two HPV genotypes. The LR HPV types were predominant compared with HR HPV types, infecting 12.5 and 9.9% of women, respectively. HPV71 was the most frequent genotype. The prevalence of type HPV16 was relatively low, while the HR HPV58, HPV51, and HPV52 were relatively frequent. This finding placed Costa Rica close to African and Asian countries, where the HPV58 and HPV52 were the most frequent. As in the areas of Latin America where a high HPV prevalence was detected, the age-specific prevalence followed a bimodal distribution with the highest peaks at the extremes of ages. HR HPV genotypes were more common in women younger than 25 years old, with a decrease in prevalence in the intermediate age group, and a minor peak in the older women. On the contrary, LR HPV genotypes showed an initial peak in prevalence among young women, a decreasing in the middle age group of women, and a highest peak among women over 60 years.

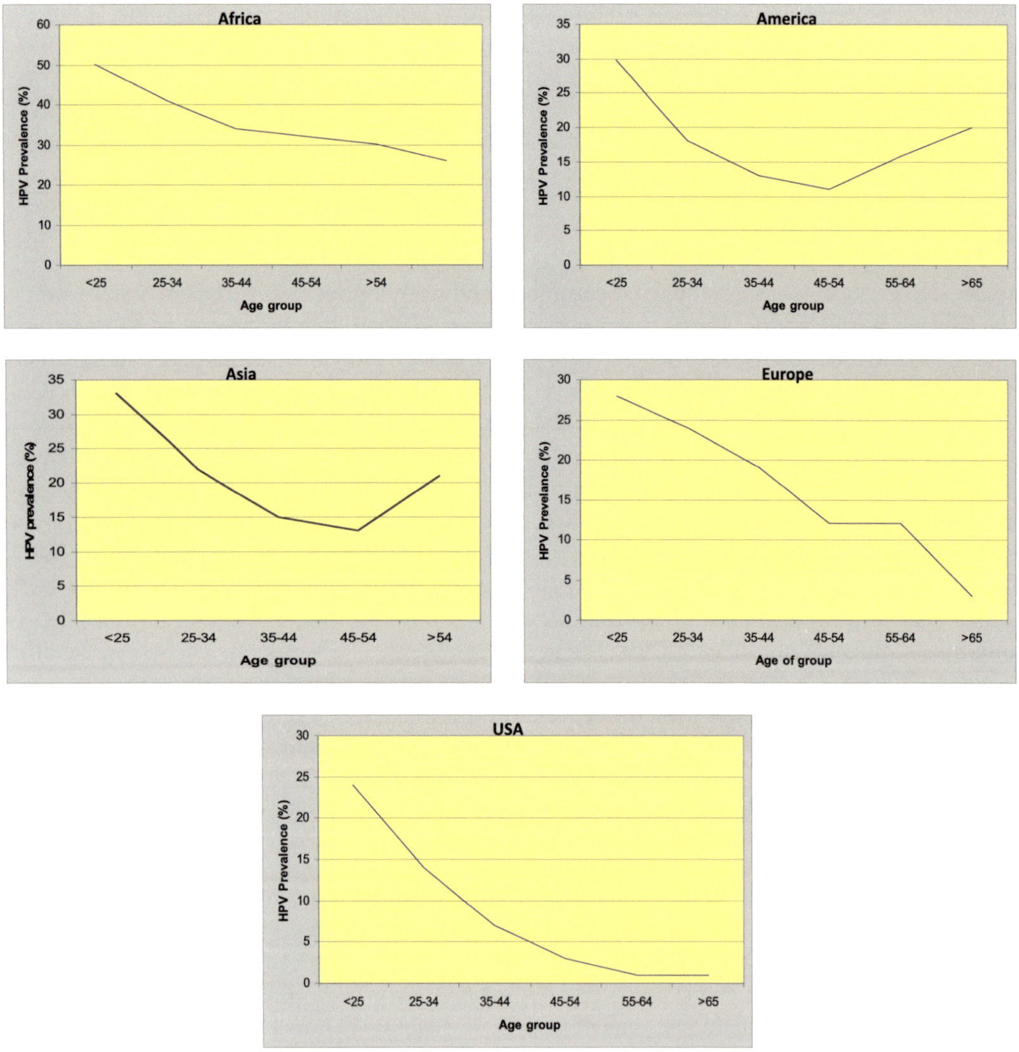

Fig. 2. HPV age-specific distribution in women without cervical cancer

In Brazil cervical cancer incidence remains among the highest in Latin America. North and Northeast regions have a higher mortality than Eastern and Southern states. Annually, 20000 cervical cancer cases were diagnosed and 8000 of Brazilian women in the general population died with the disease (WHO/ICO, 2010d). Cervical cancer is the second most frequent cancer in women in Brazil. Approximately 70 millions of women older than 15 years are at risk of developing cervical cancer (WHO/ICO, 2010d). The prevalence of HPV infection among women with normal cervical cytology was 21.1%

(Table 1). It was close to Canada and USA with 25.4% and 25.6%, respectively (Roteli-Martins et al., 2011). A decline in the HPV prevalence was found with increasing age. The most frequent HPV genotypes among healthy women were HPV16 and HPV72. The prevalence of HR types (16 ,18, 31, 33) was 5.3%, while the prevalence of LR types (72, 54, 6) was 10 fold lower (0.5%). The prevalence of HPV infection was linked to sexual behavior. HPV DNA increased with increasing number of regular partners. Women with two or more sexual partners had a higher prevalence of HPV DNA, but this finding was not statistically significant.

In Chile, cervical cancer is the sixth cause of death from malignant tumors and it represents a major public health problem (Chilean Ministry, 2005). Every year, 1500 cervical cancer cases are diagnosed in Chile and 721000 Chilean women in the general population died (WHO/ICO, 2010f). These deaths represents a major social and economic impact, because this type of cancer affects relatively young women in their reproductive age (Chilean Ministry, 2005). In fact 6.25 millions of women older than 15 years are at risk of developing cervical cancer (WHO/ICO, 2010f). The level of HPV infection (11.2%) among Chilean women with normal cytology is similar to the prevalence found in other Latin American countries, such as Mexico (14.5%), Columbia (14.9%) but higher than in many parts of Europe and Asia (Table 1). Seventy-six (73.6%) HPV infections involved a single genotype while 28 (27.1%) involved multiple types. The most common HPV genotypes were HPV16 and HPV56, followed by HPV70, HPV52, HPV58, and HPV59. The prevalence by age showed a bimodal curve with the two picks at the young and old ages and with a nadir in the middle age. For HR HPV infections the highest peak was represented by younger ages while for LR HPV by older groups. Consequently, among healthy women among 15 and 19 years of ages HR HPV was more frequent and LR HPV was less frequent. The new LR HPV increase after age 70 might be a result of the selective elimination of HR HPV by treatments. Similarly in Columbia and Costa Rica the second peak is mostly due to LR HPV while in Mexico the increase is caused by both HR and LR. Interesting, single widowed and divorced women had higher HPV infection, compared with married women. Moreover the number of partners was correlated with HPV infection. Women who reported their husbands had extramarital sexual relationships had high prevalence of HPV, but this did not reach statistical significance.

In Columbia cervical cancer is the principal cause of cancer mortality among women. Annually, 4700 cervical cancer cases are diagnosed and 2000 Colombian women in the general population died with the disease (WHO/ICO, 2010g). Approximately, 15 millions of women older than 15 years are at risk of developing cervical cancer (WHO/ICO, 2010g). The overall HPV DNA prevalence rate among healthy women was 14.9% (Table 1) which is similar to that reported in other high-risk populations. Of the HPV-positive women, 11.4% were infected with HR types and 3.2% with LR types. Similarly to Chile, the HPV age-standardized prevalence among women with normal cytological findings showed a bimodal curve, with a highest peak (26%) among women below age 20 and a lower peak among women over 55 (13.2%). HPV prevalence among women aged 45-54 was very low (2.3%). HR HPV infections were more prevalent then LR HPV infections except among women aged over 55. Mexico and Costa Rica presented some increase in HPV infection among woman in peri-and post-menopause as well. But while in Costa Rica the predominance was LR HPV, in Mexico the predominance was HR HPV with an increasing of LR HPV in younger women. This could due to a reactivation of HPV infection by decreased immune response or by hormonal changes (Ginaldi et al., 1999). The most common genotype found was HPV16 followed by HPV58. Although HPV16 is the predominant type detected worldwide, HPV58 was noted with high prevalence as well. Multiple infections were detected in 29.7% of HPV-positive women, with a high frequency among women less than 25.

Cervical cancer ranks as the second most frequent cancer in women in Argentina, and the second most frequent cancer among women between 15 and 44 years of age. Argentina has a population of 14.74 million women ages 15 years and older who are at risk of developing cervical cancer (WHO/ICO, 2010b). Current estimates indicate that every year 4000 women in the general population are diagnosed with cervical cancer and 1809 die from the disease (WHO/ICO, 2010b). The disease was not homogeneous in all the country, developed provinces of Argentina, in the northwest, had an incidence of cervical cancer nearly four times higher than Buenos Aires. The main problem is due to lack of prevention and control. For decades poor women with low education levels and less access to information were often brought into the hospital in a state of abnormal vaginal bleeding and advanced cervical cancer. In the last years, a vaccine has been developed to prevent HPV for girls from 10 to 11 years in areas at high risk. The HPV prevalence among women without cervical abnormities was 15.4% (Table 1). This value was slightly high compared with other part of the country and other geographical regions of the world (range 7.7-13.9%) (Clifford et al., 2005). Among all HPV-positive women 8.9% had an infection with a single HPV type, while 3.3% had multiple HPV types detected. The HR HPV genotypes were predominant compared to LR HPV. The most common HPV genotype was the HR HPV16, followed by LR HPV6. Differently from the other Latin American countries, the prevalence decreased consistently with the age, reaching the lowest point among women over 65 years of age.

3.2.2 North America

The incidence of cervical cancer in the United States and Canada has declined for some time until to be relatively low (Dailard, 2003). The major reason the rates are so low, despite high rates of HPV infection, is the widespread availability of Pap tests (Dailard, 2003). Pap-test can detect not only early-stage cervical cancer, but also cervical dysplasia. Since the Pap test was introduced, cases of cervical cancer in the United States have decreased dramatically (74%) between 1955 and 1992 (Dailard, 2003). HPV prevalence among healthy women in North America was high in the United States and Canada (Table 1, Figure 1). Age-specific prevalence among women with normal cytology ranged from 30% among women younger than 25 to 1% among women aged 45-54. It was very high among teen-agers and then it slowly declined until 45-54 years of age for significantly increase again among women more than 55 years (20%) (Figure 2). Only Unites States showed a significant decreasing with age (Figure 2). HPV16 was the most prevalent type among women with normal cervical cytology.

HPV was estimated to be the most common sexually transmitted infection in the United States (Winer et al., 2003, Tarkowski et al., 2004, Revzina and Diclemente, 2005, Manhart et al., 2006, Trottier and Franco, 2006). An estimated over 122 millions of women in the general population, showed that approximately 40% of the population are currently HPV-infected

(WHO/ICO, 2010l). Each year in the United States, 11000 cases of cervical cancer were diagnosed and 4000 women died with the disease (WHO/ICO, 2010l). Almost half of the infections were among women 15-25 years old. The prevalence of HPV infection among women with normal histology was 25.6% (Table 1), including 20.9% with an HR HPV type and 7.4% with an LR HPV genotype. HPV16, the most common cervical infection worldwide, was the most common prevalent type, followed by HPV52 and HPV53. It is notable that HPV18 and HPV31 were not found as commonly as in other areas of America or Asia. Similar to other studies in Europe, the prevalence of HPV increased from 14 years to 24 years, and then decreased significantly with the age. There was a 20-fold variation in the prevalence of HPV infection between young women and women over 55.

HPV is among the most common sexual transmitted disease (STD) in Canada (Public health, 2007). HPV infection affects about 550 000 Canadians in the general population annually, and at some point in their lives 80% of sexually active women will be infected by one or more of the 100 HPV types (WHO/ICO, 2010e). Of those infected, approximately 1400 women were diagnosed with cervical cancer and 544 women died with the disease (WHO/ICO, 2010e). Cervical cancer ranks as the 11th most frequent cancer among women in Canada, and the second most frequent cancer among women between 15 and 44. In September 2009, a school-based HPV vaccine program was commenced in all 14 provinces and territories of Canada (Ogilvie et al., 2010). The vaccine has the potential to change the demographics of cervical cancer among young women (Kaplan-Myrth and Dollin, 2007). The HPV prevalence among Canadian women with normal cytology was 25.4% (Table 1). The HR HPV infections were more frequent than LR HPV. The most common HPV type among HR and LR infections was HPV16 that was detected in 4.6% of the population under investigation, while HPV18 was detected only in 1.6% of the population. Similarly to Latin American countries, the HPV age-specific prevalence in healthy Canadian women showed a bimodal distribution, with about 20% of prevalence in younger and older women and a decrease among 40-49 years old. HR HPV types were common in single infections among women younger than 40 years of age but made a smaller contribution to single infections in older women.

3.3 Asia

Cervical cancer is a significant problem in developing countries and resource-insufficient areas such as Asia (Behbakht et al., 2004). This is partially related to poor availability of health care, which is induced by social and cultural barriers that decrease patient compliance and interrupt physician education (Cooper et al., 2005). It is also related to the fact that HPV vaccines will be first introduced into industrialized countries and only later in developing countries. Asia has more than 1000 million women who are at risk of developing cervical cancer (WHO/ICO, 2010c). About 313,000 cases of cervical cancer are diagnosed each year, with 160.000 women in the general population dying from the disease (WHO/ICO, 2010c). It is the second most common female cancer in the region, where a woman dies of cervical cancer every 4 minutes, often in the prime of her life. The statistics consider almost half of the world's cervical cancer cases are diagnosed in Asia, but the distribution is heterogeneous, presumably because of the ample geographical and cultural diversities of Asian population (Figure 1) (Clifford et al., 2005). For example HPV prevalence in woman with normal cytology was high in Japan and Russia but not in China or India, where the prevalence was only intermediate, or in Thailand or Vietnam, where the number of infections was the lowest (Table 1). Those data are not in agreement with historical cervical cancer incidence that showed rates of cervical cancer low for China and high for India (Parkin, 2002). The discrepancies might reflect a more liberal sexual behaviour developed in recent decades, forming new HPV epidemiology in Asian countries (Li et al., 2006). This finding could predict a rising cervical cancer epidemic in the world with a so fast growing to match the HIV epidemic. HPV prevalence tended to be lower than in other regions of the world, with the exception of Russia and Japan. Age-specific prevalence among healthy women ranged from 33% among women younger than 25 to 13% among women aged 45-54 (Figure 2). It was very high among teen-agers and then it slowly declined until 45-54 years of age for significantly raising again to 21% among women more than 55 years (Figure 2). HPV16 was the most prevalent type among women with normal cervical histology but other common HPV genotypes were HPV52, HPV58, HPV31, and HPV32. It is noteworthy that Eastern Asia (South Korea, Japan, and Thailand) had the lowest contribution of HPV16 compared with the other Asian regions. In South Korea the most frequent HPV types were HPV70 and HPV33 with 1.34% and 0.85% against 0.24% of HPV16. In Japan and in Thailand the most frequent HPV types were HPV52 and HPV72 with 6.4% and 0.78%, respectively, against 4.1% and 0.48% of HPV16. Moreover only 0.6% of woman with normal cervical histology tested positive for HPV18, which is very common in western countries.

3.3.1 Eastern Asia

In China the age standardized–HPV prevalence was similar to those areas with high incidence rates of cervical cancer like Latin America and India but lower than in the high-risk regions in Asia and South Africa (Dai et al., 2006). It was homogeneous in all the country, in urban populations in North- and South-east of China (Li et al., 2006) as well as in the rural population in Central China (Dai et al., 2006). The highest HPV prevalence in the general population was found among middle aged women even if a peak was seen among women younger than 25 years. Castle et al. suggested HPV persistence in over 45 years old women than acquisition of new infection (Castle et al., 2005). Thus, a high prevalence might indicate a reactivation of HPV infection. Furthermore, China is a conservative society, especially the central area, so it is likely that middle aged women are more frequently exposed to the HPV than young women (Dai et al., 2006). One of the limitations of HPV prevalence studies in China is the difficulty to obtain specimens from unmarried women (Dai et al., 2006). Indeed in some studies the age-specific pattern of HPV infection for the tertiary sector workers was different with a gentle decline with increasing age (Winer et al., 2003). The prevalence of HR HPV infections (8.7%) in healthy women was similar to the global average (9.2%) (Clifford et al., 2005) while the infection with LR HPV genotypes was lower (Sun et al., 2010) (Table 1). The most common identified HPV type was HPV16 but HPV52 was predominant as well, more than in non-Asian populations (Clifford et al., 2005). Only 1.80% of healthy women in China were diagnosed with HPV18 infection. The prevalence of single-type HPV infection was 9.4% while the prevalence of multiple-type HPV infection was 2.6%.

HPV infection is the most prevalent but also the least known STD in Japan. (Garland et al., 2008). Cervical cancer ranks 7th in women overall and 2nd in women aged 15-44 years (Clifford et al., 2005, WHO/ICO, 2010j). Fifteen thousand women in the general population are diagnosed with cervical cancer yearly, leading to 3500 deaths (JMH, Castellsague et al., 2007). Prevalence of HPV infection in the Japanese population has been usually conducted in small geographic areas, and little information regarding nationwide HPV prevalence was available. The proportion of HPV-positive cases among woman with normal cytology was 21.7% and decreased with aging (Table 1). Women aged 20-25 years with normal cytology and HPV infection were relatively high compared with other women from the Asian Pacific region, with the exception of Australian women (Garland et al., 2008). Although the studies were not based in the same geographic region and used different primer systems HPV DNA positivity appears to be very high in Japanese women (Onuki et al., 2009). In the most recent studies, the HPV prevalence in Japan resulted increased. The high prevalence might reflect a more liberal sexual behaviour developed in recent decades or could be due to differences in the detection methods (Onuki et al., 2009). New PCR primers used in recent studies have a higher sensitivity. Among the high-risk types, HPV52 was the most prevalent among healthy women in Japanese population, while HPV16 was more closely associated with cervical abnormalities (Konno et al., 2008). HPV16 and HPV51 were the second and the third most prevalent HPV types. The numbers of single and multiple-HPV infections were high (20.7% and 13.5%, respectively) (Table1). Several women were positive for five HPV types (0.6%).

The incidence of cervical cancer in Korea has steadily increased over the past 10 years and with a pattern of a developing country because of the increase in incidence and mortality related with cervical cancer. HPV prevalence in Korean women has been found to be diverse according to age groups, areas, socioeconomic status, and methods for detection of HPV DNA. However, most reports have shown that the prevalence of HPV infection among women with normal cervical histology was 10-15% with an average of 8.5%, in agreement with intermediate-risk developing countries (Table 1). The incidence of HPV infection was significantly higher in females between 20 and 30 years than in older women. Then it declined at age 50-59 years and increased again above 60. DNA from HR HPV types was predominant over LR HPV types below age 35, whereas LR HPV types were as equally frequent as HR HPV types in women aged 35 and older. The most common HPV genotype in either single or multiple infections was HPV70 followed by HPV33 and HPV16. Together they infected half of HPV DNA positive women. Single infections (9.8%) were more frequent than multiple infections (1.75).

3.3.2 South-eastern Asia

Vietnam is one of the poor, developing countries. Malnutrition and infectious diseases are still major health problems. Cervical cancer ranks in a relatively modest position of priority and the geographical distribution is not homogenous within the country. It used to be frequent in both the North and South but there is a gender difference between two regions: it was higher in the South than in the North. In the North the HPV detection in women without cervical abnormalities was very rare (2%); in the South the HPV detections among healthy women (10.9%) were 5-fold higher than in the North. The overall HPV prevalence was very low (5.2%), lower than worldwide average (Table 1). Infections with multiple HPV types were 9-fold more common in the South (4.5%) than in the North (0.4%). In Vietnam the most frequent HPV genotype was HPV16, followed by HPV52. A peak in the HPV prevalence among women younger than 25 years was found only in the South that then significantly decline with age. In North no clear age-pattern emerged, but the highest prevalence was found among women 35-44 years of age group. The differences between the regions cannot be due to technical reason, as women were randomly chosen in the same way and the samples were examinated in parallel. It may rather be due to the greater isolation between North and South during many decades of socialist economy.

Cervical cancer is the leading cancer in Thailand. Despite that, the prevalence of HPV infection was relatively low (4.7%) among women with normal cervical history, suggesting the spread of the infection to be relatively limited (Table 1). The vast majority of women tested reported having only one sexual partner in their lifetimes. Women who reported more than 2 sexual partners appeared to be at an increased risk of HPV detection, but only borderline statistical significance was estimated. HPV prevalence among healthy women was higher in the North area of Thailand than in South regions. This does not appear to be explained by differences in sexual habits or in HPV detection methods, as all samples were analyzed in parallel and in the same laboratory. The majority of HPV-positive women had infections with HR HPV type (61%) and the most common genotypes were HPV72 and HPV16. Multiple infections were found in 1.5% of HPV-positive women. The age-standardized prevalence among women with normal cytological findings was two fold higher in population from North Thailand than in South Thailand. In both cases, HPV DNA positivity was higher among women younger than 25 years of age and then formed a plateau among women older than 35 years of age. The prevalence of HR HPV types reached the highest value (6.5%) among women aged 25-34 years while the highest LR HPV prevalence (5.1%) was found among women younger than 25 years of age. The representativeness of HPV DNA prevalence among women younger than 25 is limited, because young women in Thailand generally were not willing to undergo a pelvic examination.

3.3.3 Western Asia

Iran is a country with a low prevalence of HPV. The incident of HPV infection among women with normal cytology in Iran was only 5,5% lower than the worldwide average but similar to that in low-prevalence areas (Table 1). Age-specific prevalence among healthy women was 4.5% among women aged between 20-40 years and gradually increased to 20% in 50-59 years old women. The prevalence of high-risk HPV was around 2% among younger women and decreased to zero in the older age group. The decreased occurrence with increasing age may suggest that the HPV infection at a young age is transient and it is eradicated by the immune-system. For the same reason not all HPV-infected women develop cervical abnomarlities (Centurioni et al., 2005, Onuki et al., 2009). The most common HPV genotype in either single or multiple infections was HPV16 followed by HPV18.

3.3.4 Southern Asia

In India the incidence of cervical cancer is high and the majority of Indian women had difficulties to access appropriate screening facilities. The country is exploring various strategies for preventing the disease and the vaccination is one of the solutions (Ghim et al., 2002, Das et al., 2008). The vaccine was found to be safe and highly immunogenic and possibly able to protect women already exposed to natural infection as well as HPV-naïve women (Swarz, 2007, Keam and Harper, 2008). In India the HPV prevalence among women with normal cervical histology was 12% which was similar to other geographical regions of the world (range 7.7-13.9%) (Clifford et al., 2005) (Table 1). Bao et al found a higher HPV infection in healthy women from hospital-based studies (25%) than from population based studies (10.9%) (Bao et al., 2008). HPV16 was the predominant type found in Indiam women without cervical abnomarlities and it was more common than HPV18 in perfectly accordance with other analysis from Asia (Clifford et al., 2005, Clifford et al., 2006). The HPV16/18–positive fraction was 32% with some variations between North and South India, with North more significant than South. After these, HPV33, HPV56, and HPV52 accounted for additional 16%. The prevalence of single-type HPV infection was 9.7% while the prevalence of multiple-type HPV infection was 2.4%. A limitation of HPV prevalence studies among women without cervical neoplastic desease in India was a reduced number of studies that fulfilled all the inclusion criteria. The few existing were not representative of each region; the Western and the central areas were not well documented.

3.4 Europe

In 2007, Europe had a population of 321.8 million and each year 59931 women are diagnosed with cervical cancer and 29812 die from the disease (WHO/ICO, 2007b). In this continent, cervical cancer is ranked as the 7th most common cancer in women, and as the second most frequent cancer among women between 15 and 44 years of age. About 6.6% of women in general population are estimated to harbor cervical HPV infection at a given time, and 73.3% of invasive cervical cancer are attributed to HPV16 and 18 (WHO/ICO, 2007b).

3.4.1 Northern Europe

The effectiveness of HPV testing in primary cervical cancer was evaluated in the United Kingdom (Kitchener et al., 2006). The HPV detection was performed on 42647 healthy women (20-64 years) by HC2 and typing through Roche reverse line blot assay. The age-specific prevalence pattern was 7.3% in the 20-29 years old group, 25.9% between 30-49 years, 11.6% in the 50-64 years of age and 44.8% in the oldest group, with ages among 50-64. Regarding HPV types, there was a 2.2% prevalence of HPV16 and HPV18 together and 8.2% of other HR HPV types, meaning that 11.3% of normal cytology samples were infected with a HR type (Table 1). In 2010, another study evaluated prevalence of type-specific HPV infections in the country (Howell-Jones et al., 2010). The Roche Linear Array test was used and the six most common HPV infections in women with normal cytology were HPV16, 61, 62, 53, CP6108 and 54, in descending order; HPV18 was only the nineteenth most common type. Infection with HR HPV was identified in 12.2% of participants.

In 1997, a population-based prospective cohort study evaluated the HPV infection in 1000 randomly chosen young Danish women (Kjaer et al., 1997). The participants were healthy women distributed over the age range (20-29 years); 30, 32 and 38% were 20-23 years old, 24-26 and 27-29 years old. Overall HPV DNA was detected in 15.4% women, 73.8% women had HR HPV types. LR HPV6, 11 was found in 30% of the women. Of the positive samples, approximately 10% contained more than one HPV type (only 3% harbored both HR and LR HPV types). Prevalence of any HPV type was associated with age: 19.4% of group age 20-23, 14.1% of 24-26 and 13.1% of 27 to 29 years old. In 2008, a study assessed the type-specific

HPV prevalence to estimate the preventive potential of an HPV 16/18 VLP vaccine in preventing cervical cancer (Kjaer et al., 2008). 11918 women with normal cytology and a mean age of 36.3 years old were tested by HC2. The HPV prevalence was 22.9%, 19.2% infected with HR HPV types and 7.4% with LR HPV types (Table 1). Multiple HPV infections (12.1%) were more prevalent than single HPV infections (9.3%). The most common HPV type was HPV16 (4.8%) followed by HPV31, 52 and 51 (3.8-3.6%).

In Sweden, Dahlstrom et al. (2010) evaluated the HPV distribution and the risk of cervical adenocarcinoma using 282 women with normal smears. The HPV prevalence was 24.8% (Table 1). Among all HPV-positive women 8.8% had an infection with a single HPV type, while 6% had multiple HPV types detected. The HR HPV genotypes were predominant compared to LR HPV. The most common HPV genotype was the HR HPV16, followed by HR HPV31 and LR HPV 42.

Keegan et al. (2007) reported an analysis of the cytological and HPV status of Irish women undergoing opportunistic cervical cancer screening. Detection of HPV was performed using MY09/MY11 consensus primers and then samples were sequenced to genotype the virus. 886 women with normal cytology were analyzed. HPV DNA was detected in 11.4% of the samples tested (Table 1). Regarding age distribution, the study samples ranged from 16 to 72 years. There were 27 HPV positive cases in women bellow 25 years, 48 cases between 25-30 and 26 cases in women with more than 35 years. The samples with normal cytological findings had HPV16 and HPV18 as the most common HPV types.

In Norway, a study investigated the cross-sectional positivity for HPV in 736 women with normal cytological findings (Trope et al., 2009). 30 years or older women were recruited from 4 Norwegian hospitals and were attending routinely administered clinical services with normal Pap smear cytology, normal cytological results from the preceding 2 years and no previous history of treatment of cervical neoplasia. A total of 10.6% women with normal cytology tested positive for HR HPV using Amplicor HPV test (Roche) (Table 1).

3.4.2 Southern Europe

Dutra et al (2008) characterized the HPV genotype distribution in 275 Portuguese women with normal cytology findings. The samples aged from 16 to 81 years old. HPV DNA was detected and typed using the commercially available Papillomavirus Clinical Arrays kit. The virus was detected in 30 women (10.9%) and it was more prevalent in age groups ranging from 25 to 34 years old and from 40 to 54 years old (Table 1). There were 1.8% cases of LR HPV infection, 6.1% cases of HR HPV and 2.5% cases of undetermined risk infection. The most common types were HPV31 (26.67%) and HPV16 (10%).

In 2011, the prevalence and distribution of HR HPV genotypes in Spanish women was studied (Lindemann et al., 2010). HC2 was carried out and all positive samples were further studied with Linear Array HPV Genotyping test (Roche). The author found 298 healthy women infected. The most prevalent type was HPV16 (17.8%) followed by HPV31 (12.8%) and HPV52 (12.4%). In total, 17 HR HPV types were identified.

Agarossi et al. (2009) studied the prevalence and the distribution of oncogenic HPV genotypes in Italy. HPVs were detected using HC2. Positive samples were genotyped by PCR. HPV 16 or 18 were present in 4% of healthy women and both were detected simultaneously in only 14 women. A study conducted by Rossi et al, analyzed the distribution of high and low risk HPV types in Italy (Giorgi Rossi et al., 2011). The presence of HR and LR types was investigated through HC2 in 3151 women with normal cytology aging from 25 to 64. The HC2 positive specimens were amplified and typed with "consensus high risk HPV genotyping test". HPV prevalence was 9.7% (Table 1). A HR HPV infection was found in 6.2% of women and LR HPV infection in 2.7%. The most common types were HPV16 found in 67 samples (2.1%) and HPV31 (0.8%).

In Greece, two molecular methods of HPV detection were used in a large sample of women (Tsiodras et al., 2010). The two methods were: commercially available HC2 and an in house PCR using consensus primers GP5+/6+. During the 4 years period, 1029 women with normal cytology were evaluated (mean age: 34,2 ± 12,1 years old). HC2 detected HPV infection in 10.2% and the PCR methodology identified 18% of infected women (Table 1). It was also possible to genotype HPV by PCR, and 2.7% multiple HPV cases were detected. The most common types were HPV33 and HPV6 with 10 cases each, HPV6 with one case and HPVX (undetermined) was identified in 159 cases. There was not any case of HPV16, 18 or 11.

Grahovac et al investigated the prevalence of HPV among Croatian women attending a regular gynecological visit (Grahovac et al., 2007). 205 women (21-37 years old) without obvious cervical changes were analyzed. HPV DNA detection and genotyping was performed by HC2 assay and additionally by consensus and type-specific primers directed PCR. The overall prevalence of HR HPV in the group of women was 35.6% with HPV16 found in 43.8% cases followed by HPV31 (17.8%), HPV33 (9.5%) and HPV18 (6.8%) (Table 1). The prevalence of HPV of undetermined type was 13.7% and 6 were the cases with multiple HPV infections (8.2%).

3.4.3 Eastern Europe

Not many studies were developed on HPV prevalence in Russia, although some reports have been released until now. In many related socio-medical aspects, Russia seem to be similar to European countries. But the sexual attitudes were long considered "inappropriate". Decades of poor knowledge on the reproductive hygiene and ignorance of the risks of STD might have been affected the distribution of HPV. The HPV prevalence among healthy women in Russia was one of the highest revealed in this study. HPV was detected in 29% of the women with normal cervical cytology (Table 1, Figure 1). The largest proportion of HPV-positive cases was regarding women on reproductive age and no significant decline of the infection was observed in older women. HPV16 was the most prevalent type being present in 21% of the infected women alone and in 5% in combinations with other HPV types. Other common types were HPV31, HPV66, and HPV39. A strong correlation between excessive number of contraceptive abortions and the presence of HPV was observed among young Russian women (Popov, 1991)

The HPV prevalence was also investigated among 3187 healthy women in the two new independent states of former Soviet Union (Kulmala et al., 2007). HPV detection, type distribution and viral load analysis in DNA samples from cervical scrapes were done with real-time PCR-based assay. The overall HPV prevalence in Belarus and Latvia were 27.5%

and 26.2% respectively and HPV16 was the most prevalent type followed by HPV31 and HPV33 in Belarus and HPV39 in Latvia (Table 1).

In 2008 the relationship between the distribution of HPV types and the outcome of cytological examination was investigated in Poland (Szostek et al., 2008). Forty-two women with normal cytology were analyzed. HPV DNA amplification and genotyping was performed with the SPF10 primer set and reverse hybridization line probe assay (INNO-LiPA). The virus was found in 21.4% women and the percentage of single and multiple infections were 9.5%. The most common HPV types were HPV51 and HPV52 while the two more worldwide common HPV16 or HPV18 were not found.

The prevalence of HPV in healthy women in Hungary was assessed in 2002 by Kornya et al (Kornya et al., 2002). The HPV DNA was detected using the Digene Hybrid Capture HPV-DNA assay and the virus could be shown in 60 out of 1018 cytology normal samples, (prevalence of 5.9%) (Table 1).

In 2010, Anton et al. analyzed the distribution of HPV genotypes in Romanian healthy women. HPV was detected and genotyped using the commercially available INNO-LiPA. From the 285 women, 43.5% had an HPV infection and the most common type was HPV16 (15.4%), followed by HPV18, 31 and 51 (Table 1).

3.4.4 Western Europe

In France, Vaucel et al (2010) assessed the HPV overall and type-specific prevalence in 980 women with normal cytological diagnosis (mean age 38.5). PCR was performed with MY09/MY11 primers and genotyping by sequence PCR products. About 13% of women were HPV positive, and 3% showed multiple HPV infection (Table 1). The proportion of HPV positive women varied significantly according to age with the highest prevalence (44%) observed bellow 20 years of age. Thereafter, the prevalence decreased with increasing age reaching about 10% above 35 years. The most prevalent HPV genotypes were, by descending order of frequency HPV16 (3.6%), HPV53 (1.4%), HPV6 (1.0%), HPV31 (0.9%) and HPV33 (0.7%).

In a study on the occurrence and distribution of HPV infection in the Flemish region (Belgium), 581 cytological normal women, ranging from 17 to 85 years old, were studied (Sahebali et al., 2003). All samples were tested with MY09/MY11 consensus primers and the HPV positive group was retested with type-specific primers for 14 HR types. HPV prevalence was 26.7% (Table 1). HR HPV and LR HPV prevalence were 17.9 and 8.8%, respectively.

The prevalence of HPV types in women screened by cytology in Germany was evaluated by Klug et al in 2007 (Klug et al., 2007). HPV detection was performed by HC2 test and all positive samples for this assay were genotyped using PGMY09/PGMY11 PCR followed by reverse line blot assay. The study included 7833 women with no cervical abnormalities aging between 30 and 60 years. 4.4% of tested women had an HPV infection, 3.1% resulted single infections and 1.2% multiple infections. (Table 1). The most HR common types were HPV16 (1.1%), HPV31 (0.5%) and HPV52 (0.4%). In the LR HPV infections, HPV73 was the commonest type (0.4%).

In the Netherlands, a study compared two molecular detection tests using 1437 women with normal cytology findings aging from 40 to 60 (Hesselink et al., 2010). The authors compared the clinical performance of Papillocheck HPV assay with that of the GP5+/6+ PCR method. The Papillocheck assay found a HPV prevalence of 5.2%. About 3.7% of the infections were HR HPV positive and 1.5% were LR HPV positive (Table 1).

In Switzerland, Dobec et al. (2009a) analyzed HPV genotype distribution in women without cervical abnormalities. It comprised 680 cervical specimens of females with ages from16 to 88 years (mean age, 40 years) tested for HPV with Linear Array HPV genotyping. Any HPV was detected in 17.2% of women and HR HPV was found in 8.1% of the study group (Table 1). The highest HPV prevalence was observed in age group 21-30 and showed a continuous decrease in older age groups. The seven most common HR HPV types were HPV16 (12%), HPV31 (9.4%), HPV52 (6%) and HPV45, 58 and 59 (4.3%, each). HPV6 was detected in 4.3% of the 117 HPV positive specimens and infection with single and multiple HPVs was found in 10.9% and 6.3%, respectively.

4. Discussion and conclusions

Our analysis included 47 countries with studies testing HPV infection in women with normal cytological findings. Figure 2 shows HPV prevalence by age and continent. In all regions, a peak in HPV infection was found at teen-agers (≤25 years), declining until middle age. In America and Asia, a modest second peak is observed at age ≥45 years, while in Europe, Africa and U.S.A. There is not an increase of infection but a continuous decline.

In HPV prevalence worldwide (Figure 1), there were significant differences not only between continents but from region to region. In America, the prevalence starts increasing from the South to the North, ranging from 11.20% to 25.60% respectively. Despite the high rates of HPV infection in North America (Canada and U.S.A.), the widespread availability of Pap tests and effective cervical screening programs, there are low rates of cervical cancer. In the South and Central American countries, the incidence of cervical cancer varies between poor and rich countries as well as the HPV prevalence rates.

In Asia the distribution is heterogeneous presumably because of the ample geographical and cultural diversities but nevertheless is lower than in other world regions. In Western and South-eastern Asia the prevalence is approximately 5% and arises to 12 and 14% in Southern and Eastern Asia with a maximum prevalence in Japan (21.7%).

In Europe, the low rates of HPV infection are located Western countries, such as Germany (4.4%) and Netherlands (5.2%) probably due to a correct vaccine implementation and high population knowledge about the virus. The prevalence starts increasing in Southern and Northern Europe countries (12.6%) and reaches the maximum European prevalence in Eastern countries (43.5%).

The highest prevalence percentages are found in the African continent (Guinea,47.9% and Mozambique, 75.9%). The Southern and Northern countries have the lowest continent prevalence, 20.4 and 23.5% respectively. The poorest countries have the highest infection rates with 24.6% in Western and 25.3% in Eastern African countries.

There is an increasing effort in generating epidemiological data on the carriage of cervical HPV in normal cytological samples. In most cases, the regions with high HPV prevalence are the ones with the highest cervical cancer incidences and the regions with lower prevalence had the lowest incidences. These findings suggest that a correct vaccination program will affect dramatically the cervical cancer incidence.

5. References

Adjorlolo-Johnson G, Unger ER, Boni-Ouattara E, Toure-Coulibaly K, Maurice C, Vernon SD, Sissoko M, Greenberg AE, Wiktor SZ, Chorba TL (2010) Assessing the relationship between HIV infection and cervical cancer in Cote d'Ivoire: a case-control study. BMC Infect Dis 10:242.

Agarossi A, Ferrazzi E, Parazzini F, Perno CF, Ghisoni L (2009) Prevalence and type distribution of high-risk human papillomavirus infection in women undergoing voluntary cervical cancer screening in Italy. J Med Virol 81:529-535.

Alhamany Z, El Mzibri M, Kharbach A, Malihy A, Abouqal R, Jaddi H, Benomar A, Attaleb M, Lamalmi N, Cherradi N (2010) Prevalence of human papillomavirus genotype among Moroccan women during a local screening program. J Infect Dev Ctries 4:732-739.

Allan B, Marais DJ, Hoffman M, Shapiro S, Williamson AL (2008) Cervical human papillomavirus (HPV) infection in South African women: implications for HPV screening and vaccine strategies. J Clin Microbiol 46:740-742.

Amrani M, Lalaoui K, El Mzibri M, Lazo P, Belabbas MA (2003) Molecular detection of human papillomavirus in 594 uterine cervix samples from Moroccan women (147 biopsies and 447 swabs). J Clin Virol 27:286-295.

Anton G, Peltecu G, Socolov D, Cornitescu F, Bleotu C, Sgarbura Z, Teleman S, Iliescu D, Botezatu A, Goia CD, Huica I, Anton AC (2011) Type-specific human papillomavirus detection in cervical smears in Romania. APMIS 119:1-9.

Bao YP, Li N, Smith JS, Qiao YL (2008) Human papillomavirus type distribution in women from Asia: a meta-analysis. Int J Gynecol Cancer 18:71-79.

Behbakht K, Lynch A, Teal S, Degeest K, Massad S (2004) Social and cultural barriers to Papanicolaou test screening in an urban population. Obstet Gynecol 104:1355-1361.

Boffetta P, Parkin DM (1994) Cancer in developing countries. CA Cancer J Clin 44:81-90. Cancer IAfRo (2003) Cancer in Africa: epidemiology and prevention. IARC Sci Publ 1-414.

Castellsague X, De Sanjose S, Aguado T (2007) HPV and cervical cancer in the world: 2007 Report (section II countries). Vaccine 25:C27-219.

Castellsague X, Klaustermeier J, Carrilho C, Albero G, Sacarlal J, Quint W, Kleter B, Lloveras B, Ismail MR, de Sanjose S, Bosch FX, Alonso P, Menendez C (2008) Vaccine-related HPV genotypes in women with and without cervical cancer in Mozambique: burden and potential for prevention. Int J Cancer 122:1901-1904.

Castellsague X, Menendez C, Loscertales MP, Kornegay JR, dos Santos F, Gomez-Olive FX, Lloveras B, Abarca N, Vaz N, Barreto A, Bosch FX, Alonso P (2001) Human papillomavirus genotypes in rural Mozambique. Lancet 358:1429-1430.

Castle PE, Schiffman M, Herrero R, Hildesheim A, Rodriguez AC, Bratti MC, Sherman ME, Wacholder S, Tarone R, Burk RD (2005) A prospective study of age trends in cervical human papillomavirus acquisition and persistence in Guanacaste, Costa Rica. J Infect Dis 191:1808-1816.

Centurioni MG, Puppo A, Merlo DF, Pasciucco G, Cusimano ER, Sirito R, Gustavino CA (2005) Prevalence of human papillomavirus cervical infection in an Italian asymptomatic population. BMC Infect Dis 5:77.

Chilean Ministry oH (2005) Department of Epidemiology.

Chu KC, Miller BA, Springfield SA (2007) Measures of racial/ethnic health disparities in cancer mortality rates and the influence of socioeconomic status. J Natl Med Assoc 99:1092-1100, 1102-1094.

Clifford G, Franceschi S, Diaz M, Munoz N, Villa LL (2006) Chapter 3: HPV type-distribution in women with and without cervical neoplastic diseases. Vaccine 24.

Clifford GM, Gallus S, Herrero R, Munoz N, Snijders PJ, Vaccarella S, Anh PT, Ferreccio C, Hieu NT, Matos E, Molano M, Rajkumar R, Ronco G, de Sanjose S, Shin HR, Sukvirach S, Thomas JO, Tunsakul S, Meijer CJ, Franceschi S (2005) Worldwide distribution of human papillomavirus types in cytologically normal women in the International Agency for Research on Cancer HPV prevalence surveys: a pooled analysis. Lancet 366:991-998.

Cooper CP, Saraiya M, McLean TA, Hannan J, Liesmann JM, Rose SW, Lawson HW (2005) Report from the CDC. Pap test intervals used by physicians serving low-income women through the National Breast and Cervical Cancer Early Detection Program. J Womens Health (Larchmt) 14:670-678.

Czegledy J, Rogo KO, Evander M, Wadell G (1992) High-risk human papillomavirus types in cytologically normal cervical scrapes from Kenya. Med Microbiol Immunol 180:321-326.

Dahlstrom LA, Ylitalo N, Sundstrom K, Palmgren J, Ploner A, Eloranta S, Sanjeevi CB, Andersson S, Rohan T, Dillner J, Adami HO, Sparen P (2010) Prospective study of human papillomavirus and risk of cervical adenocarcinoma. Int J Cancer 127:1923-1930.

Dai M, Bao YP, Li N, Clifford GM, Vaccarella S, Snijders PJ, Huang RD, Sun LX, Meijer CJ, Qiao YL, Franceschi S (2006) Human papillomavirus infection in Shanxi Province, People's Republic of China: a population-based study. Br J Cancer 95:96-101.

Dailard C (2003) HPV in the United States and Developing Nations: A Problem of Public Health or Politics? The Guttmacher Report on Public Policy. . 3.

Das BC, Hussain S, Nasare V, Bharadwaj M (2008) Prospects and prejudices of human papillomavirus vaccines in India. Vaccine 26:2669-2679.

De Marco F, Houissa-Kchouk F, Khelifa R, Marcante ML (2006) High-risk HPV types in Tunisia. A pilot study reveals an unexpectedly high prevalence of types 58 and 82 and lack of HPV 18 among female prostitutes. J Med Virol 78:950-953.

de Sanjose S, Diaz M, Castellsague X, Clifford G, Bruni L, Munoz N, Bosch FX (2007) Worldwide prevalence and genotype distribution of cervical human papillomavirus DNA in women with normal cytology: a meta-analysis. Lancet Infect Dis 7:453-459.

De Vuyst H, Parisi MR, Karani A, Mandaliya K, Muchiri L, Vaccarella S, Temmerman M, Franceschi S, Lillo F (2010) The prevalence of human papillomavirus infection in Mombasa, Kenya. Cancer Causes Control 21:2309-2313.

DeMay RM (1996) Cytopathology of false negatives preceding cervical carcinoma. Am J Obstet Gynecol 175:1110-1113.

Dobec M, Bannwart F, Kaeppeli F, Cassinotti P (2009) Automation of the linear array HPV genotyping test and its application for routine typing of human papillomaviruses in cervical specimens of women without cytological abnormalities in Switzerland. J Clin Virol 45:23-27.

Dutra I, Santos MR, Soares M, Couto AR, Bruges-Armas M, Teixeira F, Monjardino L, Hodgson S, Bruges-Armas J (2008) Characterisation of human papillomavirus (HPV) genotypes in the Azorean population, Terceira island. Infect Agent Cancer 3:6.

F.D.A. (2010) FDA licensure of bivalent human papillomavirus vaccine (HPV2, Cervarix) for use in females and updated HPV vaccination recommendations from the Advisory Committee on Immunization Practices (ACIP). MMWR Morb Mortal Wkly Rep 59:626-629.

Ferlay J, Parkin DM, Steliarova-Foucher E (2010) Estimates of cancer incidence and mortality in Europe in 2008. Eur J Cancer 46:765-781.

Fukuchi E, Sawaya GF, Chirenje M, Magure T, Tuveson J, Ma Y, Shiboski S, Da Costa M, Palefsky J, Moscicki AB, Makunike-Mutasa R, Chipato T, Smith-McCune KK (2009) Cervical human papillomavirus incidence and persistence in a cohort of HIV-negative women in Zimbabwe. Sex Transm Dis 36:305-311.

Gage JC, Ferreccio C, Gonzales M, Arroyo R, Huivin M, Robles SC (2003) Follow-up care of women with an abnormal cytology in a low-resource setting. Cancer Detect Prev 27:466-471.

Garland S, Park SN, Ngan HY, Frazer I, Tay EH, Chen CJ, Bhatla N, Pitts M, Shin HR, Konno R, Smith J, Pagliusi S, Park JS (2008) The need for public education on HPV and cervical cancer prevention in Asia. Opinions of experts at the AOGIN conference. Vaccine 26:5435-5440.

Ghim SJ, Basu PS, Jenson A (2002) Cervical Cancer: Etiology, Pathogenesis, Treatment, and Future Vaccines. Asian Pac J Cancer Prev 3:207-214.

Ginaldi L, De Martinis M, D'Ostilio A, Marini L, Loreto MF, Martorelli V, Quaglino D (1999) The immune system in the elderly: II. Specific cellular immunity. Immunol Res 20:109-115.

Giorgi Rossi P, Chini F, Bisanzi S, Burroni E, Carillo G, Lattanzi A, Angeloni C, Scalisi A, Macis R, Pini MT, Capparucci P, Guasticchi G, Carozzi FM (2011) Distribution of high and low risk HPV types by cytological status: a population based study from Italy. Infect Agent Cancer 6:2.

Grahovac M, Racic I, Hadzisejdic I, Doric A, Grahovac B (2007) Prevalence of human papillomavirus among Croatian women attending regular gynecological visit. Coll Antropol 31 Suppl 2:73-77.

Hammouda D, Clifford GM, Pallardy S, Ayyach G, Chekiri A, Boudrich A, Snijders PJ, van Kemenade FJ, Meijer CJ, Bouhadef A, Zitouni Z, Habib D, Ikezaren N, Franceschi S (2011) Human papillomavirus infection in a population-based sample of women in Algiers, Algeria. Int J Cancer 128:2224-2229.

Hassen E, Chaieb A, Letaief M, Khairi H, Zakhama A, Remadi S, Chouchane L (2003) Cervical human papillomavirus infection in Tunisian women. Infection 31:143-148.

Herrero R, Hildesheim A, Bratti C, Sherman ME, Hutchinson M, Morales J, Balmaceda I, Greenberg MD, Alfaro M, Burk RD, Wacholder S, Plummer M, Schiffman M (2000)

Population-based study of human papillomavirus infection and cervical neoplasia in rural Costa Rica. J Natl Cancer Inst 92:464-474.

Hesselink AT, Heideman DA, Berkhof J, Topal F, Pol RP, Meijer CJ, Snijders PJ (2010) Comparison of the clinical performance of PapilloCheck human papillomavirus detection with that of the GP5+/6+-PCR-enzyme immunoassay in population-based cervical screening. J Clin Microbiol 48:797-801.

Howell-Jones R, Bailey A, Beddows S, Sargent A, de Silva N, Wilson G, Anton J, Nichols T, Soldan K, Kitchener H (2010) Multi-site study of HPV type-specific prevalence in women with cervical cancer, intraepithelial neoplasia and normal cytology, in England. Br J Cancer 103:209-216.

JMH JMoH, Labour & Welfare. Vital statistical Japan. .

Kaplan-Myrth N, Dollin J (2007) Cervical cancer awareness and HPV prevention in Canada. Can Fam Physician 53:693-696, 697.

Keam SJ, Harper DM (2008) Human papillomavirus types 16 and 18 vaccine (recombinant, AS04 adjuvanted, adsorbed) [Cervarix]: profile report. BioDrugs 22:205-208.

Keegan H, Ryan F, Malkin A, Griffin M, Lambkin H (2007) Human papillomavirus prevalence and genotypes in an opportunistically screened Irish female population. Br J Biomed Sci 64:18-22.

Keita N, Clifford GM, Koulibaly M, Douno K, Kabba I, Haba M, Sylla BS, van Kemenade FJ, Snijders PJ, Meijer CJ, Franceschi S (2009) HPV infection in women with and without cervical cancer in Conakry, Guinea. Br J Cancer 101:202-208.

Kitchener HC, Almonte M, Wheeler P, Desai M, Gilham C, Bailey A, Sargent A, Peto J (2006) HPV testing in routine cervical screening: cross sectional data from the ARTISTIC trial. Br J Cancer 95:56-61.

Kjaer SK, Breugelmans G, Munk C, Junge J, Watson M, Iftner T (2008) Population-based prevalence, type- and age-specific distribution of HPV in women before introduction of an HPV-vaccination program in Denmark. Int J Cancer 123:1864-1870.

Kjaer SK, van den Brule AJ, Bock JE, Poll PA, Engholm G, Sherman ME, Walboomers JM, Meijer CJ (1997) Determinants for genital human papillomavirus (HPV) infection in 1000 randomly chosen young Danish women with normal Pap smear: are there different risk profiles for oncogenic and nononcogenic HPV types? Cancer Epidemiol Biomarkers Prev 6:799-805.

Klug SJ, Hukelmann M, Hollwitz B, Duzenli N, Schopp B, Petry KU, Iftner T (2007) Prevalence of human papillomavirus types in women screened by cytology in Germany. J Med Virol 79:616-625.

Konno R, Shin HR, Kim YT, Song YS, Sasagawa T, Inoue M, Park JS (2008) Human papillomavirus infection and cervical cancer prevention in Japan and Korea. Vaccine 26 Suppl 12:M30-42.

Kornya L, Cseh I, Deak J, Bak M, Fulop V (2002) The diagnostics and prevalence of genital human papillomavirus (HPV) infection in Hungary. Eur J Obstet Gynecol Reprod Biol 100:231-236.

Kulmala SM, Shabalova IP, Petrovitchev N, Syrjanen KJ, Gyllensten UB, Syrjanen SM (2007) Prevalence of the most common high-risk HPV genotypes among women in three new independent states of the former Soviet Union. J Med Virol 79:771-781.

Lazcano-Ponce E, Alonso P, Ruiz-Moreno JA, Hernandez-Avila M (2003) Recommendations for cervical cancer screening programs in developing countries. The need for equity and technological development. Salud Publica Mex 45 Suppl 3:S449-462.

Lazcano-Ponce EC, Castro R, Allen B, Najera P, Alonso de Ruiz PA, Hernandez-Avila M (1999) Barriers to early detection of cervical-uterine cancer in Mexico. J Womens Health 8:399-408.

Li LK, Dai M, Clifford GM, Yao WQ, Arslan A, Li N, Shi JF, Snijders PJ, Meijer CJ, Qiao YL, Franceschi S (2006) Human papillomavirus infection in Shenyang City, People's Republic of China: A population-based study. Br J Cancer 95:1593-1597.

Lindemann MLM, Calvo JMS, Antonio JC, Sanz I, Diaz E, Rubio MD, Morena ML (2010) Prevalence and distribution of high-risk genotypes of women with severe cervical lesions in Madrid, Spain: importance of detecting genotype 16 and other high-risk genotypes. Advances in Preventive Medicine 2011.

Manhart LE, Holmes KK, Koutsky LA, Wood TR, Kenney DL, Feng Q, Kiviat NB (2006) Human papillomavirus infection among sexually active young women in the United States: Implications for developing a vaccination strategy. Sex Transm Dis 33:502-508.

Markowitz LE, Dunne EF, Saraiya M, Lawson HW, Chesson H, Unger ER (2007) Quadrivalent Human Papillomavirus Vaccine: Recommendations of the Advisory Committee on Immunization Practices (ACIP). MMWR Recomm Rep 56:1-24.

Murillo R, Almonte M, Pereira A, Ferrer E, Gamboa OA, Jeronimo J, Lazcano-Ponce E (2008) Cervical cancer screening programs in Latin America and the Caribbean. Vaccine 26 Suppl 11:L37-48.

Ogedegbe G, Cassells AN, Robinson CM, DuHamel K, Tobin JN, Sox CH, Dietrich AJ (2005) Perceptions of barriers and facilitators of cancer early detection among low-income minority women in community health centers. J Natl Med Assoc 97:162-170.

Ogilvie G, Anderson M, Marra F, McNeil S, Pielak K, Dawar M, McIvor M, Ehlen T, Dobson S, Money D, Patrick DM, Naus M (2010) A population-based evaluation of a publicly funded, school-based HPV vaccine program in British Columbia, Canada: parental factors associated with HPV vaccine receipt. PLoS Med 7:e1000270.

Okolo C, Franceschi S, Adewole I, Thomas JO, Follen M, Snijders PJ, Meijer CJ, Clifford GM (2010) Human papillomavirus infection in women with and without cervical cancer in Ibadan, Nigeria. Infect Agent Cancer 5:24.

Onuki M, Matsumoto K, Satoh T, Oki A, Okada S, Minaguchi T, Ochi H, Nakao S, Someya K, Yamada N, Hamada H, Yoshikawa H (2009) Human papillomavirus infections among Japanese women: age-related prevalence and type-specific risk for cervical cancer. Cancer Sci 100:1312-1316.

Parkin DM (2002) Cancer incidence in five continents. Volume VIII. IARC Sci Publ 1-781.

Parkin DM (2006) The global health burden of infection-associated cancers in the year 2002. Int J Cancer 118:3030-3044.

Popov AA (1991) Family planning and induced abortion in the USSR: basic health and demographic characteristics. Stud Fam Plann 22:368-377. Public health Row (2007) A glance at HPV in Waterloo Region.

Raab SS, Jones BA, Souers R, Tworek JA (2008) The effect of continuous monitoring of cytologic-histologic correlation data on cervical cancer screening performance. Arch Pathol Lab Med 132:16-22.

Revzina NV, Diclemente RJ (2005) Prevalence and incidence of human papillomavirus infection in women in the USA: a systematic review. Int J STD AIDS 16:528-537.

Roteli-Martins CM, de Carvalho NS, Naud P, Teixeira J, Borba P, Derchain S, Tyring S, Gall S, Diaz A, Blatter M, Shier RM, Romanowski B, Quint WG, Issam J, Galindo C, Schuind A, Dubin G (2011) Prevalence of human papillomavirus infection and associated risk factors in young women in Brazil, Canada, and the United States: a multicenter cross-sectional study. Int J Gynecol Pathol 30:173-184.

Sahebali S, Depuydt CE, Segers K, Vereecken AJ, Bogers JJ (2003) Cervical cytological screening and human papillomavirus DNA testing in Flanders. Acta Clin Belg 58:211-219.

Sun ZR, Ji YH, Zhou WQ, Zhang SL, Jiang WG, Ruan Q (2010) Characteristics of HPV prevalence among women in Liaoning province, China. Int J Gynaecol Obstet 109:105-109.

Swarz TF (2007) Human papillomavirus -16/18 candidate vaccine adjuvanted with AS04 and its impact on the incidence of cervical cancer. . Expert Rev Obstet Gynecol 2:1320-1323.

Szostek S, Klimek M, Zawilinska B, Kosz-Vnenchak M (2008) Genotype-specific human papillomavirus detection in cervical smears. Acta Biochim Pol 55:687-692.

Tarkowski TA, Koumans EH, Sawyer M, Pierce A, Black CM, Papp JR, Markowitz L, Unger ER (2004) Epidemiology of human papillomavirus infection and abnormal cytologic test results in an urban adolescent population. J Infect Dis 189:46-50.

Thomas JO, Herrero R, Omigbodun AA, Ojemakinde K, Ajayi IO, Fawole A, Oladepo O, Smith JS, Arslan A, Munoz N, Snijders PJ, Meijer CJ, Franceschi S (2004) Prevalence of papillomavirus infection in women in Ibadan, Nigeria: a population-based study. Br J Cancer 90:638-645.

Trope A, Sjoborg K, Eskild A, Cuschieri K, Eriksen T, Thoresen S, Steinbakk M, Laurak V, Jonassen CM, Westerhagen U, Jacobsen MB, Lie AK (2009) Performance of human papillomavirus DNA and mRNA testing strategies for women with and without cervical neoplasia. J Clin Microbiol 47:2458-2464.

Trottier H, Franco EL (2006) The epidemiology of genital human papillomavirus infection. Vaccine 24:1-15.

Tsiodras S, Georgoulakis J, Chranioti A, Voulgaris Z, Psyrri A, Tsivilika A, Panayiotides J, Karakitsos P (2010) Hybrid capture vs. PCR screening of cervical human papilloma virus infections. Cytological and histological associations in 1270 women. BMC Cancer 10:53.

Tworek JA, Jones BA, Raab S, Clary KM, Walsh MK (2007) The value of monitoring human papillomavirus DNA results for Papanicolaou tests diagnosed as atypical squamous cells of undetermined significance: a College of American Pathologists Q-Probes study of 68 institutions. Arch Pathol Lab Med 131:1525-1531.

Vaucel E, Coste-Burel M, Laboisse C, Dahlab A, Lopes P (2010) Human papillomavirus genotype distribution in cervical samples collected in routine clinical practice at the Nantes University Hospital, France. Arch Gynecol Obstet.

WHO/ICO ICoHaCC-HIC (2007a) Human Papillomavirus and Related Cancers in Africa. Summary Report 2010. .

WHO/ICO ICoHaCC-HIC (2010a) Human Papillomavirus and Related Cancers in Americas. Report 2010.

WHO/ICO ICoHaCC-HIC (2010b) Human Papillomavirus and Related Cancers in Argentina. Summary Report 2010. .
WHO/ICO ICoHaCC-HIC (2010c) Human Papillomavirus and Related Cancers in Asia. Summary Report 2010.
WHO/ICO ICoHaCC-HIC (2010d) Human Papillomavirus and Related Cancers in Brazil. Summary Report 2010. .
WHO/ICO ICoHaCC-HIC (2010e) Human Papillomavirus and Related Cancers in Canada. Summary Report 2010. .
WHO/ICO ICoHaCC-HIC (2010f) Human Papillomavirus and Related Cancers in Chile. Summary Report 2010. .
WHO/ICO ICoHaCC-HIC (2010g) Human Papillomavirus and Related Cancers in Colombia. Summary Report 2010. .
WHO/ICO ICoHaCC-HIC (2010h) Human Papillomavirus and Related Cancers in Costa Rica. Summary Report 2010. .
WHO/ICO ICoHaCC-HIC (2010i) Human Papillomavirus and Related Cancers in Egypt. Summary Report 2010.
WHO/ICO ICoHaCC-HIC (2010j) Human Papillomavirus and Related Cancers in Japan.
WHO/ICO ICoHaCC-HIC (2010k) Human Papillomavirus and Related Cancers in Mexico. Summary Report 2010.
WHO/ICO ICoHaCC-HIC (2010l) Human Papillomavirus and Related Cancers in United States of America. Summary Report 2010. .
WHO/ICO ICoHaCC (2007b) HPV and cervical cancer in the 2007 report. Vaccine 25 Suppl 3:C1-230.
Winer RL, Lee SK, Hughes JP, Adam DE, Kiviat NB, Koutsky LA (2003) Genital human papillomavirus infection: incidence and risk factors in a cohort of female university students. Am J Epidemiol 157:218-226.
Womack SD, Chirenje ZM, Blumenthal PD, Gaffikin L, McGrath JA, Chipato T, Ngwalle E, Shah KV (2000) Evaluation of a human papillomavirus assay in cervical screening in Zimbabwe. BJOG 107:33-38.
Xi LF, Toure P, Critchlow CW, Hawes SE, Dembele B, Sow PS, Kiviat NB (2003) Prevalence of specific types of human papillomavirus and cervical squamous intraepithelial lesions in consecutive, previously unscreened, West-African women over 35 years of age. Int J Cancer 103:803-809.

4

Incidence of Invasive Squamous Cell Carcinoma Diagnosed with Opportunistic Screening in >70 Years-Old Women: Italy as a Case Study

Teresa Pusiol
Section of Cytopathology, Institute of Anatomic Pathology, Rovereto Hospital
Italy

1. Introduction

Cervical cancer is still one of the leading cancers worldwide (1), although there is a discrepancy between developed and developing countries. In developed countries, there is a continuous decline in incidence and mortality, whereas in developing countries, there is a more stable or even increasing pattern. The latter is more likely to be due to the lack of screening and infectious cofactors than to ethnic differences. Cervical cancer remains the only human malignancy that has been successfully reduced by medical intervention. Organised screening (OrS) for cervical cancer by the conventional Pap smear is the only means with proven efficacy of reducing the incidence and mortality of this disease in countries where it has been successfully implemented. According to the official statistics, the age standardized incidence rate of cervical cancer in Italy currently (2002) levels of at 8.1/100.000 with a mortality rate of 2.2/100.000 (2). Italy is another European country with no unified national screening programme, but each region has adopted a screening policy of its own. (3)Cervical cancer screening in Italy started as a spontaneous activity, with no national organization, which, not unexpectedly, led to incomplete population coverage. The Italian health system is managed by Italy's 20 Regions (Figure 1).

Since 1996, Italian national guidelines have recommended to Regions the implementation of organised screening programmes for cervical cancer. These recommendations, largely based on European guidelines, include personal invitations to women aged 25 to 64 years for a Pap smear every three years, a monitoring system, and quality assurance for each phase of the programme. Surveys designed to assess the level of implementation of organised programmes in Italy and to collect process indicators have been conducted by Italian Group for Cervical Screening since 1997 (4,5,6,7,8,9,10,11,12,13). Their results have been published by the Osservatorio Nazionale Screening (ONS),(National Centre for Screening Monitoring) since 2002. Since 1993 in Trentino province (North Italy) an Organized Screening (OrS) exist for women 25-65 aged. The target population comprises 146737 women. In the period 1993 - 2006 the pap-smears of OrS were examined in the Institutes of Anatomic Pathology and Cytopathology of S.Chiara Hospital Trento and Rovereto Hospital. Since 2007 the Cytopathology Section of Institute of Anatomic Pathology of Rovereto Hospital have examined only pap-tests of Opportunistic Screening (OpS), i.e. left to the woman's initiative.

OpS may be considered as all Pap-test performed outside an OrS program. For example, some women have Pap-test at their doctor's office during their physical examination independently of personal letter invitation of OrS. In Italy the complete screening history of women diagnosed with invasive cervical cancer has been performed only in Friuli Venezia Giulia - North eastern Italy -. In these region an OrS was initiated in 1999, targeting women aged 25 - 64 years, who are invited to have a Pap-test every 3 years. The screening histories of Cervical Intraepithelial Neoplasia (CIN)3 - squamous cell carcinoma in >65 years-old women may be made with study of OpS, because the OrS offers a free-of-charge Pap-test every 3 years to all women aged 25-64 years. In the present study we have examined the screening histories, treatment, human papillomavirus (HPV) detection of CIN3- invasive squamous cell carcinoma in >65 years-old women, diagnosed in the period 2007-2010 with opportunistic Pap-tests in the Cytopathology Section of Institute of Anatomic Pathology of Rovereto Hospital.

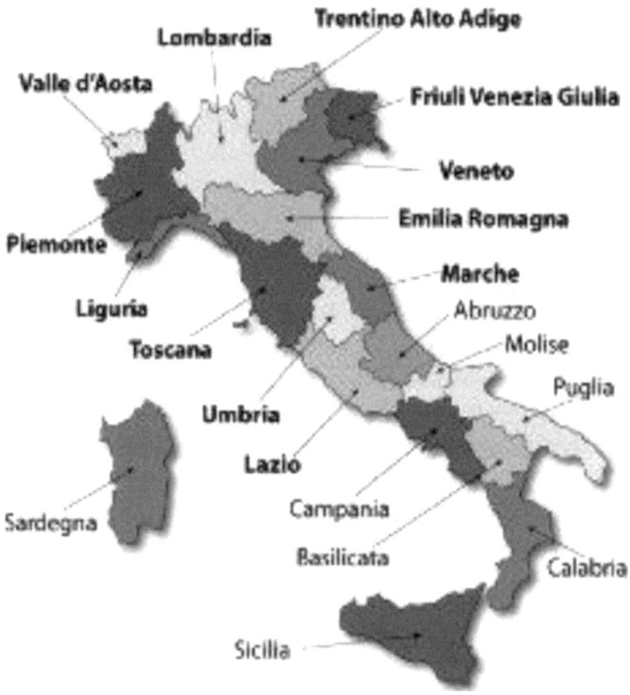

Fig. 1. Italy's regions

2. Materials and methods

In the period 2007-2010 the Cytopathology Section of Institute of Anatomic Pathology of Rovereto Hospital have been examined 28589 opportunistic Pap smears. The standard technique of conventional opportunistic Pap smears involves taking two samples (one from the endocervix with cytobrush and one from ectocervix with Ayre spatule) and smearing the cytological materials on two slides. The cytological diagnosis was performed using the 2001 Bethesda System (14). An experienced cytopathologist whose diagnostic experience exceeds 20 years have examined all abnormal smears and 10% of the normal smears previously observed a senior cytotechnologist. Colposcopic and cervical biopsies were taken by an experienced colposcopist (in practice for more than 10 years) and review by a senior colposcopist as part of the routine. HPV genotyping by PCR was performed in all histological specimens (biopsy, cone, hysterectomy) with diagnosis of low grade and high grade intraepithelial lesions and invasive cervical carcinoma.

3. Results

111 cases (0,38%) of CIN3-squamous cell carcinoma has been identified in 28589 opportunistic Pap smears. The distribution of women for decades is reported in Table 1. Between the women >64 years-old with CIN3-squamous carcinoma cytological diagnosis all were > 70 years-old and were not invited to OrS because of age > 64 years. We have reported in Table 2 the age, histological diagnosis, treatment and HPV detection of 8 patients over 70 years with CIN 3 squamous cell carcinoma cytological diagnosis.

Total number opportunistic Pap-tests	≤ 20 Years (percentage).	21 - 40 Years (percentage).	41 - 70 Years (percentage).	> 70 Years (percentage).
28.589	892 (3.2%)	11240 (39.3%)	14848 (51.9%)	1620 (5.6%)

Table 1. Opportunistic screening: decades of age of 28.589 women in the period 2007-2001

Number patients	Age	Treatment	Histological diagnosis (pT)	HPV finding
1	81	Hysterectomy with bilateral salpingo-oophorectomy	CIN3	HPV16
2	82	Cone biopsy	CIN3	Negative
3	71	Cone biopsy	CIN3	HPV58
4	79	Cone biopsy + radiotherapy	Keratinizing squamous cell carcinoma NOS	Negative
5	75	Hysterectomy with bilateral salpingo-oophorectomy	Non keratinizing squamous cell carcinoma (pT1b1)	Negative
6	82	Biopsy	Keratinizing squamous cell carcinoma NOS	Negative
7	72	biopsy + radiotherapy	Keratinizing squamous cell carcinoma NOS	HPV58
8	75	Hysterectomy with bilateral salpingo-oophorectomy + radiotherapy	Non keratinizing squamous cell carcinoma (pT1b1)	Negative

Table 2. Age, treatment, histological diagnosis, HPV detection in women over 70 years-old with CIN3-squamous cell carcinoma. NOS= not other specified

The Pap smear was performed by gynecologist to the woman's initiative. In the Pap smear of keratinizing squamous cell carcinoma the cells showed significant nuclear and cytoplasmic abnormalities, the later usually showing a marked deviation from normal cells of the same origin. The malignant keratinized cells had a characteristic bright orange or occasionally yellow cytoplasm that was dense and lack the transparent qualities of normal squamous cells. The size of keratinized cancer cells may vary from very large, comparable with normal superficial cells, to small, about the size of small parabasal cells. Their shape varies from round or polyhedral to quite irregular and bizarre (Figure 2).

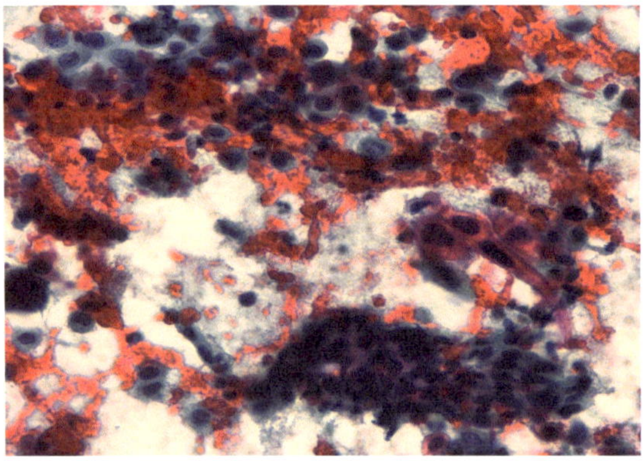

Fig. 2. Cancer cells with elongated keratinized eosinophilic cytoplasm and hyperchromatic nuclei in necrotic and hemorrhagic background. (Papanicolaou 40X).

The nuclei were usually large for the size of the cells. As is often the case in the presence of cytoplasmic keratinization, nuclear pyknosis and karyorrhexis may occur, conferring on the nucleus a dark appearance. "Tadpole" cells were present. They were elongated, club-shaped cells, with one board and one narrow end. The round or irregular hyperchromatic nucleus was eccentrically located within the larger area of the cytoplasm . The degree of cytoplasmic keratinization was variable. The spindly squamoid cells were an unusual finding in the Pap smear. These cells were narrow, elongated, and needle-shaped. Keratinization was not necessarily seen, the cytoplasm may be either eosinophilic or basophilic. The nuclei were nearly always elongated and hypercromatic (Figure 3).

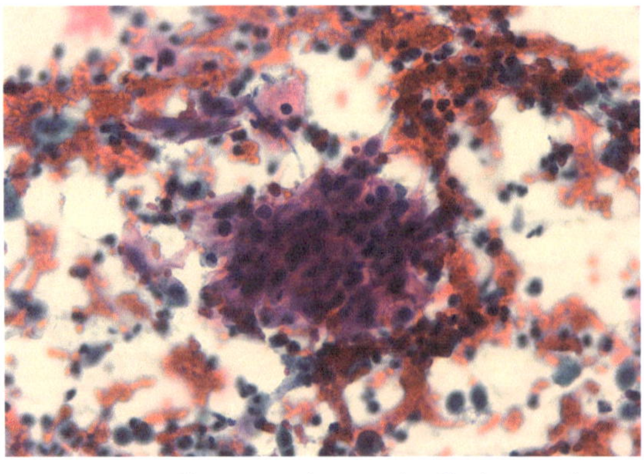

Fig. 3. Spindly squamous cancer cells. Note the markedly hyperchromatic nuclei and the cytoplasmic keratinization. (Papanicolaou 40X).

The squamous "pearls" was a very rare finding in Pap smear of squamous cell carcinoma. These were concentrically arranged clusters of being squamous cells. The difference between the benign and malignant "pearls" was in the configuration of the nuclei which, in the cancerous pearl, are enlarged and hypercromatic. In the Pap smears of non-keratinizing squamous cell carcinoma the malignant cells were solitary or arranged in syncytia (Figure 4) and show anisokaryosis. The nuclei were relatively large with unevenly distributed, coarsely granular chromatin and may have irregular nucleoli. The Pap smear of CIN-3 were characterised by cells with nuclear-to-cytoplasmatic ratio significantly increased. The cytoplasm remained well-defined resembling that of very immature metaplastic cells. Nuclei tended to be considerably hyperchromatic, and marked irregularities of nuclear envelope might be present. The cytological characteristics of menopause were found in the Pap smear with malignant cells (Figures 5-6) and CIN-3.

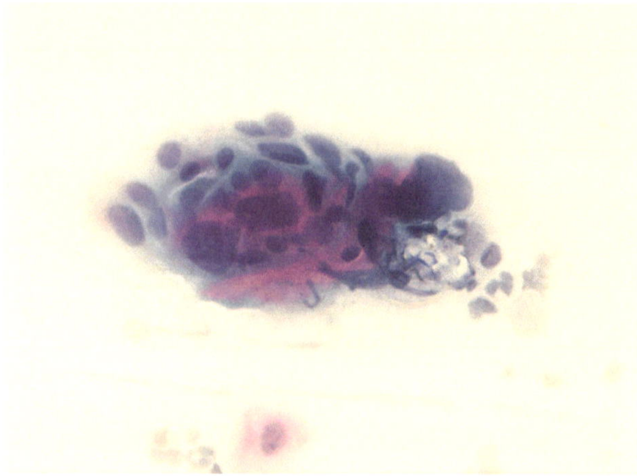

Fig. 4. A cluster concentrically arranged of undifferentiated cancer cells (Papanicolaou 40X).

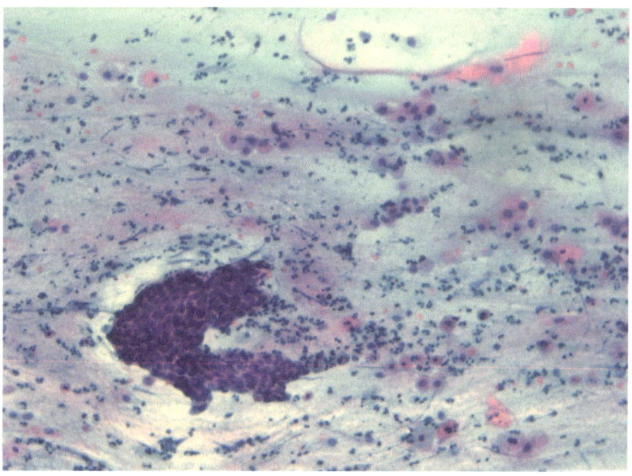

Fig. 5. Cellular pattern of advanced menopause: the cells are parabasal with filaments of nuclear material resulting from breakdown of nuclei. A cluster of undifferentiated cancer cells of invasive squamous carcinoma with dark hyperchromatic nuclei is found. (Papanicolaou 10X).

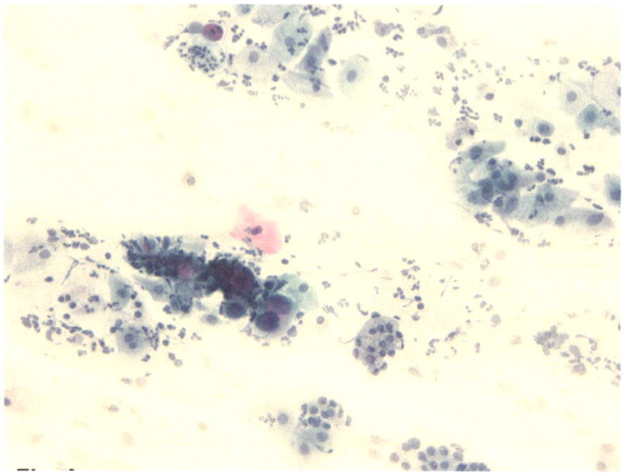

Fig. 6. Cellular pattern of intermediate menopause with cluster of neoplastic squamous cells containing hyperchromatic and irregular nuclei. (Papanicolaou 10X).

The cytologic patterns of the advanced atrophic menopause were influenced by dryness of the genital tract and scarsity of recoverable cellular material. The predominant cell was of the size and the degree of maturity corresponding to the parabasal cells. Two main effects of dryness might be observed: one was the uniform enlargement of the cell accompanied by a characteristic uniform gray discoloration of the degenerated nucleus; the second was by nuclear pyknosis and karyorrhexis. In the smear material of the eosinophilic pyknotic type there might be a striking variation in cell size and shape. Some cells might be relatively large, approaching the size of superficial cells, whereas others were the size of small parabasal cells. Sheets of spindly cells with elongated cytoplasm and large, pale nuclei may make their appearance in cervical smears and sometimes might be difficult to interpret. Nuclear pyknosis may be quite striking and often simulates the hyperchromasia of cancer cells; one must search for evidence of karyorrhexis in the form of granules of nuclear material within the cytoplasm. In some instances of extreme dryness, the cells break up during the process of smearing and will appear as standards and filaments of blue- staining nuclear material. The endocervical columnar cells in smear of the cervics were usually scarse or absent. When observed , the endocervical cells were smaller than during the childbearing age, although their columnar configuration was still preserved. The nuclei, although of normal size, may appear somewhat hypercromatic, and the cytoplasm was scanty, opaque, and shows no evidence of secretory activity except for an occasional vacuole. One Pap smear CIN-3 and one Pap smear of keratinizing squamous cell carcinoma cointained cells with koilocytotic changes (Figure 7). In the biopsies of CIN-3 maturation (including surface keratinization) was absent or confined to the superficial third of the epithelium. Nuclear abnormalities were marked throughout most or all of the thickness of the epithelium. Mitotic figures were numerous and were found at all levels if the epithelium. Abnormal mitoses were frequent. Focal koilocytosis was present in one case. Keratinizing squamous cell carcinoma were histologically characterized by mature squamous cells arranged in irregularly shaped nests or cords that varied considerably in size. The most striking feature was the present of keratine pearl within the nests of neoplastic squamous epithelium (Figures 8 and 9).

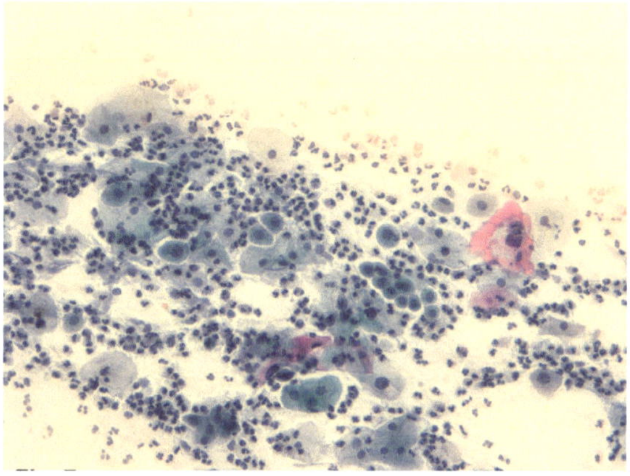

Fig. 7. Cellular pattern of intermediate menopause with nuclear enlargement of parabasal cells. Superficial squamous cell with koilocytotic atypia is present. (Papanicolaou 10X).

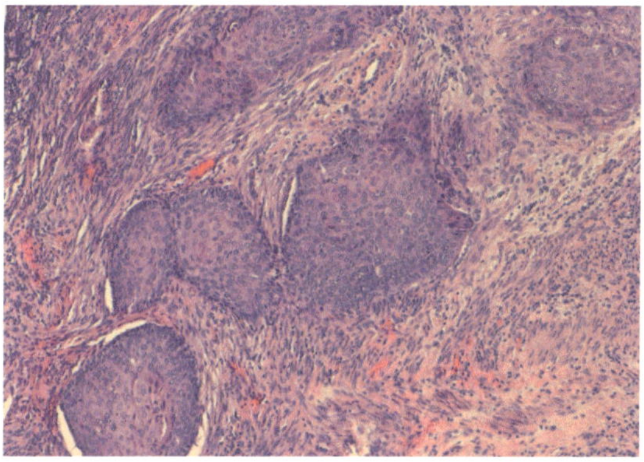

Fig. 8. Cone biopsy of keratinizing squamous invasive carcinoma of the cervix. Nests of keratinizing, markedly atypical squamous neoplastic cells are evident. (H&E 10X).

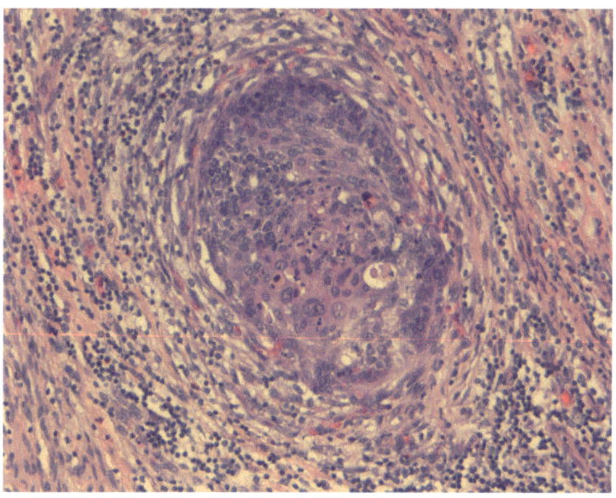

Fig. 9. Cone biopsy of keratinizing squamous invasive carcinoma of the cervix. Nest of keratinizing, markedly atypical squamous neoplastic cells is surrounded by dense inflammatory infiltrate . (H&E 10X).

Individual squamous cells were large ,with abundant eosinophilic cytoplasm, and many showed individual cell keratinization. The cells were closely apposed and often had prominent intercellular bridges. The nuclei may be enlarged or pyknotic. Mitotic activity was relatively low compared with the other tumor types.

The non-keratinizing tumors were composed of generally recognized polygonal squamous cells that might have individual cell keratinization and intercellular bridge but keratin pearls were absent (Figure 10). Cellular and nuclear pleomorphism was more obvious than in the well differentiated tumours, and mitotic figures were usually numerous.

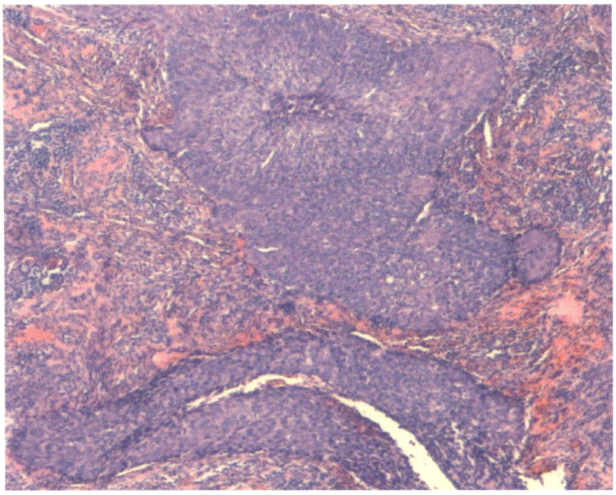

Fig. 10. Cone biopsy of non-keratinizing squamous invasive carcinoma of the cervix. The neoplasm is composed of nests of tumor cells with basaloid differentiation.(H&E 10X).

4. Discussion

In 1990 cervical cancer comprised 10% of cancers in women for a total of approximately 470,000 cancer cases world-wide (15), representing the third most common cancer in females and the most common cancer in Sub-Saharan Africa., Central America and South Central Asia. Approximately 230,000 women die annually from cervical cancer and over 190,000 of these are from developing countries. Zimbawe and India stand out not only for their high incidence, but also for an unfavourable incidence to mortality ratio. Some relatively high-incidence countries can also be found in Eastern and Central Europe (16).The incidence and mortality of invasive squamous cell cervical carcinoma have decreased dramatically in the United States over the last three decades. The incidence in the United States was 34/100,000 in 1947, 15/100,000 in1970, and 12/100,000 in 1986 (17). Although the incidence was decreased in the United States before the implementation of mass cervical cancer screening programs, screening has had an additional major impact on both the incidence and mortality (65,111). The significance of cytologic screening in reducing the incidence of cervical cancer is further underscored by comparing the 4.5/100,000 incidence per year in a screened population to the 29/100,000 incidence in an unscreened population(18). Both cohorts exhibited similar epidemiologic characteristics. In the United States, approximately half of the women who develop cervical cancer have not had a cervical smear in the preceding 3 years(19). According to the most recent global estimates, invasive squamous cell carcinoma is the second most common cancer in women world-wide, with the exception of skin cancer. There are approximately 493,000 new cases of invasive cervical cancer worldwide and 274,000 women die of the disease annually (20). The highest rates are reported in Latin America, where cervical cancer accounts for half of all female cancers. The annual incidence of invasive cervical cancer in women between 30 and 50 years of age in high-risk areas is 1/1,000. In developing countries throughout the world, cervical cancer is a major public health problem and is one of the leading causes of death (21). Recent increases in incidence and mortality rates have been observed in some Western countries including Canada, Great Britain, Sweden, and Norway (22,23,24,25). In the United States, there were 12,800 new cases and 4,600 cervical cancer deaths in 2000 (26). The incidence among blacks and Hispanics is two times higher than among whites in the United States. Moreover, in a recent study, after adjusting for a number of demographic factors, age, Federation of Gynecology and Obstetrics (FIGO) stage, other tumor characteristics, and treatment, black women had a higher mortality rate than white women, indicating that race is an independent predictor of cervical cancer survival (27). Socioeconomic, religious, sexual, obstetric, dietary factors, immunosuppression, smoking, and oral contraceptive intake have been studied in relation to cervical cancer. Studies suggest that dietary carotenoids and vitamin C have a protective effect against cervical cancer (28,29). The risk of cervical cancer is increased by the number of sexual partners, the age at which sexual intercourse is initiated, and the sexual promiscuity of the male partner. Husbands of women with cervical cancer have more sexual partners than husbands of controls (30). In a recent study, smokers had a two-fold excess risk of cancer, with the risk linked to smoking intensity and duration (31). The effect was most striking among women who had smoked continuously up to the time of cancer diagnosis and women who began smoking late in life, suggesting that smoking played a promotional role in cervical cancer rather than an initiating role. Long-duration use of hormonal contraceptives is associated with an increased risk of cervical cancer, but the public health implications depend largely on the extent to which the association remains long after the use of the contraceptives has ceased (31). Invasive squamous cell carcinoma is uncommon before the age of 30 years. Half of the patients, however, are less than 50 years old (32). In the United States, 22 percent of all women with cervical cancer are under the age of 35 years (33), but most are between 45 and 55 years of age al the time of diagnosis. Cervical cancer, however, can occur at almost any age between 17 and 90 years. The majority of the patients present with intermittent painless vagina, bleeding, often first noted after sexual intercourse or douching. With advancing disease, bleeding may become continuous, and be accompanied by a malodorous discharge and pain. Pain is frequently referred in the flank or leg as a result of tumor invasion of the pelvic wall or sciatic nerve. A cervical biopsy is mandatory for diagnosis. Although sampling problems and incorrect interpretation are partly responsible for false negative smears, necrosis and inflammation on the surface of the tumor may result in only an "atypical smear" that lacks obvious tumor cells. Consequently, the cervix that is abnormal by inspection or palpation is biopsied, even if the cytology smear is normal. In addition to biopsy of the ectocervix, an endocervical curettage Is performed as an integral part of the evaluation because invasive carcinoma, particularly adenocarcinoma, frequently involves the endocervical canal and may not be visible on the ectocervix. Cervical cancer is the most common gynecologic cancer to occur during pregnancy: about 3 lo 10 percent of cervical cancers occur in pregnant women. In these women, 83 percent present with stage I disease (34). Invasive cervical cancer can be divided in two major histological types: squamous cell carcinoma and adenocarcinoma. In terms of percentages, 80–85% of cases are squamous cell carcinoma, 10% are adenocarcinoma, and 3% are adenosquamous carcinoma and other rare tumours (35). HPV infection is the most common sexually transmitted disease, with more than 80% of the population infected at some time in their life. The main risk factor is undoubtedly genital infection with HPV. HPV infections are found in almost all pre-invasive lesions, so-called CIN and invasive squamous cell cancers (36). Based on the still-rising figures of HPV infections, one could consider it to be one of the most prevalent sexually transmitted pathogen diseases worldwide (1). From an epidemiological point of view, an HPV infection meets the criteria as a causal agent for cervical cancer (37,38). Current epidemiological and fundamental data have confirmed infection with HPV to be the basic cause of the disease (37,38). Having sexual contact is the main source of HPV infection. It is estimated that for every three people who have sex with a HPV-positive person, two will develop an infection within the next few months (1-19). In the majority of cases (75%), the infection will be asymptomatic. The peak prevalence of genital HPV infections is soon after the onset of sexual activity in women. HPV deoxyribonucleic acid (DNA) persists for about 6–12 months in the genital tract and spontaneously disappears in the majority of patients until an infection with a new type occurs. A persistent infection is the most important risk factor for initiating malignant transformation in the cervical epithelium. The time from initial infection to pre-invasive and, ultimately, invasive disease appears to be at least 10–15 years (1). Based on their association with cervical cancer, genotypes of HPV are divided into low-risk and high-risk groups, according to their presence in malignant lesions of the cervix. Functionally high risk HPV types infection contributes to carcinogenesis and tumour progression predominantly through the action of two viral oncogenes, E6 and E7. The coordinated expression of E6 and E7 has been town to transform rodent cells and immortalize primary human keratinocytes (39,49). The E6 and E7 proteins of high-risk HPVs have been demonstrated to be able to associate with the products of p53 and retinoblastoma susceptibility (Rb) genes, respectively, and inactivate the functions of these tumour suppressor proteins (40,41). The E6 protein exerts rapid degradation of p53, in corporation with E6-associated protein (E6-AP), via ubiquitin-mediated proteolysis pathway (42, 43). The E7 protein mediates the release of the E2F transcription factor from pRb-E2F complex (44). Mutational analysis of HPV 16 E6 protein revealed that a certain level of the activity to degrade p53 is required for E6 to manifest its transforming function (45). The p53 mutations are the most frequent genetic abnormalities found in a wide variety of human malignant tumours (46). Once DNA damage occurs, p53 protein is induced and arrests cells in the G1 phase to enhance DNA repair (47), or triggers apoptosis following DNA damage (48). These functions of p53 protein are important to maintain the genomic integrity. Mutant p53 proteins are devoid of these functions, because they lose the ability of DNA contact or destabilize the structure of the core domain (49). In this way, once p53 is mutated, DNA damage is fixed and subsequent genetic rearrangement progress which may be putative mechanisms to initiate cancer. Thus far, exceptionally low prevalence (0-6%) of the p53 mutations had been documented in cervical carcinomas (50, 51, 52, 53, 54). The p53 protein in cervical carcinoma is thought to be inactivated presumably due to complex formation with HPV E6 oncoprotein. Although Crook et al initially postulated that p53 mutations were confined to the HPVnegative cervical carcinomas (55,56), several recent studies implicated that p53 mutation was a very rare event and the occurrence was not strictly correlated with HPV status in primary cervical carcinomas (50,51,52,53,54). It has been also shown that p53 mutants identified in the HPV-positive anogenital cancers exhibit increased resistance to HPV E6-directed degradation, suggesting that mutation of p53 may play a role in the progression of the HPV-positive cervical cancer (56). The p53 mutation has been found only in 0–6% of cervical carcinomas. In light of recent studies demonstrating that mutation of p53 gene was found in over 20% of the patients with vulvar carcinoma (57, 58), a disease of elderly women and a known HPV- related malignancy, Nakagawa et al (59) analysed mutation of the p53 gene in 46 women with cervical carcinomas at the age of 60 or more (mean; 71 years, range; 60–96 years). Of the 46 patients, 41 had squamous cell carcinoma (keratinizing type, ten; large cell non-keratinizing type, 31) and five had adenocarcinoma (endocervical type, four; endometrioid type, one). On the basis of the FIGO criteria, 12 women had Stage I, 18 Stage II, 15 Stage III and 1 Stage IV. The presence of HPV and its type were analysed by polymerase chain reaction (PCR)-based assay using the consensus primers for L1 region. Mutation of the p53 gene was analysed by PCR-based single-strand conformation polymorphism and DNA sequencing technique. Point mutation of the p53 gene was detected in 5 out of 46 (11%) cervical carcinomas: 1 of 17 (6%) samples associated with high-risk HPVs (HPV 16 and HPV 18) and 4 of 27 samples (15%) with intermediate-risk HPVs, whereas no mutation was found in 2 HPV negative cases. The mutated residues resided in the selective sequence known as a DNA-binding domain. The immunohistochemistry revealed the overexpression in cancer tissues positive for p53 mutation. All of the observed mutations of the p53 gene were transition type, suggesting that the mutation may be caused by endogenous mutagenesis. Although falling short of statistical significance reduces the strength of the conclusion, data presented by Nakagawa et al imply that p53 gene mutation, particularly along with intermediate risk HPV types, may constitute one pathogenetic factor in cervical carcinoma affecting elderly women. To clarify the age-related genetic events in cervical cancer in elderly (>65 years) women, Saito et al (60) have analyzed for HPV typing via polymerase chain reaction, the expression of p53 via immunohistochemical study, and clinical behaviour 66 tissue specimens obtained from patients with stage Ib-IIb cervical carcinoma. Of this group, 50 women aged 64 years and younger were designated as the younger group (mean age 46.7), and 16 women aged 65 years and older were designated as the older group (mean age 67.6) The prevalence of HPV DNA was higher in the younger group than in the older group (84.0 vs. 50.0%) as was the detection rate of HPV 16 (44.0 vs. 6.3%). In contrast, HPV 18, 33, 52, 58, were frequently detected in older patients. The positive rate of p53 overexpression in the older group was similar to that in the younger group (46.7 vs. 48.8%). There was no significant difference in the incidence of lymph node metastasis, histology, and the distribution of clinical stage between the two groups. In elderly Japanese women with stage Ib-IIb, the association of HPV of types other than HPV 16 is suggested to influence the progression of cervical cancer. The most common member of the high-risk group is HPV 16, which accounts for more than 60% of all cervical cancers. The high-risk types account for more than 95% of all cases of cervical cancer. One of the main differences between high- and low-risk types is the possibility of integration in the genome. Approximately 1percent of the high-risk HPV types and only 0.1% of the low-risk HPV types will lead to the development of cervical cancer (61). In our case HPV 16 and HPV 58 were detected in two cases of CIN3 and HPV 58 in one case of squamous cell carcinoma. In one case of CIN3 and in 4 cases of squamous cell carcinoma the HPV type has been not detected. Two hypotheses may be made. There is a subset of squamous cell carcinomas that is unrelated to HPV. Other hypothesis takes into account that HPV 16 is only integrated in 72 percent of all invasive cervical cancers(62). The finding of the absence of HPV 16 DNA integration in some carcinomas implies that integration is not always required for malignant progression, but does not exclude the importance of HPV integration in the initiation of cervical cancer. Hypothetically, after the development of a carcinoma, the abnormal clone could lose the viral DNA. HPV 18, on the other hand, shows 100 percent integration. The epidermal growth factor receptor (EGFR) represents a cell membrane receptor characterized by an extracellular ligand-binding domain and an intracellular domain with tyrosine activity involved in signal transduction. EGFR receptor ligands such as epidermal growth factor (EGF) and tumor growth factor > binding to EGFR lead to a cascade of cellular events that are responsible for DNA synthesis, cell proliferation, mutation, survival maturation, and apoptosis (63). Aberrant EGFR expression results in abnormal growth, inhibition of apoptosis, angiogenesis,and the promotion of invasion/metastasis (64). EGFR overexpression has been observed in several malignancies (65). Cyclooxygenase (Cox) is the enzyme involved in the conversion of arachidonic acid to prostaglandins in the critical steps of tumor onset and progression. Two Cox isoforms have been characterized. Cox-1 is expressed constitutively in almost all tissues and serves homeostatic functions. Cox-2, which is highly inducible by growth factors, prostaglandins, and tumor promoters, plays a key role in inflammatory response (66). Cox-2 overexpression has been reported in many neoplasms; its overexpression is associated with carcinogenesis and is linked to proliferation, neoangiogenesis, high microvessel density, and inhibition of apoptosis (67). Some authors have also clarified that the aggressiveness of Cox-2 expression in different malignant neoplasms is due to the ability of this substance to modulate adhesion molecule and protease expression (68,69). To find information on invasive squamous cervical carcinoma in the elderly, Giordano et al (70) have analyzed 110 invasive squamous cervical carcinomas obtained from 2 groups of patients for HPV status by polymerase chain reaction study, for immunohistochemical EGFR, Cox-2 expression, and clinicopathologic features. In this study 64 women 60 years or younger were designated as the younger group and 46 who were 61 years or older were designated as the older group. The HPV status and the expression of Cox-2 and EGFR in the younger and older women were compared and correlated with the grading, staging neoplasm, and lymph nodal status. Overall survival curves were drawn using Kaplan-Meier estimates and were compared using log-rank tests in the whole series of 110 patients. The number of neoplasms with higher staging was significantly greater than those in the younger women. The mortality was higher in the older group than in the younger patients. In the elderly, the presence of HPV DNA in 65% of cases, and in the absence of sexual activity, could be due to reactivation of latent HPV infection. In accordance with data provided by the literature, this finding demonstrated that HPV DNA can be detected in elderly women and can be associated with cervical carcinoma (59,71,72). Thus, it is possible that, in elderly women, HPV presence, in the absence of sexual activity, could be due to reactivation of latent HPV infection because of impairment of host immunologic response (73). The overexpression of Cox-2 in a number of cases was significantly higher in the older group than in the younger group, but this immunoreactivity is not related to the staging, grading, EGFR expression, or to the presence of HPV. The simultaneous expression of Cox-2 and EGFR had a poor prognostic significance, showing lower survival rates than cases without this immunoreactivity. On multivariate analysis, Cox-2 and EGFR immunopositivity did not reveal any correlation between these markers and prognosis probably because the number of cases considered was not particularly high. Inadequate immunologic control of HPV infection resulting in viral persistence is likely an important determinant of risk of progression to cervical neoplastic disease. Previous studies have provided evidence supporting this view. Higher prevalence of HPV infection is observed in HIV-infected individuals (74, 75). Studies have also reported associations between deregulation of cytokine production and impairment of CD4+ T cell–mediated immunity and cervical precancers (76,77,78,79). Finally, the consistent association observed between HLA alleles and cervical neoplasia argue for a role of the host immune response to HPV in cervical cancer pathogenesis (80). Immunologic competence has been reported to decrease with aging (81-93). Garcia Piňeres et al (72) examined the association between lymphoproliferative responses to antigens/mitogens and persistent HPV infection in women older than 45 years. Women included in this study were participants in a 10,000-woman population-based cohort study of cervical neoplasia in Costa Rica. Women older than 45 years and HPV DNA positive at a screening visit were selected as cases (n = 283). Garcia Piňeres et al selected a comparably sized control group of HPV DNA–negative women, matched to cases on age and time since enrollment (n = 261). At an additional clinical visit, women were cytologically and virologically rescreened, and cervical and blood specimens were collected. Proliferative responses to phytohemagglutinin (PHA), influenza virus (Flu), and HPV16 virus-like particle (VLP) were lower among women with persistent HPV infection [median counts per minute (cpm): 72,849 for PHA, 1,241 for Flu, and 727 for VLP] than for the control group (median cpm: 107,049 for PHA, 2,111 for Flu, and 2,068 for VLP). The decreases were most profound in women with long-term persistence and were only observed for the oldest age group (≥65 years). The results of this study indicate that an impairment in host immunologic responses is associated to persistent HPV infection. The fact that effects were evident for all studied stimuli is suggestive of a generalized effect. Since 1993, at least 7 studies have described the screening histories of women with invasive cervical cancer (95,96,97,98). The number of cases in these studies was between 469 and 481All studies concluded that the lack of a cervical smear history is the major reason why the disease still occurs. The percentage of women with invasive cervical cancer that had no screening history varied between 28% in Connecticut, USA (99) and 54% for Maori women in New Zealand (100). This percentage strongly depends on the population coverage of screening. With a 100% coverage, the percentage will only include young women diagnosed before the starting age of the programme. In 2007 the almost 30%of the Italian population not included in organised programmes is partly the result of an implementation process still in progress in some Regions in Southern Italy, but mainly of a very limited or completely absent implementation in a few Regions in Northern Italy. In 2008 the extension of organised cervical cancer screening programmes in Italy had had a target population 13.8095.025 women, corresponding to 78,44% of Italian women aged 25-64 years vs 69% in 2006. During 2008, 39.69% of invites women were screened, vs 39.83% in the previous year. The results of single regions are not homogeneous(Table 3-13).

	2008	2007	2006
Women 25-64 yrs included in the target population of organised programmes	13.094.025	11.872.810	11.362.580
Population 25-64 yrs	78,44	71,77	69,01
Nominal extension	25,34(3.356.931/13.247.487)	25,58(3.055.353/11.943.507)	25,32(1.116.006/2.899.817)
Compliance with invitation (%)	39,69(1.332.376/3.356.931)	39,83(1.217.000/3.055.353)	38,49(1.116.006/2.899.817)
NORTHERN ITALY			
Women 25-64 yrs included in the target population of organised programmes	5.210.405	4.942.788	4.911.641
Population 25-64 yrs	68,42	65,42	65,09
Nominal extension	29,5(1.541.010/5.222.404)	28,46(1.415.361/4.972.858)	27,17(1.341.812/4.938.269)
Compliance with invitation (%)	47,67(734.577/1.541.010)	46,93(664.344/1.415.361)	45,62(612.069/1.341.812)
CENTRAL ITALY			
Women 25-64 yrs included in the target population of organised programmes	3.252.167	3.008.931	3.029340
Population 25-64 yrs	98,09	91,86	93,95
Nominal extension	26,52(890.868/3.359.359)	27,16(822.548/3.028.432)	26,84(814.208/3.033.546)
Compliance with invitation (%)	40,17(357.846/890.868)	40,23(330.925/822.548)	35,70(290.632/814.208)
SOUTHERN ITALY AND ISLANDS			
Women 25-64 yrs included in the target population of organised programmes	4.631.453	3.921.091	3.421.599
Population 25-64 yrs	80,38	68,65	60,09
Nominal extension	19,83(925.053/4.665.724)	21,38(817.444/3.942.217)	21,38(743.797/3.479.433)
Compliance with invitation (%)	27,73(239.953/925.053)	27,12(221.731/817.444)	28,68(213.305/743.797)

The data of Liguria region have not been reported.

Legend:

Nominal extension: percentage of the resident population aged 24-64 that is included in the target population of active organised programmes.
PPV = Positive predictive value.
DR = Detection rate.
ASCUS = Atypical squamous cells of undetermined significance.
CIN = Cervical Intraepithelial Neoplasia.

Table 3. Extension of organised cervical cancer screening programmes in Italy. (http://www.osservatorionazionalescreening.it)

	ABRUZZO				BASILICATA			
	2005	2006	2007	2008	2005	2006	2007	2008
Nominal extension (%)	24,9	33,5	20,2	23,8	52	64,6	54,9	54,4
Number of invitated women	87.398	118.054	73.981	88.974	90.013	111.808	96.613	95.476
Compliance to invitation (%)	24,9	33,5	20,2	23,8	52,0	64,6	54,9	54,4
Compliance with recommendation to repeat cytology%	26,9	32,9	18	31,5	32,9	36,1	36,9	33,4
Inadequate (%)	2,4	3,2	3,9		2,6	2,2	3	1,8
Recommendation to repeat cytology(%)	2,8	3,7	4,3	4,5	2,1	2,1	4,3	2,4
Compliance colposcopy with referral for ASCUS+	62,3	60,4	68,7	77,2	96,3	95,8	68,7	97,1
DR° for lesions CIN2+ unadjusted	2,7	2,5	3	4,2	1,2	1,1	1,1	0,9
PPV for CIN2+ of ASCUS+ referred to colposcopy	16,2	16,2	10,8	12,1	5,1	5,5	3,5	4,3

Table 4. Organised cervical cancer screening programmes in Italy: value of some process indicators in Abruzzo and Basilicata regions between 2005-2008(National Centre for Screening Monitoring). (http://www.osservatorionazionalescreening.it)

	CAMPANIA				**EMILIA ROMAGNA**			
	2005	2006	2007	2008	2005	2006	2007	2008
Nominal extension (%)	24	14,9	17	18,5	27,8	31,4	30,8	33,4
Number of invitated women	357.06	241.64	283.00	285.59	332.6 5	377.4 0	379.16 2	409.37 6
Compliance to invitation (%)	24,0	14,9	17,0	18,5	27,8	31,4	30,8	33,4
Compliance with recommendation to repeat cytology%	16,8	26,1	27	27,2	57,1	50,8	56	56,5
Inadequate citology (%)	2,1	2,6	2,6	2,7	1,5	1,7	2	2
Recommendation to repeat cytology(%)	2,1	1,8	2,3	1,6	2,8	2,9	2,7	3,1
Compliance colposcopy with referral for ASCUS+	75,3	63,9	40	63,4	89,1	83,2	85,9	88,8
DR° for cytologyc lesions CIN2+ unadjusted	1,6	1,3	1,4	1,5	3,6	3,8	4	4,4
PPV for CIN2+ of ASCUS+ referred to colposcopy	17,4	11,7	12,8	17,2	14,6	15,7	17,9	16,4

Table 5. Organised cervical cancer screening programmes in Italy: value of some process indicators in Campania and Emilia Romagna regions between 2005-2008(National Centre for Screening Monitoring). (http://www.osservatorionazionalescreening.it)

	LAZIO				LOMBARDIA			
	2005	2006	2007	2008	2005	2006	2007	2008
Nominal extension (%)	13,7	22,1	24,2	23,3	24,9	27,1	29,7	25,7
Number of invitated women	227.356	303.896	299.466	360.688	136.919	154.165	164.979	198.728
Compliance to invitation (%)	13,7	22,1	24,2	23,3	24,9	27,1	29,7	25,7
Compliance with recommendation to repeat cytology%	24,1	21,8	31,3	30,3	37,8	41,5	41	39,7
Inadequate citology (%)	3,5	1,9	2,6	3,9	2,2	2,4	2,5	2,4
Recommendation to repeat cytology(%)	2,9	2,4	2,7	2,7	1,5	1,4	2	1,9
Compliance colposcopy with referral for ASCUS+	92	86,6	91,3	87,6	86,3	83,9	93	86
DR° for cytologyc lesions CIN2+ unadjusted	3,2	1,8	2,4	2,7	3,3	3	4	4
PPV for CIN2+ of ASCUS+ referred to colposcopy	14,9	10,2	12,3	12	27	21,5	22,3	

Table 6. Organised cervical cancer screening programmes in Italy: value of some process indicators in Lazio and Lombardia regions between 2005-2008(National Centre for Screening Monitoring). (http://www.osservatorionazionalescreening.it)

	MOLISE				PIEMONTE			
	2005	2006	2007	2008	2005	2006	2007	2008
Nominal extension (%)	59,6	18,6	Activated only for 4 months	21,5	29,7	27	30	31,8
Number of invitated women	50	16		23	365.893	330.188	371.226	396.661
Compliance to invitation (%)	59,6	18,6		21,5	29,7	27,0	30,0	31,8
Compliance with recommendation to repeat cytology%	21,7	14,4		19,3	42,4	42,9	43	44,7
Inadequate citology (%)	6,3	6,3		12,1	2,8	2,6	3	3,2
Recommendation to repeat cytology(%)	1,4	2,2		2,5	1,8	1,9	2	2
Compliance colposcopy with referral for ASCUS+	61,5	37,1		63,1	90,7	91,6	92,2	90,5
DR° for cytologyc lesions CIN2+ unadjusted	1,5	0,62		1	2,1	2	2,2	2,3
PPV for CIN2+ of ASCUS+ referred to colposcopy	17,3	7,7		5,9	17,7	15,1	17,2	17,2

Table 7. Organised cervical cancer screening programmes in Italy: value of some process indicators in Molise and Piemonte regions between 2005-2008(National Centre for Screening Monitoring). (http://www.osservatorionazionalescreening.it)

	TRENTINO				PUGLIA			
	2005	2006	2007	2008	2005	2006	2007	2008
Nominal extension (%)	37	30	30,1	29,8			8	9,9
Number of invitated women	52.305	43.455	45.104	44.852			41.094	105.599
Compliance to invitation (%)	37,0	30,0	30,1	29,8			8,0	9,9
Compliance with recommendation to repeat cytology%	35,7	36,2	37	53,2			36,2	17,2
Inadequate citology (%)	4,8	5,7	5,5	5			3	4
Recommendation to repeat cytology(%)	1,5	1,3	1,3	1,2			4,4	1,2
Compliance colposcopy with referral for ASCUS+	75,5	78,5	79	76			45,9	59,2
DR° for cytologyc lesions CIN2+ unadjusted	3,4	2,4	3,2	2,4			0,3	0,7
PPV for CIN2+ of ASCUS+ referred to colposcopy	29,6	23,9	31,5	28,3			1,6	9,2

Table 8. Organised cervical cancer screening programmes in Italy: value of some process indicators in Trentino and Puglia regions between 2005-2008(National Centre for Screening Monitoring). (http://www.osservatorionazionalescreening.it)

	SARDEGNA				SICILIA			
	2005	2006	2007	2008	2005	2006	2007	2008
Nominal extension (%)	27	24,6	20,4	26,4	26,1	24,6	21,1	21,2
Number of invitated women	38.813	35.368	29.329	74.765	153.31	126.90	131.256	133.590
Compliance to invitation (%)	27,0	24,6	20,4	26,4	26,1	24,6	21,1	21,2
Compliance with recommendation to repeat cytology%	24	23,7	31,4	33,7	19,03	29,1	25,4	19,7
Inadequate citology (%)	6,3	5,8	6	6,1	3,4	3,5	0,3	1,9
Recommendation to repeat cytology(%)	5,2	5,6	5,7	3	2,8	3,2	3,8	4
Compliance colposcopy with referral for ASCUS+	82,6	93,1	88,2	91,1	70,5	73,4	81	83,9
DR° for cytologyc lesions CIN2+ unadjusted	3,7	4,5	5,7	4,2	1,9	2,6	3,1	3
PPV for CIN2+ of ASCUS+ referred to colposcopy	29,2	8,6	11,5	15,2	9,7	16,3	12,9	9,6

Table 9. Organised cervical cancer screening programmes in Italy: value of some process indicators in Sardegna and Sicilia regions between 2005-2008(National Centre for Screening Monitoring). (http://www.osservatorionazionalescreening.it)

	TOSCANA				UMBRIA			
	2005	2006	2007	2008	2005	2006	2007	2008
Nominal extension (%)	28,7	29,8	31,3	29,9	27,3	29,3	23,5	31,5
Number of invitated women	291.516	303.307	319.444	309.365	67.635	73.206	58.556	78.215
Compliance to invitation (%)	28,7	29,8	31,3	29,9	27,3	29,3	23,5	31,5
Compliance with recommendation to repeat cytology%	44,1	46,6	48	49,6	44,4	47,1	58,2	47,5
Inadequate citology (%)	2	2,1	1,8	1,5	1,7	3,4	1,3	2,3
Recommendation to repeat cytology(%)	1,6	1,6	1,5	1,5	2	2	1,6	1,6
Compliance colposcopy with referral for ASCUS+	78,5	77,6	81,3	82,7	68,3	70,7	66,1	78
DR° for cytologyc lesions CIN2+ unadjusted	2,6	2,9	2,8	3	3,3	4,2	2,4	4,2
PPV for CIN2+ of ASCUS+ referred to colposcopy	21,8	25,1	24,2	23,9	57,3	29,1	22,6	34,2

Table 10. Organised cervical cancer screening programmes in Italy: value of some process indicators in Toscana and Umbria regions between 2005-2008(National Centre for Screening Monitoring). (http://www.osservatorionazionalescreening.it)

	VALLE D'AOSTA				VENETO			
	2005	2006	2007	2008	2005	2006	2007	2008
Nominal extension (%)	31,8	32,6	28	26,7	22,8	24,1	24,4	25,7
Number of invitated women	11.490	11.486	9.728	9.478	305.925	315.619	321.37	346.4
Compliance to invitation (%)	31,8	32,6	28,0	26,7	22,8	24,1	24,4	25,7
Compliance with recommendation to repeat cytology%	62	63,8	59,4	73,8	44,47	43,8	44,8	41,8
Inadequate citology (%)	5,5	4,5	1	0,8	5,7	4,7	5,4	5,4
Recommendation to repeat cytology(%)	3,4	4,5	2,4	1,6	2,8	2,8	3	3,1
Compliance colposcopy with referral for ASCUS+	85	94,1	93,9	95,2	90,5	91,6	92,3	91,6
DR° for cytologyc lesions CIN2+ unadjusted	2,5	2,5	3,8	1,6	2,7	2,9	2,8	3,3
PPV for CIN2+ of ASCUS+ referred to colposcopy	12,2	12,9	20,8	13,9	12,8	13,3	13,1	14

Table 11. Organised cervical cancer screening programmes in Italy: value of some process indicators in Valle D'Aosta and Veneto regions between 2005-2008(National Centre for Screening Monitoring). (http://www.osservatorionazionalescreening.it)

	FRIULI VENEZIA GIULIA				MARCHE			
	2005	2006	2007	2008	2005	2006	2007	2008
Nominal extension (%)	30	27,8	25,2		32,4	31,8	32,7	
Number of invitated women	98,619	90,948	86,085		145,35	134,79	140,03	
Compliance to invitation (%)	30,0	27,8	25,2		32,4	31,8	32,7	
Compliance with recommendation to repeat cytology%	54,9	51,9	56,2		33	36,2	35,2	
Inadequate citology (%)		6,5	6			1,1	2	
Recommendation to repeat cytology(%)	2,3	2,2	2,1		1,9	1,8	2	
Compliance colposcopy with referral for ASCUS+	88,8	90,7	88		90,4	80	84,7	
DR° for cytologyc lesions CIN2+ unadjusted					2,1	1.05	2,1	
PPV for CIN2+ of ASCUS+ referred to colposcopy					26,4	12,1	17,1	

Table 12. Organised cervical cancer screening programmes in Italy: value of some process indicators in Friuli Venezia Giulia and Marche regions between 2005-2008(National Centre for Screening Monitoring). (http://www.osservatorionazionalescreening.it)

	ALTO ADIGE (SUDTIROL)				CALABRIA			
	2005	2006	2007	2008	2005	2006	2007	2008
Nominal extension (%)	22,4	13,4	26,1		41,4	24,2	35,6	
Number of invitated women	32,194	18,542	37,699		21,619	94,105	162,16	
Compliance to invitation (%)	22,4	13,4	26,1		41,4	24,2	35,6	
Compliance with recommendation to repeat cytology%	32,2	34	32,2		25	25	24,4	
Inadequate citology (%)	1,1	0,75	0,85			2,3	3,6	
Recommendation to repeat cytology(%)					0,6	2,2	2,7	
Compliance colposcopy with referral for ASCUS+					71,4	75,5	81,7	
DR° for cytologyc lesions CIN2+ unadjusted					0,9	2.24	1,3	
PPV for CIN2+ of ASCUS+ referred to colposcopy					25	9,5	6,3	

Table 13. Organised cervical cancer screening programmes in Italy: value of some process indicators in Alto Adige and Calabria regions between 2005-2008(National Centre for Screening Monitoring). (http://www.osservatorionazionalescreening.it)

The main examined process indicators has been not reported in all the regions. The distinction between OpS and OS screening has not been done. In the literature numerous studies has been reported the recommendations and the results of cervical cancer screening(100-101-102-103-104). With regard to screening histories of invasive cervical carcinoma, in Italy has been not published studies with exception of OrS programme of Friuli Venezia Giulia. Zucchetto et al (105) have examined the screening histories of 438 women with invasive cervical cancer diagnosed in Friuli Venezia-Giulia between 1999 and 2005. 82 cases (49.7%) were found in >65 years-old women. 165 (37.7%) women were not screening. 69 (15.8%) women were not invited to OrS because of age >64 years old. Histological type and HPV detection of invasive cervical cancers has been reported. The study of Zucchetto et al (105) shows that the lack of screening among older women and of compliance with organized programs among women in the target population are the main limitation in cervical cancer secondary prevention. The results of Zucchetto et al (105) are in agreement with research conducted in northen Europe. Bos et al (106) have analized the screening history of 3.175 women with invasive cervical cancer diagnosed in the years 1994-1997 in the Netherland. 57% of 3175 women with invasive cervical cancer had no previous smears. Given the high proportion of women with invasive cervical cancer older than 64 years at diagnosis, the possibility of inviting them to have at least one Pap smear in life after 64 years should be taken in consideration. In according to American Cancer Society Guidelines for the early detection of cancer and the guidelines of other national regional screening programme, women 70 years of age or older who have had 3 or more normal Pap-test in a know and no abnormal Pap-test results in the last 10 years may choose to stop having Pap-test. But according to National Cervical Screening program the current policy of screening women of New Zealand is to continue organized regular screening until aged 69 years with pap test every three years if the women have ever been sexually active remain in place. The present study should be support the screening policy to perform Pap test every 3 years until aged 75 years, independently to sexual activity. In older post-menopausal women the transformation zone may be difficult to see. The cervix is often much smaller and the amount of cervical cells found in the smears may be not optimal. We believe that two samples (one from the endocervix with cytobrush and one from ectocervix with Ayre spatule) and smearing the cytological materials on two slides is the procedure of choice in order to obtain adequate material.

5. Acknowledgments

The authors thank Andrea Riolfatti and Suada Musabelliu for their help in the English translation, Beatrice Ferrari and Giorgio Moretti for technical assistance.

6. References

ACS. American Cancer Society. Cervical cancer facts and figure. 2000.

Ali-Fehmi R, Morris RT, Bandyopadhyay S, Che M, Schimp V, Malone JM Jr, Munkarah AR.Expression of cyclooxygenase-2 in advanced stage ovarian serous carcinoma: correlation with tumor cell proliferation, apoptosis, angiogenesis, and survival. Am J Obstet Gynecol. 2005; 192: 819-825.

Anttila A, Ronco G; Working Group on the Registration and Monitoring of Cervical Cancer Screening Programmes in the European Union; within the European Network for Information on Cancer (EUNICE). Description of the national situation of cervical cancer screening in the member states of the European Union. Eur J Cancer. 2009; 45:2685-708. Epub 2009 Sep 8.

Arbyn M, Antoine J, Mägi M, Smailyte G, Stengrevics A, Suteu O, Valerianova Z, Bray F, Weiderpass E. Trends in cervical cancer incidence and mortality in the Baltic countries, Bulgaria and Romania. Int J Cancer. 2011; 128:1899-907.

Arbyn M, Anttila A, Jordan J, Ronco G, Schenck U, Segnan N, Wiener H, Herbert A, von Karsa L eds. European guidelines for quality assurance on cervical cancer screening. 2nd edition. Office for official publications of the European communities, Luxembourg 2008.

Arbyn M, Autiere P, Ferlay J. Burden of cervical cancer in the 27 member states of the European Union: estimates for 2004. Ann Oncol 2007;18:1425–1431.

Arbyn M, Rebolj M, De Kok IM, Fender M, Becker N, O'Reilly M, Andrae B. The challenges of organising cervical screening programmes in the 15 old member states of the European Union. Eur J Cancer. 2009 Oct;45(15):2671-8. Epub 2009 Aug 18.

Baay MF, Tjalma WA, Weyler J, Pattyn GG, Lambrechts HA, Goovaerts G, Baekelandt M, Buytaert P, Van Marck EA, Lardon F, Vermorken JB. Prevalence of human papillomavirus in elderly women with cervical cancer. Gynecol Obstet Invest. 2001; 52: 248-251.

Bastos J, Peleteiro B, Gouveia J, Coleman MP, Lunet N. The state of the art of cancer control in 30 European countries in 2008. Int J Cancer. 2010; 126:2700-15.

Bisset LR, Lung TL, Kaelin M, Ludwig E, Dubs RW. Reference values for peripheral blood lymphocyte phenotypes applicable to the healthy adult population in Switzerland. Eur J Haematol 2004; 72: 203–212.

Bos AB, Rebolj M, Habbema JD, van Ballegooijen M. Nonattendance is still the main limitation for the effectiveness of screening for cervical cancer in the Netherlands. Int J Cancer 2006;119:2372-2375.

Brinton LA, Schairer C, Haenszel W, Stolley P, Lehman HF, Levine R, Savitz DA. Cigarette smoking and invasive cervical cancer JAMA 1986; 255: 3265-3269.

Buckley JD, Harris RW, Doll R, Vessey MP, Williams PT. Case-control study of the husbands of women with dysplasia or carcinoma of the cervic uteri. Lancet 1981; 2: 1010-1015.

Carmichael JA, Clarke DH, Moher D, Ohkle ID, Karchmar EJ. Cervical carcinoma in women aged 34 and younger. Am J Obset Gynecol 1986; 66(Suppl): 82-85.

Chakravarti B, Abraham GN. Aging and T-cell-mediated immunity. Mech Ageing Dev 1999; 108: 183–206.

Chin-Hong PV, Palefsky JM. Human papillomavirus anogenital disease in HIV-infected individuals. Dermatol Ther 2005; 18: 67–76.

Chng WJ, Tan GB, Kuperan P. Establishment of adult peripheral blood lymphocyte subset reference range for an Asian population by single-platform flow cytometry: influence of age, sex, and race and comparison with other published studies. Clin Diagn Lab Immunol 2004; 11: 168–173.

Cho Y, Gorina S, Jeffrey PD and Pavletich NP. Crystal structure of a p53 tumor suppressor-DNA complex: understanding tumorigenic mutations. Science 1994; 265: 346-355.

Choo KB and Chong KY Absence of mutation in the p53 and retinoblastoma susceptibility genes in primary cervical carcinomas. Virology 1993; 193: 1042-1046.

Ciatto S, Grazzini G, Cecchini S, Iossa A. Screening history of incident cases of invasive carcinoma of the cervix. Tumori 1993; 79: 311–313.

Clerici M, Merola M, Ferrario E, Trabattoni D, Villa ML, Stefanon B, Venzon DJ, Shearer GM, De Palo G, Clerici E. Cytokine production patterns in cervical intraepithelial neoplasia: association with human papillomavirus infection. J Natl Cancer Inst 1997; 89: 245–250.

Coleman D, Day N, Douglas G, Farmery E, Lynge E, Philip J, Segnan N. European guidelines for quality assurance in cervical cancer screening. Eur J Cancer 1993; 29A (Suppl.4): 1-38.

Commissione oncologica nazionale.Proposte operative in tema di prevenzione secondaria cervico-carcinoma uterino. In: Linee guida elaborate dalla Commissione oncologica nazionale, in applicazione di quanto previsto dal Piano Sanitario Nazionale per il triennio 1994-96, relativo all'azione programmata "Prevenzione e cura delle malattie oncologiche", concernenti l'organizzazione della prevenzione e dell'assistenza in oncologia. Supplemento ordinario alla Gazzetta Ufficiale n.127, 1 June 1996.

Conferenza permanente per i rapporti tra lo Stato, le Regioni e le Province autonome di Trento e Bolzano. "Provvedimento 8 marzo 2001. Accordo tra il Ministro della sanità e le Regioni e Province autonome di Trento e Bolzano sulle linee-guida concernenti la prevenzione, la diagnostica e l'assistenza in oncologia". Gazzetta ufficiale, 2 May 2001.

Crook T and Vousden KH. Properties of p53 mutations detected in primary and secondary cervical cancers suggest mechanisms of metastasis and involvement of environmental carcinogens. EMBO J 1992; 11: 3935-3940.

Crook T, Wrede D and Vousden KH. p53 point mutation in HPV-negative human cervical carcinoma cell lines. Oncogene 1991; 6: 873-875.

De Jong A, van Poelgeest MI, van der Hulst JM, Drijfhout JW, Fleuren GJ, Melief CJ, Kenter G, Offringa R, van der Burg SH. Human papillomavirus type 16-positive cervical cancer is associated with impaired CD4+ T-cell immunity against early antigens E2 and E6. Cancer Res 2004; 64: 5449–5455.

Devesa SS, Young JL Jr, Brinton LA, Fraumeni JF Jr. Recent trends in cervix uteri cancer. Cancer 1989; 64:2184 90.

Di Bonito L. Cervical screening in Italy. Abstracts of the 35th European Congress of Cytology, Lisbon, Portugal, Sept. 27–30, 2009. Cytopathholology 2009;1:22.

Douziech N, Seres I, Larbi A, Szikszay E, Roy PM, Arcand M, Dupuis G, Fulop T Jr. Modulation of human lymphocyte proliferative response with aging. Exp Gerontol 2002; 37: 369–387.

Eide TJ. Cancer of the uterine cervix in Norway by histologic type, 1970-84. J Natl Cancer Inst 1987; 79: 199-205.

F.X. Bosch, A. Lorincz and N. Munoz, Meijer CJ, Shah KV. The causal relation between human papillomavirus and cervical cancer, J Clin Pathol 2002; 55: 244–265.

Ferlay J, Bray F, Pisani, Parkin DM (2001). Globocan 2000. Cancer Incidence, Mortality and Prevalence Worldwide. IARCPress: Lyon.

Ferlay J, Bray F, Pisani, Parkin DM. GLOBOCAN 2002: Cancer incidence, mortality and prevalence worldwide. IARC Cancer base No.5, version 2.0. Lyon: IARC Press; 2004.

Fidler HK, Boyes DA, Worth AJ. Cervical cancer detection in British Columbia. A progress report . J Obstet Gynaecol Br Commonw 1968;75:392-404.

Fujita M, Inoue M, Tanizawa O, Iwamoto S and Enomoto T. Alterations of the p53 gene in human primary cervical carcinoma with and without human papillomavirus infection. Cancer Res 1992; 52: 5323-5328.

Garcia-Pineres AJ, Hildesheim A, Herrero R, Trivett M, Williams M, Atmetlla I, Ramirez M, Villegas M, Schiffman M, Rodriguez AC, Burk RD, Hildesheim M, Freer E, Bonilla J, Bratti C, Berzofsky JA, Pinto LA. Persistent human papillomavirus infection is associated with a generalized decrease in immune responsiveness in older women. Cancer Res. 2006; 66: 11070-11076.

Giordano G, D'Adda T, Dal Bello B, Brigati F, Bersiga A, Campanini N, Berretta R, Rocco A, Merisio C. Clinicopathologic implications of the epidermal growth factor receptor, cyclooxygenase 2 expression, and human papillomavirus status in squamous cell carcinoma of the uterine cervix in the elderly. Int J Gynecol Cancer. 2011 Feb; 21: 337-348.

Green and A. Berrington de Gonzalez, Sweetland S, Beral V, Chilvers C, Crossely B, Deacon J, Hermon C, Jha P, Mant D, Peto J, Pike M, Vessey MP. Risk factors for adenocarcinoma and squamous cell carcinoma of the cervix in women aged 20–44 years: the UK National Case-Control Study of Cervical Cancer, Br J Cancer 2003; 89: 2078–2086.

Hameed A, Fox WM, Kurman RJ, Hruban RH, Podack ER. Perforin expression in human cell-mediated luteolysis. Int J Gynecol Pathol 1995; 14: 151-157.

Harris CC p53: At the crossroads of molecular carcinogenesis and risk assessment. Science 1993; 262: 1980-1981.

Helland A, Holm R, Kristensen G, Laern J, Kaern J, Karlsen F, Trope C, Nesland JM and Borresen AL. Genetic alterations of the p53 gene, p53 protein expression and HPV infection in primary cervical carcinomas. J Path 1993; 171:105-114.

Hildesheim A, Wang SS. Host and viral genetics and risk of cervical cancer: a review. Virus Res 2002; 89: 229–240.

Howell EA, Chen YT, Concato J. Differences in cervical cancer mortality among black and white women. Obset Gynecol 1999; 94: 509-515.

Huang H, Patel DD, Manton KG. The immune system in aging: roles of cytokines, T cells and NK cells. Front Biosci 2005; 10: 192–215.

Huibregtse JM, Scheffner M and Howley PM. Cloning and expression of the cDNA for E6-AP, a protein that mediates the interaction of the human papillomavirus E6 oncoprotein with p53. Mol Cell Biol; 1993; 13: 775-784.

Janerich DT, Hadjimichael O, Schwartz PE, Lowell DM, Meigs JW, Merino MJ, Flannery JT, Polednak AP. The screening histories of women with invasive cervical cancer, Connecticut. Am J Public Health 1995; 85: 762–763.

Jentsch-Ullrich K, Koenigsmann M, Mohren M, Franke A. Lymphocyte subsets' reference ranges in an age- and gender-balanced population of 100 healthy adults-A monocentric German study. Clin Immunol 2005; 116: 192–197.

Jones WB, Shingleton HM, Russell A, Fremgen Am, Clive RE, Winchester DP, Chmiel JS. Cervical carcinoma and pregnancy. A national patterns of care study of the American College of Surgeons. Cancer 1996;77: 1479-1488.

Kadish AS, Timmins P, Wang Y. Regression of cervical intraepithelial neoplasia and loss of human papillomavirus (HPV) infection is associated with cell-mediated immune responses to an HPV type 16 E7 peptide. Cancer Epidemiol Biomarkers Prev 2002; 11: 483–488.

Kam KM, Leung WL, Kwok MY, Hung MY, Lee SS, Mak WP. Lymphocyte subpopulation reference ranges for monitoring human immunodeficiency virus-infected Chinese adults. Clin Diagn Lab Immunol 1996; 3: 326–330.

Kanda T, Watanabe S and Yoshiike K. Immortalization of primary rat cells by human papillomavirus type 16 subgenomic DNA fragment controlled by SV40 promoter. Virology 1988; 165: 321-325.

Kenter GG, Schoonderwald EM, Koelma IA, Arentz N, Hermans J, Fleuren GJ. The cytological screening history of 469 patients with squamous cell carcinoma of the cervix uteri; does interval carcinoma exist? Acta Obstet Gynecol Scand 1996; 75: 400–3.

Kjellgren O. Mass screening in Sweden for cancer of the uterine cervix: effect on incidence and mortality . An overview. Gynecol Obset Invest 1986; 22: 57-63.

Kuerbitz SJ, Plunkett BS, Walsh WV and Kastan MB Wild-type p53 is a cell cycle checkpoint determinant following irradiation. Proc Natl Acad Sci USA 1992; 89: 7491-7495.

La vecchia C, Franceschi S, Decarli A, Gentile A, Fasoli M, Pampallona S, Tognoni G. Dietary vitamin A and the risk of invasive cervical cancer. Int J Cancer 1984; 34: 319-322.

Lee YY, Wilczynski P, Chumakov A, Chih D and Loeffler HP Carcinoma of the vulva: HPV and p53 mutations. Oncogene 1994; 9: 1655-1659.

Lesack D, Wahab I, Gliks CB. Radiation-induced atypia of endocervical epithelium: a histological, immunohistochemical and cytometric study. Int J Gynecol Pathol 1996; 15: 242-247.

Levi F, Lucchini F, Negri E, Franceschi S, La Vecchia C. Cervical cancer mortality in young women in Europe: patterns and trends. Eur J Cancer 2000; 36: 266-271.

Lowe SW, Schmitt EM, Smith SW, Osborne BA and Jacks T. p53 is required for radiation-induced apoptosis in mouse thymocytes. Nature 1993; 362: 847-849.

Lugada ES, Mermin J, Kaharuza F, Ulvestad E, Were W, Langeland N, Asjo B, Malamba S, Downing R. Population-based hematologic and immunologic reference values for a healthy Ugandan population. Clin Diagn Lab Immunol 2004; 11: 29–34.

M. Walboomers, M.V. Jacobs and M.M. Manos, Bosch FX, Kummer JA, Shah KV, Snijders PJ, Peto J, Meijer CJ, Munoz N. Human papillomavirus is a necessary cause of invasive cervical cancer worldwide, J Pathol 1999; 189: 12–19.

M.H. Schiffman, H.M. Bauer and R.N. Hoover RN, Glass AG, Cadell DM, Rush BB, Scott DR, Scherman ME, Kurman RJ, Wacholder S. Epidemiologic evidence showing that human papillomavirus infection causes most cervical intraepithelial neoplasia, J Natl Cancer Inst 1993; 85: 958–964.

Mendelsohn J, Baselga J. Status of epidermal growth factor receptor antagonists in the biology and treatment of cancer. J Clin Oncol. 2003; 21: 2787-2799.

Milde-Langosch KM, Albrecht K, Joram S, Schlechte H, Giessing M and Loning T. Presence and persistence of HPV infection and p53 mutation in cancer of the cervix uteri and the vulva. Int J Cancer 1995; 63: 639-645.

Ministero della salute, Direzione generale della prevenzione. Screening oncologici. Raccomandazioni per la pianificazione e l'esecuzione degli screening di popolazione per la prevenzione del cancro della mammella, del cancro della cervice uterina e del cancro del colon retto. Roma, 2006.

Miwa K, Miyamoto S, Imamura T, Nishida M, Yoshikawa Y, Nagata Y and Wake N. The role of p53 inactivation in human cervical cell carcinomadevelopment. Br J Cancer 1995; 71: 219-226.

Mubiayi N, Bogaert E, Boman F, Leblanc E, Vinarier D, Leroy JL, Querleu D. Cytological history of 148 women presenting with invasive cervical cancer [Article in French]. Gynaecol Obstet Fertil 2002; 30: 210–217.

Munger K, Werness BA, Dyson N, Phelps WC, Harlow E and Howley PM. Complex formation of human papillomavirus E7 proteins with theretinoblastoma tumor suppressor gene product. EMBO J 1989; 8: 4099-4105.

Nakagawa S, Watanabe S, Yoshikawa H, Taketani Y, Yoshiike K and Kanda T. Mutational analysis of human papillomavirus type 16 E6 protein: transforming function for human cells and degradation of p53 in vitro. Virology 1992; 212: 535-542.

Nakagawa S, Yoshikawa H, Jimbo H, Onda T, Yasugi T, Matsumoto K, Kino N, Kawana K, Kozuka T, Nakagawa K, Aoki M, Taketani Y. Elderly Japanese women with cervical carcinoma show higher proportions of both intermediate-risk human papillomavirus types and p53 mutations. Br J Cancer. 1999 Mar;79(7-8):1139-1144.

NCI.SEER Cancer Statitics Review: 1973-1996. Bethesda, MD: National Cancer Institute; 1999.

Nevins JR E2F: A link between the Rb tumor suppressor protein and viral oncoproteins. Science 1992; 258: 424-429.

Paquette RL, Lee YY, Wilczynski SP, Karmakar A, Kizaki M, Miller CW and Koeffler HP.Mutation of p53 and human papillomavirus infection in cervical carcinoma. Cancer 1993; 72: 1272-1280.

Parkin DM , Nguyen-Dinh X Day NE. The impact of screening on the incidence of cervical cancer in England and Wales. Br J Obset Gynaecol 1985; 92: 150-157.

Ratima K, Paul C, Skegg DC. Cervical smear history of Maori women developing invasive cervical cancer. NZ Med J 1993; 106: 519–521.

Rodeck U, Jost M, Kari C, Shih DT, Lavker RM, Ewert DL, Jensen PJ. EGF-R dependent regulation of keratinocyte survival. J Cell Sci. 1997; 110: 113-121.

Ronco G, Giubilato P, Naldoni C Zorzi M, Anghinoni E, Scalisi A, Dalla Palma P, Zanier L, Barca A, Angeloni C, Gaimo MD, Maglietta R, Mancini E, Pizzuti R, Iossa A, Segnan N, Zappa M. Activity level and process indicators of organised programmes for cervical cancer screening in Italy. Epidemiol Prev 2006; 30 Suppl 1: 27-40.

Ronco G, Giubilato P, Naldoni C, Zorzi M, Anghinoni E, Scalisi A, Dalla Palma P, Zanier L, Barca A, Angeloni C, Gaimo MD, Maglietta R, Mancini E, Pizzuti R, Iossa A, Segnan N, Zappa M. Livello di attivazione ed indicatori di processo dei programmi organizzati di screening in Italia. In: Roselli Del Turco M, Zappa M. Osservatorio per la Prevenzione dei Tumori femminili. Terzo rapporto. Roma 2004: 38-51.

Ronco G, Giubilato P, Naldoni C, Zorzi M, Anghinoni E, Scalisi A, Dalla Palma P, Zanier L, Barca A, Angeloni C, Gaimo MD, Maglietta R, Mancini E, Pizzuti R, Iossa A, Segnan N, Zappa M. Extension of organised cervical screening programmes in Italy and their process indicators. Epidemiol Prev 2007; 31 Suppl 2: 33-47.

Ronco G, Pilutti S, Naldoni C, Pilutti S, Anghinoni E, Zappa M, Dalla Palma P, Ciatto S, Segnan N. Stato dello screening cervicale in Italia. In: Rosselli Del Turco M, Zappa M eds. Osservatorio Nazionale per la Prevenzione dei Tumori femminili. Primo Rapporto. Roma 2002: 32-49.

Ronco G, Ricciardi V, Naldoni C et al. Livello di attivazione ed indicatori di processo dei programmi organizzati di screening cervicale in Italia. In: Rosselli Del Turco M, Zappa M. Osservatorio Nazionale per la Prevenzione dei Tumori femminili. Secondo Rapporto. Roma 2003: 36-51.

Ronco G, van Ballegooijen M, Becker N, Chil A, Fender M, Giubilato P, Kurtinaitis J, Lancucki L, Lynge E, Morais A, O'Reilly M, Sparen P, Suteu O, Rebolj M, Veerus P, Zakelj MP, Anttila A. Process performance of cervical screening programmes in Europe. Eur J Cancer. 2009; 45:2659-70. Epub 2009 Aug 25.

Saito J, Hoshiai H, Noda K. Type of human papillomavirus and expression of p53 in elderly women with cervical cancer. Gynecol Obstet Invest. 2000; 49: 190-193.

Salomon DS, Brandt R, Ciardiello F, Normanno N. Epidermal growth factor-related peptides and their receptors in human malignancies. Crit Rev Oncol Hematol. 1995; 19: 183-232.

Sansoni P, Cossarizza A, Brianti V, Fagnoni F, Snelli G, Monti D, Marcato A, Passeri G, Ortolani C, Forti E,. Lymphocyte subsets and natural killer cell activity in healthy old people and centenarians. Blood 1993; 82: 2767–2773.

Sansoni P, Fagnoni F, Vescovini R, Mazzola M, Brianti V, Bologna G, Nigro E, Lavagetto G, Cossarizza A, Monti D, Franceschi C, Passeri M. T lymphocyte proliferative capability to defined stimuli and costimulatory CD28 pathway is not impaired in healthy centenarians. Mech Ageing Dev 1997; 96: 127–136.

Santagostino A, Garbaccio G, Pistorio A, Bolis V, Camisasca G, Pagliaro P, Girotto M. An Italian national multicenter study for the definition of reference ranges for normal values of peripheral blood lymphocyte subsets in healthy adults. Haematologica 1999; 84: 499–504.

Scheffner M, Werness BA, Huibregtse JM, Levine AJ and Howley PM. The E6 oncoprotein encoded by human papillomavirus types 16 and 18 promotes the degradation of p53. Cell 1993; 63: 1129-1136J.

Shingleton HM, Orr JW. Cancer of the cervix: diagnosis and treatment. In: Monaghan J, Lind T, eds. Clinical obstretics and gynecology. New York: Churchill Livingstone; 1987.

Smith JS, Green J, Berrington de Gonzales A, Appleby P, Peto J, Plummer M, Franceschi S, Beral V. Cervical cancer and use of hormonal contraceptives: a systematic review. Lancet 2003; 361: 1159-1167.

Solomon D, Davey D, Kurman R, Moriarty A, O'Connor D, Prey M, Raab S, Sherman M, Wilbur D, Wright T Jr, Young N; The 2001 Bethesda System: terminology for reporting results of cervical cytology. JAMA. 2002;24;287:2114-2119.

Song C, Vandewoude M, Stevens W, De Clerck L, Van der Planken M, Whelan A, Anisman H, Dossche A, Maes M. Alterations in immune functions during normal aging and Alzheimer's disease. Psychiatry Res 1999; 85: 71–80.

StriFazzari M, Cu-Uvin S, Bacon M, Schuman P, Levine AM, Durante AJ, Gange S, Melnick S, Burk RD.ckler HD, Palefsky JM, Shah KV, Anastos K, Klein RS, Minkoff H, Duerr A, Massad LS, Celentano DD, Hall C . Human papillomavirus type 16 and immune status in human immunodeficiency virus-seropositive women. J Natl Cancer Inst 2003; 95: 1062–1071.

Stuart GC, Mc Gregor SE, Duggan MA, Nation JG. Review of the screening history of Alberta women with invasive cervical cancer. CMAJ 1997; 157: 513–519.

Subbaramaiah K, Dannenberg AJ. Cyclooxygenase-2 transcription is regulated by human papillomavirus 16 E6 and E7 oncoproteins: evidence of a corepressor/coactivator exchange. Cancer Res. 2007; 67: 3976-3985.

Tsegaye A, Messele T, Tilahun T, Hailu E, Sahlu T, Doorly R, Fontanet AL, Rinke de Wit TF. Immunohematological reference ranges for adult Ethiopians. Clin Diagn Lab Immunol 1999; 6: 410–414.

Tsujii M, DuBois RN. Alterations in cellular adhesion and apoptosis in epithelial cells overexpressing prostaglandin endoperoxide synthase-2. Cell. 1995; 83: 493-550.

Tsujii M, Kawano S, DuBois RN. Cyclooxygenase-2 expression in human colon cancer cells increases metastatic potential. Proc Natl Acad Sci U S A. 1997; 94: 3336-3340.

Tsukui T, Hildesheim A, Schiffman MH, Tsukui T, Hildesheim A, Schiffman MH, Tsukui T, Hildesheim A, Schiffman MH, Lucci J 3rd, Contois D, Lawler P, Rush BB, Lorincz AT, Corrigan A, Burk RD, Qu W, Marshall MA, Mann D, Carrington M, Clerici M, Shearer GM, Carbone DP, Scott DR, Houghten RA, Berzofsky JA . Interleukin 2 production in vitro by peripheral lymphocytes in response to human papillomavirus-derived peptides: correlation with cervical pathology. Cancer Res 1996; 56: 3967–3974.

W.A. Tjalma, M. Arbyn, J. Paavonen, van Waes TR, Bogers JJ. Prophylactic human papillomavirus vaccines: the beginning of the end of cervical cancer, Int J Gynecol Cancer 2004;14:751–761.

Waterhouse J, Muir C, Stranmugaratnam K, Powell J. Cancer incidence in five continent; Vol IV. IARC scientific publication series, No.42. Lyon: IARC Press; 1982.

Werness BA, Levine AJ and Howley PM. Association of human papillomavirus types 16 and 18 E6 proteins with p53. Science 1990; 248: 76-79.

Williams CS, DuBois RN. Prostaglandins endoperoxide synthase: why two isoforms? Am J Physiol. 1996; 270: 393-400.

X.B. Trinh, J.J. Bogers, E.A. Van Marck and W.A. Tjalma. Treatment policy of neuroendocrine small cell cancer of the cervix, Eur J Gynaecol Oncol 2004;25; 40–44.

Zucchetto A, Franceschi S, Clagnan E, Serraino D, Zanier L, Franzo A; Friuli Venezia Giulia Cancer Registry Working Group. Screening history of women with invasive cervical cancer in north-east Italy. Eur J Obstet Gynecol Reprod Biol. 2010; 152: 200-204.

Part 2

Novelties in Human Papillomavirus Diagnosis, Treatment and Research

5

Oligonucleotide Applications for the Therapy and Diagnosis of Human Papillomavirus Infection

María L. Benítez-Hess, Julia D. Toscano-Garibay and Luis M. Alvarez-Salas*

Laboratorio de Terapia Génica, Departamento de Genética y Biología Molecular, Centro de Investigación y de Estudios Avanzados del Instituto Politécnico Nacional, México D.F.
México

1. Introduction

Cervical cancer is the best known example of a common human malignancy with a proven infectious etiology. Clinical, epidemiological and molecular analyses have long indicated that persistent infection with high-risk human papillomaviruses (HPVs) is causally associated with cervical cancer. Although new prophylactic vaccines and highly sensitive HPV typing methods are currently available, cervical cancer continues as the most common tumor in developing countries, where most of the annual half a million new cases occur (Arbyn et al., 2011). Besides socio-cultural issues restraining professional gynecological care, the relatively high cost of these technologies has limited their availability where they are most needed. Thus, there is a pressing need for affordable and readily available detection and therapeutic tools for HPV infection and cervical cancer. In the last two decades, novel diagnostic and therapeutic approaches based on synthetic oligonucleotides and genomic information have developed into promising tools to fight human disease.

2. HPV and cervical cancer

Genital dysplasia and cervical cancer are associated with persistent infection of a subset of HPVs referred as high-risk, including HPV types 16, 18, 31, 33, 45, 52 and 58 (Clifford et al., 2003). High-risk HPVs normally replicate in keratinocytes from stratified squamous epithelia of their hosts where the 8-kb double-stranded circular DNA genome is usually retained in an episomal form. The highly conserved high-risk HPV genomes consist of six common early genes (E1, E2, E4, E5, E6 and E7) and two late genes (L1 and L2) coding for the capsid proteins (Figure 1). The early genes contribute to cellular transformation, viral regulation and DNA replication (Moody & Laimins, 2010). In addition, the HPV genome also comprises a highly variable non-coding regulatory region, the long control region (LCR), which contains the viral origin of replication and regulatory elements targeted by several cellular transcription factors and the viral E2 gene (Hebner & Laimins, 2006).

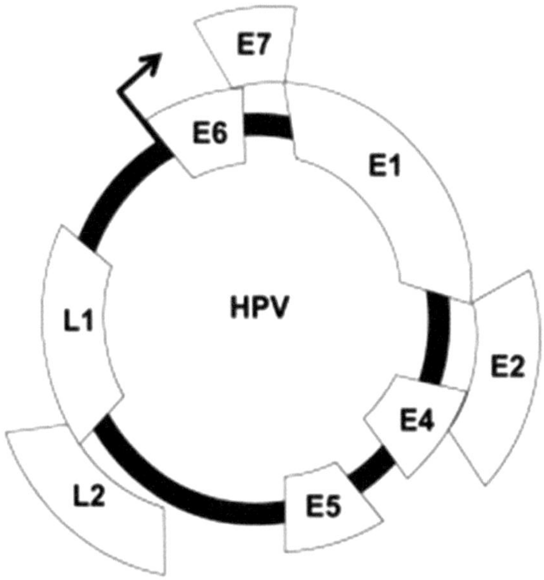

Fig. 1. Map of the HPV genome. Early (E) and ate (L) genes are indicated. The arrow indicates the early promoter.

2.1. HPV targets for diagnostic and therapeutic oligonucleotides

The relationship between cervical cancer and high-risk HPVs is related to the integration of viral DNA to the host genome with the disruption of the viral regulator E2 (Pett & Coleman, 2007; Vernon et al., 1997), and to the production of viral proteins E6 and E7 which are sufficient and necessary to acquire and maintain a transformed phenotype (Pirisi et al., 1988; Xue et al., 2010). Because E2 is usually absent in cervical tumor cells and E6/E7 genes are retained and expressed in most tumors, these features are often referred to as the hallmarks of cervical cancer (Alvarez-Salas & DiPaolo, 2007). In the absence of E2 protein, high-risk HPV E6 and E7 genes are continuously transcribed from a single promoter resulting in polycistronic mRNA containing both transcripts (Wang et al., 2011). The E6 and E7 protein products interact and functionally neutralize key cellular regulatory proteins, so that cell proliferation continues.

High-risk HPV E6 protein targets numerous cellular pathways to insure viral DNA replication and is a key oncogene in HPV associated neoplasias. E6 was first shown to interact with the p53 tumor suppressor protein (Werness et al., 1990) and the E6-AP complex to act as a ubiquitin protein ligase (Huibregtse et al., 1991) inducing the specific ubiquitination and degradation of p53 (Scheffner et al., 1993). Thus, high-risk HPV E6 results in blockage of p53-mediated apoptosis. Interestingly, E6 has been found interacting with the extrinsic apoptotic factors TNFR-1, FADD and caspase-8 (Filippova et al., 2002; Tungteakkhun et al., 2010) suggesting alternative apoptosis inhibitory functions. Although E6-mediated degradation of p53 is considered a key event for the onset of cellular transformation, it is clear that E6 possess other p53-independent transforming and anti-apoptotic activities, such as telomerase activation (Gewin et al., 2004; Klingelhutz et al., 1996; Oh et al., 2001). Many other cellular targets of high-risk E6 proteins have now been described, including PDZ domain-containing targets such as the human homologue of the tumor suppressor DLG (discs large protein) (Gardiol et al., 1999), MUPP1 (Lee et al., 2000) and MAGUK (membrane-associated guanylate kinase) proteins (Glaunsinger et al., 2000), and a number of transcription regulators (Etscheid et al., 1994; Zimmermann et al., 1999), disrupting cell adhesion, polarity, epithelial differentiation and reducing immune recognition of HPV infected cells (Howie et al., 2009).

The E7 protein plays a vital role in the viral life cycle by disrupting the tight link between differentiation and proliferation, thus allowing viral replication in normal keratinocytes that would be otherwise withdrawn from the cell cycle (McLaughlin-Drubin & Munger, 2009). E7 protein from high-risk HPVs targets pRB and disrupts the E2F-mediated transcriptional regulation resulting in the up-regulation of genes required for G1/S transition and DNA synthesis (Duensing et al., 2001; Munger & Phelps, 1993). HPV-16 E7 can directly bind the G1/S transition antagonists E2F1 (Hwang et al., 2002) and E2F6 (McLaughlin-Drubin et al., 2008) thus ensuring that the infected cells remain in an S-phase-competent state allowing HPVs to bypass negative growth signals. The steady-state level and metabolic half-life of pRB are decreased in HPV-16 E7-expressing cells, because E7 can induce the degradation of pRB through the ubiquitin-proteasome system (Berezutskaya et al., 1997; Boyer et al., 1996). High-risk HPV E7 proteins also contribute to cell cycle dysregulation through the abrogation of the growth inhibitory activities of $p21^{CIP1}$ and $p26^{KIP1}$ (Funk et al., 1997; Jones et al., 1997; Zerfass-Thome et al., 1996). Other functions associated to high-risk HPV expression include epigenetic reprogramming through induction of KDM6A and KDM6B histone demethylases (McLaughlin-Drubin et al., 2011), trophic sentinel signaling abrogation and autophagy induction (Zhou & Munger, 2009), induction of genomic instability (Duensing et al., 2000), and disruption of *Anoikis* signaling through interaction with p600 (Huh et al., 2005).

3. Oligonucleotide applications to cervical cancer and HPV infection

Although the independent E6 and E7 functions may cause genomic instability, cell immortalization and transformation by themselves, the unregulated expression of both proteins is considered the major contribution of HPVs to cervical cancer development. The demonstration of the existence of stable molecular targets in high-risk HPVs has justified the development of small oligonucleotides for cervical cancer detection and treatment. High-risk HPV-16 and 18 express E6 and E7 proteins from a single polycistronic mRNA (Schneider-Gadicke & Schwarz, 1986; Smotkin et al., 1989), suggesting that targeting of either E6 or E7 mRNA would likely impede both E6/E7 translation resulting in similar growth arrest phenotypes. Several groups have identified that inhibition of these genes translation resulted in tumor growth suppression confirming E6/E7 as attractive targets for cervical cancer therapy (Alvarez-Salas et al., 1998; Shillitoe, 2006; Venturini et al., 1999).

In the last decades, novel therapeutic approaches based on genomic information developed into promising tools to fight human disease. Therapeutic oligonucleotides are short DNA or RNA molecules designed to disrupt expression or function of disease-related genes. Approaches to therapeutic oligonucleotide technology include: 1) Blocking of gene transcription by triplex-forming oligodeoxyribonucleotides (TFOs); 2) Translation inhibition by AS-ODNs, small interfering RNAs (siRNAs) and ribozymes; 3) Inhibition of protein function by nucleic acid aptamers and 4) Immunostimulatory oligonucleotides (IM-ONS)

(Alvarez-Salas, 2008). Diagnostic oligonucleotides refer to the application of DNA or RNA oligonucleotides for diagnostic purposes. Diagnostic oligonucleotide technologies comprise oligonucleotides designed for 1) Priming polymerase chain reaction (PCR or RT-PCR) detection, 2) Hybridization-based technologies (hybrid capture or microarrays) and 3) Binding with target proteins (aptamers). Here, we will only discuss diagnostic oligonucleotides used as aptamers for HPV detection because PCR and hybridization technologies have been extensively used for HPV diagnostics for decades and the subject has been comprehensively analyzed elsewhere (Stanley, 2010).

3.1 Antigene technology

TFOs can hybridize with particular sequences in double-stranded DNA (dsDNA) through the formation of Hoogsteen or reverse-Hoogsteen hydrogen bonds between the TFOs and homopurine stretches found in the major groove of the target DNA (Letai et al., 1988; Moser & Dervan, 1987). TFOs have potential for manipulating gene structure and function in living cells, inhibiting transcription by interfering with regulatory protein binding or blocking mRNA elongation (Carbone et al., 2003) (Figure 2A). Although finding appropriate targets for TFO action in genomic DNA may be an issue, TFO technology has a potential advantage over oligonucleotide-based control of translation (antisense and siRNA technologies) because there are generally one to two targets per cell as compared with the hundreds to thousands copies of mRNA targets (Vasquez & Glazer, 2002).

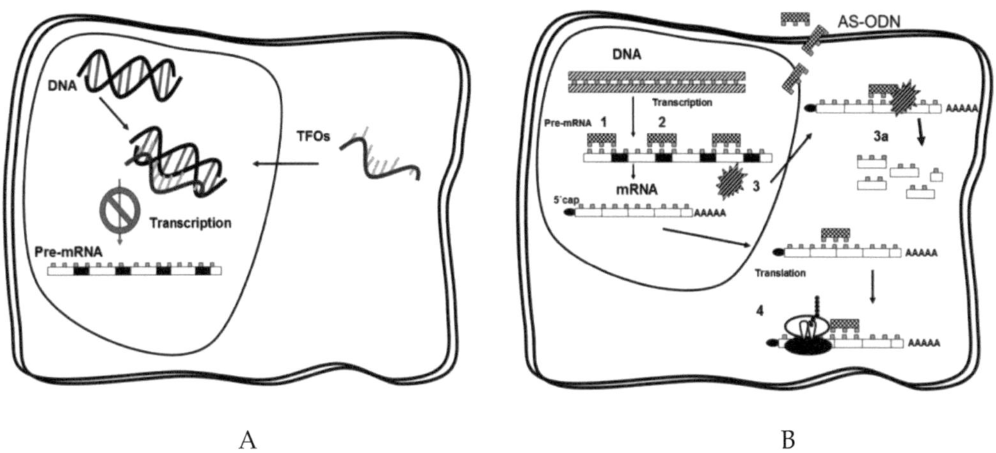

Fig. 2. A) Antigene technology. Triplex-forming oligonucleotides (TFOs) hybridize with DNA to block transcription. B) Antisense oligonucleotides (AS-ODNs) gene silencing. As-ODNs hybridize with the 5′-UTR (1) or within the coding region (2) of the target mRNA. Formation of DNA-RNA heteroduplexes induces RNaseH (3) activity over the RNA target (3a) producing degradation and thus inhibiting translation. Stable hybridization with the target 5′-UTR mRNA can inhibit ribosome anchorage (4).

3.1.1 Antigene technology on cervical cancer

Several natural triplex-forming sites have been identified within the HPV-16 genome (Malkov et al., 1993). However, only a few attempts have been reported on the use of TFOs against HPV. An initial report for the low-risk HPV-11 established an intramolecular triplex

DNA formation using a TFO directed to a 22nt-long homopurine stretch within the LCR (nt 21-42) overlapping a Sp-1 and a E2 binding site plus the origin of replication. Although the stability of the triplex DNA formation was comprehensively demonstrated, no functional effect on HPV-11 transcription/replication was reported (Hartman et al., 1992). Other report also established formation of pyrimidine-purine-pyrimidine or pyrimidine-purine-purine triplex DNA with the HPV-16 fragment nt 554-685 under favorable conditions using complementary pyrimidine or purine TFOs. The observed DNA triplexes exhibited remarkable sequence specificity (Cherny et al., 1993).

Optical DNA melting experiments and co-migration assay were used to establish stable triplex DNA formation at homopurine-homopyrimidine-rich target sites present in the HPV-16 E7 gene (nt 656-673). The target sequence was specifically recognized by several 17-mer purine TFOs designed to form antiparallel or parallel triplex DNA helices (Popa et al., 1996). Despite the reported success on triplex DNA formation using TFOs and different HPV targets, there are no reports on the application of TFOs to inhibit HPV transcription suggesting that intracellular conditions may not allow effective antigene-based therapies.

3.2 The antisense approach

Antisense inhibition uses DNA sequence information to synthesize an oligonucleotide complementary to a target mRNA and specifically inhibit or modify translation by three main mechanisms: A) Translational arrest by inhibiting ribosome binding at the 5'-UTR (Crooke, 1999); B) Induced degradation of the target mRNA by RNaseH (Agrawal et al., 1990) (Figure 2B), and C) Translational modulation by exon-skipping (Du & Gatti, 2009). The aim of all antisense approaches is to reduce the quantity of the target protein in order to revert or prevent progression of a disease process.

Two main classes of antisense oligonucleotides have been used to silence or modulate gene expression providing that the target sequences are exposed (in a single stranded form lacking secondary structure or protein binding). One class makes use of AS-ODNs complementary to the target mRNA. AS-ODN hybridization to its complementary target mRNA by Watson–Crick base pairing should provide enough specificity and affinity to produce translational arrest (physical blockage of ribosome binding) of the target mRNA. Additionally, the formation of DNA-RNA heteroduplexes leads to the activation of RNaseH thus inducing cleavage of the target mRNA (Bonham et al., 1995). The second antisense oligonucleotide technology class consists of small, catalytic RNA or DNA molecules. The catalytic core of these molecules produces cleavage of a target RNA once the catalytic moiety has hybridized with a Watson-Crick complementary sequence (Benitez-Hess & Alvarez-Salas, 2006). This mechanism may be contrasted with AS-ODNs that require cellular RNaseH activity following hybridization in order to cleave the target mRNA.

3.2.1 AS-ODNs applications as therapeutic moieties

Early use of unmodified AS-ODNs showed that they were highly unstable in biological fluids due to the presence of exonucleases thus limiting their use as therapeutic moieties. Later, several nucleotide analogues were introduced to increase ODN stability. To avoid changes in hybridization specificity, modifications were limited to the phosphate and ribose backbone of DNA/RNA oligonucleotides. First generation modified AS-ODNs consisted of sulfur-substituted DNA on the free oxygen molecules constituting a phosphodiester bond. Phosphorothioated ODNs (PS-ODNs) display a high degree of stability in biofluids while retaining the ability to form RNaseH substrates leading to efficient, highly specific degradation of the target mRNA (Agrawal & Zhang, 1997). RNaseH activity is mostly nuclear and thus would likely produce cleavage of the pre-mRNA within the nucleus before splicing (Wagner et al., 1993). However, the strongly polyanionic nature of PS-ODNs cause *in vivo* issues regarding affinity, specificity, cellular uptake, biodistribution and toxicity thus limiting their therapeutical use (Akhtar & Agrawal, 1997). Nevertheless, PS-ODNs have been the most extensively studied AS-ODNs in various animal models and humans leading to oligonucleotide-based drugs such as Fomivirsen (Vitravene™) or Affinitak (Patil et al., 2005).

The use of other modifications such as methylphosphonates, ethylphosphonates or 2'-*O*-methyl, confer high affinity for target sequences and extraordinary stability in biofluids, but they do not activate RNaseH (Mercatante & Kole, 2000). Thus, these modifications are better suited for modulating gene expression or exon-skipping approaches rather than gene silencing (Sierakowska et al., 2000). Second-generation AS-ODNs provide molecules with RNaseH activity but minimal off-target effects. Mixed-backbone oligodeoxynucleotides (MBOs) contain strategically placed segments of phosphorothioated backbones (able to induce RNaseH activity on the target mRNA) mixed with segments of either modified oligodeoxyribonucleotides or oligoribonucleotides (reducing off-target effects). The advantages of MBOs over PS-ODNs are increased biological activity, reduced polyanionic- and CG-dinucleotide-related side effects and increased *in vivo* stability (Agrawal & Zhao, 1998). A third-generation AS-ODNs contains DNA/RNA oligonucleotides with 2'-*O*-methyl modification in addition to a phosphorothioate core and methylphosphonate ends further reducing toxicity. Improved stability, high specificity and low toxicity characterize these molecules, allowing for efficient destruction of target mRNA at nanomolar concentrations (Sternberger et al., 2002).

3.2.2 Antisense technology on cervical cancer therapy

Earlier reports on high-risk HPV E6 and E7 functions used plasmid-borne full-length antisense RNA to show that inhibition of HPV-18 E6/E7 expression results in growth arrest in C4-1 cells (von Knebel Doeberitz & Gissmann, 1987; von Knebel et al., 1988). Later, plasmid-borne antisense RNA delivery was shown to induce apoptosis in CaSki cells via up-regulation of p53 and apoptosis induction (Cho et al., 2002). Delivery of antisense RNA using adenoviral vectors and retroviral vectors on SiHa and CaSki cells resulted in the reduction of HPV16 E7 protein expression and cell proliferation. These changes were accompanied by cell cycle arrest, up-regulation of RB, down-regulation of E2F-1 and BCL-2 and dose-dependent and retarded tumor growth of CaSki cells, a cervical cancer line with multiple copies of HPV-16 (Choo et al., 2000; Hayashi et al., 1997). More recently, non-neuroinvasive HSV-1 vectors, lacking the $\gamma_1 34.5$ gene, were used to express antisense RNA complementary to the first 100nt of the HPV-16 E7 gene. These recombinant viruses down-regulated E7 protein expression in CaSki cells in a dose-dependent manner (Kari et al., 2007). Overall, these results confirmed the validity of targeting high-risk HPV E6/E7 for cervical cancer therapy. Nevertheless, due to the difficulties of administrating plasmids, large antisense RNA molecules or even infectious viruses to patients, the use of small antisense moieties such as AS-ODNs, catalytic oligonucleotides or siRNAs might be a better alternative.

Pioneering attempts on E6/E7 targeting by AS-ODNs directed antisense PS-ODNs to the translational start site of E6/E7 mRNA (Steele et al., 1993; Tan & Ting, 1995). *In vivo* testing on CaSki, SiHa and HeLa cells (all cervical cancer cell lines containing high-risk HPV) showed that these PS-ODNs produced cell growth inhibition. Nevertheless, no data was provided to show growth inhibition due to a true antisense mechanism. Later, a rational approach to antisense exposed regions was applied to HPV-16 E6/E7 using fast-hybridizing RNA segments obtained from partially digested E6/E7 mRNA (Kronenwett & Sczakiel, 1997). A selection of AS-ODNs directed against such exposed sequences resulted in growth inhibition of cultured SiHa cells (Venturini et al., 1999).

Our group developed AS-ODNs covering a so-called "antisense window" within a stable HPV-16 E6 (nt 410-445) region (Alvarez-Salas et al., 1995). Two short antisense PS-ODNs complementary to nt 410-445 produced efficient growth inhibition of monolayer and agar-growth HPV-16-containing tumor cell lines in a dose-dependent manner. One of such PS-ODNs also inhibited tumor growth in nude mice (Alvarez-Salas et al., 1999; Marquez-Gutierrez et al., 2007). Interestingly, the combined use of both AS-ODNs resulted in the additive but not synergistic growth inhibition suggesting that they can be applied together to overcome issues related to genital HPV genomic variability (Marquez-Gutierrez et al., 2007). Nevertheless, the high doses used in these studies (within the micromolar range) suggest that further modifications are required to improve therapeutical efficiency avoiding off-target effects. Overall, current AS-ODN applications to high-risk HPV E6/E7 gene silencing as a therapy for cervical cancer appears promising and relatively safe, providing that the tested PS-ODNs are administered locally to control off-target issues commonly observed with phosphorothioated moieties. Nevertheless, second and third-generation AS-ODNs remain to be clinically tested as the advancement of other gene silencing technologies (i.e. siRNA and shRNAs) overcame an otherwise very effective molecular therapy.

3.3 Therapeutic catalytic oligonucleotides

Small ribozymes and DNAzymes are oligonucleotides possessing, at the very least, enzymatic RNA cleavage and ligation activities (Haseloff & Gerlach, 1988; Santoro & Joyce, 1998). Ribozymes were initially described as catalytic RNA moieties found in the self-splicing group I introns from the unicellular algae *Tetrahymena* (Kruger et al., 1982), and within the RNA active site of *Escherichia coli* RNaseP (Guerrier-Takada et al., 1983). However, the relatively large size of these two ribozymes precluded gene modulating/silencing applications. Later, small catalytic RNA cores from naturally occurring ribozymes were isolated from the circular genomes of certain pathogenic plant RNA viroids (Haseloff & Gerlach, 1989). In particular, two catalytic moieties have been intensely used as therapeutic agents; the hammerhead and hairpin ribozymes. By simply altering the native substrate recognition sequences, natural *cis*-cleaving ribozymes can be engineered to recognize and cleave any target RNA in *trans* by Watson-Crick hybridization (Michienzi & Rossi, 2001) (Figure 3A). Consequently, ribozymes received considerable attention as potentially valuable tools for the inhibition of virus replication, modulation of tumor progression, and analysis of cellular gene function (Morrissey et al., 2002).

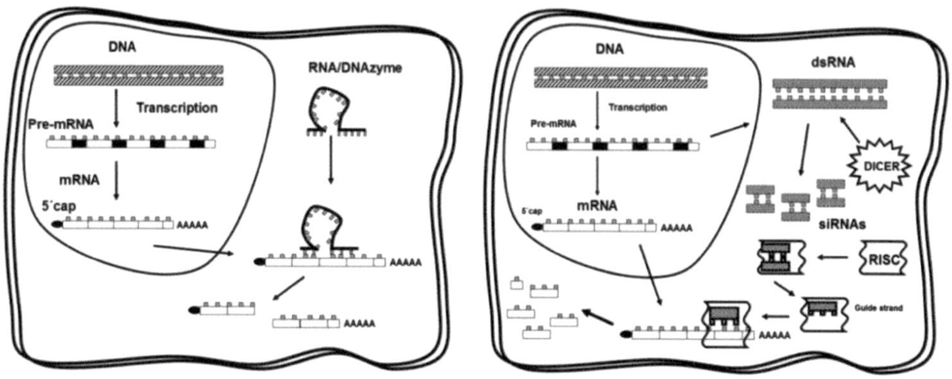

A B

Fig. 3. A) Catalytic oligonucleotides mode of action. Ribozymes or DNAzymes hybridize and cleave the target mRNA. B) RNA interference (RNAi) mechanism. Double-stranded RNA (dsRNA) found in a given mRNA are recognized and cleaved by DICER to yield small interfering RNAs (siRNAs) that in turn are incorporated into the RISC complex to cleave the mRNA from which they were derived. By administrating synthetic siRNAs the RISC complex may be manipulated to target a particular mRNA.

3.3.1 The hammerhead ribozyme

Hammerhead ribozymes are small (30-40nt) catalytic RNA moieties composed of three basic components including a highly conserved catalytic domain flanked by two base-pairing sequences and a complementary sequence within the target RNA containing the sessile phosphodiester bond. Natural catalytic centers can be formed within contiguous RNA sequences or by sequences several nucleotides apart (Epstein & Gall, 1987; Hutchins et al., 1986). Providing that the target RNA is single-stranded, hammerhead ribozymes can cleave any substrate RNA containing the triplet 5´-NUX-3´, where U is conserved, N is any nucleotide and X can be C, U or A (Vaish et al., 1998). Cleavage occurs 3′ to the 5′-NUX-3′ triplet (Uhlenbeck, 1987), generating 5′ hydroxyl termini and a 2′,3′-cyclic phosphate at the cleavage site (Hutchins et al., 1986; Prody et al., 1986).

3.3.2 The hairpin ribozyme

Hairpin ribozymes are about 60nt long and efficiently catalyze a reversible, site-specific cleavage reaction. Structurally, hairpin ribozymes are composed by the substrate recognition domain A located aside the catalytic domain B and the target RNA containing the target site. The established cleavage requirements for heterologous substrates indicate that the substrate sequence must contain a 5′-BN*GUC-3′ motif (where * is the site of cleavage) (Anderson et al., 1994; Hampel et al., 1990). Cleavage occurs at the 5′ side of guanosine and yields two products: the 3′-product containing the 5′-hydroxyl terminus newly formed within a terminal G, and the 5′-product containing the 2′,3′-cyclic phosphate (Yu & Burke, 1997).

3.3.3 Catalytic DNA

DNAzymes are small (~30nt) catalytic DNA oligonucleotides capable of cleaving target RNA molecules in a sequence specific manner (Baum & Silverman, 2008). These molecules represent a new generation of catalytic oligonucleotides artificially obtained through *in vitro* selection procedures by their capacity to catalyze the *cis*-cleavage of a target RNA sequence. Similar to ribozymes, DNAzymes hybridize substrate RNAs by Watson-Crick pairing and cleavage results in RNA fragments containing 2′,3′-cyclic phosphate and 5′-hydroxyl ends, suggesting a common mechanism (Santoro & Joyce, 1998). Therefore, the same widely tested design rules for AS-ODNs and ribozymes can be readily applied for therapeutic DNAzymes. However, unlike ribozymes, usage of DNAzymes as therapeutic moieties has the advantage of simpler and cost-effective synthesis, easier administration and higher stability in biofluids (Dass et al., 2008). So far, the 10-23 DNAzyme is the most commonly used in therapeutic applications. The 10-23 moiety structure resembles that of a hammerhead ribozyme consisting of a 15nt catalytic core flanked by two target recognition arms complementary to the target RNA (Santoro & Joyce, 1997). Cleavage is strictly dependent on Mg++ and is specifically produced at a RY (R, purine; Y, pyrimidine) junction within the target RNA (Cairns et al., 2003; Faulhammer & Famulok, 1997). Although the 10-23 DNAzyme is active at 37°C it may require nucleotide modifications to keep high activity under physiological conditions (Takamori et al., 2005). Other DNAzymes with different structural and catalytic features have been successfully used as sensors for ions, molecules and even proteins (Ali et al., 2011; Zhang et al., 2011). Thus, DNAzymes offer a wide array of possible therapeutical and diagnostic applications.

3.3.4 Hammerhead ribozymes and HPV

Early reports on ribozyme use against HPV assumed that translational start regions within mRNA are poorly structured thus allowing accessibility to antisense moieties. These reports were limited to cell-free experimentation and characterization of ribozyme cleavage on HPV target transcripts. Hammerhead ribozymes directed to HPV-16 nt 110 and 558 and expressed from plasmids showed efficient cleavage of HPV-16 E6/E7 transcripts in cell-free tests in different conditions of ionic strength, Mg^{++} concentration and temperature. Evaluation of the simultaneous activity of both ribozymes suggested a cooperative effect to disrupt HPV-16 E6/E7 gene expression (Lu et al., 1994). Similarly, targeting HPV-16 E6/E7 genes by hammerhead ribozymes specific to nt 240 and 597 showed that target size is important for catalytic activity (He et al., 1993). Chen *et al.*, developed hammerhead ribozymes targeting HPV-18 E6/E7 genes (nt 120, 309 and 671) that were initially tested by incubation of total RNA from HeLa and Vero cells with *in vitro* transcribed ribozymes resulting in the efficient and specific degradation of HPV-18 transcripts from HeLa cells. In a more unorthodox approach *E. coli* was used to co-expresses both the ribozymes and a 1266nt fragment from HPV-18 (including E6 and E7 genes). Ribozymes were induced by infection with a helper phage (T7/M13) resulting in the progressive down-regulation of the HPV-18 target. Finally, ribozyme anti-tumor activity was tested on HeLa cells resulting in a cell growth reduction, increased serum dependency, and reduced foci formation in soft agar (Chen et al., 1996; Chen et al., 1995) .

3.3.5 Hairpin ribozymes and HPV

Hairpin ribozymes are usually more efficient at 37°C than hammerhead ribozymes and co-factors are not a strict requirement for activity because the catalytic mechanism appears to rely on structural components (Walter et al., 1998). However, efficient cleavage by hairpin ribozymes requires a specific sequence within the target RNA (5′-GUC-3′ motif). We performed a comprehensive search for hairpin ribozyme target sites within HPV-16 E6/E7 genes showed six potential target sites. A hairpin ribozyme directed to site 434 (R434) was *in vivo* tested for *cis*-cleavage using a plasmid-borne HPV-16 E6/E7 transcripts containing ribozymes at the 3′-UTR. Only R434-containig transcripts caused significant delay in the growth rate of transfected cells and inhibited E6/E7 immortalization (Alvarez-Salas et al., 1998). Although this report demonstrated the feasibility of hairpin ribozyme use as a therapeutic antisense moiety for cervical cancer, the larger size of hairpin ribozymes limited their application as plasmid-borne moieties. Thus, we developed multiplex expression systems (triplex) based on hairpin ribozymes for R434. Such systems resulted in the complete release of multiple independent catalytic units from a single transcript by a self-processing mechanism, allowing individual R434 activity and increasing efficiency of degradation of E6 RNA (Aquino-Jarquin et al., 2008; Aquino-Jarquin et al., 2010). The measured activity of a single R434 unit resulted in 30% inhibition of HPV-16 E6/E7 mRNA in SiHa cells, suggesting that multiple ribozymes directed against the same or other target sites might result in complete inhibition (Aquino-Jarquin et al., 2008).

It is worth mentioning that notwithstanding the relative success on inhibiting HPV E6/E7 by ribozymes, the catalytic features from both hammerhead and hairpin ribozymes dramatically drop within the cellular environment. Intracellular variables affecting activity include Mg^{++} availability, co-localization with the target, nuclease action and protein binding (Benitez-Hess & Alvarez-Salas, 2006). Plasmid-borne ribozymes usually contain stem-loop or tRNA structures to extend intracellular life that may get targeted by several RNA-processing mechanisms thus impeding activity (Alvarez-Salas L.M., *unpublished data*). Alternatively, because of their small size (~30nt) hammerhead ribozymes may be synthesized including modified nucleotides to escape nuclease and RNA processing mechanisms but this alternative usually brings deleterious off-target effects that may mislead data interpretation and limit clinical application. The therapeutical use of ribozyme in cervical cancer has never approached to the simple, efficient and relatively safe use of AS-ODNs. Therefore, because the proven high ribozyme specificity and catalytic features for HPV transcripts it is likely that ribozymes may be better suited for diagnostic usage in cervical cancer.

3.3.6 DNAzymes on cervical cancer therapy

DNAzymes have become one of the most versatile oligonucleotide technologies available. In the last few years, DNAzymes have been used as therapeutical agents, computing DNA, biochemical analysis tools and sensors (Baum & Silverman, 2008; Stojanovic et al., 2005). However, there are only a few reports on DNAzyme application in the fields of cervical cancer and HPV. Our first report on a modified 10-23 DNAzyme directed to HPV-16 E6/E7 mRNA "antisense window" showed efficient down-regulation of E6/E7 transcripts both *in vitro* and *in vivo* resulting in specific inhibition of proliferation and cell death in a dose-dependent manner (Reyes-Gutierrez & Alvarez-Salas, 2009). To improve efficiency and intracellular stability the DNAzyme was modified with locked nucleic acids (LNAs) producing more thermostable DNAzyme-RNA complexes resulting in better cleavage efficiency (Benitez-Hess et al., 2011). In our hands, DNAzyme technology merged the relative simplicity and affordability of DNA synthesis and modification with the expected benefits of enzymatic catalysis yielding a therapeutical moiety superior in performance and specificity when compared to AS-ODNs and even siRNAs at the nanomolar range.

3.4 The small RNA revolution: siRNAs, shRNAs and miRNAs

The mechanism of RNA interference (RNAi) is a natural and wide-spread gene knockdown phenomenon induced by the formation of double-stranded RNA (dsRNA) segments in most mRNAs (Elbashir et al., 2001; Fire et al., 1998; Sharp, 1999). The RNAi process occurs in the cytoplasm where dsRNA regions within mRNAs are digested into double-stranded 21–23nt fragments, with a 2nt 3'-overhand, by the RNaseIII-like enzyme DICER (Bernstein et al., 2001). Subsequently, these small fragments, now called small interfering RNAs or siRNAs, are denatured by a helicase and one strand (leader or guide strand) is then incorporated into an RNA-induced silencing complex (RISC) that includes DICER, AGO2, TRBP and other members of the *Argonaute* family (Cullen, 2006; Hammond et al., 2001; Meister et al., 2004; Nykanen et al., 2001). The activated RISC complexes containing the guide strand hybridize and cleave the homologous mRNA from which they were derived. Therefore, there are no genes coding for particular siRNAs (Bartel, 2004). Recent reports suggest that siRNA activity exhibit serious dependence on the target site, as is the case for other antisense-based technologies, which might significantly limit the convenient use of siRNA (Miyagishi et al., 2003). Target recognition by activated RISC complexes appear to rely on the perfect matching between the target sequence and a 2-8nt region within the guide strand known as "seed" region (Lin et al., 2005).

By using synthetic siRNAs administrated exogenously, the RNAi machinery can be manipulated to silence a given mRNA (Figure 3B). These siRNAs can bypass the earlier steps in the RNAi pathway and can be loaded directly onto the RISC complex. Both synthetic siRNAs and vector-borne delivery of the equivalent short hairpin RNAs (shRNAs) have been used as potential therapeutic moieties for cervical cancer. Because shRNAs rely on the vector used, we will only focus in the developments of siRNAs as true therapeutic oligonucleotides. Although powerful, the widely reported gene silencing effects of siRNAs do not appear specific in many instances as down-regulation of unintended targets with partial sequence complementarities and stimulation of innate immune by type I interferon (IFN-I) and/or inflammatory cytokine responses have been often reported (Jackson et al., 2003; Judge et al., 2005; Kalali et al., 2008).

On the other hand, miRNAs are also small 20–25nt long non-coding dsRNAs with very specific functions modulating gene expression by hybridizing to complementary sequences present in the 3' UTR of many protein-coding mRNAs (Bartel, 2004). Unlike siRNAs, the miRNAs are coded in the genome of most metazoans (including humans) by independent loci or within intronic regions of other genes (Cullen, 2004; Kim & Kim, 2007). They are initially transcribed by the RNA polymerase II as primary miRNAs (pri-miRNAa) (Lee et al., 2004), which are cleaved into pre-miRNA hairpins by the RNaseIII-like nuclease DROSHA and PASHA/DGCR8 (Gregory & Shiekhattar, 2005). Pre-miRNAs are exported from the nucleus by the EXPORTIN-5 (Yi et al., 2003). Intronic pre-miRNAs are generated as a product of splicing of the host gene (Berezikov et al., 2007). Once in the cytoplasm, the pre-miRNA hairpins merge to the RNAi pathway and are cleaved by DICER to produce mature miRNAs that are incorporated into RISC and interact with their targets (Valencia-Sanchez et al., 2006).

3.4.1 RNAi therapeutics on HPV

Early attempts to silence high-risk HPV gene expression using siRNAs indicated selective E6/E7 mRNA. E6 silencing by a siRNA directed to HPV-16 nt 224-242 induced accumulation of cellular p53 protein, transactivation of the cell cycle control p21 gene and reduced cell growth but no apoptosis. Surprisingly, E7 silencing produced by a siRNA to nt 662-680 induced apoptotic cell death. HPV-negative cells appeared unaffected by the anti-viral siRNAs (Jiang & Milner, 2002). Because the polycistronic expression of HPV-16 E6 and E7 both siRNAs would have similar effect on E6/E7 expression and thus similar phenotypes (Butz et al., 2000). Although no explanation has been provided for this puzzling result, it is likely that the reported observations may be related to off-target effects.

Later it was reported that vector-borne and synthetic siRNAs directed against the HPV-18 E6 gene (nt 385-403) restored dormant tumor suppressor pathways in HPV-positive cancer cells that are otherwise inactive in the presence of E6. This ultimately resulted in massive apoptotic cell death, selectively in HPV-positive tumor cells (Butz et al., 2003). More recently a siRNA molecule targeting the E7 region of the bicistronic HPV-18 E6 and E7 mRNA (nt 142-160) reduced expression of E6 and E7 in HeLa cells. Application of siRNAs against E6 and E7 also inhibited cellular DNA synthesis and induced morphological and biochemical changes characteristic of cellular senescence. These results demonstrate that reducing E6 and E7 expression is sufficient to cause HeLa cells to become senescent thus establishing that targeting of E6/E7 mRNA affects synthesis and functions of both E6 and E7 (Hall & Alexander, 2003). The simultaneous targeting of HPV-18 E6/E7 has also been reported to induce apoptosis and reduce proliferation of HeLa cells (Qi et al., 2010). Interestingly, it has been shown that cellular apoptosis induced by siRNA directed to HPV-18 E6 in HeLa cells relies on the p53 and ubiquitin proteolysis pathway thus inhibiting cell proliferation and promoting cell apoptosis. Anti-oncogene and upper regulation of immunization-related genes produced regression of the malignant phenotype after E6 inhibition (Min et al., 2009).

Other synthetic siRNA decreased the levels of HPV-16 E6/E7 mRNA and induced nuclear accumulation of p53 in SiHa cells. The siRNA also suppressed monolayer and anchorage-independent growth associated with p21CIP1/WAF1 induction and hypophosphorylation of retinoblastoma protein. Furthermore, SiHa cells treated with the anti-E6 siRNA prior to subcutaneous injection, formed tumors in NOD/SCID mice that were significantly smaller than in those treated with a control siRNA (Yoshinouchi et al., 2003). Thus, sequence-specific targeting of high-risk HPV E6/E7genes, siRNAs may be developed into novel therapeutics that can efficiently inhibit growth of cervical cancer cells. Nevertheless, *in vivo* delivery of siRNAs is still a major obstacle to their clinical use.

As with other oligonucleotide-based therapeutical approaches, *in vivo* delivery of siRNA is mostly affected by ribonuclease degradation, rapid renal excretion and nonspecific uptake by the reticuloendothelial system (Whitehead et al., 2009). Additionally, siRNAs are polyanions that do not readily cross the cell membrane. In turn to avoid these issues, siRNAs are often synthesized with phosphorothioated or 2′-O-modified bases and encapsulated in delivery systems allowing enhanced stability in biofluids and cell uptake, escape immune recognition, and improve pharmacokinetics by avoiding excretion and renal filtration (Lorenz et al., 2004; Sorensen et al., 2003). Encapsulated siRNAs still need to co-localize with the appropriate target cell/tissue type leading to more complicated therapeutic strategies. Thus, several considerations regarding biodistribution, extracellular and intracellular transport must be addressed in addition to potency and biostability before clinical use of siRNAs. Nevertheless, the recent success in clinical trials using siRNA to treat age-related macular degeneration (Bevasiranib), respiratory syncytial virus infection (ALN-RSV01) and the targeted *in vivo* gene silencing via systemic delivery of siRNA using transferrin-tagged, cyclodextrin-based nanocapsules for human cancer therapy (CALAA-01) have demonstrated the therapeutic feasibility of siRNAs (Shim & Kwon, 2010).

In the last few years, siRNA use for silencing high-risk HPV E6/E7 has been widely reported although emphasis shifted from design and targeting to delivery and specificity, as highly active siRNAs are now commercially available. Many reports showed successful E6/E7 inhibition, but most of them were limited to cell culture, lacking of toxicity controls (Jonson et al., 2008; Lea et al., 2007; Sima et al., 2008; Yamato et al., 2008). A recent report, undertook a more comprehensive approach by designing and testing nine different siRNAs against either the E6 or E7 genes of HPV-16 or HPV-18 in several combinations. The siRNAs were tested on CaSki or HeLa cell lines resulting in significant cell growth and colony formation inhibition in both cell lines with a significant increase in apoptosis. The siRNAs had no effect in HPV-negative C33-A cells, demonstrating a lack of off-target effects. In addition, a xenograft study showed that intratumor injection of the siRNAs reduced tumor growth in BALB/c nude mice (Chang et al., 2010).

The transient nature of antisense technology (including siRNAs) forced research on long expression using vector-borne shRNAs. Although many reports have established the feasibility of this approach (Bai et al., 2006; Bousarghin et al., 2009; Gu et al., 2011), it is clear that prolonged siRNA expression may lead to dysfunction of the RNAi pathway (Tang et al., 2006) or other intracellular effects (Koivusalo et al., 2006) due to the sudden rise in p53 and pRB proteins after siRNA treatment (Sima et al., 2008). Thus, siRNA treatment has been used to enhance already established therapies for cervical cancer such as paclitaxel (Liu et al., 2009), cisplatin (Wu et al., 2011) and TRAIL (Eaton et al., 2011) with sometimes mixed results depending on the condition of p53 expression (Koivusalo et al., 2005).

As noted above, nucleotide modifications at specific positions enable oligonucleotides to avoid intracellular nuclease degradation and meddling with the endogenous RNAi pathway, but they also help to overcome off-targeting issues in siRNAs (Jackson et al., 2006). In addition, DNA inclusion in the seed region of the guide strand and its complementary sequence within the siRNA, so-called a double-stranded RNA-DNA chimera (dsRNA-DNA), abolishes off-target effects sacrificing some silencing activity (Ui-Tei et al., 2008). Application of dsRNA-DNA chimeras from previously reported and highly active siRNAs to nt 497, 573 and 752 within HPV-16 E6/E7 mRNA (Yamato et al., 2008), resulted in reduced cytotoxicity in two of three chimeric siRNAs (497 and 752), but not in the other (573), correlating with their reported off-target effects. Silencing activity was marginally affected in chimeric siRNAs 497 and 573 and moderately in 752. Chimeric siRNA 497 induced E6/E7-specific growth suppression of cervical cancer cells and E6/E7-immortalized human keratinocytes (Yamato et al., 2011).

The delivery of antisense moieties has also attracted much attention in siRNA research. Unlike AS-ODNs, there is a stringent requirement for transfection of siRNAs that has limited its applications as powerful cell culture inhibitors. To become truly useful therapeutic moieties, *in vivo* delivery methods have been developed for cervical cancer treatment using siRNAs besides the obvious use of vector-borne shRNAs. These approaches vary from the traditional direct intratumor injection (Fujii et al., 2006) to more innovative methods such as dendrosomal nanoparticles delivery (Dutta et al., 2010), encapsidation in HPV-16 virus-like particles (Bousarghin et al., 2005), encapsulation in lipidic particles (Wu et al., 2011) and coating of quantum dots (Zhao et al., 2011). All of these approaches showed the feasibility of *in vivo* siRNA treatment for cervical cancer. No clinical reports have been published so far.

3.4.2 MicroRNAs (miRNAs) in cervical cancer

The participation of miRNAs as regulatory molecules in differentiation, apoptosis, and proliferation strongly suggested a role in cervical cancer. Although miRNAs are not therapeutic or diagnostic oligonucleotides in strict sense, they can be used as synthetic moieties to block key biological processes leading to malignant transformation. Because the HPV life cycle is linked to epithelial differentiation and requires actively proliferating keratinocytes, it has been hypothesized that HPV proteins may modulate miRNA expression. Interestingly, high-risk HPVs do not encode for any known miRNA (Cai et al., 2006; Lui et al., 2007), although they may control expression of cellular miRNAs to regulate the activities of cellular proteins through expression of viral regulatory proteins (i.e. E5, E7 and E7) (Greco et al., 2011; Wang et al., 2009; Zheng & Wang, 2011). In the last few years, many alterations in cellular miRNA patterns in cervical cancer tissue or cervical cancer cells have been reported, suggesting that knowledge of differential miRNA expression may have a significant diagnostic and prognostic value (Lui et al., 2007).

High-risk HPV E6 may exert modulation of miRNA expression through p53 down regulation. Cervical cancer cells containing high-risk HPVs show reduced expression of miR-34a, a p53 effector with tumor-suppressor abilities. Reduction of miR-34a expression in HPV-containing human keratinocytes correlated with expression of viral E6. Furthermore, siRNA knockdown of viral E6 expression in high-risk HPV-containing cervical cancer cell lines lead to increased expression of p53 and miR-34a and accumulation of miR-34a in G0/G1 phase cells. Ectopic expression of miR-34a in HPV-containing and HPV-negative cells resulted in substantial cell proliferation inhibition and moderate apoptosis, suggesting HPV modulation of cellular miRNA expression (Wang et al., 2009). The HPV-16 E6 was also found to decrease expression of miR-23b in SiHa and CaSki cells by repressing the promoter and increased expression of its cellular target, the urokinase-type plasminogen activator (uPA), a known inductor of cell migration in cervical cancer cells. The link between HPV-16 E6 and miR-23b transcription was associated to the presence of a p53 binding site within the miR-23b promoter, suggesting a cell migration modulatory role for E6 (Au Yeung et al., 2011).

High-risk HPV E7 expression in human keratinocytes modulated expression of human miR-203 and its downstream target, ΔNp63. Although the underlying mechanism is not fully understood, E7 is sufficient for blocking miR-203 expression probably by modulation of the mitogen-activated protein kinase (MAPK) pathway signaling. The p63 family, is related to the p53 tumor suppressor. ΔNp63 isoform is expressed at high levels in proliferating undifferentiated basal keratinocytes, and its expression is down-regulated in differentiated non-proliferating cells. Down-regulation of ΔNp63 has been associated to regulation of epithelial proliferation and differentiation. Thus, inhibition of miR-203 allows HPV productive replication in differentiating cells (Melar-New & Laimins, 2010). Interestingly, expression of the high-risk HPV-16 E5 protein (considered an overall enhancer of E6/E7 activities) resulted in rapid (96 hours) alteration of miR-146a, miR-203 and miR-324-5p and their target genes in transfected keratinocytes, suggesting a miRNA regulatory role for E5 (Greco et al., 2011).

Genomic microarray analyses in normal and cervical cancer tissues using the same miRNA array platform showed increased expression miR-15b, miR-16, miR-17-5p, miR-20a, miR-20b, miR-21, miR-93, miR-106a, miR-155, miR-182, miR-185, and miR-224 and decreased expression of miR-29a, miR-34a, miR-126, miR-127, miR-145, miR-218, miR-424, miR-450, and miR-455) in cervical cancer tissues (Li et al., 2010; Wang et al., 2008). Further confirmation of miR-126, miR-143/145, miR-155, and miR-424/450 alterations was performed by deep sequencing (Witten et al., 2010). Other studies with customized miRNA arrays and different assay platforms showed increased miR-21 expression in cervical cancer, a common occurrence in cancer cells (Lui et al., 2007). More interestingly, miR-143 and miR-145 showed basically null expression in cancer samples, suggesting the potential value of these miRNAs as tumor markers (Lui et al., 2007; Pereira et al., 2010). Yet another study concluded that infection with high-risk HPV lowered miR-218 expression suggesting a role for miR-218 in the pathogenesis of cervical cancer. Nevertheless, the specific role of all these miRNAs in cervical carcinogenesis and HPV infection is unknown.

The growth inhibitory activity of miR-34c-3p was recently shown by our group in SiHa cells but not in other cell types. Although the inhibitory mechanism is not clear, transfection of a mi34c-3p mimic resulted in specific fast apoptosis induction (24 hours), inhibition of colony formation, cell migration and invasion, suggesting a potential therapeutic use for this miRNA (Lopez & Alvarez-Salas, 2011).

3.5 Aptamers

Aptamers are single-stranded oligonucleotides that, unlike AS-ODNs and siRNAs, function by folding into specific globular structures that dictate high-affinity binding to a variety of targets (Cerchia et al., 2002). They are often referred as functional homologues of the antibodies and are obtained through the use of the systematic evolution of ligands by exponential enrichment (SELEX) procedure. The SELEX method is a PCR-based *in vitro* selection procedure of large oligonucleotide libraries that recapitulates natural evolution resulting in the isolation of specific ligands that bind with high affinity to a wide variety of proteins and cell surface epitopes (Ellington & Szostak, 1990; Tuerk & Gold, 1990). These molecules have been used in flow cytometry, biosensors, affinity probe electrophoresis, capillary electrochromatography, and affinity chromatography (Yan et al., 2005).

Notwithstanding the obvious value of aptamer for diagnostics, the incorporation of modified nucleotides into RNA transcripts resulting in stability in biofluids has considerably increased the use of aptamers as probes to inhibit protein functions (Pagratis et al., 1997). Nuclease-resistant RNA and DNA aptamers to block cell adhesion events gained importance in the last years. Wang *et al.*, selected RNA aptamers that bind to infectious human cytomegalovirus and inhibit viral infection *in vitro*, showing the feasibility of the SELEX technique for the evolution of novel compounds that protect cells against infection by pathogens such HPV (Wang et al., 2000). Furthermore, combinatorial synthesized nuclease-resistant RNA and DNA aptamers are promising candidates for use in diagnostic and therapeutic onsets.

3.5.1 Aptamers on HPV detection and therapy

Even though oligonucleotide aptamer technologies have been available for a number of years, it is only beginning to be established for HPV detection. During its life cycle, HPV expresses proteins according the cellular differentiation program that is modified after E2 disruption and the onset of malignant transformation (Pett & Coleman, 2007; Xue et al., 2010). Such features offer several protein targets for the detection of HPV infection and molecular diagnosis of cervical cancer by using aptamers as diagnostic oligonucleotides. The first aptamer directed against high-risk HPV proteins was obtained using a modified SELEX in which unspecific sequences were eliminated applying an antidote-like strategy (Toscano-Garibay et al., 2011). This RNA aptamer effectively recognized the viral protein in a purified form with affinity comparable to other aptamers that bind small proteins. In addition, the interacting mechanism was common to those observed for little targets; it folds into two hairpin structures and wraps E7 making contact with independent sites located on the CR1 and CR3 protein domains. Even though its behavior with infected cell extracts showed a cross-recognition between at least two types of HPV, this aptamer constitutes an important step towards the design of reliable and affordable detection methods.

A second set of aptamers obtained against E7 has established the effect of a single nucleotide changes on the function of aptamers over the protein activity. By changing only one nucleotide (U>C) anti-E7 aptamers prevented the formation of pRB-E7 complexes, meanwhile the replacement of two bases conducted to inactive sequences (Nicol et al., 2011). These observations suggest that following a mutation-by-mutation planning process or even using error prone PCR, some of the obtained aptamers could improve intracellular stability to impede the activity E7 proteins and eventually become a complement for therapies against cervical cancer.

4. Conclusion

Over the last few years, small oligonucleotides have been proved as feasible alternatives to HPV infection and cervical cancer therapy. The most common and successful approaches appoint to antisense technology in the form of siRNAs and AS-ODNs against different target sequences within high-risk HPV E6/E7 mRNA. Above all, siRNA technology shows a higher capacity than AS-ODNs to inhibit HPV expression. However, siRNA-induced inhibition of high-risk HPV E6/E7 is still far from practical use, limiting research to cell culture applications. Several issues regarding the transient nature of siRNA-mediated inhibition and the associated and always difficult to control off-target effects have undermined the clinical application of this otherwise powerful technology. The ability to efficiently and stably produce and deliver sufficient amounts of siRNA to the proper target tissues still requires further refinement although recent advancements in siRNA delivery (encapsulation) and the use of modified nucleotides in synthetic siRNAs may finally allow clinical testing for cervical cancer. The use of vectors-borne shRNAs appears as a more distant solution due to the multiple ethical and biological issues arising from the use of viral vectors and the still impractical non-viral approaches (i.e. liposomes, dendrosomes, quantum dots, etc.).

Even though off-targeting and delivery issues might be overcome the intracellular presence of any antisense moiety or siRNA must confront the role of innate immune responses. AS-

ODNs have been shown to induce distinct classes of innate responses that can mislead data interpretation by masking true antisense effects in the clinical setup. In particular, the presence of CpG dinucleotides along the AS-ODN sequence that activate the immune system through Toll-like receptor 9 (TLR9), resulting in cytokine release and antitumor cytotoxicity (Kandimalla et al., 2005; Sivori et al., 2004). Transfection of unmodified siRNAs and shRNAs trigger a similar response through TLR3 and TLR7 (Judge et al., 2005). In fact, a whole new class of oligonucleotides known as IM-ONs that is virtually unexplored in the HPV and cervical cancer setup as therapeutical moieties or vaccine adjuvants.

The involvement of miRNAs in cervical carcinogenesis has opened a new dimension in HPV research. Although many reports establish the alteration of a myriad of miRNAs, it is becoming clear that most of these are artifacts. A more stringent protocol should be used to establish participation of miRNAs in cervical cancer including functional assays in HPV-positive and HPV-negative cervical cells and *in situ* detection in normal and tumor cervical tissues. Nevertheless, HPV modulation of miRNA expression is firmly established. The use of aptamers in cervical cancer diagnosis and HPV detection is promising as the natural history of HPV infection offers a plethora of targets previously addressed with antibodies. As SELEX-derived oligonucleotides grow in diversity and specificity, new and cost-effective aptamer-based technologies will provide fast and reliable prevention and early screening strategies that will compete with massive vaccination programs in the future. No use of aptamers in cervical cancer therapy has been reported, but the use of AS-ODNs and aptamers currently accepted by the FDA and the advent of new RNA therapeutic targets (i.e. miRNAs), suggest that the best options for the clinical application of oligonucleotides against cervical cancer are yet to come.

5. Acknowledgement

This work was partially supported by ICYTDF grant 313/2009 to LMAS.

6. References

Agrawal, S.; Mayrand, S. H.; Zamecnik, P. C. & Pederson, T. (1990). Site-specific excision from RNA by RNase H and mixed-phosphate- backbone oligodeoxynucleotides. *Proc.Natl.Acad.Sci.U.S.A.*, Vol.87, pp. 1401-1405

Agrawal, S. & Zhang, R. (1997). Pharmacokinetics of oligonucleotides. *Ciba.Found.Symp.*, Vol.209, pp. 60-75

Agrawal, S. & Zhao, Q. (1998). Mixed backbone oligonucleotides: improvement in oligonucleotide-induced toxicity in vivo. *Antisense.Nucleic.Acid.Drug Dev.*, Vol.8, pp. 135-139

Akhtar, S. & Agrawal, S. (1997). In vivo studies with antisense oligonucleotides. *Trends.Pharmacol.Sci.*, Vol.18, pp. 12-18

Ali, M.M.; Aguirre, S. D.; Lazim, H. & Li, Y. (2011). Fluorogenic DNAzyme probes as bacterial indicators. *Angew.Chem.Int.Ed Engl.*, Vol.50, pp. 3751-3754

Alvarez-Salas, L.M. (2008). Nucleic acids as therapeutic agents. *Curr.Top.Med.Chem.*, Vol.8, pp. 1379-1404

Alvarez-Salas, L.M.; Arpawong, T. E. & DiPaolo, J. A. (1999). Growth inhibition of cervical tumor cells by antisense oligodeoxynucleotides directed to the human papillomavirus type 16 E6 gene. *Antisense.Nucleic.Acid.Drug Dev.*, Vol.9, pp. 441-450

Alvarez-Salas, L.M.; Cullinan, A. E.; Siwkowski, A.; Hampel, A. & DiPaolo, J. A. (1998). Inhibition of HPV-16 E6/E7 immortalization of normal keratinocytes by hairpin ribozymes. *Proc.Natl.Acad.Sci.U.S.A.*, Vol.95, pp. 1189-1194

Alvarez-Salas, L.M. & DiPaolo, J. A. (2007). Molecular approaches to cervical cancer therapy. *Curr.Drug Discov.Technol.*, Vol.4, pp. 208-219

Alvarez-Salas, L.M.; Wilczynski, S. P.; Burger, R. A.; Monk, B. J. & DiPaolo, J. A. (1995). Polymorphism of the HPV-16 E6 gene of cervical carcinoma. *Int.J.Oncol.*, Vol.7, pp. 261-266

Anderson, P.; Monforte, J.; Tritz, R.; Nesbitt, S.; Hearst, J. & Hampel, A. (1994). Mutagenesis of the hairpin ribozyme. *Nucleic.Acids Res.*, Vol.22, pp. 1096-1100

Aquino-Jarquin, G.; Benitez-Hess, M. L.; DiPaolo, J. A. & Alvarez-Salas, L. M. (2008). A Triplex Ribozyme Expression System Based on a Single Hairpin Ribozyme. *Oligonucleotides.*, Vol.18, pp. 213-224

Aquino-Jarquin, G.; Rojas-Hernandez, R. & Alvarez-Salas, L. M. (2010). Design and function of triplex hairpin ribozymes. *Methods Mol.Biol.*, Vol.629, pp. 323-338

Arbyn, M.; Castellsague, X.; de, S. S.; Bruni, L.; Saraiya, M.; Bray, F. & Ferlay, J. (2011). Worldwide burden of cervical cancer in 2008. *Ann.Oncol.*, Vol.doi: 10.1093/annonc/mdr015, pp.

Au Yeung, C.L.; Tsang, T. Y.; Yau, P. L. & Kwok, T. T. (2011). Human papillomavirus type 16 E6 induces cervical cancer cell migration through the p53/microRNA-23b/urokinase-type plasminogen activator pathway. *Oncogene.*, Vol.30, pp. 2401-2410

Bai, L.; Wei, L.; Wang, J.; Li, X. & He, P. (2006). Extended effects of human papillomavirus 16 E6-specific short hairpin RNA on cervical carcinoma cells. *Int.J.Gynecol.Cancer.*, Vol.16, pp. 718-729

Bartel, D.P. (2004). MicroRNAs: genomics, biogenesis, mechanism, and function. *Cell.*, Vol.116, pp. 281-297

Baum, D.A. & Silverman, S. K. (2008). Deoxyribozymes: useful DNA catalysts in vitro and in vivo. *Cell Mol.Life Sci.*, Vol.65, pp. 2156-2174

Benitez-Hess, M.L. & Alvarez-Salas, L. M. (2006). Utilization of ribozymes as antiviral agents. *Letters Drug Design & Discovery.*, Vol.3, pp. 390-404

Benitez-Hess, M.L.; Reyes-Gutierrez, P. & Alvarez-Salas, L. M. (2011). Inhibition of Human Papillomavirus Expression Using DNAzymes. *Methods Mol.Biol.*, Vol.764:317-35., pp. 317-335

Berezikov, E.; Chung, W. J.; Willis, J.; Cuppen, E. & Lai, E. C. (2007). Mammalian mirtron genes. *Mol.Cell.*, Vol.28, pp. 328-336

Berezutskaya, E.; Yu, B.; Morozov, A.; Raychaudhuri, P. & Bagchi, S. (1997). Differential regulation of the pocket domains of the retinoblastoma family proteins by the HPV16 E7 oncoprotein. *Cell Growth Differ.*, Vol.8, pp. 1277-1286

Bernstein, E.; Caudy, A. A.; Hammond, S. M. & Hannon, G. J. (2001). Role for a bidentate ribonuclease in the initiation step of RNA interference. *Nature.*, Vol.409, pp. 363-366

Bonham, M.A.; Brown, S.; Boyd, A. L.; Brown, P. H.; Bruckenstein, D. A.; Hanvey, J. C.; Thomson, S. A.; Pipe, A.; Hassman, F. & Bisi, J. E. (1995). An assessment of the antisense properties of RNase H-competent and steric-blocking oligomers. *Nucleic.Acids Res.*, Vol.23, pp. 1197-1203

Bousarghin, L.; Hubert, P.; Franzen, E.; Jacobs, N.; Boniver, J. & Delvenne, P. (2005). Human papillomavirus 16 virus-like particles use heparan sulfates to bind dendritic cells and colocalize with langerin in Langerhans cells. *J.Gen.Virol.*, Vol.86, pp. 1297-1305

Bousarghin, L.; Touze, A.; Gaud, G.; Iochmann, S.; Alvarez, E.; Reverdiau, P.; Gaitan, J.; Jourdan, M. L.; Sizaret, P. Y. & Coursaget, P. L. (2009). Inhibition of cervical cancer cell growth by human papillomavirus virus-like particles packaged with human papillomavirus oncoprotein short hairpin RNAs. *Mol.Cancer Ther.*, Vol.8, pp. 357-365

Boyer, S.N.; Wazer, D. E. & Band, V. (1996). E7 protein of human papilloma virus-16 induces degradation of retinoblastoma protein through the ubiquitin-proteasome pathway. *Cancer Res.*, Vol.56, pp. 4620-4624

Butz, K.; Denk, C.; Ullmann, A.; Scheffner, M. & Hoppe-Seyler, F. (2000). Induction of apoptosis in human papillomaviruspositive cancer cells by peptide aptamers targeting the viral E6 oncoprotein. *Proc.Natl.Acad.Sci.U.S.A.*, Vol.97, pp. 6693-6697

Butz, K.; Ristriani, T.; Hengstermann, A.; Denk, C.; Scheffner, M. & Hoppe-Seyler, F. (2003). siRNA targeting of the viral E6 oncogene efficiently kills human papillomavirus-positive cancer cells. *Oncogene.*, Vol.22, pp. 5938-5945

Cai, X.; Li, G.; Laimins, L. A. & Cullen, B. R. (2006). Human papillomavirus genotype 31 does not express detectable microRNA levels during latent or productive virus replication. *J.Virol.*, Vol.80, pp. 10890-10893

Cairns, M.J.; King, A. & Sun, L. Q. (2003). Optimisation of the 10-23 DNAzyme-substrate pairing interactions enhanced RNA cleavage activity at purine-cytosine target sites. *Nucleic.Acids.Res.*, Vol.31, pp. 2883-2889

Carbone, G.M.; McGuffie, E. M.; Collier, A. & Catapano, C. V. (2003). Selective inhibition of transcription of the Ets2 gene in prostate cancer cells by a triplex-forming oligonucleotide. *Nucleic.Acids.Res.*, Vol.31, pp. 833-843

Cerchia, L.; Hamm, J.; Libri, D.; Tavitian, B. & de, F., V (2002). Nucleic acid aptamers in cancer medicine. *FEBS Lett.*, Vol.528, pp. 12-16

Chang, J.T.; Kuo, T. F.; Chen, Y. J.; Chiu, C. C.; Lu, Y. C.; Li, H. F.; Shen, C. R. & Cheng, A. J. (2010). Highly potent and specific siRNAs against E6 or E7 genes of HPV16- or HPV18-infected cervical cancers. *Cancer Gene Ther.*, Vol.17, pp. 827-836

Chen, Z.; Kamath, P.; Zhang, S.; St.John, L.; Adler-Storthz, K. & Shillitoe, E. J. (1996). Effects on tumor cells of ribozymes that cleave the RNA transcripts of human papillomavirus type 18. *Cancer Gene Ther.*, Vol.3, pp. 18-23

Chen, Z.; Kamath, P.; Zhang, S.; Weil, M. M. & Shillitoe, E. J. (1995). Effectiveness of three ribozymes for cleavage of an RNA transcript from human papillomavirus type 18. *Cancer Gene Ther.*, Vol.2, pp. 263-271

Cherny, D.I.; Malkov, V. A.; Volodin, A. A. & Frank-Kamenetskii, M. D. (1993). Electron microscopy visualization of oligonucleotide binding to duplex DNA via triplex formation. *J.Mol.Biol.*, Vol.230, pp. 379-383

Cho, C.W.; Poo, H.; Cho, Y. S.; Cho, M. C.; Lee, K. A.; Lee, S. J.; Park, S. N.; Kim, I. K.; Jung, Y. K.; Choe, Y. K.; Yeom, Y. I.; Choe, I. S. & Yoon, d. Y. (2002). HPV E6 antisense induces apoptosis in CaSki cells via suppression of E6 splicing. *Exp.Mol.Med.*, Vol.34, pp. 159-166

Choo, C.K.; Ling, M. T.; Suen, C. K.; Chan, K. W. & Kwong, Y. L. (2000). Retrovirus-mediated delivery of HPV16 E7 antisense RNA inhibited tumorigenicity of CaSki cells. *Gynecol.Oncol.*, Vol.78, pp. 293-301

Clifford, G.M.; Smith, J. S.; Plummer, M.; Munoz, N. & Franceschi, S. (2003). Human papillomavirus types in invasive cervical cancer worldwide: a meta-analysis. *Br.J.Cancer.*, Vol.88, pp. 63-73

Crooke, S.T. (1999). Molecular mechanisms of action of antisense drugs. *Biochim.Biophys.Acta.*, Vol.1489, pp. 31-44

Cullen, B.R. (2004). Transcription and processing of human microRNA precursors. *Mol.Cell.*, Vol.16, pp. 861-865

Cullen, B.R. (2006). Induction of stable RNA interference in mammalian cells. *Gene Ther.*, Vol.13, pp. 503-508

Dass, C.R.; Choong, P. F. & Khachigian, L. M. (2008). DNAzyme technology and cancer therapy: cleave and let die. *Mol.Cancer Ther.*, Vol.7, pp. 243-251

Du, L. & Gatti, R. A. (2009). Progress toward therapy with antisense-mediated splicing modulation. *Curr.Opin.Mol.Ther.*, Vol.11, pp. 116-123

Duensing, S.; Duensing, A.; Flores, E. R.; Do, A.; Lambert, P. F. & Munger, K. (2001). Centrosome abnormalities and genomic instability by episomal expression of human papillomavirus type 16 in raft cultures of human keratinocytes. *J.Virol.*, Vol.75, pp. 7712-7716

Duensing, S.; Lee, L. Y.; Duensing, A.; Basile, J.; Piboonniyom, S.; Gonzalez, S.; Crum, C. P. & Munger, K. (2000). The human papillomavirus type 16 E6 and E7 oncoproteins cooperate to induce mitotic defects and genomic instability by uncoupling centrosome duplication from the cell division cycle. *Proc.Natl.Acad.Sci.U.S.A.*, Vol.97, pp. 10002-10007

Dutta, T.; Burgess, M.; McMillan, N. A. & Parekh, H. S. (2010). Dendrosome-based delivery of siRNA against E6 and E7 oncogenes in cervical cancer. *Nanomedicine.*, Vol.6, pp. 463-470

Eaton, S.; Wiktor, P.; Thirstrup, D.; Lake, D. & Nagaraj, V. J. (2011). Efficacy of TRAIL treatment against HPV16 infected cervical cancer cells undergoing senescence following siRNA knockdown of E6/E7 genes. *Biochem.Biophys.Res.Commun.*, Vol.405, pp. 1-6

Elbashir, S.M.; Harborth, J.; Lendeckel, W.; Yalcin, A.; Weber, K. & Tuschl, T. (2001). Duplexes of 21-nucleotide RNAs mediate RNA interference in cultured mammalian cells. *Nature.*, Vol.411, pp. 494-498

Ellington, A.D. & Szostak, J. W. (1990). In vitro selection of RNA molecules that bind specific ligands. *Nature.*, Vol.346, pp. 818-822

Epstein, L.M. & Gall, J. G. (1987). Transcripts of newt satellite DNA self-cleave in vitro. *Cold Spring Harb.Symp.Quant.Biol.*, Vol.52:261-5., pp. 261-265

Etscheid, B.G.; Foster, S. A. & Galloway, D. A. (1994). The E6 protein of human papillomavirus type 16 functions as a transcriptional repressor in a mechanism independent of the tumor suppressor protein, p53. *Virology*, Vol.205, pp. 583-585

Faulhammer, D. & Famulok, M. (1997). Characterization and divalent metal-ion dependence of in vitro selected deoxyribozymes which cleave DNA/RNA chimeric oligonucleotides. *J.Mol.Biol.*, Vol.269, pp. 188-202

Filippova, M.; Song, H.; Connolly, J. L.; Dermody, T. S. & Duerksen-Hughes, P. J. (2002). The human papillomavirus 16 E6 protein binds to tumor necrosis factor (TNF) R1 and protects cells from TNF-induced apoptosis. *J.Biol.Chem.*, Vol.277, pp. 21730-21739

Fire, A.; Xu, S.; Montgomery, M. K.; Kostas, S. A.; Driver, S. E. & Mello, C. C. (1998). Potent and specific genetic interference by double-stranded RNA in Caenorhabditis elegans. *Nature.*, Vol.391, pp. 806-811

Fujii, T.; Saito, M.; Iwasaki, E.; Ochiya, T.; Takei, Y.; Hayashi, S.; Ono, A.; Hirao, N.; Nakamura, M.; Kubushiro, K.; Tsukazaki, K. & Aoki, D. (2006). Intratumor injection of small interfering RNA-targeting human papillomavirus 18 E6 and E7 successfully inhibits the growth of cervical cancer. *Int.J.Oncol.*, Vol.29, pp. 541 548

Funk, J.O.; Waga, S.; Harry, J. B.; Espling, E.; Stillman, B. & Galloway, D. A. (1997). Inhibition of CDK activity and PCNA-dependent DNA replication by p21 is blocked by interaction with the HPV-16 E7 oncoprotein. *Genes Dev.*, Vol.11, pp. 2090-2100

Gardiol, D.; Kuhne, C.; Glaunsinger, B.; Lee, S. S.; Javier, R. & Banks, L. (1999). Oncogenic human papillomavirus E6 proteins target the discs large tumour suppressor for proteasome-mediated degradation. *Oncogene,* Vol.18, pp. 5487-5496

Gewin, L.; Myers, H.; Kiyono, T. & Galloway, D. A. (2004). Identification of a novel telomerase repressor that interacts with the human papillomavirus type-16 E6/E6-AP complex. *Genes Dev.*, Vol.18, pp. 2269-2282

Glaunsinger, B.A.; Lee, S. S.; Thomas, M.; Banks, L. & Javier, R. (2000). Interactions of the PDZ-protein MAGI-1 with adenovirus E4-ORF1 and high-risk papillomavirus E6 oncoproteins. *Oncogene,* Vol.19, pp. 5270-5280

Greco, D.; Kivi, N.; Qian, K.; Leivonen, S. K.; Auvinen, P. & Auvinen, E. (2011). Human Papillomavirus 16 E5 Modulates the Expression of Host MicroRNAs. *PLoS.ONE.*, Vol.6, pp. e21646-

Gregory, R.I. & Shiekhattar, R. (2005). MicroRNA biogenesis and cancer. *Cancer Res.*, Vol.65, pp. 3509-3512

Gu, W.; Payne, E.; Sun, S.; Burgess, M. & McMillan, N. A. (2011). Inhibition of cervical cancer cell growth in vitro and in vivo with dual shRNAs. *Cancer Gene Ther.*, Vol.18, pp. 219-227

Guerrier-Takada, C.; Gardiner, K.; Marsh, T.; Pace, N. & Altman, S. (1983). The RNA moiety of ribonuclease P is the catalytic subunit of the enzyme. *Cell,* Vol.35, pp. 849-857

Hall, A.H. & Alexander, K. A. (2003). RNA Interference of Human Papillomavirus Type 18 E6 and E7 Induces Senescence in HeLa Cells. *J.Virol.*, Vol.77, pp. 6066-6069

Hammond, S.M.; Caudy, A. A. & Hannon, G. J. (2001). Post-transcriptional gene silencing by double-stranded RNA. *Nat.Rev.Genet.*, Vol.2, pp. 110-119

Hampel, A.; Tritz, R.; Hicks, M. & Cruz, P. (1990). 'Hairpin' catalytic RNA model: evidence for helices and sequence requirement for substrate RNA. *Nucleic.Acids Res.*, Vol.18, pp. 299-304

Hartman, D.A.; Kuo, S. R.; Broker, T. R.; Chow, L. T. & Wells, R. D. (1992). Intermolecular triplex formation distorts the DNA duplex in the regulatory region of human papillomavirus type 11. *J.Biol.Chem.*, Vol.267, pp. 5488-5494

Haseloff, J. & Gerlach, W. L. (1988). Simple RNA enzymes with new and highly specific endoribonuclease activities. *Nature.*, Vol.334, pp. 585-591

Haseloff, J. & Gerlach, W. L. (1989). Sequences required for self-catalysed cleavage of the satellite RNA of tobacco ringspot virus. *Gene.*, Vol.82, pp. 43-52

Hayashi, S.; Nagasaka, T.; Katayama, A.; Saito, I.; Hamada, H.; Kobayashi, T.; Yokoyama, I.; Ohtsuka, S.; Uchida, K. & Takagi, H. (1997). Adenovirus-mediated gene transfer of antisense ribozyme for alpha (1,3)galactosyltransferase gene and alpha (1, 2)fucosyltransferase gene in xenotransplantation. *Transplant.Proc.,* Vol.29, pp. 2213-2213

He, Y.K.; Lu, C. D. & Qi, G. R. (1993). In vitro cleavage of HPV16 E6 and E7 RNA fragments by synthetic ribozymes and transcribed ribozymes from RNA-trimming plasmids. *FEBS Lett.,* Vol.322, pp. 21-24

Hebner, C.M. & Laimins, L. A. (2006). Human papillomaviruses: basic mechanisms of pathogenesis and oncogenicity. *Rev.Med.Virol.,* Vol.16, pp. 83-97

Howie, H.L.; Katzenellenbogen, R. A. & Galloway, D. A. (2009). Papillomavirus E6 proteins. *Virology.,* Vol.384, pp. 324-334

Huh, K.W.; DeMasi, J.; Ogawa, H.; Nakatani, Y.; Howley, P. M. & Munger, K. (2005). Association of the human papillomavirus type 16 E7 oncoprotein with the 600-kDa retinoblastoma protein-associated factor, p600. *Proc.Natl.Acad.Sci.U.S.A.,* Vol.102, pp. 11492-11497

Huibregtse, J.M.; Scheffner, M. & Howley, P. M. (1991). A cellular protein mediates association of p53 with the E6 oncoprotein of human papillomavirus types 16 or 18. *EMBO J.,* Vol.10, pp. 4129-4135

Hutchins, C.J.; Rathjen, P. D.; Forster, A. C. & Symons, R. H. (1986). Self-cleavage of plus and minus RNA transcripts of avocado sunblotch viroid. *Nucleic.Acids Res.,* Vol.14, pp. 3627-3640

Hwang, S.G.; Lee, D.; Kim, J.; Seo, T. & Choe, J. (2002). Human papillomavirus type 16 E7 binds to E2F1 and activates E2F1-driven transcription in a retinoblastoma protein-independent manner. *J.Biol.Chem.,* Vol.277, pp. 2923-2930

Jackson, A.L.; Bartz, S. R.; Schelter, J.; Kobayashi, S. V.; Burchard, J.; Mao, M.; Li, B.; Cavet, G. & Linsley, P. S. (2003). Expression profiling reveals off-target gene regulation by RNAi. *Nat.Biotechnol.,* Vol.21, pp. 635-637

Jackson, A.L.; Burchard, J.; Leake, D.; Reynolds, A.; Schelter, J.; Guo, J.; Johnson, J. M.; Lim, L.; Karpilow, J.; Nichols, K.; Marshall, W.; Khvorova, A. & Linsley, P. S. (2006). Position-specific chemical modification of siRNAs reduces "off-target" transcript silencing. *RNA.,* Vol.12, pp. 1197-1205

Jiang, M. & Milner, J. (2002). Selective silencing of viral gene expression in HPV-positive human cervical carcinoma cells treated with siRNA, a primer of RNA interference. *Oncogene,* Vol.21, pp. 6041-6048

Jones, D.L.; Alani, R. M. & Munger, K. (1997). The human papillomavirus E7 oncoprotein can uncouple cellular differentiation and proliferation in human keratinocytes by abrogating p21Cip1-mediated inhibition of cdk2. *Genes Dev.,* Vol.11, pp. 2101-2111

Jonson, A.L.; Rogers, L. M.; Ramakrishnan, S. & Downs, L. S., Jr. (2008). Gene silencing with siRNA targeting E6/E7 as a therapeutic intervention in a mouse model of cervical cancer. *Gynecol.Oncol.,* Vol.111, pp. 356-364

Judge, A.D.; Sood, V.; Shaw, J. R.; Fang, D.; McClintock, K. & MacLachlan, I. (2005). Sequence-dependent stimulation of the mammalian innate immune response by synthetic siRNA. *Nat.Biotechnol.,* Vol.23, pp. 457-462

Kalali, B.N.; Kollisch, G.; Mages, J.; Muller, T.; Bauer, S.; Wagner, H.; Ring, J.; Lang, R.; Mempel, M. & Ollert, M. (2008). Double-stranded RNA induces an antiviral defense status in epidermal keratinocytes through TLR3-, PKR-, and MDA5/RIG-I-mediated differential signaling. *J.Immunol.*, Vol.181, pp. 2694-2704

Kandimalla, E.R.; Bhagat, L.; Li, Y.; Yu, D.; Wang, D.; Cong, Y. P.; Song, S. S.; Tang, J. X.; Sullivan, T. & Agrawal, S. (2005). Immunomodulatory oligonucleotides containing a cytosine-phosphate-2'-deoxy-7-deazaguanosine motif as potent toll-like receptor 9 agonists. *Proc.Natl.Acad.Sci.U.S.A.*, Vol.102, pp. 6925-6930

Kari, I.; Syrjanen, S.; Johansson, B.; Peri, P.; He, B.; Roizman, B. & Hukkanen, V. (2007). Antisense RNA directed to the human papillomavirus type 16 E7 mRNA from herpes simplex virus type 1 derived vectors is expressed in CaSki cells and downregulates E7 mRNA. *Virol.J.*, Vol.4, pp. 47-58

Kim, Y.K. & Kim, V. N. (2007). Processing of intronic microRNAs. *EMBO J.*, Vol.26, pp. 775-783

Klingelhutz, A.J.; Foster, S. A. & McDougall, J. K. (1996). Telomerase activation by the E6 gene product of human papillomavirus type 16. *Nature.*, Vol.380, pp. 79-82

Koivusalo, R.; Krausz, E.; Helenius, H. & Hietanen, S. (2005). Chemotherapy compounds in cervical cancer cells primed by reconstitution of p53 function after short interfering RNA-mediated degradation of human papillomavirus 18 E6 mRNA: opposite effect of siRNA in combination with different drugs. *Mol.Pharmacol.*, Vol.68, pp. 372-382

Koivusalo, R.; Mialon, A.; Pitkanen, H.; Westermarck, J. & Hietanen, S. (2006). Activation of p53 in cervical cancer cells by human papillomavirus E6 RNA interference is transient, but can be sustained by inhibiting endogenous nuclear export-dependent p53 antagonists. *Cancer Res.*, Vol.66, pp. 11817-11824

Kronenwett, R. & Sczakiel, G. (1997). Selection of fast-hybridizing complementary RNA species in vitro. *Methods Mol.Biol.*, Vol.74, pp. 281-288

Kruger, K.; Grabowski, P. J.; Zaug, A. J.; Sands, J.; Gottschling, D. E. & Cech, T. R. (1982). Self-splicing RNA: autoexcision and autocyclization of the ribosomal RNA intervining sequence of *Tetrahymena*. *Cell*, Vol.31, pp. 147-157

Lea, J.S.; Sunaga, N.; Sato, M.; Kalahasti, G.; Miller, D. S.; Minna, J. D. & Muller, C. Y. (2007). Silencing of HPV 18 oncoproteins With RNA interference causes growth inhibition of cervical cancer cells. *Reprod.Sci.*, Vol.14, pp. 20-28

Lee, S.S.; Glaunsinger, B.; Mantovani, F.; Banks, L. & Javier, R. T. (2000). Multi-PDZ domain protein MUPP1 is a cellular target for both adenovirus E4-ORF1 and high-risk papillomavirus type 18 E6 oncoproteins. *J.Virol.*, Vol.74, pp. 9680-9693

Lee, Y.; Kim, M.; Han, J.; Yeom, K. H.; Lee, S.; Baek, S. H. & Kim, V. N. (2004). MicroRNA genes are transcribed by RNA polymerase II. *EMBO J.*, Vol.23, pp. 4051-4060

Letai, A.G.; Palladino, M. A.; Fromm, E.; Rizzo, V. & Fresco, J. R. (1988). Specificity in formation of triple-stranded nucleic acid helical complexes: studies with agarose-linked polyribonucleotide affinity columns. *Biochemistry.*, Vol.27, pp. 9108-9112

Li, B.; Hu, Y.; Ye, F.; Li, Y.; Lv, W. & Xie, X. (2010). Reduced miR-34a expression in normal cervical tissues and cervical lesions with high-risk human papillomavirus infection. *Int.J.Gynecol.Cancer.*, Vol.20, pp. 597-604

Lin, X.; Ruan, X.; Anderson, M. G.; McDowell, J. A.; Kroeger, P. E.; Fesik, S. W. & Shen, Y. (2005). siRNA-mediated off-target gene silencing triggered by a 7 nt complementation. *Nucleic.Acids.Res.*, Vol.33, pp. 4527-4535

Liu, W.L.; Green, N.; Seymour, L. W. & Stevenson, M. (2009). Paclitaxel combined with siRNA targeting HPV16 oncogenes improves cytotoxicity for cervical carcinoma. *Cancer Gene Ther.*, Vol.16, pp. 764-775

Lopez, J.A. & Alvarez-Salas, L. M. (2011). Differential effects of miR-34c-3p and miR-34c-5p on SiHa cells proliferation apoptosis, migration and invasion. *Biochem.Biophys.Res.Commun.*, Vol.409, pp. 513-519

Lorenz, C.; Hadwiger, P.; John, M.; Vornlocher, H. P. & Unverzagt, C. (2004). Steroid and lipid conjugates of siRNAs to enhance cellular uptake and gene silencing in liver cells. *Bioorg.Med.Chem.Lett.*, Vol.14, pp. 4975-4977

Lu, D.; Chatterjee, S.; Brar, D. & Wong, K. K., Jr. (1994). Ribozyme-mediated in vitro cleavage of transcripts arising from the major transforming genes of human papillomavirus type 16. *Cancer Gene Ther.*, Vol.1, pp. 267-277

Lui, W.O.; Pourmand, N.; Patterson, B. K. & Fire, A. (2007). Patterns of known and novel small RNAs in human cervical cancer. *Cancer Res.*, Vol.67, pp. 6031-6043

Malkov, V.A.; Voloshin, O. N.; Soyfer, V. N. & Frank-Kamenetskii, M. D. (1993). Cation and sequence effects on stability of intermolecular pyrimidine-purine-purine triplex. *Nucleic.Acids.Res.*, Vol.21, pp. 585-591

Marquez-Gutierrez, M.A.; Benitez-Hess, M. L.; DiPaolo, J. A. & Alvarez-Salas, L. M. (2007). Effect of combined antisense oligodeoxynucleotides directed against the human papillomavirus type 16 on cervical carcinoma cells. *Arch.Med.Res.*, Vol.38, pp. 730-738

McLaughlin-Drubin, M.E.; Crum, C. P. & Munger, K. (2011). Human papillomavirus E7 oncoprotein induces KDM6A and KDM6B histone demethylase expression and causes epigenetic reprogramming. *Proc.Natl.Acad.Sci.U.S.A.*, Vol.108, pp. 2130-2135

McLaughlin-Drubin, M.E.; Huh, K. W. & Munger, K. (2008). Human papillomavirus type 16 E7 oncoprotein associates with E2F6. *J.Virol.*, Vol.82, pp. 8695-8705

McLaughlin-Drubin, M.E. & Munger, K. (2009). The human papillomavirus E7 oncoprotein. *Virology.*, Vol.384, pp. 335-344

Meister, G.; Landthaler, M.; Dorsett, Y. & Tuschl, T. (2004). Sequence-specific inhibition of microRNA- and siRNA-induced RNA silencing. *RNA.*, Vol.10, pp. 544-550

Melar-New, M. & Laimins, L. A. (2010). Human papillomaviruses modulate expression of microRNA 203 upon epithelial differentiation to control levels of p63 proteins. *J.Virol.*, Vol.84, pp. 5212-5221

Mercatante, D. & Kole, R. (2000). Modification of alternative splicing pathways as a potential approach to chemotherapy. *Pharmacol.Ther.*, Vol.85, pp. 237-243

Michienzi, A. & Rossi, J. J. (2001). Intracellular applications of ribozymes. *Methods Enzymol.*, Vol.341, pp. 581-596

Min, W.; Wen-Li, M.; Zhao-Hui, S.; Ling, L.; Bao, Z. & Wen-Ling, Z. (2009). Microarray analysis identifies differentially expressed genes induced by human papillomavirus type 18 E6 silencing RNA. *Int.J.Gynecol.Cancer.*, Vol.19, pp. 547-563

Miyagishi, M.; Hayashi, M. & Taira, K. (2003). Comparison of the suppressive effects of antisense oligonucleotides and siRNAs directed against the same targets in mammalian cells. *Antisense.Nucleic.Acid.Drug Dev.*, Vol.13, pp. 1-7

Moody, C.A. & Laimins, L. A. (2010). Human papillomavirus oncoproteins: pathways to transformation. *Nat.Rev.Cancer.*, Vol.10, pp. 550-560

Morrissey, D.V.; Lee, P. A.; Johnson, D. A.; Overly, S. L.; McSwiggen, J. A.; Beigelman, L.; Mokler, V. R.; Maloney, L.; Vargeese, C.; Bowman, K.; O'Brien, J. T.; Shaffer, C. S.; Conrad, A.; Schmid, P.; Morrey, J. D.; Macejak, D. G.; Pavco, P. A. & Blatt, L. M. (2002). Characterization of nuclease-resistant ribozymes directed against hepatitis B virus RNA. *J.Viral.Hepat.*, Vol.9, pp. 411-418

Moser, H.E. & Dervan, P. B. (1987). Sequence-specific cleavage of double helical DNA by triple helix formation. *Science,* Vol.238, pp. 645-650

Munger, K. & Phelps, W. C. (1993). The human papillomavirus E7 protein as a transforming and transactivating factor. *Biochim.Biophys.Acta.,* Vol.1155, pp. 111-123

Nicol, C.; Bunka, D. H.; Blair, G. E. & Stonehouse, N. J. (2011). Effects of single nucleotide changes on the binding and activity of RNA aptamers to human papillomavirus 16 E7 oncoprotein. *Biochem.Biophys.Res.Commun.,* Vol.405, pp. 417-421

Nykanen, A.; Haley, B. & Zamore, P. D. (2001). ATP requirements and small interfering RNA structure in the RNA interference pathway. *Cell,* Vol.107, pp. 309-321

Oh, S.T.; Kyo, S. & Laimins, L. A. (2001). Telomerase activation by human papillomavirus type 16 E6 protein: induction of human telomerase reverse transcriptase expression through Myc and GC-rich Sp1 binding sites. *J.Virol.,* Vol.75, pp. 5559-5566

Pagratis, N.C.; Bell, C.; Chang, Y. F.; Jennings, S.; Fitzwater, T.; Jellinek, D. & Dang, C. (1997). Potent 2'-amino-, and 2'-fluoro-2'-deoxyribonucleotide RNA inhibitors of keratinocyte growth factor. *Nat.Biotechnol.,* Vol.15, pp. 68-73

Patil, S.D.; Rhodes, D. G. & Burgess, D. J. (2005). DNA-based therapeutics and DNA delivery systems: a comprehensive review. *AAPS.J.,* Vol.7, pp. E61-E77

Pereira, P.M.; Marques, J. P.; Soares, A. R.; Carreto, L. & Santos, M. A. (2010). MicroRNA Expression Variability in Human Cervical Tissues. *PLoS.ONE.,* Vol.5, pp. e11780-

Pett, M. & Coleman, N. (2007). Integration of high-risk human papillomavirus: a key event in cervical carcinogenesis? *J.Pathol.,* Vol.212, pp. 356-367

Pirisi, L.; Creek, K. E.; Doniger, J. & DiPaolo, J. A. (1988). Continuous cell lines with altered growth and differentiation properties originate after transfection of human keratinocytes with human papillomavirus type 16 DNA. *Carcinogenesis.,* Vol.9, pp. 1573-1579

Popa, L.M.; Schutz, H.; Winter, S.; Kittler, L. & Lober, G. (1996). Specific targeting of human papillomavirus type 16 E7 oncogene with triple-helix forming purine oligodeoxyribonucleotides. *Biochem.Mol.Biol.Int.,* Vol.38, pp. 285-295

Prody, G.A.; Bakos, J. T.; Buzayan, J. M.; Schneider, I. R. & Bruening, G. (1986). Autolytic processing of dimeric plant virus satellite RNA. *Science,* Vol.321, pp. 1577-1580

Qi, Z.; Xu, X.; Zhang, B.; Li, Y.; Liu, J.; Chen, S.; Chen, G. & Huo, X. (2010). Effect of simultaneous silencing of HPV-18 E6 and E7 on inducing apoptosis in HeLa cells. *Biochem.Cell Biol.,* Vol.88, pp. 697-704

Reyes-Gutierrez, P. & Alvarez-Salas, L. M. (2009). Cleavage of HPV-16 E6/E7 mRNA mediated by modified 10-23 deoxyribozymes. *Oligonucleotides.,* Vol.19, pp. 233-242

Santoro, S.W. & Joyce, G. F. (1997). A general purpose RNA-cleaving DNA enzyme. *Proc.Natl.Acad.Sci.U.S.A.,* Vol.94, pp. 4262-4266

Santoro, S.W. & Joyce, G. F. (1998). Mechanism and utility of an RNA-cleaving DNA enzyme. *Biochemistry.,* Vol.37, pp. 13330-13342

Scheffner, M.; Huibregtse, J. M.; Vierstra, R. D. & Howley, P. M. (1993). The HPV-16 E6 and E6-AP complex functions as a ubiquitin-protein ligase in the ubiquitination of p53. *Cell.,* Vol.75, pp. 495-505

Schneider-Gadicke, A. & Schwarz, E. (1986). Different human cervical carcinoma cell lines show similar transcription patterns of human papillomavirus type 18 early genes. *EMBO J.,* Vol.5, pp. 2285-2292

Sharp, P.A. (1999). RNAi and double-strand RNA. *Genes Dev.,* Vol.13, pp. 139-141

Shillitoe, E.J. (2006). Papillomaviruses as targets for cancer gene therapy. *Cancer Gene Ther.,* Vol.13, pp. 445-450

Shim, M.S. & Kwon, Y. J. (2010). Efficient and targeted delivery of siRNA in vivo. *FEBS J.,* Vol.277, pp. 4814-4827

Sierakowska, H.; Agrawal, S. & Kole, R. (2000). Antisense oligonucleotides as modulators of pre-mRNA splicing. *Methods Mol.Biol.,* Vol.133, pp. 223-233

Sima, N.; Wang, W.; Kong, D.; Deng, D.; Xu, Q.; Zhou, J.; Xu, G.; Meng, L.; Lu, Y.; Wang, S. & Ma, D. (2008). RNA interference against HPV16 E7 oncogene leads to viral E6 and E7 suppression in cervical cancer cells and apoptosis via upregulation of Rb and p53. *Apoptosis.,* Vol.13, pp. 273-281

Sivori, S.; Falco, M.; Della, C. M.; Carlomagno, S.; Vitale, M.; Moretta, L. & Moretta, A. (2004). CpG and double-stranded RNA trigger human NK cells by Toll-like receptors: induction of cytokine release and cytotoxicity against tumors and dendritic cells. *Proc.Natl.Acad.Sci.U.S.A.,* Vol.101, pp. 10116-10121

Smotkin, D.; Prokoph, H. & Wettstein, F. O. (1989). Oncogenic and nononcogenic human genital papillomaviruses generate the E7 mRNA by different mechanisms. *J.Virol.,* Vol.63, pp. 1441-1447

Sorensen, D.R.; Leirdal, M. & Sioud, M. (2003). Gene silencing by systemic delivery of synthetic siRNAs in adult mice. *J.Mol.Biol.,* Vol.327, pp. 761-766

Stanley, M. (2010). Pathology and epidemiology of HPV infection in females. *Gynecol.Oncol.,* Vol.117, pp. S5-S10

Steele, C.; Cowsert, L. M. & Shillitoe, E. J. (1993). Effects of human papillomavirus type 18-specific antisense oligonucleotides on the transformed phenotype of human carcinoma cell lines. *Cancer Res.,* Vol.53, pp. 2330-2337

Sternberger, M.; Schmiedeknecht, A.; Kretschmer, A.; Gebhardt, F.; Leenders, F.; Czauderna, F.; von, C., I; Engle, M.; Giese, K.; Beigelman, L. & Klippel, A. (2002). GeneBlocs are powerful tools to study and delineate signal transduction processes that regulate cell growth and transformation. *Antisense.Nucleic.Acid.Drug Dev.,* Vol.12, pp. 131-143

Stojanovic, M.N.; Semova, S.; Kolpashchikov, D.; Macdonald, J.; Morgan, C. & Stefanovic, D. (2005). Deoxyribozyme-based ligase logic gates and their initial circuits. *J.Am.Chem.Soc.,* Vol.127, pp. 6914-6915

Takamori, K.; Kubo, T.; Zhelev, Z.; Rumiana, B.; Ohba, H.; Doi, K. & Fujii, M. (2005). Suppression of bcr/abl chimeric gene by conjugate DNA enzymes in human cells. *Nucleic.Acids.Symp.Ser.(Oxf.).,* Vol.333-334

Tan, T.M. & Ting, R. C. (1995). In vitro and in vivo inhibition of human papillomavirus type 16 E6 and E7 genes. *Cancer Res.,* Vol.55, pp. 4599-4605

Tang, S.; Tao, M.; McCoy, J. P. J. & Zheng, Z. M. (2006). Short-term induction and long-term suppression of HPV16 oncogene silencing by RNA interference in cervical cancer cells. *Oncogene.,* Vol.25, pp. 2094-2104

Toscano-Garibay, J.D.; Benitez-Hess, M. L. & Alvarez-Salas, L. M. (2011). Isolation and characterization of an RNA aptamer for the HPV-16 E7 oncoprotein. *Arch.Med.Res.,* Vol.42, pp. 88-96

Tuerk, C. & Gold, L. (1990). Systematic evolution of ligands by exponential enrichment: RNA ligands to bacteriophage T4 DNA polymerase. *Science,* Vol.249, pp. 505-510

Tungteakkhun, S.S.; Filippova, M.; Fodor, N. & Duerksen-Hughes, P. J. (2010). The full-length isoform of human papillomavirus 16 E6 and its splice variant E6* bind to different sites on the procaspase 8 death effector domain. *J.Virol.*, Vol.84, pp. 1453-1463

Uhlenbeck, O.C. (1987). A small catalytic oligoribonucleotide. *Nature.*, Vol.328, pp. 596-600

Ui-Tei, K.; Naito, Y.; Zenno, S.; Nishi, K.; Yamato, K.; Takahashi, F.; Juni, A. & Saigo, K. (2008). Functional dissection of siRNA sequence by systematic DNA substitution: modified siRNA with a DNA seed arm is a powerful tool for mammalian gene silencing with significantly reduced off-target effect. *Nucleic Acids Res.*, Vol.36, pp. 2136-2151

Vaish, N.K.; Kore, A. R. & Eckstein, F. (1998). Recent developments in the hammerhead ribozyme field. *Nucleic.Acids Res.*, Vol.26, pp. 5237-5242

Valencia-Sanchez, M.A.; Liu, J.; Hannon, G. J. & Parker, R. (2006). Control of translation and mRNA degradation by miRNAs and siRNAs. *Genes Dev.*, Vol.20, pp. 515-524

Vasquez, K.M. & Glazer, P. M. (2002). Triplex-forming oligonucleotides: principles and applications. *Q.Rev.Biophys.*, Vol.35, pp. 89-107

Venturini, F.; Braspenning, J.; Homann, M.; Gissmann, L. & Sczakiel, G. (1999). Kinetic selection of HPV 16 E6/E7-directed antisense nucleic acids: anti-proliferative effects on HPV 16-transformed cells. *Nucleic Acids Res.*, Vol.27, pp. 1585-1592

Vernon, S.D.; Unger, E. R.; Miller, D. L.; Lee, D. R. & Reeves, W. C. (1997). Association of human papillomavirus type 16 integration in the E2 gene with poor disease-free survival from cervical cancer. *Int.J.Cancer,* Vol.74, pp. 50-56

von Knebel Doeberitz, M. & Gissmann, L. (1987). Analysis of the biological role of human papilloma virus (HPV)- encoded transcripts in cervical carcinoma cells by antisense RNA. *Hamatol.Bluttransfus.*, Vol.31, pp. 377-379

von Knebel, D.; Oltersdorf, T.; Schwarz, E. & Gissmann, L. (1988). Correlation of modified human papilloma virus early gene expression with altered growth properties in C4-1 cervical carcinoma cells. *Cancer Res.*, Vol.48, pp. 3780-3786

Wagner, R.W.; Matteucci, M. D.; Lewis, J. G.; Gutierrez, A. J.; Moulds, C. & Froehler, B. C. (1993). Antisense gene inhibition by oligonucleotides containing C-5 propyne pyrimidines. *Science,* Vol.260, pp. 1510-1513

Walter, F.; Murchie, A. I.; Thomson, J. B. & Lilley, D. M. (1998). Structure and activity of the hairpin ribozyme in its natural junction conformation: effect of metal ions. *Biochemistry.*, Vol.37, pp. 14195-14203

Wang, J.; Jiang, H. & Liu, F. (2000). In vitro selection of novel RNA ligands that bind human cytomegalovirus and block viral infection. *RNA.*, Vol.6, pp. 571-583

Wang, X.; Meyers, C.; Wang, H. K.; Chow, L. T. & Zheng, Z. M. (2011). Construction of a full transcription map of human papillomavirus type 18 during productive viral infection. *J.Virol.*, Vol.85, pp. 8080-8092

Wang, X.; Tang, S.; Le, S. Y.; Lu, R.; Rader, J. S.; Meyers, C. & Zheng, Z. M. (2008). Aberrant expression of oncogenic and tumor-suppressive microRNAs in cervical cancer is required for cancer cell growth. *PLoS.ONE.*, Vol.3, pp. e2557-

Wang, X.; Wang, H. K.; McCoy, J. P.; Banerjee, N. S.; Rader, J. S.; Broker, T. R.; Meyers, C.; Chow, L. T. & Zheng, Z. M. (2009). Oncogenic HPV infection interrupts the expression of tumor-suppressive miR-34a through viral oncoprotein E6. *RNA.*, Vol.15, pp. 637-647

Werness, B.A.; Levine, A. J. & Howley, P. M. (1990). Association of human papillomavirus types 16 and 18 E6 proteins with p53. *Science,* Vol.248, pp. 76-79

Whitehead, K.A.; Langer, R. & Anderson, D. G. (2009). Knocking down barriers: advances in siRNA delivery. *Nat.Rev.Drug Discov.*, Vol.8, pp. 129-138

Witten, D.; Tibshirani, R.; Gu, S. G.; Fire, A. & Lui, W. O. (2010). Ultra-high throughput sequencing-based small RNA discovery and discrete statistical biomarker analysis in a collection of cervical tumours and matched controls. *BMC.Biol.*, Vol.8, pp. 58-72

Wu, S.Y.; Singhania, A.; Burgess, M.; Putral, L. N.; Kirkpatrick, C.; Davies, N. M. & McMillan, N. A. (2011). Systemic delivery of E6/7 siRNA using novel lipidic particles and its application with cisplatin in cervical cancer mouse models. *Gene Ther.*, Vol.18, pp. 14-22

Xue, Y.; Bellanger, S.; Zhang, W.; Lim, D.; Low, J.; Lunny, D. & Thierry, F. (2010). HPV16 E2 is an immediate early marker of viral infection, preceding E7 expression in precursor structures of cervical carcinoma. *Cancer Res.*, Vol.70, pp. 5316-5325

Yamato, K.; Egawa, N.; Endo, S.; Ui-Tei, K.; Yamada, T.; Saigo, K.; Hyodo, I.; Kiyono, T. & Nakagawa, I. (2011). Enhanced specificity of HPV16 E6E7 siRNA by RNA-DNA chimera modification. *Cancer Gene Ther.*, Vol.18, pp. 587-597

Yamato, K.; Yamada, T.; Kizaki, M.; Ui-Tei, K.; Natori, Y.; Fujino, M.; Nishihara, T.; Ikeda, Y.; Nasu, Y.; Saigo, K. & Yoshinouchi, M. (2008). New highly potent and specific E6 and E7 siRNAs for treatment of HPV16 positive cervical cancer. *Cancer Gene Ther.*, Vol.15, pp. 140-153

Yan, A.C.; Bell, K. M.; Breeden, M. M. & Ellington, A. D. (2005). Aptamers: prospects in therapeutics and biomedicine. *Front.Biosci.*, Vol.10:1802-27., pp. 1802-1827

Yi, R.; Qin, Y.; Macara, I. G. & Cullen, B. R. (2003). Exportin-5 mediates the nuclear export of pre-microRNAs and short hairpin RNAs. *Genes Dev.*, Vol.17, pp. 3011-3016

Yoshinouchi, M.; Yamada, T.; Kizaki, M.; Fen, J.; Koseki, T.; Ikeda, Y.; Nishihara, T. & Yamato, K. (2003). In vitro and in vivo growth suppression of human papillomavirus 16-positive cervical cancer cells by E6 siRNA. *Mol.Ther.*, Vol.8, pp. 762-768

Yu, Q. & Burke, J. M. (1997). Design of hairpin ribozymes for in vitro and cellular applications. *Methods Mol.Biol.*, Vol.74, pp. 161-169

Zerfass-Thome, K.; Zwerschke, W.; Mannhardt, B.; Tindle, R.; Botz, J. W. & Jansen-Durr, P. (1996). Inactivation of the cdk inhibitor p27KIP1 by the human papillomavirus type 16 E7 oncoprotein. *Oncogene*, Vol.13, pp. 2323-2330

Zhang, L.; Han, B.; Li, T. & Wang, E. (2011). Label-free DNAzyme-based fluorescing molecular switch for sensitive and selective detection of lead ions. *Chem.Commun.(Camb.).*, Vol.47, pp. 3099-3101

Zhao, M.X.; Li, J. M.; Du, L.; Tan, C. P.; Xia, Q.; Mao, Z. W. & Ji, L. N. (2011). Targeted cellular uptake and siRNA silencing by quantum-dot nanoparticles coated with beta-cyclodextrin coupled to amino acids. *Chemistry.*, Vol.17, pp. 5171-5179

Zheng, Z.M. & Wang, X. (2011). Regulation of cellular miRNA expression by human papillomaviruses. *Biochim.Biophys.Acta.*, Vol.

Zhou, X. & Munger, K. (2009). Expression of the human papillomavirus type 16 E7 oncoprotein induces an autophagy-related process and sensitizes normal human keratinocytes to cell death in response to growth factor deprivation. *Virology.*, Vol.385, pp. 192-197

Zimmermann, H.; Degenkolbe, R.; Bernard, H. U. & O'Connor, M. J. (1999). The human papillomavirus type 16 E6 oncoprotein can down-regulate p53 activity by targeting the transcriptional coactivator CBP/p300. *J.Virol.*, Vol.73, pp. 6209-6219

6

The Human Papilloma Virus – Ion Channel Link in Cancer: *An Alternative Opportunity for Diagnosis and Therapy*

Ana Ramírez and Javier Camacho
Department of Pharmacology,
Centro de Investigación y de Estudios Avanzados
Mexico City
Mexico

1. Introduction

Despite hundreds of clinical trials being conducted for cancer patients, the overall response is below 4% and cancer remains a major health problem worldwide (Roberts, 2007; Kamb et al., 2007). Indeed, early detection of the disease should help improve diagnosis and treatment leading to a reduction in cancer mortality. The arising link between human papilloma virus (HPV) and ion channels presents a very interesting opportunity for the early diagnosis and therapy of different types of cancer, including cervical, head and neck, oral cavity and lung cancer, some of them within those of the highest incidence in the world.

HPV infection has been proposed as the main etiological factor for cervical cancer (Walboomers et al., 1999; zur Hausen, 2002). Nevertheless, HPV infection has been also suggested to be associated with head, neck and oral cavity cancer (Anaya-Saavedra et al, 2008). Interestingly, in a population of taiwannesse women, more than 90% of lung cancer cases were not associated to cigarrette smoke (Chen et al., 1990). Analysis of HPV expression and its E6 oncoprotein in lung cancer biopsies from non-smoker taiwannesse women, led to suggest HPV as a lung cancer risk factor in such population (Cheng et al., 2001; 2007). Therefore, HPV presence might be used as an early marker for several types of cancer.

Ion channels play important roles in cell physiology, including excitability, neural transmission, cardiac contraction, pancreatic cell metabolism, apoptosis and cell proliferation. Accordingly, alterations in either channel activity or expression are associated to several diseases (Ashcroft, F. 2006), and cancer is not an exception. Actually, several ion channels are suggested as tumor markers and therapeutic targets for different types of cancer, including those malignancies associated to HPV infection.

Ion channels are integral membrane proteins transfering small ions through the hydrophobic lipid bilayer of the cell membrane, such as potassium (K^+), sodium (Na^+), chloride (Cl^-) and calcium (Ca^{2+}). They are present in the plasma and intracellular membranes of every cell type in the human body. Most ion channels require the presence of a stimulus to be activated (*gated*), this can be accomplished by changes in the membrane potential (*voltaged-gated ion channels*), neurotransmitters or other molecules (*ligand-gated ion channels*), as well as light, temperature, mechanical forces, etc. Ion channels play an important role in a variety of cellular functions regulating every aspect of the cell physiology, the voltage-gated channels provide the ionic currents to generate and spread neuronal activity, calcium channels trigger synaptic transmission, hormonal secretion, and muscle contraction, and some channels participate in the regulation of cell migration, cell cycle progression, apoptosis and gene transcription. An increased number of human diseases has been found to result from defects in ion channel function or expression, including epilepsy, cardiac arrhythmias, skeletal muscle disorders and diabetes (Hübner, C. & Jentsch, T. 2002; Ashcroft, F. 2006). Since channels play an important role in proliferation and growth, and because cancer is a multifactorial disease, these membrane proteins also participate in tumor development. Many types of human cancers show alterations on ion channel expression presumably to help to transform healthy cells into malignant, invasive, and fast growing tissue (Schönherr, R. 2005).

In this Chapter, we begin with a general overview of ion channels in cancer followed by the specific description of the participation of potassium, calcium, sodium and chloride channels in tumor cells. Then we focus on cervical cancer as the best example of a malignancy in which a link between HPV and ion channels can be found. Lastly, we describe in detail the regulation of human oncogenic *ether à-go-go-1* (Eag1) channels by HPV oncogenes and estradiol.

2. Ion channels in cancer

The control of cell proliferation involves diverse signaling pathways, growth factors, and receptors, which have a restrict regulation in order to maintain the cell homeostasis (Vermeulen, et al., 2003). From a general view, the eukaryotic cell cycle consists of four phases (Figure 1) and some checkpoints (Norbury, C. & Nurse, P. 1992; Massagué, J., 2004). Ion channels coordinate the upstream and downstream signals that converge on the cell cycle machinery. Both voltage- and ligand-gated channels have been implicated in the control of different cell cycle checkpoints in normal as well as neoplastic cells. Cell proliferation involves at some point the activation of Cl^- channels, K^+ channels and Ca^{2+} channels; these channels appear to play an active role in the pathways leading to duplication of any given cell (Kunzelmann, K. 2005).

There are more than 400 genes encoding ion channel subunits that regulate the flow of ions across the plasma membrane and the intracellular organelle membrane. In tumor cells, during the change from normal to cancer phenotype, a series of genetic alterations occur in which genes encoding ion channels might be affected. This might lead to changes in either channel expression or activity, which may be responsible, in part, of the pathophysiological features that cause malignant growth.

Many types of ion channels have been described to play a potential role in the development and growth of cancer cells, some of them are listed in Table 1. Hallmarks of cancer have been recently reviewed and include altered cell cycle progression, self sufficiency in growth signals, insensitivity to antigrowth signals, evasion of apoptosis, adaptation to harsh conditions, sustained angiogenesis, tissue invasion and metastasis (Hanahan, D. & Weinberg, R., 2011). Most of the ion channels that contribute to the development of cancer have the capacity to induce proliferation by regulating the cell cycle at some point. Cell proliferation is a highly regulated process in which ion channels participate as regulators of the cell cycle, but surprisingly, the same ion channel mechanisms that regulate cell proliferation are involved in the control of apoptosis (programmed cell death) (Wang, Z. 2004). Cell proliferation and apoptosis are two counterparts that are responsible for maintaining normal cellular functions. Abnormal enhanced proliferation and/or impaired apoptosis alters the cell homeostasis leading to loss of control of the cellular growth.

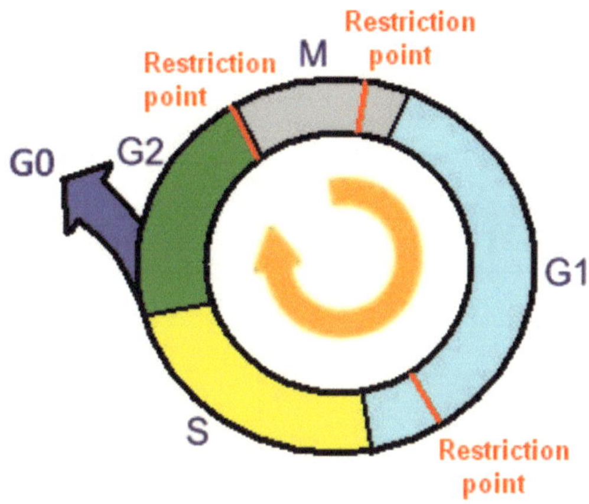

Fig. 1. Phases of the eukayotic cell cycle.

Details of the different types of ion channels involved in proliferation or invasion of tumor cells are described in Table 1.

2.1 Potassium channels

Potassium channels are the most extense family of ion channels and some of the most studied in cancer. Several potassium channels are overexpressed in tumors as compared to the corresponding healthy tissues. Some types of these channels include Kv´s (voltage-gated potassium channels), K_{Ca} (calcium-activated potassium channels), K_{2P} (two-pore domain) and K_{ir} (inward rectifier). All of these classes of potassium channels are further subdivided into subfamilies (Chandy & Gutman, 1993), and they regulate a vast diversity of functions in the cells including maintenance of the cell membrane potential, regulation of the cell volume (Lang, 2007), and cell cycle progression (Blackiston et al., 2009).

Potassium ions are important for the osmotic regulation of cell volume by working in concert with the Na^+-H^+ exchanger and the Na^+-K^+ ATPase, contributing to the regulation of intracellular pH (pH_i) (Ikuma et al., 1998). Thus, K^+ channels participate in physiological and pathological proliferation by playing a role in membrane potential, cell volume and pH_i change during cell-cycle progression. K^+ channels also provide a hyperpolarizing effect on membrane voltage during cell cycle and therefore stimulate calcium influx. This increase in intracellular Ca^{2+} concentration is needed during progression through G1 phase and the G1/S transition (Wonderlin and Strobl, 1996; Kulzenmann, 2005). Usually, cancer cells have less negative voltage membrane than normal cells (Marino et al., 1994); therefore, it is likely that they would require a higher expression of certain types of K^+ channels to produce the transient hyperpolarization required to proceed with cell cycle progression. Therefore, K^+

Channels name IUPHAR	Type of cancer	Reference
K^+ channels		
K_v 1.3	Breast, Colon, Prostate	Abdul, M., et al. (2003) ; Abdul, M. & Hoosein, N. (2002a) ; Abdul, M. & Hoosein, N. (2002c)
K_v 1.5	Glioma	Preussat, K., et al. (2003)
K_v 3.4	Oral Squamous cell carcinoma	Chang, K., et al. (2003)
K_{ca} 1.1	Cervical, Ovarian, Breast, Glioma	Han, et al. (2007); Ouadid, H., et al. (2004a); Liu, X., et al. (2002)
K_{ca} 3.1	Prostate, Breast, Melanoma, Pancreas	Parihar, A., et al. (2003); Ouadid, H., et al. (2004b); Jäger, H., et al. (2004); Gavrilova, O., et al. (2002)
K_v 10.1	Breast, Colon, Cervix, Gastric, Prostate, Sarcoma, Ovarian	Pardo, L., et al. (1999); Hemmerlein, B., et al. (2006); Ousingsawat, J., et al (2007); Farias, L., et al. (2004); Ding, X., et al. (2007); Mello, F., et al. (2006); Asher, V., et al. (2010)
K_v 11.1	Colon, Endometrial, Glioma, Leukemia, Stomach	Lastraioli, E., et al. (2004); Cherubini, A., et al. (2000); Masi, et al., (2008); Smith, G., et al. (2002); Pillozzi, S., et al. (2002); Shao, X., et al. (2008)
K_{2p} 9.1	Breast, Lung	Mu, D., et al. (2003); Pei, L., et al. (2003)
K_{ir} 3.1	Lung	Plummer, H., et al. (2005)
Ca+2 Channels		
Ca_v 1.2	Colon	Wang, X., et al. (2000)
Ca_v 3.2	Prostate	Mariot, P., et al. (2002)
Na+ Channels		
Na_v 1.2	Prostate	Anderson, J., et al. (2003)
Na_v 1.4	Prostate	Bennett, E., et al. (2004)
Na_v 1.5	Breast, Ovarian	Roger, S., et al. (2003); Gao, R., et al. (2010)
Na_v 1.6	Cervical, Glioma	Hernandez, E., et al. (2011); Schrey, M., et al. (2002)
Na_v 1.7	Prostate	Diss, J., et al. (2205)
Other channels		
Cl channels	Breast, Cervical, Hepatoma, Glioma, Prostate	Abdel, M., et al. (2003); Mao, et al. (2009); Roman, R., et al. (2001); Olsen, M., et al. (2003) ; Shuba, Y., et al. (2000).
TRPC1	Prostate	Vanden, F., et al. (2003)
TRPV6	Breast, Colon, Ovarian, Prostate, Thyroid	Bolanz, K., et al. (2008); Vanden, F., et al. (2003); Zhuang, L., et al. (2002); Fixemer, T., et al. (2003)
TRPM8	Breast, Colon, Lung, Melanoma, Prostate	Tsavaler, L., et al. (2001); Yamamura, H., et al. (2008)
P2X7	Cervical, Leukemia, Neuroblastoma,	Feng, Y., et al. (2006); Wiley, J., et al. (2002); Per Larsson, K., et al. (2002)

Table 1. Examples of ion channels involved in cancer.

channel activation is particularly important for the early G1 phase of the cell cycle. During G1/S transition and S phase, cells swell and activate a regulatory volume decrease (RVD) mechanism, which allows shrinkage of the cell after mitosis. RVD requires efflux of water and solutes, which is due to simultaneous opening of K^+ and Cl^- channels (Kulzenmann, 2005), allowing the cell to proliferate. Another evidence associating K^+ channels with proliferation is that voltage-gated K^+ channels blockers inhibit proliferation in many cell types; this has been observed in normal physiological proliferation (lymphocytes) and in pathological conditions (as in cancer cells). Thus the cells require K^+ channels in order to proceed with cell cycle progression (Wonderlin and Strobl, 1996).

Most studies are devoted to the impact of voltage-gated potassium channels on proliferation of tumor cells, particularly those of epithelial origin (Abdul & Hoosein, 2002; Farias et al., 2004; O'Grady & Lee, 2005; Pardo, 2004; Pardo et al, 2005; Arcangeli et al., 2009). One of the most studied voltage-gated potassium channel in cancer is the Eag1 channel. Eag1 displays oncogenic properties and shows a very restricted distribution in normal tissues (Pardo et al., 1999; Hemmerlein et al., 2006) but it is expressed in many types of tumors including cervical, breast, lung, prostate, liver and colon carcinoma (Farías et al., 2004; Hemmerlein et al., 2006; Ousingsawat et al., 2007). Inhibition of either channel activity or expression leads to decreased tumor cell proliferation both *in vitro* and *in vivo* (Pardo et al., 1999; Gómez-Varela et al., 2007; Ousingsawat et al., 2007). The restricted distribution of Eag1 and its role in proliferation have converted this ion channel in an attractive tool for diagnose and therapy of many cancers.

It has also been shown that several K^+ channels associate with other proteins related to proliferation, for instance Kv11.1 channels associate with 14-3-3 (Kagan et al., 2002), Src (Cayabyab, 2002), or TNF-_ receptors (Wang et al., 2002), Kv1.3 associate with integrins (Levite et al., 2000) and p56lck (Hanada et al., 1997), and Kv10.1 associates with calmodulin (Schönherr et al., 2000). Increased expression of K^+ channels in tumors offers an additional tool for cancer diagnose and treatment.

2.2 Calcium channels

Calcium entry via different channels activates intracellular signalling cascades. Calcium channels play pivotal roles in many human diseases, particularly of the cardiac and nervous systems, for example, epilepsy, hypertension and migraine. In addition, these channels have been involved in pain and cancer. Cytosolic Ca^{2+} activity is necessary throughout the cell cycle since it plays a critical role on the regulation of cell proliferation (Whitfield et al., 1995; Parekh & Penner, 1997; Berridge et al., 1998, 2000, 2003). It has been shown that decreased levels of extracellular Ca^{+2} inhibit the progression through the G1 phase, causing cells to remain at the G1/S boundary. Moreover, Ca^{2+} is highly concentrated in intracellular stores and is released from the endoplasmic reticulum or mitochondria upon mitogenic stimulation (Nilius et al., 1993; Lepple et al., 1996). In excitable tissues, Ca^{2+} influx occurs through voltage-gated Ca^{2+} channels depending on the cell type. In non-excitable tissues, hyperpolarization of the membrane voltage is important for the increase of intracellular Ca^{2+}, providing the driving force for Ca^{2+} entry from the extracellular space.

Among voltage-gated Ca^{2+} channels, members of the Ca_v3 subfamily, and in particular $Ca_v3.2$ channels, are implicated in proliferation. It has been observed that voltage-gated calcium channels Ca_V1 (L-type currents), are expressed in non-proliferative phases, while expression of Ca_V3 channels (T-type currents) often increases during the proliferative phases. This is observed in both normal and cancer cells, although the precise physiological significance is uncertain. $Ca_v3.2$ channels are expressed in several cancer-derived cell lines, and blockage of the channel generates antiproliferative action (Roger et al., 2006, Panner & Wurster, 2006). T-type calcium channels have been found in lung carcinoma cells (Oguro-Okano et al., 1992) and calcium influx through different ion channels has been suggested to participate in migration and invasion of prostate, breast and fibrosarcoma cells (Monet et al., 2009; Yang et al., 2009; Huang et al., 2004).

Other types of calcium channels have also been involved in cancer progression and prognosis. For instance, expression of the Ca^{+2} channel TRPV6 was correlated with prostate cancer grade, in which patients with positive TRPV6 prostate cancer had a poor prognosis (Fixemer et al., 2003).

2.3 Sodium channels

Voltage gated sodium channels (VGSCs) that selectively conduct sodium due to changes in membrane potential, allow sodium entry and thus the propagation of depolarization along the plasma membrane of nerve, muscle and other electrically excitable cells. Non-voltage-gated sodium channels like the degenerin/epithelial sodium channel (ENaC) superfamily, which are permeable also to lithium and potassium, is a group of proteins involved in diverse biological processes, including sodium homeostasis, salt taste, nociception, pain transduction, touch sensation and mechanotransduction (Goldin et al., 2000). Sodium channels have various functional and pharmacological properties in different tissues and species, and VGSCs in particular play an important role in generating action potentials. There are ten genes that encode VGSCs α subunits, from which nine constitute a single family named Na_V1 ($Na_V1.1$ to $Na_V1.9$), whose members associate with one or more auxiliary β subunits ($Na_V\beta1$ to $Na_V\beta4$) to form the whole channel protein complex (Yu et al., 2003). The remaining isoform, Na_X, shows a structure diverging from the Na_V1 family and seems to be gated by sodium concentration and not by voltage.

VGSCs have been suggested as participants in the development of cancer. Enhanced metastasis correlates with the appearance of membrane channels and currents that are characteristic of excitable membranes. Metastasis is a process where cells escape from a primary tumor, enter circulation (blood or lymph), migrate and invade other tissues, proliferate and form secondary tumors. In *in vitro* experiments, it has been shown that VGSCs are associated to proliferation, motility, and invasion of breast, lung, ovary and prostate cancer (Roger et al., 2003; Gao et al., 2010; Diss et al. 2005; Chioni et al., 2010; Roger et al., 2007; House, et al., 2010; Bennett et al., 2004). In prostate cancer cells, the main VGSC overexpressed is the $Na_V1.7$ subunit, while in breast, colon and ovary the $Na_V1.5$ subunit is the predominant subunit overexpressed. In addition, functional expression of VGSCs (mainly $Na_V1.7$, $Na_V1.6$ and $Na_V1.5$) is often associated with metastasis and VGSCs have been found in biopsies from prostate and breast metastatic cancer (Roger et al., 2006). The mechanisms responsible for VGSCs upregulation and for their pro-invasive roles are still poorly understood, but diverse hypothesis exists. One hypothesis strongly suggests that there is a regulation of growth factors release and/or activity which is common to all the cancers described, highly malignant cancer cell types that overexpress VGSCs also express growth factors such as epidermal growth factor (EGF) and nerve growth factor (NGF) (Brackenbury & Djamgoz, 2007; Uysal & Djamgoz, 2007), empasizing that growth factors could play a major role in upregulating VGSCs. Another hypothesis describes that embryonic genes, which are silent in the cells of the mature organ, are re-expressed in cancer cells (Monk & Holding, 2001). This might be the case for VGSCs, since highly metastatic cancers (prostate and breast) mostly express embryonic isoforms of VGSCs (Diss et al., 2005; Fraser et al., 2005). Hence overexpresion of VGSCs contributes to the physiological and pathophysiological invasive processes in several metastatic cancers, representing a potential target to inhibit invasion and metastasis.

2.4 Chloride channels

Cl^- channels play a crucial role in controlling the ionic composition of the cytoplasm and the volume of cells. According to their gating mechanisms there are five classes of chloride channels:

- Voltage-gated chloride channels (CLC).
- Volume/swell-regulated/sensitive anion/chloride channels (VRAC).
- Cystic fibrosis transmembrane conductance regulator (CFTR).
- Calcium-activated chloride channels (CLCA).
- Ligand-activated chloride channels, which mainly form synaptic channels.

Cl^- channels play a crucial role in controlling the ionic composition of the cytoplasm and the cell volume. Cl^- channels are expressed in a variety of tumor cells and participate in cell proliferation, invasion and migration. Proliferation is associated with volume increase along the G1 phase, but non-specific cell swelling can inhibit proliferation. To regulate their volume, cells are endowed with various ions and organic osmolyte transport proteins that become activated upon cell swelling or shrinkage. In the presence of a significant water permeability of the plasma membrane, water follows osmotically, resulting in a regulated change of cell volume. This is called regulatory volume increase (RVI) or regulatory volume decrease (RVD). RVI most often involves the uptake of Na^+ and Cl^-, for instance, by the concomitant activation of Na^+/H^+ and Cl^-/HCO_3^- exchangers. Na^+ is replaced by K^+ through the Na^+-K^+-ATPase, resulting in a net intracellular accumulation of KCl. In RVD, intracellular KCl may be extruded by KCl cotransporters or by the concerted activation of swelling-activated Cl^- channels and K^+channels (Jentsch et al., 2002). Cell proliferation has been shown to correlate with increases in cell volume in fibroblasts, mesangial cells, lymphocytes, human promyelocytic leukemia cells (HL-60 cells), hybridoma cells (GAP A3), smooth muscle cells and cervical carcinoma cells (HeLa cells). The signaling of cell proliferation needs at some stage transient cell shrinkage, which may require the activation of Cl^- channels. Usually, intracellular Cl^- is above electrochemical equilibrium and activation of Cl^- channels leads to Cl^- efflux and thus depolarization. As long as K^+ channels are active, the Cl^- outward movement is paralleled by K^+ efflux. The loss of KCl and water shrinks the cells (Lang et al., 1998).

It has been observed that pharmacological inhibition of Cl^- channnels impairs the cell ability to migrate and limits tumor progression in experimental tumor models (McFerrin & Sontheimer, 2006). The outer membrane of mitochondria contains a Cl^- selective porin, the so-called voltage-dependent anion channel (VDAC). On the other hand, VRAC´s modulate progression of nasopharyngeal carcinoma cells through the G1 restriction point and endow nasopharyngeal carcinoma cells with enhanced proliferation ability. In addition, it is reported that VRAC displays cell cycle-dependent expression in tumor cells. Also CLC-3, an important member of the CLC superfamily, plays a crucial role in a variety of cellular processes, including cell proliferation and cell cycle progression, and it has been demonstrated that inhibition of CLC-3 protein expression down-regulates invasion and migration ability of tumor cells.

3. Ion Channels in apoptosis

Cell homeostasis requires a delicate balance between formation of new cells by cell proliferation and cell elimination by apoptosis (programmed cell death). Apoptosis eliminates abundant and potentially harmful cells (Green & Reed, 1998). Apoptotic pathways involve several proteins with great enzymatic cell degrading potential including Bcl-2, caspases and cytochrome C. This process is initiated by death-promoting molecules such as TNF-α or CD95 Fas ligand, DNA damage, lack of growth factors, or cell exposure to genotoxics like radiation or oxidants. Apoptosis evasion might be one of the first steps for the transformation of nomal cells into cancerous cells, and it is a tightly regulated and highly efficient cell death program which requires the interplay of multiple factors. Upon receving specific signals instructing the cell to enter apoptosis, distinctive changes occur in the cell including shrinkage, nuclear condensation, DNA fragmentation, formation of sub-cellular apoptotic bodies, and mitochondrial depolarization. Ion channels have been involved in the regulation of apoptosis.

Potassium ions must leave the cell as an obligatory step in the apoptotic pathway. Activation of K+ channels and loss of intracellular K+ has been directly correlated to trigger apoptosis (Wang, 2004). Therefore, inhibition of apoptosis might take place by either increasing extracellular K+ concentration (Prehn et al., 1997; Colom et al., 1998) or inhibiting K+ channels (Lang et al., 2003). In any case, cellular K+ loss seems to be an important trigger of apoptosis in a wide variety of cells. Activation of K+ channels leads to hyperpolarization of the cell membrane, thus increasing the electrical driving force for Cl- outflow into the extracellular space. Then, if K+ channel activity is paralleled by Cl- channel activity, it leads to cellular loss of KCl with osmotically obliged water and hence to cell shrinkage, a hallmark of apoptosis (Lang et al., 1998). Subsequently, metabolic enzymes are activated, such as caspases and nucleases, which further propagate death signals. Remarkably, all these enzymes are controlled by the intracellular K+ concentration and while the concentration of various ions may change during apoptotic cell shrinkage, that of K+ plays a necessary and probably pivotal role in the cell death program. Cl- and K+ conductances must stay within a certain values in order to support proliferation, otherwise programmed cell death is triggered (Lang et al., 2004).

Sustained increase of cytosolic Ca2+ activity has been shown to trigger apoptosis in a variety of cells (Green & Reed, 1998; Spassova et al., 2004; Parekh & Putney, Jr., 2005). Cytosolic Ca2+ may trigger mechanisms required for cell proliferation and stimulate enzymes executing apoptosis. Ca2+ signal convergence results in activation of intracellular channels that leads to cytochrome C release from mitocondria. During apoptosis, small amounts of mitochondrial cytochrome C translocate to the endoplasmic reticulum and trigger Ca2+ release via IP3R channels. This leads to a bursting Ca^{2+} overload, which coordinates massive cytochrome C release from mitochondria, leading to activation of the caspase cascade, essential for the development of apoptosis (Boehning, D. *et al.*, 2003). Both the magnitude, space- and time- occurrence of Ca^{2+} entry is a major determinant to trigger apoptosis.

Both cell proliferation and apoptosis involve at some point activation of Cl^- channels, K^+ channels and Ca^{2+} channels. Due to complex interaction with other signaling pathways, a given ion channel may play a dual role in both cell proliferation and apoptosis.

At this point we focus on cervical cancer, a very well recognized cancer type strongly associated to HPV infection and ion channel expression. A potential link between HPV and ion channel expression has been also proposed for this type of cancer.

4. Overview of ion channels in cervical cancer

Expression of several ion channels has been reported in cervical cancer suggesting these proteins as potential markers and/or therapeutic targets for this malignancy. Large Ca^{2+}-activated K^+ (BK) channels are ion channels activated by changes in membrane electrical potential and/or by increases in the intracellular concentration of Ca^{2+}, contributing to cell proliferation and migration (Yuan et al., 2010). BK channels are expressed in HeLa cells, and it has been observed that they play a significant role in the regulation of proliferation of this cell line. Blockage of BK channels in HeLa cells results in tumor cell apoptosis and cycle arrest at G1 phase. The transduction pathway underlying such anti-proliferative effects is linked to the increased expression of apoptotic protein p53 and the decreased expression of its chaperone heat shock proteins (Hsp). Heat shock proteins function as intra-cellular chaperones (proteins that bind to and stabilize an otherwise unstable conformer of another protein) for other proteins, such as p53 (Zylicz M, King FW, Wawrzynow A., 2001); upon cell stress, the levels of these proteins increase dramatically. Other K^+ channels induce expression of heat shock proteins to exert tissue protective effects (Shinohara et al. 2004), suggesting that the intracellular potassium homeostasis may play a certain role in modulating heat shock proteins. The tumor suppressor gene p53 is involved in a variety of cellular processes including induction of G1 arrest and apoptosis by transactivating a number of downstream genes (Jin S, Levine A., 2001). One of those genes is p21 Cip1 (cyclin-dependent kinase inhibitor 1A), which is a cell-cycle regulatory protein that interacts with cyclin-CDK2 and -CDK4, inhibiting cell cycle progression at G1. The expression of p21 is tightly controlled by p53, through which this protein mediates the p53-dependent cell cycle arrest at G1 phase (Zamzami N, Kroemer G., 2005). Blockage of BK channels increases p53, p21Cip1, and Bax protein levels inducing cell arrest and apoptosis. In adition, inhibition of BK channels decreased the expression levels of some Hsp´s, which could be an upstream signaling of the BK channel-mediated p53 change. This would keep p53 under negative control by the activity of BK channels, inhibiting apoptosis in cervical cancer (Han et al., 2007).

Purinergic ATP-gated nonselective ion channels (P2X receptors) have been also suggested to participate in cervical cancer. These channels are permeable to Ca^{2+}, $Na^+$and K^+ (Burnstock, 2004) and several members have been identified and termed P2X1 through P2X7. Extracellular ATP is a physiological ligand that activates P2X7 receptor (Surprenant et al., 1996). Under normal conditions, extracellular ATP is present in only low concentrations, but increases significantly under inflammatory conditions and in response to tissue trauma (e.g., ischemia/hypoxia). The ionotropic purinergic P2X7 receptors activate a diverse range of cellular responses thay play a role in evading apoptosis of cervical cancer cells. In normal cervical epithelial cells, the activation of P2X7 receptors forms a pore that increases calcium influx and induces apoptosis via the Ca^{2+}-dependent mitochondrial pathway. Human cervical cancer cells express a P2X splice variant (P2X7j) that do not mediates P2X7-dependent apoptosis, causing downregulation of the functional P2X7 receptor, thereby preventing the Ca^{2+} influx required to trigger apoptosis and leading to defective apoptosis and enhanced growth of cervical cancer cells (Feng, et al., 2006).

Voltage-gated sodium channels (VGSC) have also been detected in cervical carcinoma cells that may be involved in metastasis. Expression of $Na_V1.4$, $Na_V1.6$ and $Na_V1.7$ channels has been detected in biopsies from cervical cancer (Díaz et al., 2007). Whether the activity of the sodium channel participates in the invasiveness of cervical cancer cells remains to be determined, but the pharmacological blockade of VGSCs commonly results in the reduced migration of highly metastatic cell lines, whereas the facilitation of channel opening by agonists enhances migration without impairing cell proliferation or viability (Roger et al., 2007). The abnormal expression of these VGSCs might be used as a tumor marker and a potential therapeutic target for cervical carcinoma.

It has been suggested that the expression of volume-activated current ($I_{Cl,vol}$) in HeLa cells contributes to the cell cycle dependent regulation of cell migration. The density of $I_{Cl,vol}$ was positively correlated to the rate of cell migration during cell-cycle progression indicating that volume-activated Cl^- channels are involved in the cell-cycle-dependent migratory behaviour of HeLa cells. Moreover, expression inhibition of the voltage-gated chloride channel ClC-3 arrested HeLa cells in S phase (Mao et al., 2009). The capacity of Cl^- channels to participate in migration could be associated to cell volume regulation, since regulatory volume decrease plays an important role in migration of tumor cells. Cl^- channels helps the cell to undergo changes in their shape and volume, facilitating tumors cells to move trough the extracellular space. In the following section we describe the very interesting oncogenic Eag channels, which are to our best knowledge the only known channels regulated by HPV oncogenes.

5. Oncogenic Eag1 K^+ channels in cervical cancer and regulation by HPV oncogenes

Ether à go go (Eag1) K^+ channel has gained great interest in cervical cancer diagnosis and therapy (Farias et al., 2004). Eag1 is a voltage gated K^+ channel first described as a cell-cycle regulated channel (Brüggemann et a., 1997; Camacho et al., 2000), and was the first ion channel identified to display oncogenic properties (Pardo et al., 1999). These channels are widely distributed in the central nervous system, but their expression in peripheral tissues is very restricted, finding the channel only in placenta, transiently in myoblasts, testis and adrenal glands (Occhiodoro et al., 1998; Pardo et al., 1999; Hemmerlein et al., 2006). This restricted distribution in normal tissues is one of the most attractive features of Eag1 as a potential tumor marker. Eag1 channels are overexpressed in various cancer cell lines including IGR1, IPC298, and IGR39 from melanoma, SH-SY5Y from neuroblastoma, MCF-7 from breast cancer and HeLa from cervical cancer. Eag1 channels have transforming properties, they confer lose of contact inhibition and sustained growth in the absence of serum. Cells transfected with Eag1 channel and implanted into inmunosuppreseed mice induce formation of aggressive tumors (Pardo et al. 1999). Eag1 has been found to be overexpressed in many types of tumors including breast, lung, prostate, liver and colon (Hemmerlein et al., 2006). Thus, Eag is a promising tumor marker. On the other hand, inhibition of either channel activity or expression decreases proliferation of tumor cells both *in vitro* and *in vivo* (Pardo et al., 1999; Ousingsawat et al., 2007; Gómez-Varela et al. 2007; Downie et al., 2008; Díaz et al., 2009). Therefore, Eag is also a promising therapeutic target for many types of cancer (Camacho, 2006; Pardo & Stühmer, 2008).

Eag1 mRNA expression was found in 100% of cervical cancer human biopsies while only in 33% of normal control samples (Farias et al., 2004). Interestingly, in this study it was observed that in one of the patients that was submitted to hysterectomy without any previous evidence of cervical malignancy (negative pap smears), postsurgery pathological studies showed an unexpected endocervical adenocarcinoma expressing Eag1. This case, although unique in such study, emphasizes the potential significance of Eag1 as a tumor marker in cervical cancer (Farías et al., 2004; Camacho, 2006). In addition, one of the normal cervical samples that were positive for Eag1 expression was correlated with HPV infection. This led to suggest that Eag1 expression in normal cervix could be an early sign of tumor development associated to HPV infection.

The primary transforming activity of high-risk HPVs is provided by the E6 and E7 oncoproteins which act cooperatively in the development of HPV-induced cancers. A primary target of E7 is the retinoblastoma (Rb) family of proteins that control the activity of E2F transcription factors, which are key regulators of S phase genes. The efficient abrogation of Rb function by E7 leads to increased levels of p53 and, consequently, the E6 proteins have evolved to target p53 for degradation. Researchers investigated the potential link between HPV infection and Eag oncogenic channels by transfecting normal human keratinocytes with E6 and/or E7 HPV oncogenes (Díaz et al., 2009). They observed that normal human keratinocytes do not express Eag channels. Interestingly, keratinocytes transfected with either E6, E7 or both HPV oncogenes, displayed a strong Eag channel expression. This finding suggests a novel mechanism by which HPV induces tumor formation, namely, up-regulation of the oncogenic Eag1 channel.

Regulation of Eag1 channels by E6/E7 HPV oncogenes suggests that the regulation of Eag1 in cervical cancer might be via p53 and Rb pathways. A novel signaling pathway has been described that might explain how Eag is regulated by p53. It appears that Eag1 is a terminal component in the p53-miR-34-E2F1 pathway. miR-34 is a micro RNA, which silences expression of target genes through the RNA interference pathway and is commonly downregulated in human cancers; one example is miR-34, which is a direct target of p53. miR-34 transcription is activated by p53, and expression of miR-34 inhibits proliferation by inducing cellular senescence and cell cycle arrest at G1. When cellular stress or damage exist, p53 increases, causing the miR-34 transcription to increase, and the increased miR-34 will decrease the trancription factor E2F1. One of the target genes for transcription of E2F1 is the K^+ channel Eag1. Supression of E2F1 will repress Eag1, this will diminish Eag1 expression and function, resulting in a shut down of the cell proliferation or a cell cycle arrest, thus upregulation of miR-34 represses E2F1 and Eag1. Therefore, p53 negatively regulates Eag1 expression by a negative feed forward mechanism through the p53-miR-34-E2F1 pathway (Lin et al., 2011). This pathway might also help to explain the effect of the E7 oncogene on Eag regulation. E7 binds to Rb disrupting the Rb–E2F complexes, resulting in the constitutive expression of E2F1-responsive genes including Eag1.

6. Effect of estrogens on HPV and eag channels

HPV infection has been suggested as a necessary but not sufficient factor to induce cervical cancer. Thus other contributing factors have been proposed, especially estrogens. The uterine cervix is highly responsive to steroidal hormones and the use of oral contraceptives and multiple pregnancies have been shown to significantly increase the risk for cervical cancer in HPV-infected women (Moreno et al., 2002; Muñoz et al., 2002). In mice models for HPV-associated cancers, estrogen is required for the development of cervical and vaginal cancers (Brake & Lambert, 2005). The estrogen receptor alpha (ERα) is also required in mice for these cancers to develop and ER antagonists can cause efficient regression of cancer, dysplasia, and atypical squamous metaplasia, preventing malignant progression (Chung & Lambert, 2009). Other studies also suggest the relevance of estrogen in the carcinogenesis of cervical cancer. Growth stimulation of SiHa cervical cancer cells by estrogens appeared to be related to the increased expression of HPV E6/E7 oncogenes, estradiol stimulated both cell growth and transcription of E6/E7 viral oncogenes (Rosembaum, et al., 1989; Kim, et al., 2000). In addition, overexpression of aromatase, the enzyme that transforms testosterone into estrogen, is known to increase estrogen activity in breast tissue, and in cervical cancers it has been reported that 35% of human cervical cancer tested express aromatase, but

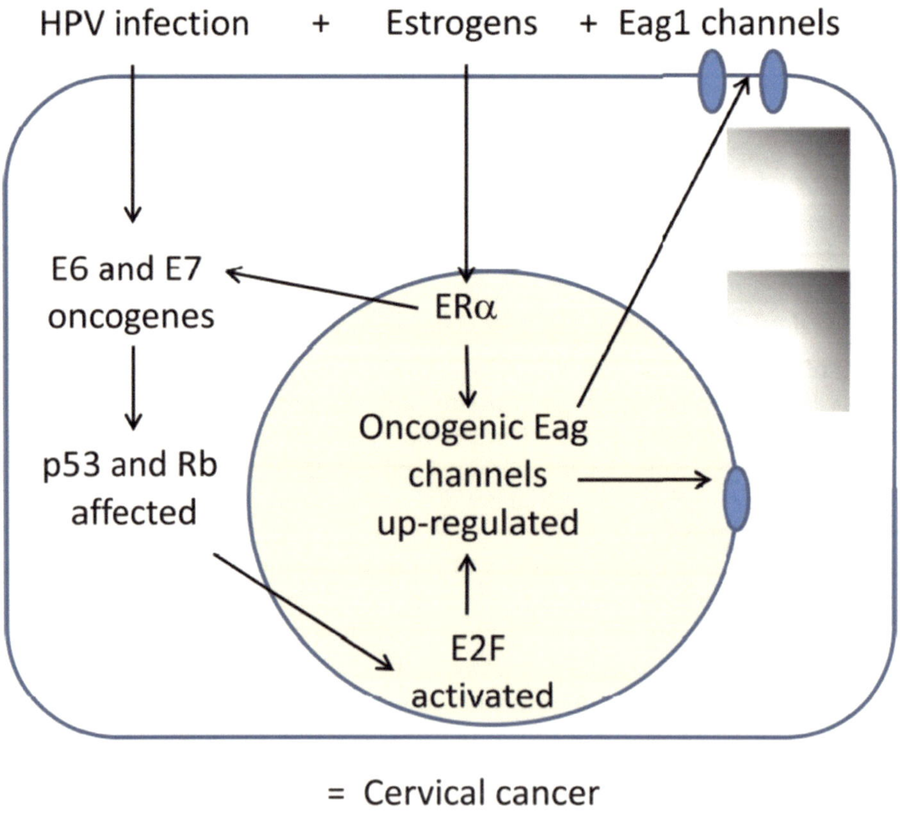

Fig. 2. Regulation of Eag1 oncogenic Eag1 channels by HPV oncogenes and estradiol. Eag1 might become extremely up-regulated since HPV oncogenes are in turn regulated by estradiol, leading cervical cells to cancer.

aromatase expression was not detected in precancerous or normal cervical tissue samples. Aromatase overexpression induced the expression of cyclin D1, proliferating cell nuclear antigen and HPV oncogenes (Nair, et al., 2005). It was also observed that women that expressed higher levels of estrogen receptors transcripts were significantly more likely to have cervical HPV infection; it may be that the presence of the receptor allows cellular acquisition of HPVand increased viral transcription (Shew, M., et al. 2005). These data suggest that a mechanism of synergistic cooperation exist between estrogen exposure and viral oncogenes, so it raises the possibility that steroidal hormones, such as estrogen, might affect cancers of the cervix, much like that of other hormonally responsive female organs. In summary, several studies suggest that estrogens play a critical role not only in the genesis of cervical cancer but also in its persistence and continuous development.

Eag1 channel expression is also up-regulated by estrogens. HeLa cells transfected with ERα and treated with 17-β estradiol, induce a strong up-regulation of Eag1 channels. These results suggest ERα activation as one of the mechanisms of the estrogenic regulation of Eag1. Thus the regulation of the Eag1 channel in cervical cancer is mediated by HPV oncogenes and estrogens (Diaz, L., et al., 2009). HPV-infection in cervical cells might lead to a very significant increase in oncogenic Eag channels. Since estrogens might regulate both HPV-oncogens and Eag1 channels, these related pathways might easily drive the cell into a tumor phenotype (Figure 2).

7. Conclusion

Ion channels are emerging as potential tools for diagnosis and treatment of many types of cancer including those where HPV infection plays a major role. Particularly, up-regulation of the oncogenig human Eag channel by HPV oncoogens offers a novel mechanism by which HPV associates to some types of cancer. Since several ion channels are up-regulated by HPV oncogenes and/or factors closely associated to HPV, for instance estrogens, simultaneous detection of HPV infection and ion channel expression should provide an alternative option for early detection of tumors. Besides, HPV detection might also serve to target ion channels involved in tumor progression. This combined approach should help reduce cancer mortality.

8. Acknowledgment

We thank all of our collaborators participating in our publications. The current research project on cervical cancer in the laboratory of JC is partially funded by Conacyt, Mexico (Grant No. 141126).

9. References

Abdel, M., Cheng, H., Elble, R., Lin, H., DiBiasio, J. & Pauli, B. (2003). The interacting binding domains of the beta (4) integrin and calcium-activated chloride channels (CLCAs) in metastasis. *The Journal of Biological Chemistry*. Vol. 278, pp. 49406-49416.

Abdul, M., & Hoosein, N. (2002a). Voltage-gated potassium ion channels in colon cancer. *Oncology Reports,* Vol. 9, pp. 961-964.

Abdul, M., & Hoosein, N. (2002b). Voltage-gated sodium ion channels in prostate cancer: expression and activity. *Anticancer Research,* Vol. 22, pp. 1727–1730.

Abdul, M. & Hoosein, N. (2002c). Expression and activity of potassium ion channels in human prostate cancer. *Cancer Letters.* Vol. 186, pp. 99-105.

Abdul, M., Santo, A. & Hoosein, N. (2003). Activity of potassium channel-blockers in breast cancer. *Anticancer Research.* Vol. 23, pp. 3347-3351.

Anaya-Saavedra, G. Ramírez-Amador V, Irigoyen-Camacho ME, García-Cuellar CM, Guido-Jiménez M, Méndez-Martínez R, & García-Carrancá A. (2008). High association of human papillomavirus infection with oral cancer: a case-control study. *Archives of Medical Research,* Vol. 39, pp. 189-197.

Anderson, J., Hansen, T., Lenkowski, P., Walls, A., Choudhury, I., Schenck, H., Friehling, M., Höll, G.,Patel, M., Sikes, R. & Brown, M. (2003). Voltage-gated sodium channel blockers as cytostatic inhibitors of the androgen-independent prostate cancer cell line PC-3. *Molecular Cancer Therapeutics.* Vol. 11, pp. 1149-1154.

Arcangeli, A., Crociani, O., Lastraioli, E., Masi, A., Pillozzi, S., & Becchetti A., (2009). Targeting ion channels in cancer: a novel frontier in antineoplastic therapy. *Current Medicinal Chemistry,* Vol. 16, pp. 66–93.

Ashcroft, F. (2006). From molecule to malady. *Nature,* Vol. 440, pp. 440-447.

Asher, V., Khan, R., Warren, A., Shaw, R., Schalkwyk, G., Bali, A. & Sowter, H. (2010). The Eag potassium channel as a new prognostic marker in ovarian cancer. *Diagnostic Pathology.* Vol. 7.

Bennett, E., Smith, B., & Harper, J. (2004). Voltage-gated Naþ channels confer invasive properties on human prostate cancer cells. *Pflügers Archiv European Journal of Physiology.* Vol. 447, pp. 908- 914.

Berridge, M., Bootman, M., & Lipp, P. (1998). Calcium–a life and death signal. *Nature,* Vol. 395, pp. 645- 648.

Berridge, M., Lipp, P., & Bootman, M. (2000). The versatility and universality of calcium signalling. *Nature Reviews Molecular Cell Biology,* Vol. 1, pp. 11–21.

Berridge, M., Bootman, M., & Roderick, H. (2003). Calcium signalling: dynamics, homeostasis and remodelling. *Nature Reviews Molecular Cell Biology,* Vol. 4, pp. 517–529.

Blackiston, D.J., McLaughlin, K.A., & Levin, M. (2009). Bioelectric controls of cell proliferation: ion channels, membrane voltage and the cell cycle. *Cell Cycle,* Vol. 8, No. 21, pp. 3519-3528.

Boehning, D., Patterson, R., Sedaghat, L., Glebova, N., Kurosaki, T., & Snyder, S. (2003). Cytochrome c binds to inositol (1,4,5) trisphosphate receptors, amplifying calcium-dependent apoptosis. *Nature Cell Biology.* Vol. 5, No. 12, pp. 1051-1061.

Bolanz, K., Hediger, M. & Landowski, C. (2008) The role of TRPV6 in breast carcinogenesis. *Molecular Cancer Therapeutics.* Vol. 7, pp. 271–279.

Brackenbury, W. & Djamgoz, M. (2007) Nerve growth factor enhances voltage-gated Na+ channel activity and Transwell migration in Mat-LyLu rat prostate cancer cell line. *Journal of Cell Physiology,* Vol. 210, pp. 602–608.

Brüggemann A., Stühmer W., & Pardo L. (1997). Mitosis-promoting factormediated suppression of a cloned delayed rectifier potassium channel expressed in Xenopus oocytes. *Procedings of the National Academic of Sciences,* Vol. 94, pp. 537-542.

Brake, T. & Lambert, P. (2005) Estrogen contributes to the onset, persistence, and malignant progression of cervical cancer in a human papillomavirus-transgenic mouse model. *Proceedings of the National Academy of Sciences USA.* Vol. 102, pp. 2490–2495.

Burnstock, G. (2004). Introduction: P2 receptors. Current Topics in Medicinal *Chemistry,*Vol. 4, pp. 793- 803.

Camacho, J. (2006). Ether à go-go potassium channels and cancer. *Cancer Letters,* Vol. 233, pp. 1-9.

Camacho J., Sánchez A., Stühmer W., & Pardo, L., (2000). Cytoskeletal interactions determine the electrophysiological properties of human EAG potassium channels. *Pflügers Archiv European Journal Physiology*, Vol. 441, pp. 167-174.

Cayabyab, F., & Schlichter, L., (2002). Regulation of an ERG K+ current by *Src* tyrosine kinase. *Journal of Biological Chemistry,* Vol. 277, pp. 13673–13681.

Chandy, K., & Gutman, G. (1993). Nomenclature for mammalian potassium channel genes. *Trends in Pharmacological Sciences,* Vol. 14, No. 12, Dec, 1993, pp. 434.

Chang, K., Yuan, T., Fang, K., Yang, F., Liu, C., Chang, C. & Lin, S. (2003). The increase of voltage-gated potassium channel Kv3.4 mRNA expression in oral squamous cell carcinoma. *Journal of Oral Pathology and Medicine.* Vol. 32, pp. 606-611.

Chen CJ, Wu HY, Chuang YC, Chang AS, Luh KT, Chao HH, Chen KY, Chen SG, Lai GM, Huang HH, et al. (1990). Epidemiologic characteristics and multiple risk factors of lung cancer in Taiwan. *Anticancer Research,* Vol. 10, pp. 971-979.

Cheng, YW, Chiou HL, Sheu GT, Hsieh LL, Chen JT, Chen CY, Su JM, & Lee H. (2001). The association of human papillomavirus 16/18 infection with lung cancer among non-smoking Taiwanese women. *Cancer Research,* Vol. 61, pp. 2799-2803.

Cheng, YW, Wu MF, Wang J, Yeh KT, Goan YG, Chiou HL, Chen CY, & Lee H.(2007). Human papillomavirus 16/18 E6 oncoprotein is expressed in lung cancer and related with p53 inactivation. *Cancer Research,* Vol. 67, pp. 10686-10693.

Cherubini, A., Taddei, G., Crociani, O., Paglierani, M., Buccoliero, A., Fontana, L., Noci, I., Borri, P., Borrani,

E., Giachi, M., Becchetti, A., Rosati, B., Wanke, E., Olivotto, M. & Arcangeli, A. (2000). HERG potassium channels are more frequently expressed in human endometrial cancer as compared to non- cancerous endometrium. *British Journal of Cancer.* Vol. 83, pp. 1722-1729.

Chioni, A., Shao, D., Grose, R. & Djamgoz, M. (2010). Protein kinase A and regulation of neonatal Nav1.5 expression in human breast cancer cells: activity-dependent positive feedback and cellular migration. *International Journal of Biochemistry and Cell Biology,* Vol. 42, pp. 346-358.

Chung, S., & Lambert, P. (2009). Prevention and treatment of cervical cancer in mice using estrogen receptor antagonists. *Procedings of the National Academic of Sciences* Vol. 106, pp. 19467–19472

Colom, L., Diaz, M., Beers, D., Neely, A., Xie, W., & Appel, S. (1998). Role of potassium channels in amyloid-induced cell death. *Journal of Neurochemistry*, Vol. 70, pp. 1925–1934.

Diaz, D., Delgadillo, D., Hernández, E., Ramírez, M., Hinojosa, L., Ortiz, C., Berumen, J., Camacho, J. & Gomora, J. (2007) Functional expression of voltage-gated sodium channels in primary cultures of human cervical cancer. *Journal of Cell Physiology*, Vol. 210, pp. 469–478.

Díaz, L., Ceja, I., Restrepo, I., Larrea, F., Avila, E., García, R., Borja, E., Barrera, D., Ahumada, E., Gariglio, P., Alvarez, E., Ocadiz, R., Garcia, E., Hernandez, E., Camacho, I., Morales, A., Ordaz, D., Garcia, E., Escamilla, J., Sanchez, L., Saqui, M., Gamboa, A.,Vera, E., Uribe, M., Murbartian, J., Ortiz, C., Rivera, C., De Vizcaya, A. & Camacho, J. (2009). Estrogens and human papilloma virus oncogenes regulate Human Ether-à -go-go-1 Potassium Channel Expression. *Cancer Research,* Vol. 69, pp. 3300-3307.

Ding, X., Luo, H., Jin, X., Yan, J. & Ai, Y. (2007). Aberrant expression of Eag1 potassium channels in gastric cancer patients and cell lines. *Medical Oncology*. Vol. 24, pp. 345-350.

Diss, J., Stewart. D., Pani, F., Foster, C., Walker, M., Patel, A. & Djamgoz, M. (2005). A potential novel marker for human prostate cancer: voltage-gated sodium channel expression in vivo. *Prostate Cancer and Prostatic Diseases,* Vol. 8, pp. 266-273.

Downie, B., Sánchez. A., Knötgen, H., Contreras, C., Gymnopoulos, M., Weber, C., Stühmer, W. & Pardo, L., (2008). Eag1 expression interferes with hypoxia homeostasis and induces angiogenesis in tumors. *Journal of Biological Chemistry*, Vol. 283, pp. 36234-36240.

Farias, L., Ocana, D., Diaz, L., Larrea, F., Avila, E., Cadena, A., Hinojosa, L., Lara, G., Villanueva, L., Vargas, C., Hernandez, E., Camacho, I., Duenas, A., Perez, E., Pardo, L., Morales, A., Taja, L., Escamilla, J., Sanchez, C., & Camacho, J. (2004). Ether à go-go potassium channels as human cervical cancer markers. *Cancer Research,* Vol. 64, pp. 6996–7001.

Feng, Y., Li, X., Wang, L., Zhou, L. & Gorodeski GI. (2006). A truncated P2X7 receptor variant (P2X7-j) endogenously expressed in cervical cancer cells antagonizes the fulllength P2X7 receptor through hetero-oligomerization. *Journal of Biological Chemistry,* Vol. 281, pp. 17228–17237.

Fixemer, T., Wissenbach, U., Flockerzi, V. & Bonkhoff, H. (2003) Expression of the Ca2+-selective catión channel TRPV6 in human prostate cancer: a novel prognostic marker for tumor progression. *Oncogene*, Vol. 22, pp. 7858–7861

Fraser, S., Diss, J., Chioni, A., Mycielska, M., Pan, H., Yamaci, R., Pani, F., Siwy, Z., Krasowska, M., Grzywna, Z., Brackenbury, W., Theodorou, D., Koyutürk, M., Kaya, H., Battaloglu, E., De Bella, M., Slade, M., Tolhurst, R., Palmieri, C., Jiang, J., Latchman, D., Coombes, R. & Djamgoz, M. (2005) Voltage-gated sodium channel expression and potentiation of human breast cancer metastasis. *Clinical Cancer Research,* Vol. 11, pp. 5381–5389.

Gao, R., Shen, Y., Cai, J., Lei, M. & Wang, Z. (2010). Expression of voltage-gated sodium channel alpha subunit in human ovarian cancer. *Oncology Reports*, Vol. 23, pp. 1293-1299.

Gavrilova, O., Schönherr, K., Gessner, G., Schönherr, R., Klapperstück, T., Wohlrab, W. & Heinemann, S. (2002). Effects of imipramine on ion channels and proliferation of IGR1 melanoma cells. *Journal of Membrane Biology*. Vol. 188, pp. 137-149.

Goldin, A., Barchi, R., Caldwell, J., Hofmann, F., Howe, J., Hunter, J., Kallen, R., Mandel, G., Meisler, M., Netter, Y., Noda, M., Tamkun, M., Waxman, S., Wood, J. & Catterall, W. (2000). Nomenclature of voltage-gated sodium channels. *Neuron*, Vol. 28, pp. 365-368.

Gómez-Varela, D., Zwick, E., Knötgen, H., Hettmann, T., Ossipov, D., Weseloh, R., Contreras, C., Rothe, M., Stühmer, W. & Pardo, L. (2007). Monoclonal antibody blockade of the human Eag1 potassium channel function exerts antitumor activity. *Cancer Research*, Vol.67, pp. 7343-7349.

Green, D. & Reed, J. (1998). Mitochondria and apoptosis. *Science*, Vol. 281, pp. 1309-1312.

Han, X., Wang, F., Yao, W., Xing, H., Weng, D., Song, X., Chen, G., Xi, L., Zhu, T., Zhou, J., Xu, G., Wang, S., Meng, L., Ladecola, C., Wang, G., & Ma, D. (2007). Heat shock proteins and p53 play a critical role in K^+ channel-mediated tumor cell proliferation and apoptosis. *Apoptosis*, Vol. 12, pp. 1837-1846.

Hanada, T., Lin, L., Chandy, K., Oh, S., & Chishti, A., (1997). Human homologue of the *Drosophila Discs Large* tumor suppressor binds to p56lck tyrosine kinase and Shaker type Kv1.3 potassium channel in T lymphocytes. *Journal of Biological Chemistry*, Vol. 272, pp. 26899-26904.

Hanahan, D. & Weinberg, RA. (2011). Hallmarks of cancer: the next generation. *Cell*, Vol. 144, pp. 646-674.

Hemmerlein B., Weseloh R., Mello F., Knötgen H., Sánchez A., Rubio M., Martin S., Schliephacke T., Jenke M., Joachim H., Stühmer W., & Pardo L., (2006). Overexpression of Eag1 potassium channels in clinical tumours. *Molecular Cancer*, Vol. 5.

Hernández, E., Ortiz, C., Marquina, B., Medina, I., Alfaro, A., Berumen, J., Rivera, M. & Gomora, J.(2011). Over expression of Na (V) 1.6 channels is associated with the invasion capacity of human cervical cancer. *International Journal of Cancer*. DOI: 10.1002/ijc.26210

House, C., Vaske, C., Schwartz, A., Obias, V., Frank, B., Luu, T., Sarvazyan, N., Irby, R., Strausberg, R., Hales, T.,Stuart, J. & Lee, N. (2010). Voltage-Gated Na+ Channel SCN5A Is a Key Regulator of a Gene Transcriptional Network That Controls Colon Cancer Invasion. *Cancer Research*, Vol. 70., pp. 6957-6967.

Huang, J.B., Kindzelskii, A.L., Clark, A.J. and Petty, H.R. 2004. Identification of channels promoting calcium spikes and waves in HT1080 tumor cells: Their apparent roles in cell motility and invasion. *Cancer Research*, Vol. 64, pp. 2482-2489.

Hübner, C. & Jentsch, T. (2002). Ion channel diseases. *Human Molecular Genetics*, Vol. 11, pp. 2435-2445.

Ikuma, M., Binder, H.J., & Geibel, J. (1998). Role of apical H-K exchange and basolateral K channel in the regulation of intracellular pH in rat distal colon crypt cells. *Journal of Membrane Biology*, Vol. 166, December, pp. 205–212.

Jager, H., Dreker, T., Buck, A., Giehl, K., Gress, T., & Grissmer, S. (2004). Blockage of intermediate-conductance Ca2+- activated K+ channels inhibit human pancreatic cancer cell growth in vitro. *Molecular Pharmacology,* Vol. 65, pp. 630–638.

Jentsch, T., Stein, V., Weinreich, F., & Zdebik, A. (2002). Molecular Structure and Physiological Function of Chloride Channels. *Physiological Reviews*, Vol. 82, pp. 503–568.

Jin, S., & Levine, A. (2001). The p53 functional circuit. *Journal of Cell Science*, Vol. 114, pgs. 4139–4140.

Kagan, A., Melman, Y., Krumerman A., & McDonald, T., (2002). 14-3-3 amplifies and prolongs adrenergic stimulation of HERG K+ channel activity. *EMBO Journal,* Vol. 21, pp. 1889–1898.

Kamb, A. et al. (2007). Why is cancer drug discovery so difficult? *Nature Reviews Drug Discovery*. 6:115-120.

Kim, C., Um, S., Kim, T., Kim, E., Park, T., Kim, S., Namkoong, S., & Park, J. (2000). Regulation of cell growth and HPV genes by exogenous estrogen in cervical cancer cells. *International Journal of Gynecological Cancer,* Vol. 10, pp. 157-164.

Kunzelmann, K., 2005. Ion channels and cancer. *Journal of Membrane Biology,* Vol. 205, pags. 159-173.

Lang, F., Busch, G., Ritter, M., Volkl, H., Waldegger, S., Gulbins, E., & Haussinger, D. (1998). Functional significance of cell volume regulatory mechanisms. *Physiological Reviews,* Vol. 78, pp. 247–306.

Lang, F., Gulbins, E., Szabo, I., Lepple, A., Huber, S., Duranton, C., Lang, K., Lang, P., & Wieder, T. (2004). Cell volume and the regulation of apoptotic cell death. *Journal of Molecular Recognition*, Vol. 17, pp. 473–480.

Lang, F. (2007). Mechanisms and significance of cell volume regulation. *Journal of the American College of Nutrition*, Vol. 26, No. 5, Oct .,(5 Suppl):613S-623S.

Lang, P., Warskulat, U., Heller, B., Huang, D., Grenz, A., Myssina, S., Duszenko, M., Lang, F., Haussinger, D., Vallon, V., & Wieder, T. (2003). Blunted apoptosis of erythrocytes from taurine transporter deficient mice. *Cell Physiology Biochemistry,* Vol. 13, pp. 337–346.

Lastraioli, E., Guasti, L., Crociani, O., Polvani, S., Hofmann, G., Witchel, H., Bencini, L., Calistri, M., Messerini, L., Scatizzi, M., Moretti, R., Wanke, E., Olivotto, M., Mugnai, G. & Arcangeli, A. (2004). herg1 gene and HERG1 protein are overexpressed in colorectal cancers and regulate cell invasion of tumor cells. *Cancer Research.* Vol. 15, pp. 606-611.

Lepple, A., Berweck, S., Bohmig, M., Leo, C., Meyling, B., Garbe, C., & Wiederholt, M. (1996). K+ channels and the intracellular calcium signal in human melanoma cell proliferation. *Journal of Membrane Biology,* Vol. 151, pp. 149–157

Levite, M., Cahalon, L., Peretz, A., Hershkoviz, R., Sobko, A., Ariel, A., Desai, R., Attali, B., & Lider, O. (2000). Extracellular K+ and opening of voltage-gated potassium channels activate T cell integrin function: physical and functional association between Kv1.3 channels and b1 integrins. *The Journal of Experimental Medicine*, Vol. 191, pp. 1167–1176.

Lin, H., Li, Z., Chen, C., Luo, X., Xiao, J., Dong, D., Lu, Y., Yang, B. & Wang, Z. (2011) Transcriptional an Post-Transcriptional Mechanisms for Oncogenic Overexpression of Ether A` Go-Go K+ Channel. *PLoS One*, Vol. 6, pg. e20362

Liu, X., Chang, Y., Reinhart, P., & Sontheimer, H. (2002). Cloning and Characterization of Glioma BK, a Novel BK Channel Isoform Highly Expressed in Human Glioma Cells. *The Journal of Neuroscience*. Vol. 22, pp. 1840–1849.

Lu, F., Chen, H., Zhou, C., Liu, S., Guo, M., Chen, P., Zhuang, H., Xie, D., & Wu, S. (2008). T-type Ca2+ channel expression in human esophageal carcinomas: A functional role in proliferation. *Cell Calcium*, Vol. 43, pp. 49–58

Mc Ferrin, M. & Sontheimer, H. (2006) A role for ion channels in glioma cell invasion. *Neuron Glia Biology*, Vol. 2, pp. 39–49.

Mao, J., Chen, L., Xu, B., Wang, L., Wang, W., Li, M., Zheng, M., Li, H., Guo, J., Li, W., Jacob, T. & Wang L. (2009).Volume-activated chloride channels contribute to cell-cycle-dependent regulation of HeLa cell migration. *Biochemical Pharmacology*, Vol. 15, pp. 159-168.

Marino, A., Iliev, I., Schwalke, M., Gonzalez, E., Marler, K., & Flanagan, C. (1994). Association between cell membrane potential and breast cancer. *Tumour Biology*, Vol. 15, pp. 82–89.

Mariot, P., Vanoverberghe, K., Lalevee, N., Rossier, M. & Prevarskaya, N. Overexpression of an alpha 1H (Cav3.2) T-type calcium channel during neuroendocrine differentiation of human prostate cancercells. *The Journal of Biological Chemistry*. Vol. 277, pp. 10824-10833.

Masi, A., Becchetti, A., Restano, R., Polvani, S., Hofmann, G., Buccoliero, A., Paglierani, M., Pollo, B., Taddei, G., Gallina, P., Di Lorenzo, N., Franceschetti, S., Wanke, E. & Arcangeli, A. (2008) hERG1 channels are overexpressed in glioblastoma multiform and modulate VEGF secretion in glioblastoma cell lines. *Journal of Biological Chemistry*. Vol. 283, pp. 36234–36240.

Massagué, J. (2004). G1 cell-cycle control and cancer. *Nature*, Vol. 432, pp. 298-306.

Mattson, M., & Chan, S. (2003). Calcium orchestrates apoptosis. *Nature Cell Biology*, Vol. 5, No. 12, pp. 1041-1043.

Mello, F., Suarez, G., Stühmer, W. & Pardo, L. (2006). Ether à go-go potassium channel expression in soft tissue sarcoma patients. *Molecular Cancer*. Vol. 5.

Monet, M., Gkika, D., Lehen´kyi V., Pourtier,A., Abeela, F.V., Bidaux, G., Juvin., Rassendren, F., Humez, S. & Prevarskaya, N. (2009). Lysophospholipids stimulate prostate cancer cell migration via TRPV2 channel activation. *Biochimica et Biophysica Acta-Molecular Cell*, Vol. 1793, pp. 528-539.

Monk, M. & Holding, C. (2001). Human embryogenic genes re-expressed in cancer cells. *Oncogene*, Vol. 20, pp. 8085-8091.

Moreno, V., Bosch, F., Muñoz, N., Meijer, C., Shah, K., Walboomers, J., Herrero, R. & Franceschi, S. (2002). Effect of oral contraceptives on risk of cervical cancer in women with human papillomavirus infection: The IARC multicentric case-control study. *Lancet*, Vol. 359, pp. 1085–1092.

Mu. D., Chen, L., Zhang, X., See, L., Koch, C., Yen, C., Tong, J., Spiegel, L., Nguyen, K., Servoss, A., Peng, Y., Pei, L., Marks, J., Lowe, S., Hoey, T., Jan, L., McCombie, W., Wigler, M. & Powers, S. (2003). Genomic amplification and oncogenic properties of the KCNK9 potassium channel gene. *Cancer Cell.* Vol. 3, pp. 297-302.

Munoz, N., Franceschi, S., Bosetti, C., Moreno, V., Herrero, R., Smith, J., Shah, K., Meijer, C., & Bosch, F. (2002). Role of parity and human papillomavirus in cervical cancer: The IARC multicentric case-control study. *Lancet,* Vol. 359, pp. 1093–1101.

Nair, H., Luthra, R., Kirma, N., Flowers, L., Evans, D., & Tekmal, R. (2005). Induction of aromatase expression in cervical carcinomas: effects of endogenous estrogen on cervical cancer cell proliferation. *Cancer Research,* Vol 65, pp. 11164-11173.

Nilius, B., Schwarz, G., & Droogmans, G. (1993). Control of intracellular calcium by membrane potential in human melanoma cells. *American Journal of Physiology,* Vol. 265, pp. C1501–C1510.

Norbury, C. & Nurse, P. (1992). Animal cell cycles and their control. *Annual Review of Biochemistry,* Vol. 61, pp. 441-470.

Occhiodoro TL, Bernheim L, Liu JH, Bijlenga P, Sinnreich M, Bader CR, Fischer-Lougheed J: Cloning of a human ether-a-go-go potassium channel expressed in myoblasts at the onset of fusion. *FEBS Lett* 1998, 434:177-182.

Oguro-Okano M., Griesmann G.E., Wieben, E.D., Slaymaker, S.J., Snutch, T.P. & Lennon, V.A. (1992). Molecular Diversity of neuronal-type calcium channels identified in small cell lung carcinoma. *Mayo Clinic Proceedings,* Vol. 67, pp. 1150-1159.

O'Grady, S., & Lee, S. (2005). Molecular diversity and function of voltage-gated (Kv) potassium channels in epithelial cells. *International Journal of Biochemistry and Cell Biology,* Vol. 37, pp. 1578–1594.

Olsen, M., Schade, S., Lyons, S., Amaral, M. & Sontheimer, H. (2003) Expression of voltage-gated chloride channels in human glioma cells. *Journal of Neuroscience.* Vol. 23, pp. 5572-5582.

Ouadid, H., Roudbaraki, M., Ahidouch, A., Delcourt, P., Prevarskaya, N. (2004a). Cell-cycle-dependent expression of the large Ca^{2+}-activated K^{+} channels in breast cancer cells. *Biochemical and Biophysical Research Communications.* Vol. 316, pp. 244–251.

Ouadid, H., Roudbaraki, M., Delcourt, P., Ahidouch, A., Joury, N., & Prevarskaya, N. (2004b). Functional and molecular identification of intermediate-conductance $Ca^{(2+)}$- activated $K^{(+)}$ channels in breast cancer cells: association with cell cycle progression. *American Journal of Physiology, Cell Physiology,* Vol. 287, pp. C125–C134.

Ousingsawat J, Spitzner M, Puntheeranurak S, Terraciano L, Tornillo L, Bubendorf L, Kunzelmann K and Schreiber R. (2007). Expression of voltage-gated potassium channels in human and mouse colonic carcinoma. *Clinical Cancer Research,* Vol. 13, pp. 824-831.

Panner, A., & Wurster, R. (2006). T-type calcium channels and tumor proliferation. *Cell Calcium,* Vol. 40, pp. 253-259.

Pardo, L., Camino D., Sánchez A., Alves F., Brüggemann A., Beckh S., & Stühmer W., (1999). Oncogenic potential of EAG K+ channels. *EMBO Journal,* Vol. 18, pp. 5540-5547.

Pardo, L. (2004). Voltage-gated potassium channels in cell proliferation. *Physiology (Bethesda),* Vol.19, pp. 85-292.

Pardo, L., Contreras, C., Zientkowska, M., Alves, F., & Stühmer W. (2005). Role of Voltage-gated Potassium Channels in Cancer. *Journal of Membrane Biology,* Vol. 205, pp. 115–124.

Pardo, L. & Stühmer, W. (2008) Eag1: an emerging oncological target. *Cancer Research,* Vol. 68, pp. 1611–1613.

Parekh, A., & Penner, R. (1997). Store depletion and calcium influx. *Physiological Reviews,* Vol. 77, pp. 901–930.

Parekh, A., & PutneyJW Jr. (2005). Store-operated calcium channels. *Physiological Reviews,* Vol. 85, pp. 757–810.

Parihar, A., Coghlan, M., Gopalakrishnan, M. & Shieh, C. (2003). Effects of intermediate-conductance Ca2+-activated K+ channel modulators on human prostate cancer cell proliferation. *The European Journal of Pharmacology.* Vol. 471, pp. 157-164.

Pei, L., Wiser, O., Slavin, A., Mu, D., Powers, S., Jan, L. & Hoey, T. (2003). Oncogenic potential of TASK3 (Kcnk9) depends on K+ channel function. *The Proceedings of the National Academy of Sciences USA.* Vol. 100, pp. 7803-7807.

Per Larsson, K., Hansen, A. & Dissing, S. (2002). The human SH-SY5Y neuroblastoma cell-line expresses a functional P2X7 purinoceptor that modulates voltage-dependent Ca2+ channel function. *Journal of Neurochemistry.* Vol. 83, pp. 285–298.

Pillozzi, S., Brizzi, M., Balzi, M., Crociani, O., Cherubini, A., Guasti, L., Bartolozzi, B., Becchetti, A., Wanke, E., Bernabei, P., Olivotto, M., Pegoraro, L. & Arcangeli, A. (2002). HERG potassium channels are constitutively expressed in primary human acute myeloid leukemias and regulate cell proliferation of normal and leukemic hemopoietic progenitors. *Leukemia.* Vol. 16, pp. 1791-1798.

Plummer, H., Dhar, M., Cekanova, M. & Schuller, H. (2005). Expression of G-protein inwardly rectifying potassium channels (GIRKs) in lung cancer cell lines. *BMC Cancer.* Vol. 5.

Prehn, J., Jordan, J., Ghadge, G., Preis, E., Galindo, M., Roos, R., Krieglstein, J., & Miller, R.(1997). Ca2+ and reactive oxygen species in staurosporine-induced neuronal apoptosis. *Journal of. Neurochemistry,* Vol. 68, pp. 1679–1685.

Preussat, K., Beetz, C., Schrey, M., Kraft, R., Wölfl, S., Kalff, R. & Patt, S. (2003).Expression of voltage-gated potassium channels Kv1.3 and Kv1.5 in human gliomas. *Neuroscience Letters.* Vol. 346, pp. 33-36.

Roberts, T.G., Goulart, B.H., Squitieri, L., Stallings, S.C., Halpern, E.F., Chabner, B.A., Gazelle, G.S., Finkelstein, S.N, & Clark J.W. 2004. Trends in the risk and benefits to patients with cancer participating in phase 1 clinical trials. *The Journal of the American Medical Association,* 292, 2130-2140.

Roger S, Besson P, & Le Guennec JY. (2003). Involvement of a novel fast inward sodium current in the invasion capacity of a breast cancer cell line. *Biochimica et Biophysica Acta,* Vol. 1616, pp. 107–111.

Roger, S., Potier, M., Vandier, C., Besson, P., & Le Guennec, J. (2006) Voltage-gated sodium channels: new targets in cancer therapy? *Current Pharmaceutical Design,* Vol. 12, pp. 3681–3695

Roger, S., Rollin, J., Barascu, A., Besson, P., Raynal, P., Iochmann, S., Lei, M., Bougnoux, P., Gruel, Y. & Le Guennec, J. (2007) Voltage-gated sodium channels potentiate the invasive capacities of human non-small-cell lung cancer cell lines. Int. J. Biochem. *Cell Biology,* Vol. 39, pp. 774–786.

Roman, R., Smith, R., Feranchak, A., Clayton, G., Doctor, R. & Fitz, J. (2001). ClC-2 chloride channels contribute to HTC cell volume homeostasis. *American Journal of Physiology - Gastrointestinal and Liver Physiology.* Vol. 280, pp. G344-G353.

Rosenbaum, S., Tsvieli, R., & Kaspa, R. (1989). Oestrogen stimulates differential transcription of human papillomavirus type 16 in SiHa cervical carcinoma cells. *Journal of General Virology,* Vol. 70, pp. 2227- 2232.

Shao, X., Wu, K., Guo, X., Xie, M., Zhang, J. & Fan, D. (2008). Expression and significance of HERG protein in gastric cancer. *Cancer Biology and Therapy.* Vol. 7, pp. 45-50.

Shew, M., McGlennen, R., Zaidi, N., Westerheim, M., Ireland, M., & Anderson, S. (2002). Oestrogen receptor transcripts associated with cervical human papillomavirus infection. *Sexually Transmited Infections,* Vol. 78, pp. 210-214.

Schönherr, R., Lober, K., & Heinemann, S. (2000). Inhibition of human ether à go-go potassium channels by Ca2+/calmodulin. *EMBO Journal,* Vol. 19, pp. 3263–3271.

Schönherr, R. (2005). Clinical Relevance of Ion Channels for Diagnosis and Therapy of Cancer. *Journal of Membrane Biology,* Vol. 205, pp. 175–184.

Schrey, M., Codina, C., Kraft, R., Beetz, C., Kalff, R., Wölfl, S. & Patt, S. (2002). Molecular characterization of voltage-gated sodium channels in human gliomas. *Neuroreport.* Vol. 13, pp. 2493-2498.

Shuba, Y., Prevarskaya, N., Lemonnier, L., Van, F., Kostyuk, P., Mauroy, B. & Skryma, R. (2000). Volume-regulated chloride conductance in the LNCaP human prostate cancer cell line. *American Journal of Physiology - Cell Physiology.* Vol. 279, pp. C1144-C1154.

Shinohara, T., Takahashi, N., Ooie, T., Ichinose, M., Hara, M., Yonemochi, H., Saikawa, T., & Yoshimatsu, H. (2004). Estrogen inhibits hyperthermia-induced expression of heat-shock protein 72 and cardioprotection against ischemia/reperfusion injury in female rat heart. *Molecular Cell Cardiology,* Vol. 37, pp. 1053–1061.

Smith, G., Tsui, H., Newell, E., Jiang, X., Zhu, X., Tsui, F., Schlichter, L. (2002).Functional up-regulation of HERG K+ channels in neoplastic hematopoietic cells. *The Journal of Biological Chemistry.* Vol. 277, pp. 18528-18534.

Spassova,M., Soboloff, J., He, L., Hewavitharana, T., Xu, W., Venkatachalam, K., van Rossum, D., Patterson, R., & Gill, D. (2004). Calcium entry mediated by SOCs and TRP channels: variations and enigma. *Biochimica et Biophysica Acta,* Vol. 1742, pp. 9–20.

Surprenant, A., Rassendren, F., Kawashima, E., North, R. A., & Buell, G. (1996).The cytolytic P2Z receptor for extracellular ATP identified as a P2X receptor (P2X7). *Science.* Vol. 272, pp. 735–738

Tsavaler, L., Shapero, M., Morkowski, S. & Laus, R. (2001). Trp-p8, a novel prostate-specific gene, is up-regulated in prostate cancer and other malignancies and shares high homology with transient receptor potential calcium channel proteins. *Cancer Research.* Vol. 61, pp. 3760-3769.

Uysal, P. & Djamgoz, M. (2007) Epidermal growth factor potentiates in vitro metastatic behavior of human prostate cancer PC-3 M cells: involvement of voltage-gated sodium channel. *Molecular Cancer,* Vol. 6, pg., 76.

Vanden, F., Shuba, Y., Roudbaraki, M., Lemonnier, L., Vanoverberghe,K., Mariot, P., Skryma, R. &Prevarskaya, N. (2003). Store-operated Ca2+ channels in prostate cancer epithelial cells: function,regulation, and role in carcinogenesis. *Cell Calcium.* Vol. 33, pp. 357-373.

Vermeulen, K., Van, D. & Berneman Z. (2003). The cell cycle: a review of regulation, deregulation and therapeutic targets in cancer. *Cell Proliferation,* Vol. 36, pp. 131–149.

Walboomers JMM, Jacobs MV, Manos MM, Bosch FX, Kummer JA, Shah KV, Snijders PJF, Peto J, Meijer CJLM, & Munoz N (1999). Human papillomavirus is a necessary cause of invasive cervical cancer worldwide *Jorunal of Pathology,* Vol. 189, pp. 12-19.

Wang, H., Zhang, Y., Cao, L., Han, H., Wang, J., Yang, B., Nattel, S., & Wang, Z., (2002). HERG K+ channel, a regulator of tumor cell apoptosis and proliferation. *Cancer Research,* Vol. 62, pp. 4843–4848.

Wang, Z. (2004). Roles of K(+) channels in regulating tumour cell proliferation and apoptosis. *Pflügers Archiv: European Journal of Physiology,* Vol. 448, pp. 274–286.

Wang, Q., Li, X., Wang, L., Feng, Y. H., Zeng, R., & Gorodeski, G. (2004). Antiapoptotic effects of estrogen in normal and cancer human cervical epithelial cells. *Endocrinology,* Vol. 145, pp. 5568–5579.

Wang, X., Nagaba, Y., Cross, H., Wrba, F., Zhang, L. & Guggino, S. (2000). The mRNA of L-type calcium channel elevated in colon cancer: protein distribution in normal and cancerous colon. *American Journal of Pathology.* Vol. 157, pp. 1549-1562.

Whitfield, J., Bird, R., Chakravarthy, B., Isaacs, R., & Morley, P. (1995). Calcium-cell cycle regulator, differentiator, killer, chemopreventor, and maybe, tumor promoter. *Journal of Cellular Biochemistry,* Vol 22, pp. 74–91.

Wiley, J., Dao, L., Gu, B., Sluyter, R., Shemon, A., Li, C., Taper, J., Gallo, J. & Manoharan, A. (2002). A loss-of- function polymorphic mutation in the cytolytic P2X7 receptor gene and chronic lymphocytic leukaemia: a molecular study. *Lancet.* Vol. 359, pp. 1114-1119.

Wonderlin, W., & Strobl, J. (1996). Potassium channels, proliferation and G1 progression. *Journal of Membrane Biology,* Vol. 154, pp. 91–107.

Yamamura, H., Ugawa, S., Ueda, T., Morita, A. & Shimada, S. (2008). TRPM8 activation suppresses cellular viability in human melanoma. *American Journal of Physiology - Cell Physiology.* Vol. 295, pp. C296-C301.

Yang, S.Y., Zhang, J.J.L. & Huang, X.Y. (2009). Orai1 and STIM1 are critical for breast tumor cell migration and metastasis. *Cancer Cell,* Vol. 15, pp. 124-134.

Yu, F. & Catterall, W. (2003). Overview of the voltage-gated sodium channel family. *Genome Biology,.* Vol. 4, pp. 207.

Yuan, P., Leonetti, M., Pico, A., Hsiung, Y., & MacKinnon, R. (2010). Structure of the Human BK Channel Ca^{2+}- Activation Apparatus at 3.0 a Resolution. *Science.* Vol. 329, pp. 182-186.

Zamzami, N., & Kroemer, G. (2005). p53 in apoptosis control: an introduction. *Biochemical and Biophysical Research Communications*, Vol. 331, pp. 685–687.

Zhuang, L., Peng, J., Tou, L., Takanaga, H., Adam, R., Hediger, M. & Freeman, M. (2002).Calcium-selective ion channel, CaT1, is apically localized in gastrointestinal tract epithelia and is aberrantly expressed in human malignancies. *Laboratory Investigations*. Vol. 82, pp. 1755-1764.

zur Hausen H (2002) Papillomaviruses and cancer: from basic studies to clinical applications *Nature Reviews Cancer,* Vol. 2, pp. 342-350.

Zylicz, M., King, F.W., & Wawrzynow, A. (2001). Hsp70 interactions with the p53 tumour suppressor protein. *EMBO Journal,* Vol. 20, pp. 4634–4638

7

Analysis Models for HPV-Related Pathobiology

Águeda Buitrago-Pérez, Jesús M. Paramio and Ramón García-Escudero
Molecular Oncology Unit, Dept. of Basic Research, CIEMAT, Madrid
Spain

1. Introduction

Human papillomaviruses (HPV) are involved in the aetiology of human carcinomas arising in different anatomical locations such as skin, anogenital region and oropharynx (Marur et al., 2010; Pfister, 2003; zur Hausen, 2002). The virus infects stratified epithelia of these locations, producing new infectious viral particles. HPV life cycle is intimately dependant of a proper squamous cell differentiation, so simple cell culture systems are unable to recapitulate essential processes for a complete virus replication. Mucosal HPVs are responsible of benign lesions and carcinomas of the anogenital region and oropharynx. There are a few types of mucosal HPVs that are present in cancers in these anatomical locations, and they are called high-risk types (mainly HPV types 16 and 18) (de Sanjose et al., 2010). Furthermore, low-risk mucosal HPV types are responsible of frequent benign lesions in the same locations (mainly HPV types 6 and 11) (zur Hausen, 2002). Although these HPV-lesions (condylomas and respiratory papillomatosis) do not evolve normally to overt tumours, they are difficult to treat.

Cervical cancer is the second leading cause of deaths by cancer in women worldwide, representing an important disease in developing countries. The vast majority of cervical carcinomas (about 85%) are infected with high-risk HPVs, so viral infection is considered the major main etiological agent of this malignancy (de Sanjose et al., 2010). Head and neck squamous cell carcinoma (HNSCC) is the sixth most common cancer worldwide. An important proportion of human HNSCC are infected with high-risk HPV (about 20%), especially in the oropharynx, where about 50% of the cancers have been found to harbour viral DNA (Marur et al., 2010). HNSCC is etiologically associated with tobacco use and alcohol consumption. Epidemiological and molecular studies have suggested than HPV-negative and HPV-positive tumours represent different subtypes of HNSCC with different clinical consequences. The infected HNSCC display a better clinical outcome after treatment with radio or chemotherapy.

Cutaneous HPVs, similarly to mucosal viruses, are associated to benign lesions (such as skin warts) or premalignant actinic keratosis or squamous cell carcinomas (SCC), especially in patients of the rare genodermatosis Epidermodysplasia verruciformis (EV) or in organ transplant recipients (OTRs) (Pfister, 2003). In these patient populations, the infection with certain HPV types, belonging to the beta family (beta-HPVs), is clearly associated with the appearance of those skin pathologies, mostly in sun exposed areas of the body. Although the majority of cervical carcinomas are produced by 2 major HPV types (HPV16 and

HPV18), epidemiological studies have demonstrated that SCCs arising in papillomavirus-infected skin are associated to diverse HPV types, and that multiple infections frequently appear in a single sample (Berkhout et al., 2000; Harwood et al., 2000). Collectively these epidemiological data show that the infection with HPV is associated with a relevant number of human malignancies, and the finding of effective anti-HPV therapies represents an important medical challenge.

The most important high-risk HPV genes involved in carcinogenesis are the E6 and E7 early genes, as they are expressed in pretumoral and invasive cervical carcinomas. Importantly, a number of cellular targets for E6 and E7 have been described so far, some of which may be functionally inactivated *in vivo*, giving to the appearance of malignant cervical tumours. Tumour suppressors targeted by virus oncogenes are the retinoblastoma protein (pRb) and p53, which are inhibited by high-risk HPV E7 and E6 virus oncogenes, respectively (Dyson et al., 1989; Werness et al., 1990). E7 protein from HPV16 binds directly the 3 members of the retinoblastoma protein family: pRb, p107 and p130. Upon interaction, these proteins are targeted for degradation (Boyer et al., 1996; Gonzalez et al., 2001), releasing the transcription factor complex E2F that induces the expression of genes involved in G1-S transition, thereby activating cellular proliferation. HPV16 E7 protein can also inhibit other negative regulators of the cell cycle, such as $p21^{cip1}$ thought direct binding (Funk et al., 1997; Helt et al., 2002; Jones et al., 1997). Although the virus DNA is normally maintained in the basal cells as an episome, during the malignant transformation of cervical lesions both E6 and E7 are integrated into the cellular genome (Smith et al., 1992), concomitantly with a more efficient oncogene expression. The interaction with pRb, p53 and $p21^{cip1}$ tumour suppressors, and additional targets or/and genetic alterations may eventually transform infected cells and induce the formation of invasive carcinomas. Cutaneous betaHPVs are thought to act by potentiating the harmful effects of UV radiation, for example by impairing DNA repair and apoptosis following UV-induced damage through E6 molecular activities (Akgul et al., 2005; Giampieri et al., 2004; Jackson et al., 2000; Jackson & Storey, 2000). Mucosal high-risk HPVs could possibly act together with steroid hormone signalling and/or tobacco consumption (Moreno et al., 2002; Munoz et al., 2002). Finally, immunosupression also contributes to carcinoma progression, especially for skin SCCs.

2. HPV analysis models

In order to recapitulate virus life cycle towards virion production, or to analyze the phenotypical and molecular consequences of the expression of HPV genes in stratified epithelia, several models have been described. Organotypic (raft) cultures of skin where first described in 1988 to partially recapitulate the differentiation defects of human biopsies of cervical intraepithelial neoplasia (CIN) lesions, which are the precursor lesions of invasive HPV-related cervical cancers (McCance et al., 1988). The system provides an *in vitro* assay where primary human foreskin epithelial cells, seeded onto a collagen matrix, are forced to differentiate and reconstitute human skin (Asselineau & Prunieras, 1984; Kopan et al., 1987). On the other hand, transgenic mouse models expressing HPV genes have demonstrated the oncogenic activities of some early viral genes, mainly E6 an E7 (Griep et al., 1993). Viral transgenes have been expressed under the control of the K14 promoter, normally expressed in the basal layer of mouse stratified epithelia (Arbeit et al., 1994). Advantages and disadvantages of both model systems will be described below. Furthermore, we perform a comparison of the HPV-mouse models with transgenic mice with conditional expression of the host genes normally targeted by virus oncogenes, and whose functional inactivation is essentially involved in virus carcinogenesis, such as retinoblastoma proteins or $p21^{cip1}$ (targeted by E7) and p53 (targeted by E6).

2.1 Organotypic (raft) cultures and HPV

Raft cultures allow primary human keratinocytes (PHK) to achieve stratification and differentiation morphologically similar to foreskin (Asselineau & Prunieras, 1984; Kopan et al., 1987). In this system, PHK cells are seeded on a dermal equivalent consisting of a porous collagen gel containing fibroblasts. At confluence, the assembly is raised to the medium-air interface. The keratinocytes stratify and exhibit a differentiated morphology, generating a living skin equivalent. This system was originally used to study the features of HPV-immortalized cell lines or cell lines obtained from cervical pathological biopsies (Blanton et al., 1991; McCance et al., 1988; Woodworth et al., 1992). These early studies demonstrated altered differentiation patterns and morphological features resembling human cervical neoplasia such as suprabasal mitosis, enlarged nuclei, abnormal mitotic figures, or koilocytosis. Later, rafts were used to produce virus particles using different strategies. Thus, Meyers et al. were able to produce virions using raft cultures of the cell line CIN-612 treated with TPA (Meyers et al., 1992). Similarly, mature particles were obtained from condyloma containing HPV11 explanted on rafts (Dollard et al., 1992).

The raft culture system has been an essential tool to analyze some of the molecular functions and consequences of the expression of E6 and E7 oncogenes from high-risk mucosal HPVs. Using retrovirally infected PHKs, it was demonstrated that E7 was able to induce DNA replication in suprabasal differentiated keratinocytes (Cheng et al., 1995), an activity directly linked to the capacity of binding retinoblastoma family or "pocket" proteins, as demonstrated by using E7 mutant proteins. Furthermore, most of the morphological features observed using HPV-cell lines where reproduced expressing E7 protein, and more clearly, with the combined expression of E6 and E7 oncogenes.

Recently, a system to produce autonomous HPV-18 genomes and high titer, mature virus particles was described using Cre-loxP-mediated recombination and organotypic cultures of PHKs (Wang et al., 2009). Interestingly, the method showed that E6 protein, and thus p53 degradation, was necessary to obtain a productive HPV program, including viral DNA amplification and production of virus capsid protein L1.

2.2 Mouse models of HPV-mediated carcinogenesis

Transgenic mouse models have been frequently used to analyze the molecular and phenotypic consequences of the expression of oncogenes in tumour development. Early studies demonstrated that E6 and E7 early genes from HPV16 induced tumours when the expression was targeted to the ocular lens (Griep et al., 1993), or the skin of transgenic mice (Arbeit et al., 1994; Lambert et al., 1993). These studies contributed importantly to the establishment that E6 and E7 genes are directly implicated in the carcinogenic potential of HPV16 in an animal model. Furthermore, they opened new and important research areas that have significantly contributed to the understanding of the molecular activities of both oncogenes in the context of HPV-associated carcinogenesis. Additionally, similar mouse models using early genes from cutaneous HPVs, associated with human skin SCC, have also helped to demonstrate their carcinogenic potential (Dong et al., 2005; Schaper et al., 2005).

Transgenic mouse containing the E6 and E7 genes from HPV16 under the control of the human keratin 14 (K14) allow expression of the virus genes in stratified epithelia, such as skin or mucosal tissues. Reproducible multi-stage progression from hyperplastic and/or dysplastic lesions to squamous cell carcinomas of the epidermis was observed in K14-16E6E7 animals (Arbeit et al., 1994; Coussens et al., 1996). Concomitant with tumour progression, a disorganization of the normal differentiation was observed based of histological analysis and expression patterns of keratin markers such as keratin 5 (K5, normally expressed in basal cells), keratin 10 (K10, normally expressed in spinous cells) and filaggrin (normally expressed in granular cells). Furthermore, proliferative cells appeared ectopically in suprabasal cells and the mitotic index was augmented in premalignant and malignant skin lesions.

Herber et al reported in 1996 the first experimental evidence that the E7 protein from HPV16 is able to induce carcinogenesis in an animal model (Herber et al., 1996). Histological analysis of K14-16E7 mice demonstrated that E7 causes epidermal hyperplasia in skin, but also in mouth palate, oesophagus, forestomach and exocervix. Late in life, K14-16E7 animals develop highly differentiated and locally invasive skin carcinomas. Also, expression of E6 in K14-16E6 mice not only increased cell proliferation and induced epidermal hyperplasia, but also leads the development of skin tumours (Song et al., 1999). In contrast to the tumours derived from K14-16E7 transgenic mice, which were primarily benign, those appearing in K14-16E6 transgenic mice were mostly malignant, indicating that E6 alone not only is sufficient to induce tumour development but it also confers increased malignant potential *in vivo*.

The mouse models above described recapitulated in the skin the pathological features observed in human CIN lesions and cervical carcinomas. Moreover, these models demonstrate that most of these features are due to the expression of E6 and E7 HPV16 oncogenes. However, the K14-HPV16 animals did not develop spontaneous tumours in the cervix nor in the head and neck region. Importantly, Arbeit et al demonstrated that chronic estrogen administration induced cervico-vaginal squamous carcinomas in K14-16E6E7 animals (Arbeit et al., 1996). Previous epidemiological analyses already showed that the prolonged use of contraceptives, most of which contain estrogen, did double the risk of HPV neoplasia and malignancy (Brisson et al., 1994). Importantly, no control animals neither K14-16E6E7 mice develop pathological neoplasias or carcinomas, demonstrating for the first time a synergism between estrogens and HPV oncogenes in cervical carcinogenesis.

Human HNSCC is associated with tobacco use, and an important proportion of tumours are HPV-infected. Strati et al demonstrated that K14-HPV16 animals, when treated with the chemical carcinogen 4-nitroquinoline 1-oxide (4NQO), increased dramatically the animal's susceptibility to HNSCC (Strati et al., 2006). 4NQO causes a spectrum of DNA damage similar to that caused by tobacco-associated carcinogens, and it induces cancers in the oral cavity in rodents when it is supplied in their drinking water. 4NQO-treated, HPV16-transgenic mice developed HNSCC at a much higher frequency than no transgenic mice, and display tumours with molecular characteristics similar to the human counterparts.

Cutaneous beta-HPVs are associated with actinic keratosis and skin SCCs in immunocompetent but mainly in immunosupressed patients, such as OTR. Some of these viruses (HPV5 and HPV8) were originally described in EV patients (Jablonska & Majewski, 1994; Lutzner et al., 1984), but these and other beta-HPVs have been generally associated to human skin cancer. As for high-risk mucosal HPVs, transgenic mouse models have been generated in order to analyze the carcinogenic properties of cutaneous HPVs. Schaper et al demonstrated that the early region of HPV8, containing the E2, E6 and E7 genes, was able to induce single or multifocal tumours in 91% of K14-HPV8 animals and skin carcinomas in 6% of all examined mice (Schaper et al., 2005). This report was the first experimental proof of the carcinogenic potential of an EV-associated HPV type *in vivo*. A few months later, Dong et al described skin hyperproliferation and susceptibility to chemical carcinogenesis in transgenic mice expressing the E6 and E7 genes of HPV38 (another EV-associated beta-HPV) under the control of the bovine homolog of human keratin 10 (K10) promoter (Dong et al., 2005). Although transgenic K10-HPV38 mice did not develop spontaneous tumours, two-stage carcinogenesis protocols led to a high incidence of papillomas, keratoacanthomas and SCC in the transgenic mouse skin compared with nontransgenic control mice. These results showed HPV38 E6 and E7 display transforming properties *in vivo*.

3. Synergism and individual contribution of E6 and E7 oncogenes to HPV16-induced carcinogenesis

K14-HPV16 transgenic animals have been valuable tools to demonstrate the essential role of virus E6 and E7 oncogenes in stratified epithelia carcinogenesis. The individual contribution of both genes as well as the synergism has been studied for carcinoma models in skin, cervix and head and neck. Thus, E6 is the most important oncogene in skin cancer as the tumours arising are more malignant than those that appeared in K14-16E7 animals (Song et al., 2000; Song et al., 1999) (Fig. 1). An analysis including chemical carcinogenesis with DMBA/TPA demonstrated that E6 acts weakly at the promotion stage of carcinogenesis in the formation of benign tumours, but strongly at the progression stage, which involves the malignant conversion of these benign tumours (Song et al., 1999). In contrast, E7 primarily affected the promotion stage of carcinogenesis. These results provide direct evidence that E6 and E7 contribute differently to carcinogenesis; E7 promotes the formation of benign tumours, and E6 acts primarily to accelerate progression of these benign tumours to the malignant stage. Consistent with this model, the authors found that E6 and E7 cooperated in inducing tumour formation in mice expressing both oncogenes.

In the case of estrogen induced cervical carcinomas in K14-HPV16 animals, E7 was found to be the most important oncogene (Fig. 1). Importantly, although p53 levels were eliminated in cervical epithelium of estrogen treated K14-16E6 mice, neither neoplasia nor cancer was observed. Again, a synergism was observed with both E6 and E7 oncogenes, giving rise to large, extensively invasive cancers (Riley et al., 2003).

Similarly, the individual contribution of each virus oncogene was analyzed in the HNSCC model of K14-HPV16 animals. The results demonstrated that E7 is the major transforming oncogene in HPV-associated HNSCC, whereas E6 is more likely to play a secondary role in contributing to later stages of carcinogenesis (Strati & Lambert, 2007) (Fig. 1). As described above for skin and cervical carcinogenesis, again both E6 and E7 oncogenes act synergistically to produce a higher grade of disease and slightly increased tumour multiplicity.

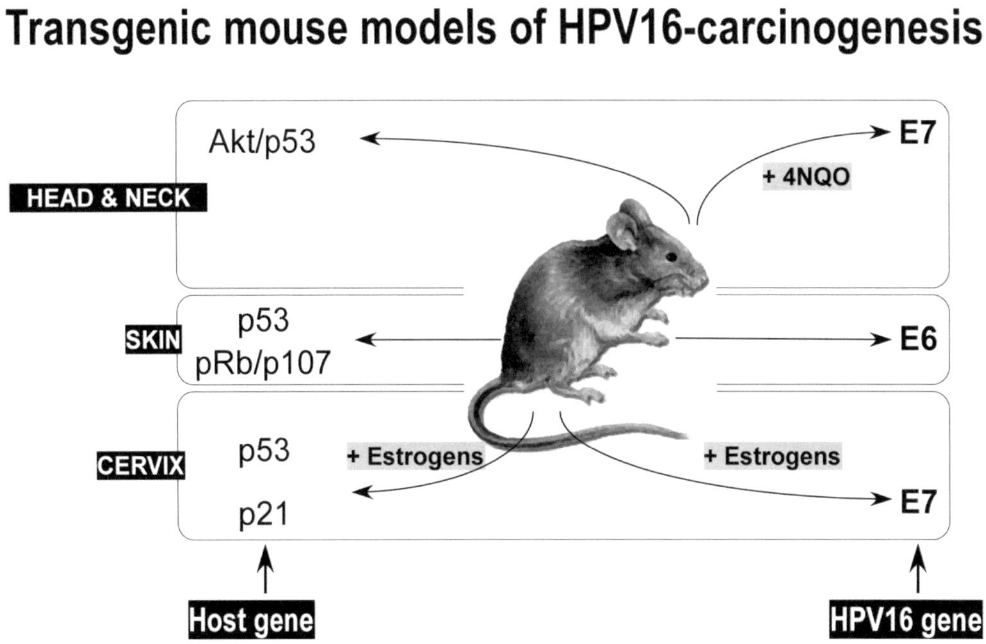

Fig. 1. Transgenic mouse models of HPV16-carcinogenesis. K14-HPV16 mouse models develop carcinomas in the head and neck region, skin, and cervix. While spontaneous tumors arise in the skin, HNSCCs appear in cooperation with the 4NQO carcinogen, and cervical carcinomas in cooperation with estrogens. Characterization of K14-16E6, K14-16E7, and K14-16E6E7 mice have demonstrated that E6 is the main virus oncogene in skin SCC, and E7 in HNSCC and cervical carcinoma. On the other hand, transgenic animals with deletion in HPV-cellular targets have demonstrated that p53 or pRb/p107 are major tumor supressors in skin. In the presence of estrogens, deletions of p53 or p21 give rise to carcinogenesis in the mouse cervix. Finally, continuous activation of Akt in the absence of p53 induces spontaneous carcinomas in the head and neck region. For references, see text.

4. Role of cellular targets of HPV oncogenes in carcinogenesis

A number of cellular proteins are targets of HPV oncogenes. However, the real contribution of these targets in human pathology during the carcinogenesis process is not completely understood. Compelling evidences have demonstrated that p53 and pRb are the major cellular targets of high-risk HPV E6 and E7 oncogenes, respectively. The role of both cellular proteins as tumour suppressors in the vast majority of human cancer has been fully established. However, the importance of their inhibition during the carcinogenesis associated to HPV-infection has not been completely characterized. K14-HPV16 models have demonstrated that E7 is the main oncogene in HNSCC and cervical cancer, but in skin tumour formation only participated at the initiation step. Interestingly, both E6 and E7 oncogenes act synergistically to induce tumour formation and malignancy in the three types of cancer.

4.1 Skin cancer

In relation with skin cancer, mouse models with conditional somatic deletion of pRb and/or p53 have been characterized. The elimination of pRb in the epidermis of transgenic mice using the Cre-lox system (K14Cre;Rb$^{loxP/loxP}$) produces hyperplasia, altered differentiation and ectopic suprabasal proliferation in the skin (Balsitis et al., 2003; Ruiz et al., 2004) but not spontaneous tumours. This phenotype resembles the epidermal histological features of K14-16E7 animals, which is in line with the inactivation of pRb due to E7 expression (Balsitis et al., 2003). However, when both E7 was expressed and Rb was deleted in the same tissue, increased hyperplasia and dysplasia were observed, suggesting that E7 possesses pRb-independent effects. E7 protein from HPV16 is also able to inactivate the other two members of the retinoblastoma family, p107 and p130. It is tempting to speculate that the epidermal phenotype observed in K14-16E7 animals could be partially due to inactivation of pRb, but also of p107 and/or p130. Interestingly, we have previously demonstrated that the absence of p107 alleles in K14Cre;Rb$^{loxP/loxP}$ mice (K14Cre;Rb$^{loxP/loxP}$;p107-/-) increased the K14Cre;Rb$^{loxP/loxP}$ epidermal phenotype with augmented hyperplasia, proliferation and altered differentiation (Lara et al., 2008a; Ruiz et al., 2004), which was associated to a equivalent increase in the expression of pRb-dependent gene expression program (Lara et al., 2008a; Ruiz et al., 2004). However, we were not able to observe an increase in the K14Cre;Rb$^{loxP/loxP}$ epidermal phenotype in K14Cre;Rb$^{loxP/loxP}$;p130-/- animals, suggesting that p107 (and not p130) could functionally compensate some of the pRb-dependent functions. Although K14Cre;Rb$^{loxP/loxP}$;p107-/- animals died soon after birth, thus precluding analysis of phenotype in adult animals, we were able to analyze the consequences of somatic inactivation of both pRb and p107 by transplanting K14Cre;Rb$^{loxP/loxP}$;p107-/- neonatal skin onto immunodeficient *NOD/Scid* mice. The grafted transgenic skin develops well differentiated SCC, characterized by a reduced apoptosis possibly due to a defective p53 pathway (Lara et al., 2008b) (Fig. 1). Moreover, the K14Cre;Rb$^{loxP/loxP}$;p130-/- mice do not develop spontaneous tumours with age. Altogether, these data suggest that the spontaneous skin SCCs that appear in K14-16E7 animals could be due to simultaneous inactivation of pRb and p107 in the epidermis, although inactivation of all three pocket proteins cannot be discarded. In this regard, the elimination of p130 and p107 also produces severe skin defects, indicating that these two proteins also exert overlapping functions that cannot be carried out by pRb in epidermis (Ruiz et al., 2003).

In relation with p53, others and we have demonstrated that p53 is a major tumour suppressor in skin (Jonkers et al., 2001; Martinez-Cruz et al., 2008) (Fig. 1). When K14Cre;Rb$^{loxP/loxP}$ animals were treated with the DMBA/TPA chemical carcinogenesis protocol, they display reduced number and smaller tumours than the control, Rb$^{loxP/loxP}$ littermates. However, these tumours also displayed a more malignant phenotype partially due to the absence of p53 (Ruiz et al., 2005). These results strongly suggested that p53, in the absence of pRb, had compensatory tumour suppressor activities. The essential role of p53 as a tumour suppressor in skin was fully demonstrated when analyzing K14Cre;p53$^{loxP/loxP}$ and K14Cre;Rb$^{loxP/loxP}$;p53$^{loxP/loxP}$ animals. Both transgenic animals developed spontaneous tumours in the skin with full penetrance, although the onset was earlier in the case of double conditional knock-out (Martinez-Cruz et al., 2008). No major differences were observed in overt tumours, which were characterized as moderately differentiated or undifferentiated, locally aggressive and metastatic. Interestingly, the gene expression pattern of tumours from both mouse genotypes resembles that of human tumours with mutations in p53 (Garcia-Escudero et al., 2010). As previously described, K14-16E6 mice develop spontaneous tumours with a more aggressive behaviour than K14-16E7 tumours. Altogether the results would indicate that E6 is the most important HPV oncogene in skin as it is able to inhibit p53, a predominant tumour suppressor in skin.

Finally, p53-independent activities have been described for E6 in skin. Numerous cellular proteins interact with E6. One group of proteins, the PDZ partners (including hDLG, hSCRIBBLE, MUPP1, and MAGI) interact to the C-terminal four amino acids of E6 through their PDZ domains, leading to their degradation. Additionally, E6's binding to PDZ proteins may explain the E6 ability to transform cells in tissue culture and to confer tumorigenicity to cells in xenograft experiments (Kiyono et al., 1997). Mice with a mutant of E6 lacking the last six amino acids of its carboxyl terminus (K14-16E6$^{\Delta 146\text{-}151}$) were generated, and allowed to demonstrate that the ability of E6 to bind PDZ domain partners is necessary for E6 to confer epithelial hyperproliferation *in vivo*. The K14-16E6$^{\Delta 146\text{-}151}$ mice exhibit a radiation response similar to that of the K14-16E6 mice, demonstrating that this protein, as predicted, retained an ability to inactivate p53.

4.2 Cervical cancer

Using K14-HPV16 transgenic mice and estrogen treatment, mouse models have demonstrated an essential contribution of the E7 oncogene in cervical cancer. Furthermore, repression of the E7 oncogene efficiently cleared already established carcinomas. In order to elucidate the role of pRb in suppression of cervical cancer, K14Cre;Rb$^{loxP/loxP}$ animal were hormone treated. The results demonstrated no carcinoma formation, suggesting that pRb-independent activities are exerted by E7. Further evidence was provided by the generation of Rb$^{\Delta L/\Delta L}$ mice. This gene construct bears three alanine mutations in pRb that interact with E7, thereby producing a mutant pRb protein that fails to bind E7 (Lee et al., 1998). On the other hand pRb$^{\Delta L}$ retains the ability to bind E2Fs, induces G1 arrest in pRb-negative SAOS2 cells, and is phosphorylated and inactivated by cyclin D/cdk4 complexes similarly to wt pRb (Dick et al., 2000). pRb$^{\Delta L}$ also represses gene expression from E2F-responsive promoter constructs, although incrementally less effectively than wt pRb. On the other hand, pRb$^{\Delta L}$ fails to bind cellular LxCxE motif-containing proteins, and pRb$^{\Delta L}$ -induced G1 arrest cannot be reversed by expression of HPV-16 or HPV-18 E7 (Dick et al., 2000; Isaac et al., 2006). K14E7Rb$^{\Delta L/\Delta L}$ mice were used to analyze cervical carcinoma formation. The development of spontaneous tumours indicates, again, that other molecular activities of E7, independent of pRb, make critical contributions to cervical carcinogenesis. Although the role in cervical carcinogenesis has not been tested, it is possible that p107 may act as a tumour suppressor in this tissue in the absence of pRb, as we have been demonstrated for skin SCC (Lara et al., 2008b). However, we cannot discard an essential role of other tumour suppressors, such as p130 or p21^{Cip1}, also targeted by high-risk E7.

Using knock-out animals, Shin et al described that cervical disease was significantly increased in p21 -/- mice compared with p21+/+ mice, showing that p21^{Cip1} can function as a tumour suppressor in this tissue (Shin et al., 2009) (Fig. 1). Importantly, the induction of cervical cancers by E7 was not increased in the absence of p21^{Cip1}, arguing against the hypothesis that the ability of E7 to inhibit p21^{Cip1} contributes to carcinogenesis. However, cervical carcinogenesis in mice expressing a mutant form of HPV-16 E7, $E7^{CVQ}$, which cannot inactivate $p21^{Cip1}$, was reduced when compared with that in K14-16E7 mice. Nonetheless, K14-16$E7^{CVQ}$ mice still displayed augmented levels of cervical carcinogenesis compared with non-transgenic mice, indicating that activities of E7, besides its capacity to inactivate $p21^{Cip1}$, also contribute to cervical carcinogenesis.

The interaction of E6 with many cellular proteins, including p53, leads to their destabilization. This property is mediated, at least in part, through the ability of E6 to recruit the ubiquitin ligase E6-associated protein (E6AP) into complexes with these cellular proteins, resulting in their ubiquitin-mediated degradation by the proteasome pathway. Shai et al addressed the requirement for E6AP in mediating acute and oncogenic phenotypes of E6, including induction of epithelial hyperplasia, abrogation of DNA damage response, and induction of cervical cancer (Shai et al., 2010). Loss of E6AP had no discernible effect on the ability of E6 to induce hyperplasia or abrogate DNA damage responses. Nevertheless, in cervical carcinogenesis studies, there was a complete loss of the oncogenic potential of E6 in E6AP-null mice. Thus, E6AP is absolutely required for E6 to cause cervical cancer. However, when K14Cre;$p53^{loxP/loxP}$ were treated with estrogen, nearly all mice developed cervical cancer, in sharp contrast to its complete absence in treated K14-16E6; $p53^{loxP/loxP}$ mice, indicating that HPV16 E6 must only partially inactivate p53 (Shai et al., 2008) (Fig. 1). p53-independent activities of E6 also contributed to carcinogenesis, but these activities were manifested only in the presence of the HPV16 E7 oncogene.

4.3 Head and neck squamous cell carcinoma

Individual and synergistic contributions of E6 and E7 oncogenes were also determined in a mouse model for human HNSCC where K14-HPV16 animals are treated with the 4NQO carcinogen. The results showed that E7 is the major oncogene (Strati & Lambert, 2007) in HPV-associated HNSCC, whereas E6 is more likely to play a secondary role in contributing to later stages of carcinogenesis. Mutations in p53 have been described in about 50% of human HNSCC, demonstrating that the inactivation of the p53 pathway is a highly relevant molecular event for carcinogenesis in this region. In the case of HPV-infected HNSCC, the frequency of mutations is very low as E6 would be able to inhibit p53 function. However, we have recently described a mouse model where an active form of the Akt1 kinase (myr-Akt) expressed in stratified epithelia under the control of the keratin 5 (K5) promoter is able, in the absence of p53 (K5myrAkt;K14Cre;$p53^{loxP/loxP}$), to induce HNSCC (Moral et al., 2009) (Fig. 1). This mouse model recapitulates most of the pathological features of human HNSCC, such as local lymph node metastasis. The results corroborate the epidemiological studies about the role of p53 in human HNSCC, as K5myrAkt animals display significant reduction in the development of overt tumours although they display high number of pretumoral lesions and also display increased susceptibility to chemical carcinogenesis protocols (Moral et al., 2009; Segrelles et al., 2007). Possibly, the treatment with 4NQO induces mutations that inactivate the p53 pathway, thus explaining the secondary role of E6 in the HPV-associated HNSCC mouse model. Alternatively, the E6 protein may not completely inactivate p53 in head and neck, as suggested before in the case of cervical cancer (Shai et al., 2008).

Furthermore, a conditional deletion of pRb did not recapitulate all E7-mediated cancer phenotypes in HNSCC (Strati & Lambert, 2007). As in the case of cervical cancer mouse models, the results highlight the importance of pRb-independent functions of E7 in head and neck carcinogenesis, although do not preclude an important role for the E7-pRb interaction.

5. Analysis of preclinical therapies in the mouse cervical cancer model

Interfering with the expression of E7 in HPV-positive cell lines derived from human cervical cancers inhibits their ability to proliferate, indicating that the expression of E7 is important in maintaining the transformed phenotype *in vitro*. Accordingly, *in vivo* experiments using transgenic mice with inducible repression of the E7 oncogene of HPV16 demonstrated that E7 expression in estrogen induced cervical carcinomas is necessary to maintain established tumours and high-grade cervical dysplasia (Jabbar et al., 2009). The results obtained suggest that E7 is a relevant target nor only for anticancer therapy but also for the treatment of HPV-positive dysplastic cervical lesions.

Mouse models of human cancer are necessary tools to understand basic processes of carcinogenesis in a living organism, but also as tools to analyze preclinical therapies. In this sense, Chung et al have recently described that estrogen receptor antagonists are effective preventive and therapeutic drugs in mouse models of cervical cancer (Chung & Lambert, 2009). The authors demonstrated that ICI 182, 780 (a complete ER antagonist) and raloxifene (a selective ER modulator) efficiently clear cancer and precursor lesions in both the cervix and the vagina. Importantly, these findings suggest that ER antagonists could help to control this gynecological disease of the women lower reproductive tract.

6. Conclusion

Analysis models of HPV based on organotypic cultures of human skin or transgenic mice have helped to understand the function and carcinogenesis role of HPV oncogenes. Thus, the role of E6 and E7 as major oncogenes has been established and the contribution of each of them, as well other cofactors, has been analyzed. Human cancers associated with HPV-infection are multifactorial diseases, in which genetic predisposition, tobacco or estrogen consumption, radiation exposure, or immunosuppression are factors that could contribute to its appearance or development. In K14-HPV16 animal models, E7 is the most important virus oncogene for cervical cancer and HNSCC. Although pRb is the major E7 target, there are pRb-independent functions for E7-mediated carcinogenesis. In the case of skin SCC, E6 gives rise to more malignant tumours that E7, which coincides with a role of p53 as an important tumour suppressor in K14Cre;p53$^{loxP/loxP}$ animals. Furthermore, these p53 mutant mice develop aggressive tumours in skin and cervical cancer models with high penetrance, showing that E6 from HPV16 is not able to completely inactivate p53. On the other hand, transgenic mice have helped to demonstrate tumorigenic activity of cutaneous beta-HPV oncogenes *in vivo*, for the first time.

Human papillomaviruses are infectious agents with clinical importance. Although already developed vaccines are a preventive treatment against non-malignant and malignant virus-associated lesions, new HPV therapies are necessary for already infected people. In this sense, raft cultures have the advantage that they are done with PHKs (the proper cellular target and species of HPV-infection), but the disadvantage that the time window to test therapies is limited to a few days. On the other hand, mouse models allow testing long-term effects of new possible anti-HPV treatments in a living organism, but the differences between mouse and human species must to be taken into account. Future models, able to bypass these drawbacks must be developed in the future for a better success in preclinical analysis, thus delivering new effective treatments to HPV-pathologies in the future.

7. Acknowledgments

Grant support: Ministerio de Ciencia e Innovación (MICINN) grant SAF2008-0121, Comunidad Autónoma de Madrid Oncocycle Program Grant S2006/BIO-0232, Ministerio de Sanidad y Consumo grant ISCIII-RETIC RD06/0020/0029 and from Fundación Sandra Ibarra Para la Investigación del Cáncer de Mama.

8. References

Akgul, B., Lemme, W., Garcia-Escudero, R., Storey, A. & Pfister, H. J. (2005). UV-B irradiation stimulates the promoter activity of the high-risk, cutaneous human papillomavirus 5 and 8 in primary keratinocytes. *Arch Virol* 150(1), 145-51.

Arbeit, J. M., Howley, P. M. & Hanahan, D. (1996). Chronic estrogen-induced cervical and vaginal squamous carcinogenesis in human papillomavirus type 16 transgenic mice. *Proc Natl Acad Sci U S A* 93(7), 2930-5.

Arbeit, J. M., Munger, K., Howley, P. M. & Hanahan, D. (1994). Progressive squamous epithelial neoplasia in K14-human papillomavirus type 16 transgenic mice. *J Virol* 68(7), 4358-68.

Asselineau, D. & Prunieras, M. (1984). Reconstruction of 'simplified' skin: control of fabrication. *Br J Dermatol* 111 Suppl 27, 219-22.

Balsitis, S. J., Sage, J., Duensing, S., Munger, K., Jacks, T. & Lambert, P. F. (2003). Recapitulation of the effects of the human papillomavirus type 16 E7 oncogene on mouse epithelium by somatic Rb deletion and detection of pRb-independent effects of E7 in vivo. *Mol Cell Biol* 23(24), 9094-103.

Berkhout, R. J., Bouwes Bavinck, J. N. & ter Schegget, J. (2000). Persistence of human papillomavirus DNA in benign and (pre)malignant skin lesions from renal transplant recipients. *J Clin Microbiol* 38(6), 2087-96.

Blanton, R. A., Perez-Reyes, N., Merrick, D. T. & McDougall, J. K. (1991). Epithelial cells immortalized by human papillomaviruses have premalignant characteristics in organotypic culture. *Am J Pathol* 138(3), 673-85.

Boyer, S. N., Wazer, D. E. & Band, V. (1996). E7 protein of human papilloma virus-16 induces degradation of retinoblastoma protein through the ubiquitin-proteasome pathway. *Cancer Res* 56(20), 4620-4.

Brisson, J., Morin, C., Fortier, M., Roy, M., Bouchard, C., Leclerc, J., Christen, A., Guimont, C., Penault, F. & Meisels, A. (1994). Risk factors for cervical intraepithelial neoplasia: differences between low- and high-grade lesions. *Am J Epidemiol* 140(8), 700-10.

Cheng, S., Schmidt-Grimminger, D. C., Murant, T., Broker, T. R. & Chow, L. T. (1995). Differentiation-dependent up-regulation of the human papillomavirus E7 gene reactivates cellular DNA replication in suprabasal differentiated keratinocytes. *Genes Dev* 9(19), 2335-49.

Chung, S. H. & Lambert, P. F. (2009). Prevention and treatment of cervical cancer in mice using estrogen receptor antagonists. *Proc Natl Acad Sci U S A* 106(46), 19467-72.

Coussens, L. M., Hanahan, D. & Arbeit, J. M. (1996). Genetic predisposition and parameters of malignant progression in K14-HPV16 transgenic mice. *Am J Pathol* 149(6), 1899-917. de Sanjose, S., Quint, W. G., Alemany, L., Geraets, D. T., Klaustermeier, J. E., Lloveras, B., Tous, S., Felix, A., Bravo, L. E., Shin, H. R., Vallejos, C. S., de Ruiz, P. A., Lima, M. A., Guimera, N., Clavero, O., Alejo, M., Llombart-Bosch, A., Cheng-Yang, C., Tatti, S. A., Kasamatsu, E., Iljazovic, E., Odida, M., Prado, R., Seoud, M., Grce, M., Usubutun, A., Jain, A., Suarez, G. A., Lombardi, L. E., Banjo, A., Menendez, C., Domingo, E. J., Velasco, J., Nessa, A., Chichareon, S. C., Qiao, Y. L., Lerma, E., Garland, S. M., Sasagawa, T., Ferrera, A., Hammouda, D., Mariani, L., Pelayo, A., Steiner, I., Oliva, E., Meijer, C. J., Al-Jassar, W. F., Cruz, E., Wright, T. C., Puras, A., Llave, C. L., Tzardi, M., Agorastos, T., Garcia-Barriola, V., Clavel, C., Ordi, J., Andujar, M., Castellsague, X., Sanchez, G. I., Nowakowski, A. M., Bornstein, J., Munoz, N. & Bosch, F. X. (2010). Human papillomavirus genotype attribution in invasive cervical cancer: a retrospective cross-sectional worldwide study. *Lancet Oncol* 11(11), 1048-56.

Dick, F. A., Sailhamer, E. & Dyson, N. J. (2000). Mutagenesis of the pRB pocket reveals that cell cycle arrest functions are separable from binding to viral oncoproteins. *Mol Cell Biol* 20(10), 3715-27.

Dollard, S. C., Wilson, J. L., Demeter, L. M., Bonnez, W., Reichman, R. C., Broker, T. R. & Chow, L. T. (1992). Production of human papillomavirus and modulation of the infectious program in epithelial raft cultures. OFF. *Genes Dev* 6(7), 1131-42.

Dong, W., Kloz, U., Accardi, R., Caldeira, S., Tong, W. M., Wang, Z. Q., Jansen, L., Durst, M., Sylla, B. S., Gissmann, L. & Tommasino, M. (2005). Skin hyperproliferation and susceptibility to chemical carcinogenesis in transgenic mice expressing E6 and E7 of human papillomavirus type 38. *J Virol* 79(23), 14899-908.

Dyson, N., Howley, P. M., Munger, K. & Harlow, E. (1989). The human papilloma virus-16 E7 oncoprotein is able to bind to the retinoblastoma gene product. *Science* 243(4893), 934-7.

Funk, J. O., Waga, S., Harry, J. B., Espling, E., Stillman, B. & Galloway, D. A. (1997). Inhibition of CDK activity and PCNA-dependent DNA replication by p21 is blocked by interaction with the HPV-16 E7 oncoprotein. *Genes Dev* 11(16), 2090-100.

Garcia-Escudero, R., Martinez-Cruz, A. B., Santos, M., Lorz, C., Segrelles, C., Garaulet, G., Saiz-Ladera, C., Costa, C., Buitrago-Perez, A., Duenas, M. & Paramio, J. M. (2010). Gene expression profiling of mouse p53-deficient epidermal carcinoma defines molecular determinants of human cancer malignancy. *Mol Cancer* 9, 193.

Giampieri, S., Garcia-Escudero, R., Green, J. & Storey, A. (2004). Human papillomavirus type 77 E6 protein selectively inhibits p53-dependent transcription of proapoptotic genes following UV-B irradiation. *Oncogene* 23(34), 5864-70.

Gonzalez, S. L., Stremlau, M., He, X., Basile, J. R. & Munger, K. (2001). Degradation of the retinoblastoma tumor suppressor by the human papillomavirus type 16 E7 oncoprotein is important for functional inactivation and is separable from proteasomal degradation of E7. *J Virol* 75(16), 7583-91.

Griep, A. E., Herber, R., Jeon, S., Lohse, J. K., Dubielzig, R. R. & Lambert, P. F. (1993). Tumorigenicity by human papillomavirus type 16 E6 and E7 in transgenic mice correlates with alterations in epithelial cell growth and differentiation. *J Virol* 67(3), 1373-84.

Harwood, C. A., Surentheran, T., McGregor, J. M., Spink, P. J., Leigh, I. M., Breuer, J. & Proby, C. M. (2000). Human papillomavirus infection and non-melanoma skin cancer in immunosuppressed and immunocompetent individuals. *J Med Virol* 61(3), 289-97.

Helt, A. M., Funk, J. O. & Galloway, D. A. (2002). Inactivation of both the retinoblastoma tumor suppressor and p21 by the human papillomavirus type 16 E7 oncoprotein is necessary to inhibit cell cycle arrest in human epithelial cells. *J Virol* 76(20), 10559-68.

Herber, R., Liem, A., Pitot, H. & Lambert, P. F. (1996). Squamous epithelial hyperplasia and carcinoma in mice transgenic for the human papillomavirus type 16 E7 oncogene. *J Virol* 70(3), 1873-81.

Isaac, C. E., Francis, S. M., Martens, A. L., Julian, L. M., Seifried, L. A., Erdmann, N., Binne, U. K., Harrington, L., Sicinski, P., Berube, N. G., Dyson, N. J. & Dick, F. A. (2006). The retinoblastoma protein regulates pericentric heterochromatin. *Mol Cell Biol* 26(9), 3659-71.

Jabbar, S. F., Abrams, L., Glick, A. & Lambert, P. F. (2009). Persistence of high-grade cervical dysplasia and cervical cancer requires the continuous expression of the human papillomavirus type 16 E7 oncogene. *Cancer Res* 69(10), 4407-14.

Jablonska, S. & Majewski, S. (1994). Epidermodysplasia verruciformis: immunological and clinical aspects. *Curr Top Microbiol Immunol* 186, 157-75.

Jackson, S., Harwood, C., Thomas, M., Banks, L. & Storey, A. (2000). Role of Bak in UV-induced apoptosis in skin cancer and abrogation by HPV E6 proteins. *Genes Dev* 14(23), 3065-73.

Jackson, S. & Storey, A. (2000). E6 proteins from diverse cutaneous HPV types inhibit apoptosis in response to UV damage. *Oncogene* 19(4), 592-8.

Jones, D. L., Alani, R. M. & Munger, K. (1997). The human papillomavirus E7 oncoprotein can uncouple cellular differentiation and proliferation in human keratinocytes by abrogating p21Cip1-mediated inhibition of cdk2. *Genes Dev* 11(16), 2101-11.

Jonkers, J., Meuwissen, R., van der Gulden, H., Peterse, H., van der Valk, M. & Berns, A. (2001). Synergistic tumor suppressor activity of BRCA2 and p53 in a conditional mouse model for breast cancer. *Nat Genet* 29(4), 418-25.

Kiyono, T., Hiraiwa, A., Fujita, M., Hayashi, Y., Akiyama, T. & Ishibashi, M. (1997). Binding of high-risk human papillomavirus E6 oncoproteins to the human homologue of the Drosophila discs large tumor suppressor protein. *Proc Natl Acad Sci U S A* 94(21), 11612-6.

Kopan, R., Traska, G. & Fuchs, E. (1987). Retinoids as important regulators of terminal differentiation: examining keratin expression in individual epidermal cells at various stages of keratinization. *J Cell Biol* 105(1), 427-40.

Lambert, P. F., Pan, H., Pitot, H. C., Liem, A., Jackson, M. & Griep, A. E. (1993). Epidermal cancer associated with expression of human papillomavirus type 16 E6 and E7 oncogenes in the skin of transgenic mice. *Proc Natl Acad Sci U S A* 90(12), 5583-7.

Lara, M. F., Garcia-Escudero, R., Ruiz, S., Santos, M., Moral, M., Martinez-Cruz, A. B., Segrelles, C., Lorz, C. & Paramio, J. M. (2008a). Gene profiling approaches help to define the specific functions of retinoblastoma family in epidermis. *Mol Carcinog* 47(3), 209-21.

Lara, M. F., Santos, M., Ruiz, S., Segrelles, C., Moral, M., Martinez-Cruz, A. B., Hernandez, P., Martinez-Palacio, J., Lorz, C., Garcia-Escudero, R. & Paramio, J. M. (2008b). p107 acts as a tumor suppressor in pRb-deficient epidermis. *Mol Carcinog* 47(2), 105-13.

Lee, J. O., Russo, A. A. & Pavletich, N. P. (1998). Structure of the retinoblastoma tumour-suppressor pocket domain bound to a peptide from HPV E7. *Nature* 391(6670), 859-65.

Lutzner, M. A., Blanchet-Bardon, C. & Orth, G. (1984). Clinical observations, virologic studies, and treatment trials in patients with epidermodysplasia verruciformis, a disease induced by specific human papillomaviruses. *J Invest Dermatol* 83(1 Suppl), 18s-25s.

Martinez-Cruz, A. B., Santos, M., Lara, M. F., Segrelles, C., Ruiz, S., Moral, M., Lorz, C., Garcia-Escudero, R. & Paramio, J. M. (2008). Spontaneous squamous cell carcinoma induced by the somatic inactivation of retinoblastoma and Trp53 tumor suppressors. *Cancer Res* 68(3), 683-92.

Marur, S., D'Souza, G., Westra, W. H. & Forastiere, A. A. (2010). HPV-associated head and neck cancer: a virus-related cancer epidemic. *Lancet Oncol* 11(8), 781-9.

McCance, D. J., Kopan, R., Fuchs, E. & Laimins, L. A. (1988). Human papillomavirus type 16 alters human epithelial cell differentiation in vitro. *Proc Natl Acad Sci U S A* 85(19), 7169-73.

Meyers, C., Frattini, M. G., Hudson, J. B. & Laimins, L. A. (1992). Biosynthesis of human papillomavirus from a continuous cell line upon epithelial differentiation. *Science* 257(5072), 971-3.

Moral, M., Segrelles, C., Lara, M. F., Martinez-Cruz, A. B., Lorz, C., Santos, M., Garcia-Escudero, R., Lu, J., Kiguchi, K., Buitrago, A., Costa, C., Saiz, C., Rodriguez-Peralto, J. L., Martinez-Tello, F. J., Rodriguez-Pinilla, M., Sanchez-Cespedes, M., Garin, M., Grande, T., Bravo, A., DiGiovanni, J. & Paramio, J. M. (2009). Akt activation synergizes with Trp53 loss in oral epithelium to produce a novel mouse model for head and neck squamous cell carcinoma. *Cancer Res* 69(3), 1099-108.

Moreno, V., Bosch, F. X., Munoz, N., Meijer, C. J., Shah, K. V., Walboomers, J. M., Herrero, R. & Franceschi, S. (2002). Effect of oral contraceptives on risk of cervical cancer in women with human papillomavirus infection: the IARC multicentric case-control study. *Lancet* 359(9312), 1085-92.

Munoz, N., Franceschi, S., Bosetti, C., Moreno, V., Herrero, R., Smith, J. S., Shah, K. V., Meijer, C. J. & Bosch, F. X. (2002). Role of parity and human papillomavirus in cervical cancer: the IARC multicentric case-control study. *Lancet* 359(9312), 1093-101.

Pfister, H. (2003). Chapter 8: Human papillomavirus and skin cancer. *J Natl Cancer Inst Monogr*(31), 52-6.

Riley, R. R., Duensing, S., Brake, T., Munger, K., Lambert, P. F. & Arbeit, J. M. (2003). Dissection of human papillomavirus E6 and E7 function in transgenic mouse models of cervical carcinogenesis. *Cancer Res* 63(16), 4862-71.

Ruiz, S., Santos, M., Lara, M. F., Segrelles, C., Ballestin, C. & Paramio, J. M. (2005). Unexpected roles for pRb in mouse skin carcinogenesis. *Cancer Res* 65(21), 9678-86.

Ruiz, S., Santos, M., Segrelles, C., Leis, H., Jorcano, J. L., Berns, A., Paramio, J. M. & Vooijs, M. (2004). Unique and overlapping functions of pRb and p107 in the control of proliferation and differentiation in epidermis. *Development* 131(11), 2737-48.

Ruiz, S., Segrelles, C., Bravo, A., Santos, M., Perez, P., Leis, H., Jorcano, J. L. & Paramio, J. M. (2003). Abnormal epidermal differentiation and impaired epithelial-mesenchymal tissue interactions in mice lacking the retinoblastoma relatives p107 and p130. *Development* 130(11), 2341-53.

Schaper, I. D., Marcuzzi, G. P., Weissenborn, S. J., Kasper, H. U., Dries, V., Smyth, N., Fuchs, P. & Pfister, H. (2005). Development of skin tumors in mice transgenic for early genes of human papillomavirus type 8. *Cancer Res* 65(4), 1394-400.

Segrelles, C., Lu, J., Hammann, B., Santos, M., Moral, M., Cascallana, J. L., Lara, M. F., Rho, O., Carbajal, S., Traag, J., Beltran, L., Martinez-Cruz, A. B., Garcia-Escudero, R., Lorz, C., Ruiz, S., Bravo, A., Paramio, J. M. & DiGiovanni, J. (2007). Deregulated activity of Akt in epithelial basal cells induces spontaneous tumors and heightened sensitivity to skin carcinogenesis. *Cancer Res* 67(22), 10879-88.

Shai, A., Pitot, H. C. & Lambert, P. F. (2008). p53 Loss synergizes with estrogen and papillomaviral oncogenes to induce cervical and breast cancers. *Cancer Res* 68(8), 2622-31.

Shai, A., Pitot, H. C. & Lambert, P. F. (2010). E6-associated protein is required for human papillomavirus type 16 E6 to cause cervical cancer in mice. *Cancer Res* 70(12), 5064-73.

Shin, M. K., Balsitis, S., Brake, T. & Lambert, P. F. (2009). Human papillomavirus E7 oncoprotein overrides the tumor suppressor activity of p21Cip1 in cervical carcinogenesis. *Cancer Res* 69(14), 5656-63.

Smith, P. P., Friedman, C. L., Bryant, E. M. & McDougall, J. K. (1992). Viral integration and fragile sites in human papillomavirus-immortalized human keratinocyte cell lines. *Genes Chromosomes Cancer* 5(2), 150-7.

Song, S., Liem, A., Miller, J. A. & Lambert, P. F. (2000). Human papillomavirus types 16 E6 and E7 contribute differently to carcinogenesis. *Virology* 267(2), 141-50.

Song, S., Pitot, H. C. & Lambert, P. F. (1999). The human papillomavirus type 16 E6 gene alone is sufficient to induce carcinomas in transgenic animals. *J Virol* 73(7), 5887-93.

Strati, K. & Lambert, P. F. (2007). Role of Rb-dependent and Rb-independent functions of papillomavirus E7 oncogene in head and neck cancer. *Cancer Res* 67(24), 11585-93.

Strati, K., Pitot, H. C. & Lambert, P. F. (2006). Identification of biomarkers that distinguish human papillomavirus (HPV)-positive versus HPV-negative head and neck cancers in a mouse model. *Proc Natl Acad Sci U S A* 103(38), 14152-7.

Wang, H. K., Duffy, A. A., Broker, T. R. & Chow, L. T. (2009). Robust production and passaging of infectious HPV in squamous epithelium of primary human keratinocytes. *Genes Dev* 23(2), 181-94.

Werness, B. A., Levine, A. J. & Howley, P. M. (1990). Association of human papillomavirus types 16 and 18 E6 proteins with p53. *Science* 248(4951), 76-9.

Woodworth, C. D., Cheng, S., Simpson, S., Hamacher, L., Chow, L. T., Broker, T. R. & DiPaolo, J. A. (1992). Recombinant retroviruses encoding human papillomavirus type 18 E6 and E7 genes stimulate proliferation and delay differentiation of human keratinocytes early after infection. *Oncogene* 7(4), 619-26. zur Hausen, H. (2002). Papillomaviruses and cancer: from basic studies to clinical application. *Nat Rev Cancer* 2(5), 342-50.

8

Overview on Molecular Markers to Implement Cervical Cancer Prevention: Challenges and Perspectives

Sandra Rosini and Roberta Zappacosta
Oncology and Experimental Medicine Department, Cytopathology Unit, G. d'Annunzio University of Chieti-Pescara
Italy

1. Introduction

A decline in the incidence and mortality of cervical cancer has been observed in most Western countries since the first third of the past century. This may be mainly attributed to the introduction of Pap test, that is considered one of the milestones in medicine. Nevertheless, worldwide burden of cervicocarcinoma is still enormous. This fact is well known among the scientific community, and has led to an extensive search for optional screening tools and predictive markers, currently under testing in different countries.

2. A brief history

Modern research on Papillomavirus and Papillomaviruses began more than 150 years ago. In a famous paper, the Italian physician Rigoni-Stern analyzed death certificates of woman in Verona, during the period 1760-1839. He noted that cervical cancer was common among prostitutes, married women and widows but rare in virgins and nuns. He concluded that the development of this cancer should be related to sexual contacts. Later, in 1898, McFadyean and Hobday successfully transmitted canine oral papillomatosis, while Codeac transmitted warts from horse to horse, in 1901. In spite of a limited number of studies on Papillomavirus in subsequent decades, it was almost 80 more years later when this area of research engendered broad interest. In 1934 Rous and Beard noted that papillomas of domestic rabbits frequently converted to squamous-cell carcinomas. Although Rous conceptually preceded his contemporaries by several decades, the importance of his ponderous work was only acknowledged in 1966, when he received the Nobel Prize. Rous's research was not specifically driven towards the agent causing rabbit papillomas, but using the frequent progression of rabbit papillomas to squamous-cell carcinomas, he provided an universal model to analyse cervical cancer development. From this point, a number of anecdotal reports of the malignant conversion of genital warts appeared in the medical literature and resulted in a persistent interest about the possible role of HPV infection in cervical cancer. This interest began more concrete with the failures in finding traces of Herpes simplex virus type 2 (HSV2) DNA in cervical cancer biopsies. These fails prompted the search for other potential infectious etiology. In the mild-1970s, within precancerous cervical lesions, Meisels and Fortin firstly observed areas of koilocytic atypia, which they considered to be the cytopathic effect of HPV infection (Meisels & Fortin, 1976).

In 1978, Della Torre et al., in Italy, and Laverty et al. in Australia, firstly demonstrated the presence of HPV virions within dense bodies of koilocytes, but deeper investigations were limited by the inability to propagate HPV in cultured cells or in simple animal models. By the end of 1970s, the revolutionary advent of recombinant DNA technologies and molecular cloning techniques, provided the key for advanced investigation on HPV biology, in order to confirm the role of Papillomavirus in cervical cancer etiology (Zur Hausen et al., 1977). Topically, in 1983, Harald zur Hausen et al., for the first time isolated HPV-16 from a cervical cancer biopsy and cloned its genome. Using HPV-16 sequence and Southern blotting technology, zur Hausen detected this genotype in about one-half of cervicocarcinoma biopsies (Boshart et al., 1984) and demonstrated the selective transcription of viral E6 and E7 oncoproteins in cervical cancer derived cell lines (Schwartz et al, 1985). zur Hausen's findings indirectly demonstrated the heterogeneity of the Human Papillomavirus family; this fact consequently led to the classification of genital HPVs into low-risk and high-risk oncogenic groups, in dependence of the ability to induce cancer. In 2008, Dr. zur Hausen will receive the Nobel prize for medicine. Actually, there is uniform agreement regarding the central role of high-risk HPV-infection in cervical cancer and the necessary but far from sufficient etiopathogenetic role of the virus in causing cervicocarcinomas (Solomon, 2003).

The practical implication of this long series of studies is evident: an enormous increase in the quality of diagnostic approach of precursor lesions of cervical cancer and the development of preventive vaccine (Zur Hausen, 2002).

3. HPV and its life cycle

Papillomavirus are small, non-enveloped, epitheliotropic, double-stranded DNA viruses that can infect basal epithelial cells of the skin or inner lining of tissue and induce cellular proliferation in a specie-specific manner. More than 100 genotypes of Papillomavirus have been isolated and branded molecularly; they were categorized as cutaneous or mucosal type.

Basing on their association with cervical cancer and precursor lesions, HPVs can be grouped in: "high risk" (HR) or "oncogenic" types (16, 18, 26, 31, 33, 35, 39, 45, 51, 53, 56, 58, 59, 66, 68, 73, 82, and "low-risk" (LR) or "non-oncogenic" types (6, 11, 40, 42, 44, 54, 61, 70, 72, 81, 89), related to benign epithelial proliferation but not with cancer (Munõz et al., 2004, 2006). Among the nineteen oncogenic HPV types, five are most often found to be associated with cervical cancer; particularly, virus 16 is accountable for about half of cervicocarcinoma cases discovered in Northern America, Europe and Australia; viruses 18, 31, 33 and 45 are responsible for additional 30% of cases (Cliffort et al., 2003; De Sanjosè et al., 2007; Kraus et al., 2006). All papillomaviruses show a common genetic structure: a single molecule of double-stranded circular DNA of about 7900 base-pairs genome, enclosed in a non-evenloped icosahedral capsid. HPV-DNA encodes for eight open-reading frames (ORFs) which are transcribed from the single encoding DNA strand. The genome is functionally divided into three regions. The first is a non-coding one, referred as Long Control Region (LCR) or Upper Regolatory Region (URR). This section of HPV's genome includes enhancer and silencer sequences that regulate DNA replication by controlling the transcription of the ORFs. The second is the Early (E) Region, consisting of ORFs E1, E2, E4, E5, E6 and E7, which are implicated in viral replication and oncogenesis. The third is the Late (L) region, that encodes the L1 and L2 structural proteins.

4. A silent but epidemic virus

The global burden of HPV-associated disease is very high. At present, HPV infections represent the most common sexually transmitted disease (SMT) in the world (Snijders et al., 2006). In the United States alone, it was estimated that 6.2 million of new infections occur annually, with an approximately prevalence of 20 million (Clifford et al., 2005).

Within population, the prevalence of HPV infection in asymptomatic women is estimated to range from 2% to 44%; the highest peak was reported in women younger than 25 years of age.

The vast majority of HPV infection is transient and resolves within 2 years without necessarily led to clinically significant cervical lesions. Only 10% of infected women remain HPV-positive within 5 years. In 2008 (the most recent year for which statistics are available), 12,280 women in the United States had cervical cancer, and 4,021 died from the disease (Arbyn M et al., 2011). Rates of infection appears actually to be in incessant and rapidly increasing.

Interest in HPV and cervical pathology is primarily justified by the morbidity and mortality caused by cervical epithelial cancer: cervicocarcinomas represents the second most common cancer among women worldwide. Its worldwide burden is enormous, with over 500,000 new cases of cervical cancer diagnosed each year, and 280,000 deaths recorded (Jemal A et al., 2010; Parkin D et al., 2002). While in developed Western countries screening programmes have significantly reduced the incidence of disease, about 80% of cervicocarcinomas cases still occur in underdeveloped countries.

The natural history of cervical cancer is characterized by a well-defined pre-malignant phases. These pre-malignant changes represent a spectrum of abnormalities ranging from Low-grade Squamous Intraepithelial Lesion (LSIL) to High-grade Squamous intraepithelial Lesions (HSIL). In the United States, about five hundred thousand high-grade precursors and 2-3 milion cases of low-grade lesions are referred for colposcopic assessment each year. The attendant costs for the management of these lesions was estimated in 3-6 billion dollars (Stoler, 2004).

Prospective studies showed that infection with oncogenic HPVs precedes the development of cervical neoplasia, and that it's necessary, even if not sufficient, to have HR-HPV infection to develop squamous intraepithelial lesion (SIL) or invasive cervical cancer (ICC). Virtually all cervical cancers test positive for HR-HPV DNA. Surprisingly, the etiopathogenetic role of HPV for cervical cancer is higher than smoke is for lung cancer and than Human Epatitis B (HBV) is for liver cancer (Carter JR et al., 2011).

HR-HPVs increased the risk of developing cervical cancer in the order of 50-300 fold. A meta-analysis of Smith et al. shows that the overall prevalence of HR-HPVs in ICC is on the order of 87%, ranging from 86% to 94% by region. Overall, HR-HPVs prevalence in HSIL ranges from 78% in Asia to 88% in Europe (Smth et al., 2007).

There is a broad variation between the most prevalent HR-HPV types around the world. However, types 16 and 18 remain the most common in cervical lesions, causing 60-80% of all cervical cancers. HPV-16 ranges from 52% in Asia to 58% in Europe; HPV-18 ranges from 13% in South-Central America to 22% in North America (Smith et al., 2007).

It was originally believed that there was an irreversible progression of cervical disease from low-grade to high-grade lesions and then invasive cervical cancer. However, through a much greater understanding of the natural history of HPV infection, we actually know that the majority of low-grade lesions would regress without treatment. To the necessary activity of HR-HPV, other co-factors such as smoking, long-term oral contraceptive pill use, human immunodeficiency virus (HIV) co-infection, high parity, Chlamydia Trachomatis and HSV infections, immune suppression as well as nutritional and dietary factors may be associated to induce cervical cancer. Generally, the vast majority of these condition adversely affects antigen-processing Langerhans cells, needed for cell-mediated immunity, or enhances HPV gene expression in the cervix, thus promoting the integration of the virus into the host genome.

5. Molecular basis of the transformation: Knowledge is power

HPV life cycle is linked to the differentiation of the infected epithelial cell; it starts with the penetration of virions in the basal cells layers (stratum germinativum), through micro-abrasions of the transformation zone of the cervix. The ability of HPVs to establish their genome in basal cells relies mainly upon E1, E2, E6 and E7 genes. Normally, when basal cells undergo cell division , it loses contact with the basement membrane and migrates into the suprabasal compartment, where it withdraws from the cell cycle and initiates a programme of terminal differentiation. In HPV infection, suprabasal cells fail to withdraw from the cell cycle.

During acute infection, to replicate its genome and successfully produce infectious virions, HPV switches to amplify its DNA at high copy number, synthesises capsid protein and causes viral assembly, within the differentiated keratinocytes of the suprabasal layers of cervical epithelium. In this context many viral gene products are implicated. E7 has been shown to be necessary to induce suprabasal DNA synthesis, assisted by E5. E4 gene is essential for HPV-DNA replication and for the expression of L1 and L2 genes. E4 also interrupts cytoplasmic cytokeratin network, causing condentation of tonofilaments at the cell periphery, and perinuclear cytoplasmic halo; the results is the koilocyte. Encapsidation of viral DNA, to generate viral progeny into differentiated cellular compartment, is qualitatively dependent upon L2 gene. L2 may be also play a role during intracellular transport of virions, and in the localization of viral DNA within host nucleus.

During latent infection, HPV stays as non-productive within the basal layer of the epithelium and establish itself as a low copy number episome, usually once molecule/cell cycle (Doorbar, 2005). At the basal and parabasal cellular levels only very little, if any, gene expression of the virus can be observed. Conversely, expression of early E1, E2, E4, E5, E6 and E7 genes is evident within differentiated cells of the upper layers of the epithelium, which have lost the capacity to replicate their genome and are at no further risk of acquiring functional mutations. The above mentioned mechanism is a meticulous HPV strategy that allows maximal production of virions, causing almost no injury to infected host. The situation changes radically if regulatory intracellular mechanisms driving the control of the viral are disturbed and deregulated. In this case, the expression of genes involved in the replication of viral genome occurs also in epithelial stem cells, which lost their capacity to differentiate. The inhibition of the differentiation process leads to a cellular state that cannot support the full viral life cycle. Interference of viral genes with cellular pathways that control replication and life cycle of epithelial cell might result in chromosomal instability. In epithelial stem cells with chromosomal instability, HPV DNA integrates into the host genome. HPV integration sites are randomly distributed over the whole genome, with a clear predilection for fragile sites (Wentzensen et al., 2004). Whether any property of the virus drives this integration event or whether it reflects random recombination events remain still unclear; however, two consequences of integration are certain: the loss of E2 regulatory gene and the selective up-regulation of viral E6 and E7 oncogenes. Disruption or deletion of E2 gene, occurring during HPV-DNA integration, interferes with down-regulation of E6/E7 transcription genes and leads to an increased and selective expression of E6/E7 oncoproteins, in replicating epithelial stem cells. As result, E6/E7 proteins bind to cell cycle regulators, stimulate cell-cycle progression and induce cellular instability (Doorbar, 2005). When E6 gene product binds to p53, physiological activities of p53, which governs G1 arrest and DNA repair or apoptosis, are abrogated (Doorbar, 2006; Tang et al., 2006). E6 protein of non-oncogenic HPV types does not bind p53 at detectable levels and has no effect on p53 stability, *in vivo*. When E7 gene product binds to the hypophosphorilated form of the pRb, the result is the disruption of pRb-cellular transcription factor E2F-1 complex, the release of E2F-1 and the transcription of genes whose products are required to enter in phase S of cellular cell cycle. Non-oncogenic E7 protein binds to pRb with a decreased affinity (Litchtig, 2006). Together E6/E7 proteins deregulate cell cycle checkpoints G1/S and G2/M.

Host cells showing viral E6/E7 expression may acquire defects in differentiations, immortal phenotype, chromosomal instability and an increased probability of mutation allowing to invasion. Such described are obviously extraordinary molecular accidents occurring during HPV cell cycle and, in view of many HPV-infected cells, are extremely rare events. On the other hand, the continuous and deregulated E6/E7 activity in cervical stem cells compartments, enhances the selection and the growth of mutated cell clones. Then persistence represents the essential and indispensable requisite to develop cervical cancer.

Numerous studies concerning HPV infection in immunocompromised population, reported that E6/E7 would also play an important role in the inhibition of the host cell immune response (Kraus et al., 2006), particularly by down-regulating the expression of Interleukin-8 (IL-8). IL-8 is a T-cell chemoattractive molecule (Guess & Mc Cance, 2005), that also suppresses the expression of the Monocyte Chemoattractant Protein 1 (MCP-1) in epithelial cells of female genital tract (Biswas & Sodhi, 2002). E6/E7 would also favour the evasion of infected cells from the antiviral and antiproliferative activities of Tumor Necrosis Factor Alpha (TNF-α) (Scott et al., 2001).

6. The ancient Pap test

The concept of utilizing exfoliative cytology to identify women with cervical cancer was introduced by Papanicolaou and Babes, in 1920s. Next, Papanicolaou refined the technique and demonstrated that conventional cytology could also be used to identify precancerous lesions of the cervix. The shift from using cytology as a way to identify cases of invasive cervical cancer to using it to identify women with pre-neoplastic lesions was extremely significant. It meant that cervical cytology could be used to prevent cervical cancer, over than to identify cases in early phases.

In the 1960s, cervical cytology began to be extensively used. In about 30 years, cytology-based screening reduced the incidence of cervicocarcinomas by up to 75% in countries that have been able to realize quality-controlled screening programs (Arbyn et al., 2011). No improvements or modifications of the Pap test were instituted during this time, as there was no doubt that well-organized screening programs, realizing high compliance and good quality control, were effectual in saving lives.

The process of change began when the article "Lax Laboratories" was published in the Wall Street Journal in 1987 (November, 2), by Bogdanich. The phrase "The Pap Test Misses Much Cervical Cancer Through Labs Errors", implying that false negative Pap tests resulted largely from carelessness of doctors, alerted the public. The accuracy of cervical cytology began to be questioned. The article led to increased people awareness, and climaxed with the introduction, in 1988, of the governmental regulatory document known as CLIA 88 (Clinical Laboratory Improvement Act). CLIA 88 enforced regulations to ensure high quality testing

At the same time, in 1988, the National Cancer Institute sponsored a workshop to address the standardization of diagnosis in cervical cytology. The workshop introduced a new classification system designated as "The Bethesda System" (TBS). TBS, further revised in 1991 and 2001, provided a uniform format and offered a standardized terminology, specifically emphasizing communication of clinically relevant information (National Cancer Institute Group, 1989). TBS has been widely accepted and is endorsed by both Pathology and Gynecological Societies.

In the 1990s, it was realized that the efficacy of Pap test have reached a nadir, and meta-analyses indicated that both sensitivity and specificity of a single Pap test in detecting cervical intraepithelial neoplasia or invasive cancer is in the order of 80-85% and 76%, respectively (Stoler et al., 2001). A review of the UK program found that, within women developing invasive cervical cancer, 47% had an apparently adequate screening history during the previous 5 years (Sasieni et al., 1996); some of these patients also had a history of negative smear results. These considerations suggested that the frontiers of effectiveness of conventional cytology have been reached and that was imperative to improve the diagnostic assessment of the Pap test. This fact has been well recognized among the scientific community that emphasize the necessity to find other solutions to cope with this increasing problem.

Prerequisites for an effective screening program is a high quality in sampling technique, in processing and in reporting. Basing on these considerations, technology entered in cytology practice with a variety of optional screening tolls to replace or complement conventional Pap test; among these, monolayer cytology and computer-assisted cytology .

7. Challenges with conventional screening methods

7.1 Monolayer cytology

The low sensitivity of a single cervical smear is due to a variety of factors, including: incorrect or inadequate sampling of cervix; poor transfer of cells to the glass slide; non-representative sample placed on the slide; poor fixation. Particularly, sampling and preparing are together guilty for about two-third of false-negative tests (Cibas et al., 2008).

To minimize false-negative cytology results and to improve the diagnostic accuracy of cervical cytology, some programs proposed to repeat the Pap test every year, to balance the relative limited sensitivity of conventional cytology; however, this conduct would compromise cost-efficacy of Pap test and the possibility to use an algorithm with greater screening intervals and similar safety. New methods of collection and processing would need to surmount all these problems.

Liquid-based cytology (LBC) was introduced in the mid-1990s, as a way to improve the performances of Pap test. By this technology, clinician does not prepare the specimen at the bedside by spreading the exfoliated cells onto a glass slide, but the cervical sampling device (i.e. spatula or brush) is rinsed in a vial containing a fixative-transport medium. In laboratory, slides are prepared using an instrument that mixes the specimen and transfers an exact number of cells onto a filter membrane, with minimal cellular overlap. Then, the filter with the cells are transferred onto a slide and stained using the Pap stain (Abulafia et al., 2003). The automated process of such slides preparation prevents drying artefacts (very common in conventional Pap slides) and eliminates non-diagnostic debris, such as blood, mucus and inflammatory cells. Background material such as inflammatory exudates, cytolysis, microorganisms and tumor diathesis can still be identified but it does not obscure the epithelial cells (Davey et al., 2006).

To date, there are three currently FDA-approved LBC techniques, These include: SurePath™ System (TriPath Imaging Inc., Burlington, NC, USA), ThinPrep® System (Hologic, Crawley, UK) and MonoPrep System (MonoGen, Lincolnshire, IL) (Cibas et al., 2008).

ThinPrep and SurePath methods are the most widely studied technologies in literature; their underlying principles are similar, the only difference being that ThinPrep collects samples into methanol-based preservative solution, while SurePath dispenses cells into ethanol-based fluids.

More than forty publications promote the use of these preparation methods. In particular, all the authors show statistically significant improvement (about 10% or more) of the diagnostic sensitivity of conventional cytology in all categories of cervical disease (Bernstein et al., 2001; Davey at al., 2007; Nance et al, 2007; Papillo et al., 2008.).

Currently, LBC constitutes over 80% of cervical screening tests in USA. In 2003, the UK National Institute for Clinical Excellence (NICE) recommended the introduction of LBC as primary way to process samples in cervical cancer screening programs (Stoykova et al., 2008). The National Health Service of the United Kingdom agreed to introduce LBC throughout the country, in view of the reduction of inadequate specimens from 9% with conventional cytology to 1-2% with LBC (Nance et al., 2007).

LBC techniques improved the quality of the smear, being cytological evaluation and interpretation facilitated by the thin layer of evenly distributed cells. Abnormal cells are not hidden in thick areas of the slide; Then, will follow an increased detection of the lesions (such as HSIL lesions), a reduction of the number of false-negative diagnosis and the diminution of unsatisfactory specimens. Moreover, the availability of residual cellular material, preserved for several week at room temperature, is usefulness for additional investigations, such as immunocytochemistry or molecular procedures. In the USA, the Consensus Guidelines for the Management of Women with Cytologic Abnormalities considered HPV-DNA testing on residual LBC specimen to be the preferred approach to managing women with ASC-US cytological results. This suggestion was based on the grounds that HPV-DNA reflex testing could offer the advantage that women do not need to return to additional clinical examination (Wright at al., 2002).

7.2 Computer-assisted cytology

Screening of Pap smears is monotonous. It was recognised that the monotony of screening large numbers of normal slides promotes periods of lack of attention during which abnormal cells may be disregarded. Among women who have cervical cancer and have been screened, 14% to 33% of the cases represent failure to detect abnormalities. It is therefore not surprising that great efforts have been made to automate also this aspect of cervical cancer screening. The aim of computer-assisted reading of cervical smears is to increase the sensitivity of cytological testing by finding cells known to be very difficult to detect in conventional slides. This technology should also increase productivity by excluding normal slides or part of the slides from manual screening and by selecting most atypical images to be checked by cytologists (Dunton, 2000).

In the mid-1990s two automated devices, based on traditional computer image technology and neural network software, have been subjected to extensive multicentre trials and subsequently approved by the American Food and Drug Agency for screening cervical smears: PAPNET system (Neuromedical Sciences Inc, Amsterdam) and AutoPap 300 (NeoPath Inc, Redmond Washington USA). Both are interactive systems, which select smears for manual review by the screener. They were initially approved for quality control or supplementary screening of cervical smears. Subsequently they were admitted for primary screening.

PAPNET was introduced as a pre-screening method of conventional Pap smears. The smears were analysed using a combination of algorithmic and neural network programs; then, 128 images of the most abnormal looking cells or cell groups were selected for inspection by the screener.

The images were stored on compact disc and viewed by the screener on a video monitor placed in the laboratory. The screener triages the images and decides whether the slide is negative or requires manual review. Those slides which were triaged negative were not subjected to manual microscopic review.

AutoPap was also designed to also pre-screen conventional slides. This technology uses a computer algorithm method to classify and score glass slides to overall level of abnormality. All slide were processed through the device and then, on the basis of "abnormality index", they were ranked in descending order of potential abnormality and broken into quintiles. This system, now manufactured by TriPath inc. and called FocalPoint®, was designed to look for abnormalities slide by slide and to rule out the 25% of slides with the lowest risk. These slides were automatically excluded from the list of those requiring manual microscopic review thus reducing the screener's workload by 25%. Slides with the most severe abnormalities were completely reviewed by scientists.

FocalPoint is intended to be used on both conventionally-prepared and SurePath™ cervical cytology slides. This system analyses the samples using a series of algorithms and assigns a score to the sample. The sample is then graded into a group called "No Further Review" (NFR) or into one of 5 risk categories. The purpose of this assignation is to make unnecessary to look at the NFR category. Cytoscreeners can instead concentrate themselves on looking at the slides graded as abnormal. The operator is guided to the areas containing the cells of interest (Fields of View/FOV) which have been detected by the system.

Recently, Cytic Corporation developed its computer assisted system, the ThinPrep Imager®, which received FDA approval for use with ThinPrep slides. A bench-op image processor analyses ThinPrep slides, which were reviewed by cytotechnologists, by using a microscope with a motorized stage. Special software drives the reviewer to the 22 most abnormal fields on the slides. Full manual review is required only if any of the 22 fields contain a suspicious or abnormal cell.

Devices of computer-assisted screening were tested in extensive multicentre trials comparing automated and manual screening of the same slides. All trials found that automated systems were at least as sensitive as manual screening; however, in automation more smears could be analysed per unit of time. On the other hand, due to high development costs, these systems were not found to be cost effective for the use in laboratories processing less than 50,000 smears per annum; this fact excluded many laboratories in the USA and Europe.

8. The revolution: Molecular diagnosis

The awareness of the viral origin of cervicocarcinoma, the refinement of the techniques for cytological diagnosis and the introduction of liquid-based medium for collection of cytological specimens has open new and interesting options to improve cervical cancer screening programs.

The consciousness that cervical cancer is a multistep process and that it occurs in women who have been infected with oncogenic HPVs, led to the development of molecular techniques able to identifying carcinogenic Papillomavirus in cervical sample (Bosch et al., 2002). The era of diagnosis based on aetiology was beginning.

Serological assays to detect antibodies against HPV capsid or against functional protein received attention as investigational tools, both in epidemiological and clinical studies (Jochmus-Kudielka et al, 1989; Galloway, 1992). However, serology detected humoral immune response to HPV antigens, which may reflect cumulative exposure to HPV infection acquired in mucosal sites other than genital; moreover, it was unreliable to determine whether an HPV infection was present or past (Dillner J, 1999), by using serological tests. So, an accurate diagnosis of HPV infection could only be based on the detection of viral nucleic acid.

Testing for Human Papillomavirus by different molecular tools has been proposed as an adjunct or as an independent screening tool, with several potential advantages. Testing for the etiological agent of cervical cancer offers the opportunity to detect women at increased risk of cervical cancer at the stage of latent and subclinical infection, preceding by several months to years the clinical stages detectable by the Pap test.

Wide range of methods to detect HPV-DNA in cytological specimens are available. They evolved considerably in the last 25 years. Initial methods were based on direct probe hybridation technology, such as dot blot and Southern blot. Besides being labor-intensive and time-consuming, these techniques showed low sensitivity and required large amounts of DNA in clinical samples. So they have largely been superseded by amplification technology. Amplification techniques can be further classified into two separate categories:(i) target amplification assays (i.e., PCR, in which a target nucleic acid is amplified) and (ii) signal amplification assays (in which the signal generated from each probe is increased by a compound-probe or branched-probe technology). To date, all the above methodologies (Figure 1) have been applied to HPV detection field (Zappacosta et al., 2008).

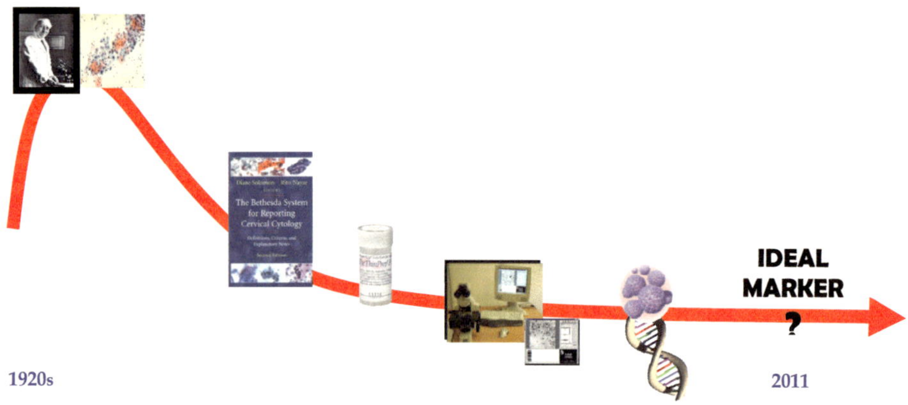

Fig. 1. Technology assessment in cervical cancer screening

8.1 Southern blot

The first method for HPV detection was the Southern blot (Sb). Sb utilizes enzymes to break HPV-DNA chain extracted from the specimen. The product, integrated into a gel, is subjected to electrophoresis, that separates viral DNA basing on the size of each fragment. DNA fragments are next transferred to a nitrocellulose membrane and hybridized with HPV genomic probes, which are labelled with radioisotopes. In addition to poor labour applicability (reliance on radiolabelled probes) and high time-consuming, Sb procedures showed low sensitivity, mainly due to the need of large amounts of DNA in clinical samples. For all these reasons, Sb technique has now largely been superseded by amplification technologies.

8.2 Direct hybridization

In situ hybridization (ISH) is a direct probe method that assess the presence of a target nucleic acid or gene expression within either paraffin-embedded tissue or cervical smear. The nucleic acid probes used in ISH are derivatized, typically with biotin, in multiple sites. Detection is frequently achieved employing a sandwich approach, involving streptavidin-chromogen complexes. Improvements in sensitivity of ISH have been reached with fluorescent probe (FISH) utilization, in order to add a further amplification of the signal. The major advantages of ISH/FISH techniques is that HPV-DNA can be identified inside specific cells (normal, koilocytes, neoplastic) and that viral physical status may also be determined (integration *versus* episomal) (Hopman et al., 2005). Low sensitivity and specificity (30% and 72%, respectively), nucleic acid degradation during sample processing, and high time-consuming (due to multiple assays which must be carried out for HPV genotyping), are the main factors that make these techniques troublesome in its performances (Seedlacek, 1999).

Laboratories using molecular assays for detection of infectious organisms should use standardized tools. In this context, the World Health Organization (WHO) has initiated an International Collaborative Study enrolling several laboratories worldwide (Pagliusi & Garland, 2007). The aim of developing HPV international standard reagents is to capacitate diagnostic laboratories to be able to validate their own assays and to determine their analytical sensitivity. Within surveillance studies, this standardization will allow comparison of HPV-DNA detection between different geographic localization, populations and anatomical sites over time. Standardization is particularly important in view of post-vaccine population responses data.

High-throughput assays suitable for large-scale cervical cancer screening are currently based on two different amplification technologies: Polymerase Chain Reaction (PCR) and hybridization-based assays (i.g., Hybrid Capture 2 assay). The advantages and disadvantages of these basically different assays will be extensively discussed below together with the analysis of several recent studies comparing the performances of both techniques.

8.3 Polymerase chain reaction

PCR is a selective target amplification assay capable of exponential and reproducible increase in the HPV sequences present in biological specimens. The amplification process can theoretically produce one billion HPV-DNA copies from a single double-stranded molecule. after 30 cycles of amplification, For this reason, PCR has very high level of molecular sensitivity and permits the detection of less than 10 copies of HPV-DNA in a mixture

There are two main approaches to detect HPV-DNA by PCR: type-specific PCR and consensus PCR. The latter are able to amplify sequences from several different HPV types, because they target conserved DNA regions in the HPV genome. The most extensively used PCR assay utilizes consensus primers that target a highly conserved region of HPV L1 genome, thus amplifying a vast spectrum of HPV types in one reaction. Initially, most laboratories used PCR assay with degenerated primers pair MY09/11. These primers are now been replaced by a new set of oligonucleotides pool: GP5/6 and modified GP5+/GP6+, PGMY09/11 (modified MY09/11), SPF1/2, the last one especially appropriated for formalin-fixed paraffin-embedded tissue samples, which often offer a small amount of amplifiable DNA (Boulet et al., 2008; Perrons et al., 2005). Amplification with each of these primers provides different size amplification products, resulting in varying sensitivity for HPV-DNA detection. Although discrimination of sequence homology is better for longer sequences, and would theoretically permit improved HPV types resolution, shorter fragments tend to confer better sensitivity when potentially degraded specimens, such as paraffin-embedded tumor tissue, are used.

Up to date literature reports clinical sensitivity of PCR protocols varying from 75% to 95% (Kulusingam et al., 2002), with a median of 82%. Of interest is the PCR versus HC2 data obtained from ALTS study: on 278 cases of CIN3/cancer, PCR test employing the PGMY09/11 primers achieved clinical sensitivity and specificity of 87.4% and 55.6% respectively, while the corresponding value for HC2 test were 95.5 and 51.1% (Belinson et al., 2001; Zappacosta et al., 2010.

The commercial assay by Roche Diagnostics, Amplicor® HPV test (Roche Molecular Systems, Inc., Branchburg, NJ, USA) has been recently released, although not yet FDA approved. The test is designed to amplify HPV DNA from 13 high-risk genotypes (16, 18, 31, 33, 35, 39, 45, 51, 52, 56, 58, 59, and 68), by using biotinylated primers to define a sequence of approximately 165 bp in length within the polymorphic L1 region of the HPV genome, and to simultaneously assess the presence of human β-globin gene as a positive control. The test do not discriminate HPV genotypes specifically. In the International Papillomavirus Congress which took place in Mexico City during 2004, several studies showed data related to the utilization of Amplicor® test in two different LBC media (ThinPrep® and Surepath™) and illustrated the performance of the test in different clinical settings. Particularly, van den Brule at al., (Hessenlink et al., 2005) compared Amplicor® test with the GP5+/GP6+ PCR assay in cervical samples collected in PreservCyt® medium. The two tests gave similar results, but the sensitivity of Amplicor® appeared slightly higher. Roche assay and HC2 test gave identical results in detecting high-grade CIN (Monsonego J et al., 2005).

The scenario changes when HPV genotyping is needed. HPV genotyping is now considered a relevant tool for women management, in order to identify persistent type-specific oncogenic HPV infection, and for the stratification of cancer risk. Among HPV-positive women, 20% to 40% harbour at least two genotypes (Mendez et al., 2005). Interest in multiple HPV infections has recently increased as prophylactic vaccines against HPV have been introduced (Jenkins, 2008). Moreover, the correct profiling of HPV types in patients with multiple infections is important to learn more about the natural history of cervical cancer. Constant progress in HPV typing based on PCR methods has been made over the past few years. The majority of available protocols uses degenerate and/or consensus primers, followed by the examination of the generated PCR product through sequence analysis, restriction fragments length polymorphisms analysis or hybridization with type-specific probes in different formats (such as the reverse line blot assay [van den Brule et al., 2002] or bead-based multiplex HPV genotyping method [Schmitt et al., 2006]). The use of these technologies offers the advantage of detecting a large spectrum of HPV types by a single PCR. However, they may be less efficient in detecting specific HPV types, in cases of multiple infections (Schmitt et al., 2010).

Generally, amplification-based methods, mainly PCR, are currently the most sensitive methods for the detection of HPV-DNA. They are ideal instruments for research and epidemiological purposes, since they allow the detection of low viral load infections, also minimizing the risk of misclassification of HPV infection status. However, due to the frequent contamination problems and consequent false-positive results as well as to the costs which are still too high, they are not routinely applicable in diagnostic laboratories. In order to overcome these problems, Digene Diagnostics developed Hybrid Capture System DNA detection.

8.4 Hybrid capture 2

Hybrid Capture 2 (HC2, Qiagen, Valencia, CA) is a simple, high-throughput, semi-automated HPV-DNA test, operating on the principle of signal amplification. HC2 is the only HPV test currently approved by the US FDA. The method utilizes long (> 1 kb) single-strained RNA probes which are complementary to the entire HPV-DNA genomic sequence. DNA is firstly denatured and subsequently mixed with RNA probe pool in a buffered solution. Two RNA probe pool are used. The test can be performed using both probe pool together or separately. Probe A recognizes non-oncogenic HPV types (6, 11, 42, 43, and 44); pool B identifies oncogenic HPVs (16, 18, 31, 33, 35, 39, 45, 51, 52, 56, 58, 59 and 68). DNA-RNA complexes are immobilized onto microplates which has been coated with polyclonal IgG antibody that recognize specific DNA-RNA hybrids, at room temperature. The immobilized hybrids are then identified by a second DNA-RNA antibody, conjugated to alkaline phosphatise and bounded to a chemiluminescent substrate, CDP Star (Figure 2). Microplates are then transferred into a software program where results are analysed; in particular, CDP Star ligh is measured by a luminometer. The intensity of the light emitted by each specimen is expressed on a scale as RLUs (Relative Light Units), relative to the average reactivity measured in triplicate wells with a positive control containing 1.0 pg of HPV-16 DNA/ml.

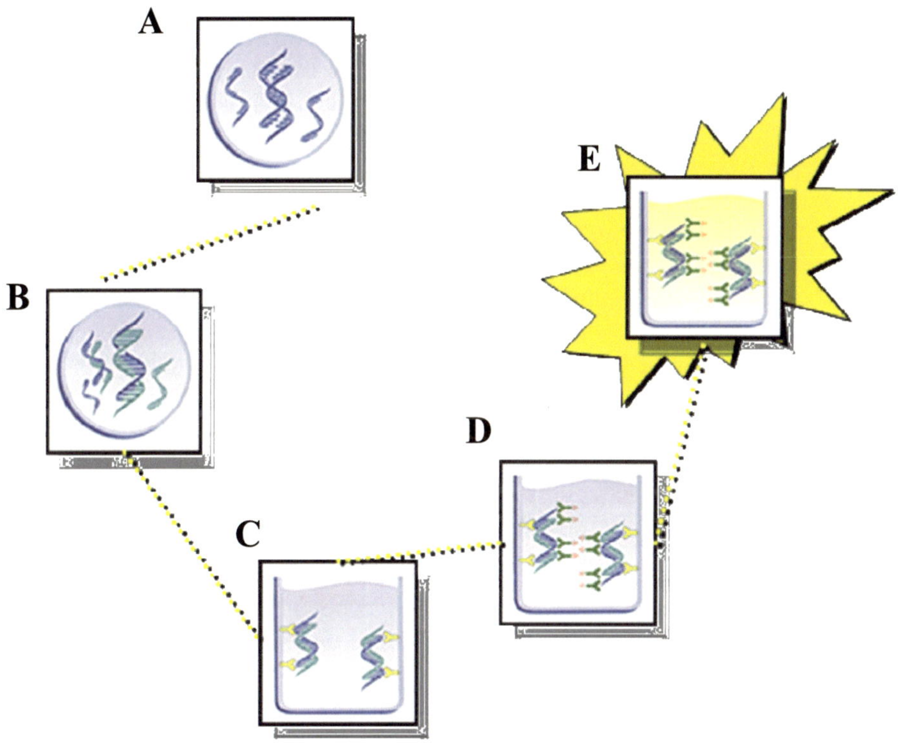

Fig. 2. Hybrid Capture 2 Technology. A - HPV-DNA denaturation; B – single-stranded RNA probes recognizes oncogenic HPV-DNA; C - DNA-RNA complexes are immobilized onto microplates coated with polyclonal IgG antibody; D – identification of immobilized hybrids by a second DNA-RNA alkaline phosphatise conjugated antibody, bounded to CDP star; E – a luminometer measures light emitted by the specimen (Digene-Qiagen website, modified)

The first generation of HC assay (HC1) was a tube-based detection system and probed for only nine HR-HPV types. The analytical sensitivity of the assay was 50,000 copies of HPV-16 DNA.

Several studies evaluated the clinical sensitivity and specificity of this first generation assay mainly against PCR and histology (Cavuslu et al., 1996; Cope et al., 1997; Shah et al., 1997). As expected, HC1 was less sensitive than PCR and other application techniques, but its specificity and positive predictive value (PPV) were higher than those of PCR. To improve the sensitivity of HC1, the Digene Corporation modified the first generation assay. The improved second-generation assay (Hybrid capture 2) is commercially available from the beginning of 1998. In this technology, the analytical sensitivity was increased to 1,000 HPV-DNA copies. Studies comparing first and second generation of Hybrid Capture technology shoved concordance in 96.8%. Interestingly, in all discordant samples containing HPV-DNA types covered by the probes included in both assay generation, the RLU/cutoff value ratios obtained in the second-generation assay were very low, which would indicate that low HPV viral load was the reason that produced false-negative results in the first-generation assay. HC2 assay is actually considered more sensitive than HC1, as well as more rapid, easier to perform and thus more appropriate for the routinary detection of HPV infection. In addition, as RLU signal is proportional to the amount of HPV-DNA present in the specimen, HC2 assay could be occasionally used to deduce viral load, on a semi-quantitative basis. The main advantage of HC2 test is the high sensitivity and the abundant clinical data which allowed to its FDA approval. Moreover, since HC2 test is less affected by cross-specimen contamination than PCR, it don't need for special laboratory (Carozzi et al., 2005; Cubie et al., 2005). On the other hand, there are many limitation to this techniques which have to be taken into account. First, the test cannot determine the specific HPV type present in the sample; this fact limits the recognition of persistent infection by the same viral type, which is the most important risk factor that induce cervical lesion to progress to invasive cancer. Second, at the standard FDA-approved cut-off of 1 pg/ml (RLU ≥1.0) and even at higher discriminating levels, RNA probes suffers from a cross-reactivity with non-oncogenic viral types and with certain oncogenic untargeted HPV types (53, 66, 67, 73) (Howard et al., 2004). Cross-reactivity with other oncogenic-HPV types might be beneficial for test sensitivity. On the other hand, cross-reactivity with non-cancer-causing types would have an adverse impact on clinical specificity and positive predictive value of the test, especially in population with a high prevalence of non-oncogenic types (Castle et al., 2003).

During 2003, a prototype version of Hybrid Capture 3® (HC3), possibly the next generation of HC2, has been evaluated for the detection of CIN3 and cancer. HC3 was designed to minimize cross-reactivity with untargeted HPV types. HC3 showed slightly higher sensitivity that HC2 for the detection of CIN2+ lesions but equal specificity. Actually, HC3 has not been marketed yet.

HC2 technology is amenable to automation, in case of high-volume screening use. The next-generation Hybrid Capture® (NextGen, QIAensemble™, Qiagen Inc., Gaithesburg, MD), consists of a fully automated platform (JE2000™) which utilizes a reengineered HC2 test. The implementation of analytical specificity, the maintenance of comparable levels of analytical sensitivity, the longer on-instrument stability of reagents, the detection of HPV-16 and 18 at lower copy number, the reduction of assay time (< 2.5 hrs compared to up to 5 hrs for HC2), as well as the reduction of the cross-reactivity with non-oncogenic HPV types (Eder et al., 2009), are the main advantages of NextGen. To validate the use of NextGen within screening context, pre-clinical studies using specimens from patients with histologically confirmed CIN2+ lesions are needed.

9. New paradigms in cervical cancer screening

Detection of oncogenic-HPV DNA is considered to be potentially useful in three clinical application: in population screening, as a primary test or in combination with cytology to detect cervical cancer precursors; in triaging, to select which cytological lesions must to be referred for colposcopy; in follow-up of women treated for high-grade intraepithelial lesion, to accurately identify patients with residual or recurrent lesion.

In adjunct to cytology, the purpose of HPV-DNA assay is the detection of latent or subclinical infection among symptoms-free women. In 2001, Belinson et al., performed a large cross-sectional study (1997 women ageing 35-45) in order to compare the sensitivity of LBC and HC2 test for the detection of CIN2+ lesions (Belinson et al., 2001). Essentially, the rationale of the use of adjunctive HPV-DNA testing is based on the accepted concept of necessary causality of HPV in determining cervical cancer and on the basis of the very high negative predictive value (90-100%) of the combination HPV-DNA test/LBC. Combining HPV-DNA test with LBC improves the performance of Pap test alone, especially when cervical cytology is ambiguous (*i.e.*, ASC-US and LSIL lesions). Using mathematical models to evaluate clinical and economics outcomes. Goldie at al., concluded that using HPV-DNA test plus cytology in women ≥ 30 years of age were more effective in reducing cancer incidence. Combining molecular biology and LBC could also result in increasing the screening interval for women testing negative at both cytology and DNA testing. Longer screening intervals with more sensitive tests would be the strategy providing the most advantageous balance between benefits and costs (Goldie et al., 2004).

In triage, the goal is to guide the management of patients with borderline or mildly diskaryotic smears (ASC-US and LSIL, respectively). ASC-US/LSIL Triage Study, a multicenter and randomized clinical trial sponsored by National Cancer Institute (NCI), evaluated three management strategies for women with ASC-US and LSIL cytological results: (i) immediate colposcopy; (ii) repeated cytology with referral to colposcopy if cytological findings showed HSIL lesion; (iii) HPV triage, with referral to colposcopy in case of HPV-DNA positivity (Rodriguez et al., 2008; Solomon et al., 2001).

ALTS established that: (a) HPV-DNA triage is as sensitive as immediate colposcopy in HSIL+ detection; however, molecular testing would spare all HPV-negative women from emotional and financial weight of colposcopy. (b) repeating cytology, would refer more than two-third of ASC-US/LSIL abnormalities to colposcopy. ALTS study attested that HPV-DNA method represents the best triage (Munoz et al., 2003). In the USA, HPV-DNA testing has been definitively integrated into cervical cancer screening programs and has become the standard of care in the triage of women over the age of 30, having minor cytological abnormalities (Wright et al., 2002); the rationale is the high proportion of HPV-DNA negative women (about 50%) among ASC-US group and the consequent extremely low risk of developing high-grade lesions. In this context, the role of DNA testing is to focus on those women ASC-US/DNA-positive in which colposcopic assessment is justified.

Following treatment with cryosurgery, laser ablation or LEEP for HSIL cervical lesion, 5-25% of patients may develop residual or recurrent high-grade disease (Kocken et al., 2011). Standard of care has been close cytological and colposcopic follow-up at 6, 12 and 24 months after treatment. However, since follow-up Pap test has a low specificity in detecting residual HSIL and given that HPV is cleared from the cervix following adequate treatment, DNA testing has been evaluated to predict the presence of residual dysplasia (Nam et al., 2009). In a recent meta-analysis, Zielinski et al. considered 11 studies evaluating HR-HPV DNA testing in monitoring women after treatment of CIN2+ lesions. It has been shown that the association HPV-DNA testing/cytology reached a NPV of 99% (Zielinski et al., 2004). The adoption of such algorithm of surveillance would mean to focus colposcopy only on women positive for both Pap and DNA test.

The consciousness of the necessary causality of HPV in determining cervical cancer defined new possible approaches to screen and prevent cervical cancer. In population screening, as a primary test, the purpose of HPV-DNA assay is the detection of latent or subclinical infection among symptom-free women (Rebolj et al., 2011).

Most authors evaluated the performances of cytology (conventional or LBC) and HPV testing (PCR or HC2) in detecting CIN2+ lesions or cervical cancer in several populations. Despite various study design, various ranges of age, various HPV detection techniques, various cervical lesions prevalence rates, the global survey of results leads to three main conclusions: for CIN2+ or greater (CIN2+), HPV testing is more sensitive (88-98% *versus* 51-86%) and has an higher negative predictive value (NPV) than cytology; specificity of DNA testing is lower than that of cytology (83-94% *versus* 92-99%); The sensitive and NPV of combined testing is near to 100%. The objective is then to start the primary screening by the most sensitive and automated test, HPV testing, and in second time to use the best specificity of cytology for diagnosis and triage (Arbyn et al., 2009). Women with abnormal smears would be immediately refer to colposcopy. Since a single negative HPV-DNA test reliably predicts a low risk of subsequent CIN2+, it would be justified to extend screening intervals. (Bulkmans et al., 2007).

Current European Guidelines for quality assurance in cervical cancer screening recommend implementation of pilot program with a validated HPV-DNA test within national organized cervical cancer screening programs and, if effective, permanent implementation of such programs (Arbyn et al., 2008). Longitudinal studies assessing the incidence of CIN2+ lesions are then essential to define the role of HPV testing in cervical cancer screening policies (Leinonen et al., 2009). Actually only baseline results of large randomized controlled trials are available.

Anttila et al., evaluated the impact of primary HPV-DNA screening plus conventional cytology triage of HPV-DNA positive women and compared this cohort with cytology-based screening cohoort. The study incorporated the population enrolled in organised screening programme for cervical cancer in Finland (Anttila et al., 2010). The evaluation was based on the total number of CIN3+ cases detected within five years after the invitation. The study, adding longitudinal information based on cancer registry files, showed that a single round of HPV primary test has been able to reduce the number of cases of invasive cervical cancer. These data suggest that using HPV DNA testing in primary screening, followed by cytology to triage HPV-DNA positive women, would represent an approach more sensitive than that based on cytology alone, in identifying CIN2+ lesions.

In Sweden Naucler et al., explored the efficacy of 11 different screening strategies based on HPV DNA testing alone, cytology alone, and HPV DNA testing combined with cytology (Naucler et al., 2009). They showed that using HPV DNA testing as primary screening followed by cytological triage and repeating HPV DNA testing on DNA-positive/ cytology negative women after at least 1 year would be a feasible strategy in primary cervical screening.

The Italian NTCC (New Technology for Cervical Cancer) randomized controlled trial compared Human Papillomavirus testing (HC2) alone with conventional cytology as the primary cervical cancer screening test, in a total of about 49,200 having a median age of 42 years (Ronco et al., 2008). Among women aged 35-60 years, HPV testing did not show a statistically significant extent *vs* conventional cytology for the detection of CIN2+ lesion. Vice versa, increasing the cut-off for HPV-DNA positive results from 1 to 2 pg/ml, molecular testing arm showed a statistically significant increase in sensitivity, associated to a non statistically significant reduction of PPV. The sensitivity of HPV testing compared with conventional cytology was much larger among women aging 25-34 than among older women. Ronco et al., recommended the use of HPV testing as primary screening in women older than 35 years of age and a preferable 2 pg/ml cut-off for HC2. In women aged less than 35 years, to avoid colposcopic overtreatment in HPV-positive/cytology negative patients, NTCC suggested 1 year molecular retesting (Figure 3).

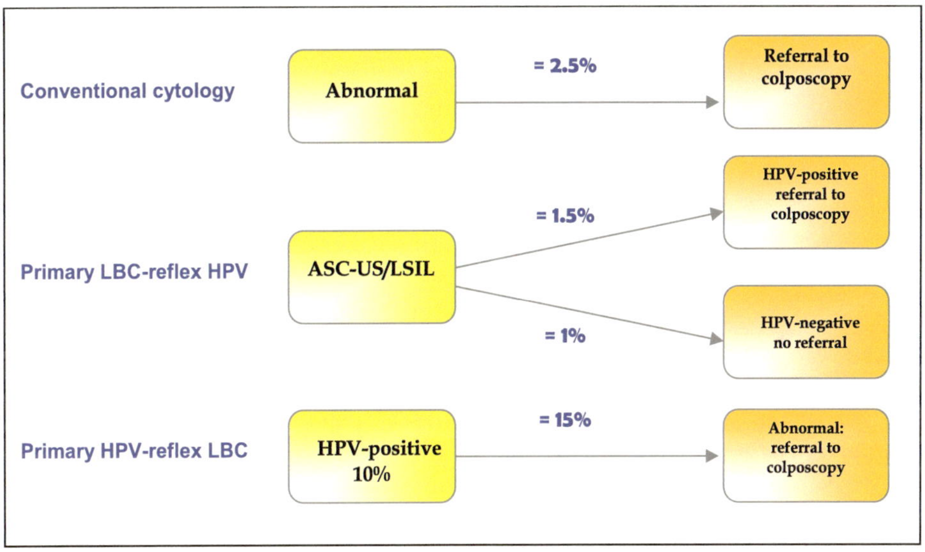

Fig. 3. Three different approaches to cervical cancer screening (Dillner J et al., BMJ 2008, modified)

The consultation of the Medline database by formulating the queries "HPV testing", "cervical cancer screening", "cervical cancer", "HPV testing in primary screening", "HPV-DNA screening test" allows to the following consideration:

1. all the trials (except for NTCC) found that sensitivity of HPV-DNA testing was higher than that of cytology, in detecting CIN2+ lesion;
2. all the trials state that NPP is higher for HPV testing than that for cytology. On the other hand, DNA testing is less specific than Pap test (89% *vs* 95%);
3. HPV testing alone might induce an overtreatment, especially in the youngest population. The specificity for both HPV testing and cytology are clearly lower below 30 years of age;

4. several studies showed that HPV-negativity alone or in combination with negative cytology triage would signify a longer disease interval against CIN2+ lesions than that being for cytology alone. In this context, it seems that a screening interval of five years, would be best choice. After five years, women testing DNA-negative would have a considerable lower risk for CIN2+ (0.25%) than woman having a normal Pap test (0.83%);
5. cytology triage of HPV-DNA positive women, would be the best strategy for referring to colposcopy patients who were DNA-positive/cytology positive;
6. it's meaningless to perform cytology on DNA-negative women; in this case, double testing adds negligible protection compared to HPV testing alone;
7. the better protection but the lower specificity of DNA testing implies that it should only be used in well-organized screening programs, in which the test is not used too frequently, or at too younger age (Dillner et al., 2008; Naucler et al., 2007; Naucler et al., 2009).

It's our opinion that further evaluation of the risk of CIN2+ lesions with different combination of test and in relation to women's age, would be the next step; then, it's important to choose the best primary screening tool, taking in account costs and logistics of the single countries.

The next step in research could be to improve the specificity of HPV-DNA testing by validating adjunctive markers, predictive of HPV persistence, in liquid-based cytology biobanks.

10. New ways to use existing technologies

From the meta-analyses summarised above, it is clear that HPV-DNA testing is substantially more sensitive than cytology at detecting CIN2+ lesions. However, molecular testing is rather less specific than cytology. The main problem with DNA testing is the high prevalence of HPV-DNA positivity among female population, compared with the low number of women with transient infection which spontaneously would regress. These considerations suggest that the more sensitive test should be applied firstly (i.e. DNA testing), while the more specific test should be used only in HPV-positive women, in order to establish the correct management strategy.

The approach of using HPV-DNA test as the sole primary screening modality has several advantages: HPV-DNA detection assays is an objective and automatable test with a dichotomous result; his allows for better quality of screening. Cytology can thus to be reserved for the 5-15% of women who are DNA-positive. This protocol would obtain cost savings through reductions in staff numbers, would reduce turnaround time of diagnosis, would avoid overtreatment and could permit a longer screening interval. For DNA testing, the requirement for adequate specimen sampling is less rigorous, when compared to cytology. Several studies evaluated the diagnostic accuracy of self-collected cervico-vaginal specimens (Ogilvie et al., 2005). With an overall sensitivity of 74% and specificity of 84%, self-taken sampling appears to be favourable in settings where sensitivity of cytology is typically less than 70%. Göh M et al., found that women prefer self-sampling to a clinician taken-sampling (Gök et al., 2010). These results suggest that self-sampling for HPV-DNA testing could be a valuable screening method to recruit women who refuse to attend clinician-based screening, and to improve population coverage of screening.

11. Screening in low-resource settings: changing the paradigm of cervical cancer prevention and control

In developing countries, it seems unrealistic to introduce cytological screening and histopathological follow-up because of financial, technical and human limitations. Alternative methods of screening that would surmount barriers consisting in the "three-visit cytology-based approach" are needed which accurately predict the presence of cervical cancer or precursors (Table). Three requisites are essential in effective screening program: screening diagnosis and treatment should be provided on-site or in clinics accessible to the vast majority of women at risk of developing cancer; reproducible, validated, low-cost screening test should be available; screening should ensure high participation of women at risk for cervical cancer, by using appropriate educational programmes direct towards both health workers and population. While the first two conditions are essential in low-resource settings, the third is an universal requirement.

In low-resource settings, a wide number of tests have been investigated over the years, as alternative screening tests to cytology. The four most widely studied alternative approaches are VIA (visual inspection with acetic acid), VILI (visual inspection with Lugol's iodine), self-sampling and HPV testing.

Screening test	Sensitivity*	Specificity*	Characteristics
Conventional cytology	44%-78%	91%-96%	Requires adequate laboratory-based healthcare infrastructure, stringent training and quality control
HPV testing	66%-100%	61%-96%	High throughput, objective, reproducible and robust but currently expensive
VIA	62%-80%	77%-84%	Low cost, strict linkage to immediate treatment
VILI	92%	85%	Low cost, strict linkage to immediate treatment
Colposcopy	44%-77%	85%-90%	Expensive, inappropriate for low-resource settings

Table. Ranges of sensitivity and specificity and characteristics of some screening methods. VIA: visual inspection with acetic acid; VILI: visual inspection with Lugol's iodine

11.1 Visual inspection with acetic acid

This technique involves the examination of the cervix with the naked eye and a bright light source, one minute after the application of 3-5% diluted acetic acid. Detection of well-defined aceto-white areas close to the squamocolonnar junction, indicates a positive test. CIN and microinvasive cancer switch-on white following acetic acid application. Aceto-whitening is essentially due to a reversible coagulation of intracellular proteins. The high concentration of intracellular proteins in neoplasia led to the dense aceto-whitening appearance. The main advantage of VIA is that it yields an immediate result, thus making it possible for treatment of abnormalities at the same visit ("screen-and-treat"approach). This method is also inexpensive and can be carried out by using modest equipments, without the need for laboratory infrastructures. Moreover, health workers can be rapidly trained to perform VIA (about ten days of courses duration). Several cross-sectional studies evaluated the accuracy of VIA in developing countries. Pooled estimates of the sensitivity of the test in detecting CIN2+ lesions vary from 62 to 80%, and the specificity from 77 to 84% (Arbyn et al., 2008; Gaffikin et al., 2008; Hovland et al., 2010). The greatest reduction in incidence and mortality rates are observed for the 30-39 years of age group.

11.2 Visual inspection with Lugol's iodine

VILI involves the examination of the cervix the naked eye, in order to identify yellow areas after the application of Lugol's iodine. A multi-centre study conducted in Africa and India showed a pooled sensitivity and specificity to detect CIN2+ lesions of 92% and 85% respectively, thus indicating a higher sensitivity than VIA but a similar specificity (Sarian et al., 2005).

11.3 Self-sampling

Self-sampling method using self-collected vaginal samples is another alternative approach for primary screening in developing countries. The aim would be to try to increase the coverage of population when women do not undergo a gynaecological examination and when cytology screening is not available. Prevalence of oncogenic HPV types on self-sampled vaginal material is about 5-10%, lower than for cervical smear; sensitivity for detecting CIN is also decreased in respect to cytology (Bekkers et al., 2006). However, for women not participating in programs of screening, vaginal self-sampling could be a good alternative and could reduce the risk of cervical cancer.

11.4 HPV-DNA testing

Screening must be linked to treatment to ensure its efficacy. This can be done using the traditional approach (screen, diagnosis, confirm and treat), intermediate approach (screen, diagnose and treat, with post-treatment biopsy confirmation) or screen-and-treat approach (treatment is based on the result of screening alone). A number of studies have investigated the screen-and-treat approach, and its safety and feasibility has been always confirmed. Basing on these studies, primary screening with HPV testing was considered an attractive approach.

The use of HPV-DNA testing may prove more practical, especially when incorporated into strategies less dependent on existing laboratory infrastructure, such as low-resource setting and developing countries. This "single-visit HPV-DNA testing strategy" requires screening sites to run the test on the day in which the sample is received and to allow for treatment of cervical lesion during the same visit (Levin et al., 2010). "See and treat' approach would reduce the number of non-compliance to treatment and improve the efficiency of the program.

No HPV-DNA existing test was deemed appropriate for the use in low-resources settings. For this reason, PATH (Seattle, WA, USA) and Qiagen entered into collaborative agreement and developed a new rapid, simple and affordable HPV-DNA test, specifically designed for developing countries. CareHPV™ is a signal-amplification assay that detects 14 different carcinogenic HPV types (16, 18, 31, 33, 35, 39, 45, 51, 52, 56, 58, 59, 66 and 68) in 2-5-hrs processing time. The assay needs only a footprint, no mains electricity or running water. The short time-consuming would permit a same-day diagnostic evaluation, with treatment in a second visit, or even screening and treatment in the same day. CareHPV can be performed by inexperienced, newly trained and minimally educated technicians, under suboptimal condition of temperature, humidity, lightning and space. CareHPV use would be associated to fewer visits and transportation costs, and would reduce loss to follow-up. The rapid HPV-DNA, with its lower cost per test and greater sensitivity than conventional cytology now dominates other screening methods in developing countries. Levin CE et al., showed that accuracy for the detection of CIN2+ lesions was higher for careHPV test than for VIA. No differences has been detected between CareHPV and HC2, when screening women 30 years of age and older (Levin et al., 2010).

With the availability of vaccine against HPV-16 and 18, there has been enthusiasm for vaccination of young adolescent girls, also in disadvantage settings. Although preadolescent vaccination offers great hope for future generation, there exist a number of uncertainties that will persist for the next decades, including the need for drastically lower vaccine prices and creative financing sources to support vaccination costs. For the older women, the best option to reduce deaths from cervical cancer will still be the secondary prevention. Rapid HPV-DNA testing, 3 time per lifetime, would have excellent potential to be and effective and cost-effective strategy. Particularly, the strategy of vaccinating targeting young adolescent and screening and treat older women, could address social, economic and political organization to contribute in reducing cervical cancer incidence and mortality in developing countries (Tsu et al., 2008).

12. Molecular surrogate markers

The sensitivity of HPV-DNA assays for the detection of CIN2+ is high, although they cannot discriminate transient infections from persistent infections, thus lacking in specificity. Consequently, there is motivation to evaluate more disease-specific biomarkers, able to identify women susceptible to progression. Ideally the candidate marker, defining the different stages (clearance, persistence, progression) of cellular changes associated with HPV infection, should give a high positive predictive value in predicting progression to cervical cancer. Recently, guidelines have been proposed for the development of biomarker-based screening toll for early detection of cancer, which can be categorized into five phases: 1) preclinical exploratory studies for marker discovery; 2) clinical assay development and validation; 3) retrospective longitudinal repository studies; 4) prospective screening; 5) cancer control studies, including cost-benefit analysis.

Potential markers of progression include HPV viral load, DNA methylation, HPV-DNA sequences integrated into the host genome, over-expression of cell-cycle regulator proteins or proliferation markers, telomerase and messenger RNA for E6 and E7 oncoproteins. Here, we will restrict the discussion to the markers which have been evaluated in large clinical trials and reached some level of clinical applicability.

12.1 HPV VIral load

HR-HPV viral load has been suggested to be a useful marker in distinguishing infection of clinical relevance (48, 49). Among women with HPV-DNA positivity, cytological abnormalities are more common in those having high viral load (Lilli et al., 2005; Xi et al., 2011).

However, it is now clear that the liaison between viral load and cervical disease is more complex that it was previously thought. (De Oer et al., 2007). Many cross-sectional studies reported an increased viral load with growing disease severity, but others found no association (50). There are some probable reasons for these contradictions: HPV integrated status increases with enhancing of disease severity; integration status is characterized by a declined viral replication. Thus paradoxically, the risk of disease progression is not associated to the rate of viral replication but is sometimes just the opposite! (Denis et al., 2008). In our retrospective longitudinal analysis, we did not observe a significant association between semi-quantitative value of viral load and low-grade cervical lesions outcome (Zappacosta R et al, data not shown). In addition, the relationship between viral load and cervical disease varies among oncogenic HPV types. Studies using quantitative type-specific PCR for HR-HPV 16, 18, 31, 33 and 45 and LR-HPV 6 and 11 showed that HPV-16 can reach a much higher viral load than the other above listed types and that only HPV-16 viral load might correlate with increased severity of cervical disease (Saunier et al., 2008). Then, all oncogenic HPV types but 16 are able to provoke cervical cancer, even when they are present at low levels (Boulet et al., 2008).

12.2 DNA methylation markers

More recently, epigenetic alteration of genome of HPV-infected cells have been considered as diagnostic marker for cervical cancer. Aberrant presence of CpG-rich DNA sequences (the so-called CpG islands) in the promoter region of tumor suppressor genes, represents one of the several epigenetic changes that contribute to carcinogenesis (Esteller et al., 2002). DNA methylation involves the covalent addition of a methyl (-CH3) group at the carbon-5 position of a cytosine that precedes a guanosine. Usually, DNA methylation plays a role in maintaining genome stability and in regulating gene expression (Jung et al., 2011). However, global hypermethylation of CpG clusters located in the promoter region of multiples genes have been associated with malignancy (Ehrlich, 2002). Numerous clinical studies demonstrated that these epigenetic methylation changes are often present in a variety of cancer. In this framework, silencing of the Tumor Suppressor Lung Cancer 1 (TSLC1) gene by promoter hypermethylation may be a valuable biomarker to detect cervical lesions with high malignancy potential. TSLC1 was found to be silenced in 91% of cervical cancer cell lines, primarily resulting from promoter hypermethylation (Yang et al., 2006). Moreover, such hypermethylation was detected in 58% of cervical carcinomas and in 35% of CIN2+ lesions, but not in low-grade CIN or in normal cervix (Fenq et al., 2005). The high frequency of TSLC1 methylationin in cervical cancer was confirmed by studies of Li et al., (Li et al., 2005) and Gustafson et al. (Gustafson et al., 2004). These data suggest that the analysis of methylation patterns of TSLC1 gene maight be a valuable tool in forthcoming screening programs; however, they appear more likely to play a role in detecting cervical cancer cell clones rather than cells in early initiating events of cervical carcinogenesis.

12.3 Markers of viral DNA integration

Viral integration often occurs at the E2 gene of the HPV genome. Disruption of the E2 gene is believed to result in more intensive transcription of the oncogenes E6 and E7. In the episomal state, E2 and E6 DNA are present in equal amounts, while in the integrated form, less intact E2 is present (zur Hausen, 2002). Then, a decrease in E2/E6 DNA ratio assessed with real-time PCR would be a valuable potential progression marker.

12.4 Ki-67 and other markers of proliferation or regulation of cell cycle

Expression of Ki-67 protein occurs in proliferating cells and its presence is normally confined to the basal or suprabasal epithelial cells layers. Expression of Ki-67 allows distinction of negative atrophic cells and positive neoplastic cells in menopausal women. Expression beyond the inner third of the cervical epithelium is observed in case of CIN and cancer. Several authors have found a significant correlation between the presence/intensity of Ki-67 and the severity of cytological abnormality in cytological preparation (Luzzatto et al., 2004; Sahebali et al., 2003). However, deeper analysis did not confirm the initially hopeful results and showed that these markers did not have adequate sensitivity and specificity to supply the request of additive prognostic markers, in cytological screening (Wentzensen & von Knebel Doeberitz, 2007).

Several other proteins are overexpressed in proliferating cells. So, certain cell progression regulators have been proposed as potential markers for cervical neoplasia: Proliferating Cell Nuclear Antigen (PCNA), Mcm5, Cdc6 and Cyclin E. Proliferation markers are physiologically present in basal and parabasal cells, and are an objective indicator of neoplasia when observed beyond the lower cell layers. In cervical smears, lacking architectural information, the presence of proliferation markers is less informative and can easily yield false-positive results.

12.5 Telomerase

Telomerase are repeated arrays of six nucleotides (TTAGGG) at the chromosome ends that protects chromosomes against degradation, aberrant fusion or recombination. They become progressively shorter as cells multiply, resulting in chromosomal instability and senescence when a critical short length is reached. The enzyme telomerase is a ribo-nucleoprotein composed of two parts: an RNA part (hRT) and a catalytic part (hTERT), which controls telomere length. hTERT is believed to play a role in cells immortalization. Its activity in increased in CIN and cancer (Barbosa et al., 2011). The intensity of telomerase activity is reported to be correlated with the severity of the abnormality, both in cervical biopsies and cytology. However, reliable detection of hTR, hTERT and telomerase activity is still limited by analytical deficiencies (Xiang et al., 2011).

12.6 p16 ^{INK4a}

Cyclin-dependent kinases (CDKs), cyclins and CDK inhibitors are key molecules that control the cell cycle and coordinate DNA synthesis, chromosome separation and cell division. The cyclin-dependent kinase inhibitor p16 ^{INK4a} prevent the CDK4/6 interaction with cyclin D1, thus stopping progression of cell cycle through the G1/S checkpoint. Usually, HPV-E7 oncoprotein is expressed only in terminally differentiated superficial cell layers of the cervical epithelium, Several factors, such as loss of cellular inhibiting factors and integration of HPV genome into the host genome, can lead to the expression of E7 in basal cell layers. The result is the cellular transformation and the massive accumulation of p16 ^{ink4A} into cells. Accumulation of p16 mRNA and related protein has been reported in response to inactivation of the retinoblastoma gene product (pRb), through binding with viral E7 oncoprotein. p16 is then overexpressed at very low levels in normal cells, while it is strongly over-expressed in cervical cancer cell lines, in which pRB has been inactivated by E7 (Lambert et al., 2006).

The usefulness of immunocytochemical detection of p16 overexpression in cervical samples has been shown in many trials and has been widely accepted, especially as reflex test for the triage of equivocal or mildly abnormal Pap cytologic results. In triaging ASC-US and LSIL cases, it has been shown that p16 immunocytochemical analyses might provide similar sensitivity for the detection of underlying CIN2+ lesions as HPV testing, but at significantly higher specificity level (Denton et al., 2010). A recent meta-analysis (Tsoumpou et al., 2009), showed a substantial variability in the literature regarding the cut-off for positive p16 results; this variability was probably due to the wide range of colorbased qualitative (nuclear or cytoplamatic positivity, staining intensity, etc.) and quantitative parameters (ie, number of immunoreactive cells), which singly or in combinations could be use for the evaluation of results. The purely colour-based approaches to identify abnormal cells in cervical smears using $p16^{INK4a}$, is hampered by the fact that some normal endocervical, endometrial, intercalated, squamous metaplastic or atrophic cells may also display p16-immunoreactivity. For this reason, it was proposed the evaluation of a score based on a four-tiered classification of nuclear abnormalities of p16-positive cells, to discriminate between no abnormal nuclei (score 1), slightly abnormal nuclei (score 2), clearly abnormal nuclei (score 3), and severely abnormal nuclei (score 4). Nuclei from normal-intermediate cells or polymorphonuclear granulocytes were used as an internal size, shape, staining, and texture standard (Wentzenses et al., 2005). Despite NS classification, there are still disagreement in literature regarding the utility of $p16^{INK4a}$ tool, both as locator of high-grade cervical cells-positive cell as well as interpreter, for the predictive assessment of potential abnormal cells. Disagreements are based on the common conviction about the poor feasibility of $p16^{INK4a}$ immunocytochemical assay.

13. Novel approaches with prognostic significance in cervical cancer prevention

13.1 *p16/Ki-67* dual stain

Under physiological conditions, the simultaneous expression of a protein with a tumor-suppressive function (p16) and a proliferation marker (Ki-67) mutually excludes each other. Vice versa, simultaneous detection of p16 overexpression and expression of proliferation marker K1-67 within the same cervical epithelial cell indicates deregulation of the cell cycle. In this context, it has been proposed the use of the immunocytochemical evaluation of p16-Ki-67 coexpression to identify esocervical cells with deregulated cell cycle, independently from morphology-based interpretation parameters (Galgano et al., 2010). The presence of one or more double-immunoreactive cell may be considered positive and indicative of underlying CIN2+ lesion (Schmidt D et al., 2011). The European Equivocal or Mildly Abnormal Papanicolaou Cytology Study (EEMAPS) evaluated the performance of the new immunocytochemical p16/Ki-67 dual-stain protocol (CINtec+ assay, mtm laboratories AG, Heidelberg, Germany) in the triage of ASC-US and LSIL lesions. Results from this study showed a high sensitivity of CINtec+ test for the detection of underlying CIN2+ lesions in women with ASC-US and LSIL cytology, comparable to sensitivity showed by HPV testing and p16 single-stain cytology. Particularly, Schmidt et al., showed that, in ASC-US triage, p16/Ki-67 dual-stain identified the same proportion of underlying CIN2+ lesions as HPV testing, but significantly reducing the number of women which would need referral to colposcopy, especially in younger population. Regarding CINtec+ dual-stain specificity, this was significantly improved in comparison with that of p16 single-stain approach.

In a recent retrospective analysis, conducted within the regional organized screening program of Abruzzo region (Italy), in which Hybrid Capture 2 test is used in primary screening, we analyzed the diagnostic performances of p16^{INK4a}/Ki67 dual-stained cytology in identifying CIN2+ lesion in 372 HPV-DNA positive women triaged for LSIL-or-worse (LSIL+) Pap cytology (unpublished data). Preliminary results showed that reflex CINtec+ test improved significantly sensitivity and NPV of cytology alone in triaging LSIL+ lesions (90.8% *vs* 62% and 77.2% *vs* 88.3%, respectively), but reduced triage cytology specificity and PPV (42.6% *vs* 79.6% and 49.4% *vs* 65.2%, respectively). In this context we believe that p16/Ki67 cytology, as a reflex test, may efficiently complement HPV-based screening programs to prevent cervical cancer, but follow-up studies are needed to assess its effective value in terms of predictive marker.

13.2 Direct detection of cervical carcinogenesis: mRNA markers

As previously described, one of the key consequences of HPV-induced chromosomal instability is the integration of HPV genome into the host-cell genome together with the continuous and deregulated expression of E6/E7 viral oncogenes. Then persistent expression of E6/E7 is a necessary step for HPV-induced carcinogenesis.

E6 expression is regulated at transcriptional or post-transcriptional level. HPV-16 E6 ORF encodes for three different variants of E6 protein, which may have dissimilar roles in the viral cell cycle. These transcripts are either unspliced (full length-FL- E6 transcripts) or spliced (Figure 4). Interestingly, only FL E6 protein has been found to be powerfully bound to p53, thus promoting its degradation. Moreover, only the unspliced E6 form was found to be more strongly associated with tumorigenicity. Studies carried out on cervical cancer samples show that FL transcripts are always present (Wise-Draper, & Wells, 2008). These studies indicate FL transcripts as being the most important biomarkers for the carcinogenic process (Asadurian et al., 2007). Then, tests for the detection of E6/E7 mRNA seems to be promising in increasing HPV testing specificity.

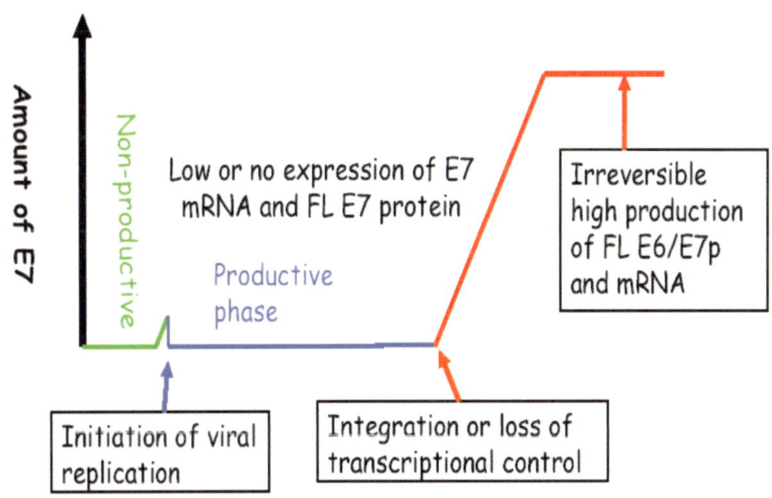

Fig. 4. Full length E7 transcripts in relation to HPV life cycle

13.2.1 Nuclisens® EasyQ HPV mRNA test and PreTect™ HPV- Proofer mRNA test

Various in-house assays for E6/E7 mRNA detection have been described, most of which have employed a reverse transcription PCR approach, focusing on HPV-16 and -18. Now, two commercial RNA assays are available: the Nuclisens EasyQ HPV assay (biomérieux S.A., France), in certain countries distribuited as the PreTect HPV-Proofer® assay (Norchip AS, Klokkarstua, Noway), and the Aptima® HPV Assay (Gen-Probe Incorporated, San Diego, CA) .

Both assays are compatible with samples collected in cytology media.

Nuclisens EasyQ HPV assay is a multiplex nucleic acid sequence amplification (NASBA) method, detecting FL transcripts of E6/E7 oncoproteins in a DNA background is commercially available from two companies; they are the and (Boulet et al., 2008). The test is based on the molecular beacon probe technology and on the real-time detection of five oncogenic HPV types (16, 18, 31, 33 and 45). Molecular beacons are oligonucleotide probes consisting of stem-loop structure and of two regions: loop region, is a single-stranded 18-30 base pair sequence that is complementary to the target sequence; stem region, typically consists of 5-7 base pair long double-stranded sequences that lie on both arms of loop region; 5′ sequences are labeled with a fluorescent dye (fluorophore) while 3′ sequences are covalently labeled with a non-fluorescent quencher. In absence of a complementary target sequence, molecular beacon remains closed and in a nonhybridized state; in this situation, the quencher captures the fluorescent signal. When beacon unfolds the presence of the complementary target (E6/E7 mRNA), loop region hybridizes with this sequence, fluorophore separates itself from the quencher, and the fluorescent signal is transmitted (Figure 5).

In Nuclisens procedure, two different labeled molecular beacon probes for each multiplex reaction are used. Fluorescein (FAM) is used as fluorophore for the detection of HPV-16, 31, and 33; Texas Red (TxR) as fluorophore for the detection of U1A gene, HPV-18, and HPV-45.

U1A is a small nuclear specific ribonucleoprotein A included in HPV-Proofer kit to avoid false-negative results, and to monitor sample mRNA integrity. NASBA amplification is achieved through coordinated activities of three enzymes (Avian Myeloblastosis Virus Reverse Transcriptase, *E.Coli* Rnase H and T7 RNA polymerase) and two DNA oligonucleotide primers that are specific for the target sequence of interest. RNA amplification is performed for one hundred and fifty minutes at isothermal temperature of 41 °C. In presence of the target sequences, a fluorescent signal is observed. A fluorescent analyzer measures, in real-time, the emitted fluorescence from molecular beacon hybridized with amplified mRNA (Varnai et al., 2008).

Cuschieri et al., carried out a follow-up study on 54 HPV-DNA positive samples obtained from 3,444 cytologically normal women. Samples which were PreTect HPV-Proofer-positive over 9 months (persistence), were proven to have CIN3 in most cases (Cuschieri et al., 2004). This study showed the strict correlation between E6/E7 mRNA expression and oncogenic HPV-DNA persistence, moreover detecting a mRNA test specificity higher (81%) than DNA-based methods (44%). Cuschieri concluded that mRNA test (PreTech or Nuclisens) would find persistent HPV infection and would reduce the need for follow-up or repeated test, that will be sometime necessary if DNA-based technology is used.

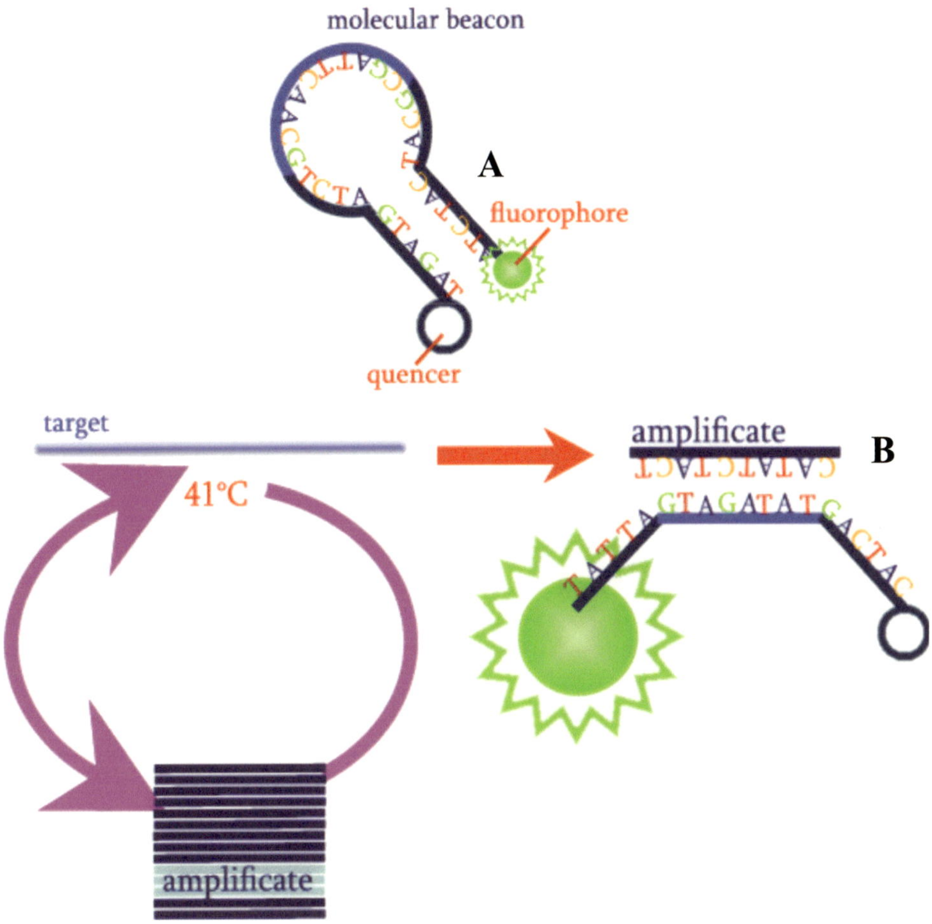

Fig. 5. NASBA technology. A – molecular beacon in absence of target sequence; B – molecular beacon unfolds the presence of the complementary target and transmits fluorescent

The high clinical accuracy of E6/E7 mRNA test has been confirmed by a large cross-sectional study, carried out on about 4,000 women older than 30 years assessed longitudinally for a minimum of 2 years, based on detection of HPV-DNA and E6/E7 mRNA. Cytological and histological data related to follow-up were also included (Molden et al., 2005). DNA and RNA test showed identical sensitivity to detect CIN2+ lesion, but the specificity for RNA and DNA test was 85% and 50% respectively. Benevolo et al carried out a retrospective study to evaluate the performance of mRNA test as a triage test for cytology and HPV DNA testing. The study analyzed 1,201 women, 688 of whom had a colposcopy follow-up and 195 of whom had histology-confirmed CIN2+ lesion. Diagnostic accuracy for CIN2+ were determined for mRNA test in comparison to HPV-DNA test and cytology. Stratifying by cytological grades, mRNA test sensitivity ranged from 62% to 83%. The corresponding figures for DNA testing ranged from 91% to 96%. Specificity values for mRNA test and DNA test ranged from 45% to 82% and from 4% to 29%, respectively. Used as a triage test for ASC-US and L-SIL, mRNA test reduced colposcopies by 69-79%, while

DNA testing reduced colposcopies by 15-38%. As a HPV-DNA positivity triage, mRNA test reduced colposcopies by 63%, whereas cytology at the ASC-US+ threshold reduced colposcopies by 23% (Benevolo et al., 2011).

These data, combined with others 15 extensive studies carried out in many countries, show that mRNA test might reduce the number of ASCUS and LSIL cases to be followed by colposcopy-directed biopsies by more than 70% (Nakagawa et al., 2000). Then, overexpression of E6/E7 for carcinogenic HPV types might prove a specific and predictive marker of precancerous lesions that need clinical attention. At present, only the above listed five oncogenic HPV types are detectable by Nuclisens technology; at the first sight this may be considered a disadvantage in comparison with the available DNA genotyping strategies. However, studies carried out to find E6/E7 mRNA in cervical smears of women with cervical cancer, demonstrated a 100% coverage by these genotypes (Kraus et al., 2006; Skomedal et al., 2006).

13.2.2 Aptima® HPV mRNA test

APTIMA® HPV Assay (Gen-Probe Incorporated, San Diego, CA) is a target amplification nucleic acid probe test for the in vitro qualitative detection of E6/E7 mRNA from 14 oncogenic HPV types (16, 18, 31, 33, 35, 39, 45, 51, 52, 56, 58, 59, 66, 68), in LBC specimens. The assay provides a qualitative result (positive/negative) for the presence/absence of these oncogenic HPV types, but does not determine the specific HPV type present in the specimen.This technology amplifies target mRNAs using transcription-mediated amplification (TMA) and detects the amplification products using nucleic acid probes without specific distinction among the specific HPV types implicated.

APTIMA HPV Assay involves three main steps, which take place in a single tube: capture, amplification and detection. To capture the target mRNA, HPV-specific capture oligomers and magnetic microparticles are used. Target mRNA is amplified by transcription-mediated amplifications (TMA) and using two enzymes: Moloney murine leukemia virus reverse transcriptase and T7 RNA polymerase. Targeted amplification is achieved using primers that hybridize to conserved regions of oncogenic E6/E7 mRNA. The detection of the amplification products (amplicons) is carried out through dual kinetic assay . Specifically, analyte amplicons are detected using 2-methyl acridinium ester-labeled probes, which hybridized to conserved region of carcinogenic HPV types. An fluoro-acridium ester-labeled probe is used to detect internal control amplicon added to each reaction to verify the performance of each step of the assay.

Positive and negative calibrators are used to determine the validity of the run and to establish the assay cut-off values for the internal control and analyte signals. Chemiluminescent signal observed for each reaction is measured using a luminometer, and compared to the cut-off values. Specimens with cut-off (S/CO) ratio ≥1.00 are considered positive. Samples with S/CO ratio <1.00 must have an internal control signal greater than or equal to the internal control cut-off value and may be considered a valid negative result.

FASE (French APTIMA Screening Evaluation) study was the first trial comparing Aptima mRNA test with LBC and HC2 (Monsonego et al., 2011). Data from about 4,500 Parisian women have been analyzed. Results showed that the sensitivity of Aptima mRNA test for detecting CIN2+ lesions was similar to that offered by HC2 test but is significantly higher than that of LBC. In addition, the specificity of Aptima was significantly higher than that of both HC2 and cytology.

Actually, for its characteristics, Aptima test is considered to be the ideal assay for primary cervical cancer screening, offering good specificity without losing sensitivity. The use of APTIMA HPV Assay would reduce the number of false positive results compared to DNA assays, helping limit the number false positive results leading to inappropriate and costly diagnostic procedures, over-treatment and needless anxiety in women.

On the other hand, PreTect HPV-Proofer/Nuclisens EasyQ HPV mRNA tests with their high specificity and PPV, is considered helpful in the clinical work-up of DNA-positive women, particularly of those with ASC-US/LSIL cervical abnormalities, also in consideration of its flexibility when used in LBC samples, stored at room temperature in cytological biobanks.

Basing on these consideration, mRNA-based technology would certainly increase the diagnostic accuracy of cervical abnormalities, through a better identification of HPV infection which are more likely to persist and induce CIN2+ lesions in future, and by reducing psychological distress and costs for women who only have a transient infection.

14. Conclusions

Persistent HPV infection has proven to be important in predicting cell abnormalities. Hence, a supplementary method should reveal HPV persistence and preferentially give additional information about the outcome of the disease. The ideal test should then reveal optimal analytical and clinical accuracies. Analytical accuracy of a test merely refers to the ability of detection of an endpoint. Clinical accuracy is a parameter which is more related to medical practice: it expresses the ability of the test to detect a relevant phase of disease.

Studies summarized above resulted in a long list of candidate tools which may improve Pap test in the early detection of cervical cancer. Most of these markers have not yet passed the first phases of validation but surely, their number is expected to expand, as more genomic and proteomic studies will appear in the near future.

Before integrating the ideal marker into clinical practice, deeper clinical validation studies are needed, particularly longitudinal assessment to prospectively evaluate its clinical performances. At the moment, it is difficult to predict which of those markers or marker panels are ultimately the most promising candidates, also considering the shift to primary HPV screening.

Currently, most national vaccination program are primarily aimed to preadolescents and adolescents. It is an extremely positive fact to hope in use of a vaccine capable to prevent a neoplasia with so strong social impact such as cervicocarcinoma. However, there are several issues that still need to be addressed before the fully appreciation of HPV vaccination in matter of overall potential and impact for public health (Psirry & Di Maio, 2008; Stanley et al., 2006). First, the duration of protection is unknown. Second, bivalent vaccination will only protect against HPV-16 and 18. Third, prophylactic vaccines are likely to provide limited benefits to women previously infected with oncogenic HPVs. Fourth, vaccines are relatively expensive and vaccine delivery in developing world is more difficult. Fifth, the effects of vaccination on the female psychology could be dangerous: if vaccinated women will believe to be at no further risk of developing HPV-induced cancer and will leave screening programs, the last impact of vaccination on the incidence of cervicocarcinoma will be invalided (Welters et al., 2008).

It is therefore important that both, women and healthcare professionals, do not perceive HPV vaccination as an immediate alternative to cervical cancer screening, because only integrating HPV vaccination into screening programs will maximize the benefits offered by vaccine and will lead to a greater reduction of cervical cancer prevalence, incidence, and mortality. It was recently reported that , if both HPV testing and vaccination are performed, the total number of annual number of Pap tests is predicted to be reduced by 43% (Logatto-Filho & Schmitt, 2007). In this context, the nature of the screening and the management of women must to be adapted to the new technologies.

In conclusion, moving the diagnostics from the cellular level into the molecular level allows not only to better identify cervical precancerous states, but also to prevent cervical pathology in the stage of molecular changes. In this context, the management of women with HPV infection would be based on risk categories rather than on specific assay results. This tailored cervical cancer risk assessment give hope for the improvement of effectiveness of cervical cancer prevention and for a significant reduction of screening costs.

15. References

Abulafia, O., Pezzullo, J.C. & Sherer, D.M. (2003). Performance of ThinPrep liquid-based cervical cytology in comparison with conventionally prepared Papanicolaou smears: a quantitative survey. *Gynecol Oncol* 90: 137-144.

Anttila, A., Kotaniemi-Talonen, L., Leinonen, M., Hakama, M., Laurila, P., Tarkkanen, J., Malila, N. & Nieminen, P. (2010). Rate of cervical cancer, severe intraepithelial neoplasia, and adenocarcinoma in situ in primary HPV DNA screening with cytology triage: randomised study within organised screening programme. *BMJ* 27; 340-350.

Arbyn, M., Sankaranarayanan, R., Muwonge, R., Keit,a N., Dolo, A., Mbalawa, C.G., Nouhou, H., Sakande. B., Wesley, R., Somanathan, T., Sharma, A., Shastri, S. & Basu, P. (2008). Pooled analysis of the accuracy of five cervical cancer screening tests assessed in eleven studies in Africa and India. *Int J Cancer* 1; 123(1): 153-160.

Arbyn, M., Martin-Hirsch, P., Buntinx, F., Van Ranst, M., Paraskevaidis, E. & Dillner, J. (2009). Triage of women with equivocal or low-grade cervical cytology results: a meta-analysis of the HPV test positivity rate. *J Cell Mol Med* 13(4):648-659.

Arbyn, M., Castellsagué, X., de Sanjosé, S., Bruni, L., Saraiya, M., Bray, F. & Ferlay, J. (2011). Worldwide burden of cervical cancer in 2008. *Ann Oncol* 6, in press.

Asadurian, Y., Kurilin, H., Lichtig, H., Jackman, A., Gonen, P., Tommasino, M., Zehbe, I. & Sherman, L. (2007). Activities of human papillomavirus 16 E6 natural variants in human keratinocytes. *J Med Virol* 79: 1751-1760.

Barbosa, L.C., da Silva, I.D., Corrêa, J.C. & Ribalta, J.C. (2011). Survivin and telomerase expression in the uterine cervix of women with human papillomavirus-induced lesions. *Int J Gynecol Cancer* 21: 15-21.

Bekkers, R.L., Meijers, C.J., Massunger, L.F., Snijders, P.J. & Melchers, W.J. (2006). Effects of HPV detection in population-based screening programmes for cervical cancer: a Dutch moment. *Gynecol Oncol* 100: 451-454.Belinson, J., Qiao, Y.L., Pretorius, R., Zhang, W.H., Elson, P., Li, L., Pan, Q.J., Fischer, C., Lorincz, A. & Zahniser, D. (2001). Shanxi Province cervical cancer study: a cross-sectional comparative trial of multiple techniques to detect cervical neoplasia. *Gynecol Oncol* 83: 439-444.

Benevolo, M., Vocaturo, A., Caraceni, D., French, D., Rosini, S., Zappacosta, R., Terrenato, I., Ciccocioppo, L., Frega, A. & Giorgi Rossi, P. (2011) Sensitivity, Specificity, and Clinical Value of Human Papillomavirus (HPV) E6/E7 mRNA Assay as a Triage Test for Cervical Cytology and HPV DNA Test. *J Clin Microbiol* 49(7): 2643-2650.

Bernstein, S. J., Sanchez-Ramos, L. & Ndubisi, B. (2001). Liquid-based cervical cytologic smear study and conventional Papanicolaou smears: A metaanalysis of prospective studies comparing cytologic diagnosis and sample adeguacy. *Am J Obstet Gynecol* 185: 308-317.

Biswas, S.K. & Sodhi, A. (2002). Effect of monocyte chemoattractant protein-1 on murine bone marrow cells: proliferation, colony-forming ability and signal transduction pathway involved. *Int J Immunopathol Pharmacol* 15: 183-187.

Boshart, M., Gissmann, L., Ikenberg, H., Kleinheinz, A., Scheurlen, W. & zur Hausen, H. (1984). A new type of papillomavirus DNA, its presence in genital cancer biopsies and in cell lines derived from cervical cancer. *EMBO J* 3(5): 1151-1157.

Boulet, G.A.V., Horvath, C.A.J., Berghmans, S. & Bogersn, J. (2008). Human papillomavirus in cervical cancer screening: important role as biomarker. *Cancer Epidemiol Biomarkers Prev* 17: 810-817.

Bulkmans, N.W., Berkhof, J. & Rozendaal, L. (2007). Human Papillomavirus DNA testing for the detection of cervical intraepithelial neoplasia grade 3 and cancer: 5-year follow-up of a randomized controlled implementation trial. *Lancet* 370(9601): 1764-1772.

Carozzi, F.M., Del Mistro, A., Confortini, M., Sani, C., Puliti, D. & Trevisan, R. (2005). Reproducibility of HPV DNA testing by Hybrid Capture 2 in a screening setting: intralaboratory and interlaboratory quality control in seven laboratories partecipating in the same clinical trial. *Am J Clin Pathol* 124: 1-6.

Carter, J.R., Ding, Z. & Rose, B.R. (2011). HPV infection and cervical disease: a review. Aust N Z J Obstet Gynaecol. 51(2): 103-108.

Castle, P.E., Lorincz, A.T., Scott, D.R., Sherman, M.E., Glass, A.G., Rush, B.B., Wacholder, S., Burk, R.D., Manos, M.M., Schussler, J.E., Macomber, P. & Schiffman, M. (2003). Comparison between prototype hybrid capture 3 and hybrid capture 2 human papillomavirus DNA assays for detection of high-grade cervical intraepithelial neoplasia and cancer. *J Clin Microbiol* 41(9): 4022-4030.

Cavuslu, S., Mant, C., Starkey, W. G., Bible, J.M., Biswas, C., Kell, B., Rice, P., Best, J.M. & Cason, J. (1996). Analytic sensitivities of hybrid-capture, consensus and type-specific polymerase chain reactions for the detection of human papillomavirus type 16 DNA. *J Med Virol* 49: 319–324.

Cibas, E.S., Alonzo, TA., Austin, RM., Bolick, DR., Glant, MD., Henry, MR., Moriarty, AT., Molina, JT., Rushing, L., Slowman, SD., Torno, R. & Eisenhut, C.C. (2008). The MonoPrep Pap test for the detection of cervical cancer and its precursors. Part I: results of a multicenter clinical trial. *Am J Clin Pathol* 129: 193-201.

Clifford, G.M., Smith, J.S., Plummer, M., Muñoz, N., & Franceschi, S. (2003). Human papillomavirus types in invasive cervical cancer worldwide: a meta-analysis. *Br J Cancer* 88: 63-73.

Clifford, G.M., Gallus , S. & Herrero, R. (2005). Worldwide distribution of human Papillomavirus types in cytologically normal women in the International Agency for Research on Cancer HPV Prevalence Survey: a pooled analysis. *Lancet* 366: 991-998.

Cope, J.U., Hildesheim, A., Schiffman, M.H., Manos, M.M., Lörincz, A.T., Burk, R.D., Glass, A.G., Greer, C., Buckland, J., Helgesen, K., Scott, D.R., Sherman, M.E., Kurman. R.J. & Liaw, K.L. (1997). Comparison of the Hybrid Capture tube test and PCR for detection of human papillomavirus DNA in cervical specimens. *J Clin Microbiol* 35:2262–2265.

Cubie, H.A., Moore, C., Waller, M. & Moss, S., on behalf of the National Cervical Screening Committee LBC/HPV Pilot Steering Group. (2005). The development of a quality assurance program for HPV testing with the UK NHS cervical screening LBC/HPV studies. *J Clin Virol* 33: 287-292.

Cuschieri, K.S., Whitley, M.J. & Cubie, H.A. (2004). Human papilloma virus type specific DNA and RNA persistence. Implication for cervical disease progression and monitoring. *J Med Virol* 73: 65-70.

Dalstein, V., Merlin, S., Bali, C., Saunier, M., Dachez, R. & Ronsin, C. (2009). Analytical evaluation of the PapilloCheck test, a new commercial DNA chip for detection and genotyping of human papillomavirus. *J Virol Methods* 156(1-2): 77-83.

Davey, E., Barratt, A., Irwing, L., Chan, S.F., Macaskill, P., Mannes, P. & Saville, A.M. (2006). Effect of study design and quality on unsatisfactory rates, cytological classifications, and accuracy in liquid-based versus conventional cervical cytology: a systematic review. *Lancet* 367: 122-132.

Davey, E., d'Assuncao, J., Irwig, L., Macaskill, P., Chan, S.F., Richards, A. & Farnsworth, A. (2007). Accuracy of reading liquid based cytology slides using the ThinPrep Imager compared with conventional cytology: prospective study. *BMJ* 335: 28-35.

Denis, F., Hanz, S. & Alain, S.(2008). Clearance, persistence and recurrence of HPV infection. *Gynecol Obstet Fertil* 36: 430-440.

Denton, K.J., Bergeron, C., Klement, P., Trunk, M.J., Keller, T. & Ridder. R., European CINtec Cytology Study Group. (2010). The sensitivity and specificity of p16(INK4a) cytology vs HPV testing for detecting high-grade cervical disease in the triage of ASC-US and LSIL pap cytology results. *Am J Clin Pathol* 134(1): 12-21.

De Oer, M.A., Jordanova, E.S., Kenter, G.G., Peters, A.A., Corver, W.E., Trimbos, J.B. & Fleuren, G.J. (2007). High Human Papillomavirus oncogene mRNA expression and not viral load is associated with poor prognosis in cervical cancer patients. *Clin Cancer Res* 13: 132-138.

De Sanjosé, S., Diaz, M., Castellsagué, X., Clifford, G., Bruni, L., Muñoz, N. & Bosch, F. X. (2007). Worldwide prevalence and genotype distribution of cervical human papillomavirus DNA in women with normal cytology: a meta-analysis. *Lancet Infect Dis* 7: 453-459.

Dillner, J. (1999). The serological response to Papillomavirus. *Sem Cancer Biol* 9: 423-430.

Dillner, J., Rebolj, M., Birembaut, P., Petry, K.U., Szarewski, A., Munk, C., de Sanjose, S., Naucler, P., Lloveras, B., Kjaer, S., Cuzick, J., van Ballegooijen, M., Clavel, C. &

Iftner, T., for Joint European Cohort Study. (2008). Long term predictive values of cytology and human papillomavirus testing in cervical cancer screening: joint European cohort study. *BMJ* 13: 337-347.

Doorbar, J. (2005). The papillomavirus life cycle. *J Clin Virol* 32S: S7-S15.

Doorbar, J. (2006). Molecular biology of human papillomavirus infection and cervical cancer. *Clin Sci (Lond)* 110: 525-541.

Dunne, E.F., Unger, E.R.., Sternberg, M., McQuillan, G., Swan, D.C. & Patel, S.S. (2007). Prevalence of HPV infection among females in the United States. *J Am Med Assoc* 297: 813-819.

Dunton, C.J. (2000). New technology in Papanicolaou smear processing. *Clin Obstet Gynecol* 43(2):410-417.

Eder, P.S., Lou, J., Huff, J. & Macioszek, J. (2009). The next- generation Hybrid Capture® High-Risk HPV DNA assay on a fully automated platform. *J Clin Virol* 45(S1): S85-S92.

Ehrlich, M. (2002). DNA methylation in cancer: too much, but also too little. *Oncogene* 21, 5400-5413.

Esteller, M. & Herman, J.G. (2002). Cancer as an epigenetic disease: DNA methylation and chromatin alterations in human tumours. *J Pathol* 196: 1-7.

Fenq, Q., Balasubramanian, A., Hawes, S.E., Tiure, P., Sow, P.S. & Dem, A. (2005). Detection of hypermethylated genes in women with and without cervical neoplasia. *J Natl Cancer Inst* 97: 273-282.

Gaffikin, L., McGrath, J., Arbyn, M. & Blumenthal, P.D. (2008). Avoiding verification bias in screening test evaluation in resource poor settings: a case study from Zimbabwe. *Clin Trials* 5(5): 496-503.

Galgano, M.T., Castle, P.E., Atkins, K.A., Brix, W.T., Nassau, S.R. & Stoler, M.H. (2010). Using biomarkers as objective standards in the diagnosis of cervical biopsies. *Am J Surg Pathol* 34: 1077-1087.

Gök, M., Heideman, D.A., van Kemenade, F.J., Berkhof, J., Rozendaal, L., Spruyt, J.W., Voorhorst, F., Beliën, J.A., Babovic. M., Snijders. P.J. & Meijer, C.J. (2010). HPV testing on self collected cervicovaginal lavage specimens as screening method for women who do not attend cervical screening: cohort study. *BMJ* 11; 340-351.

Goldie, S.J., Kim, J. & Wright, T.(2004). Cost-effectiveness of human papillomavirus DNA testing for cervical cancer screening in women aged 30 years or more. *Obstet Gynecol* 103: 619-631.

Guess, J.C. & McCance, D.J. (2005). Decreased Migration of Langerhans Precursor-Like Cells in Response to Human Keratinocytes Expressing Human Papillomavirus Type 16 E6/E7 Is Related to Reduced Macrophage Inflammatory Protein-3 Production. *Virol* 79: 14852-14857.

Gustafson, K.S., Furth, E.E., Heiyjan, D.F., Fansler, Z.B. & Clark, D.P. (2004). DNA methylation profiling of cervical squamous intraepithelial lesions using liquid-based cytology specimens: an approach that utilizes receiver-operating characteristic analysis. *Cancer* 102: 259-268.

Hesselink, A.T., van den Brule, A.J., Groothuismink, Z.M., Molano, M., Berkhof, J., Meijer, C.J. & Snijders, P.J. (2005). Comparison of three different PCR methods for quantifying human papillomavirus type 16 DNA in cervical scrape specimens. *J Clin Microbiol* 43(9): 4868-4871.

Hopman, A.H., Kamps, M.A., Smedts, F., Speel, E.J., Herrington, C.S. & Ramaekers, F.C. (2005). HPV in situ hybridization: impact of different protocols on the detection of integrated HPV. *Int J Cancer* 115: 419-428.

Hovland, S., Arbyn, M., Lie, A.K., Ryd, W., Borge, B., Berle, E.J., Skomedal, H., Kadima, T.M., Kyembwa, L., Billay, E.M., Mukwege, D., Chirimwami, R.B., Mvula, T.M., Snijders, P.J., Meijer, C.J. & Karlsen, F. (2010). A comprehensive evaluation of the accuracy of cervical pre-cancer detection methods in a high-risk area in East Congo. *Br J Cancer* 16; 102(6): 957-965.

Howard, M., Sellors, J., Kaczorowsky, J. & Lõrincz, A. (2004). Optimal cut-off of the Hybrid Capture II human papillomavirus test for self-collected vaginal, vulvar and urine specimens in a colposcopy referral population. *J Lower Gen Tract Dis* 8: 33-37.

Jenkins, D. (2008). A review of cross-protection against oncogenic HPV by an HPV-16/18 AS04-adjuvanted cervical cancer vaccine: importance of virological and clinical endpoints and implications for mass vaccination in cervical cancer prevention. *Gynecol Oncol* 110: S18–S25.

Jordan, J., Arbyn, M., Martin-Hirsch, P., Schenck, U., Baldauf, J.J., Da Silva, D., Anttila, A., Nieminen, P. & Prendiville, W. (2008). European guidelines for quality assurance in cervical cancer screening: recommendations for clinical management of abnormal cervical cytology, part 1. *Cytopathology* 19(6): 342-354.

Jung, S., Yi, L., Jeong, D., Kim, J., An, S., Oh, T.J., Kim, C.H., Kim, C.J., Yang, Y., Kim, K.I., Lim, J.S. & Lee, M.S. (2011). The role of ADCYAP1, adenylate cyclase activating polypeptide 1, as a methylation biomarker for the early detection of cervical cancer. *Oncol Rep* 25(1): 245-252.

Kocken, M., Helmerhorst, T.J., Berkhof, J., Louwers, J.A., Nobbenhuis, M.A., Bais, A.G., Hogewoning, C.J., Zaal, A., Verheijen, R.H., Snijders, P.J. & Meijer, C.J. R(2011). Risk of recurrent high-grade cervical intraepithelial neoplasia after successful treatment: a long-term multi-cohort study. *Lancet Oncol* 12(5): 441-450.

Kraus, I.., Molden, T., Holm, R., Lie, A.K., Karlsen, F., Kristensen, G.B. & Skomedal, H. (2006). Presence of E6 and E7 mRNA from human papillomavirus types 16, 18, 31, 33, and 45 in the majority of cervical carcinomas. *J Clin Microbiol* 44:1310-1317.

Kulusingam, S.L., Hughes, J.P., Kiviat, N.B., Mao, C., Weiss, N.S. & Kuypers, J.M. (2002). Evaluation of human papillomavirus testing in primary screening for cervical abnormalities: comparison of sensitivity, specificity, and frequency of referral. *JAMA* 288: 1749-1757.

Lambert, A.P., Anschau, F. & Schmitt, V.M. (2006). p16INK4a expression in cervical premalignant and malignant lesions. *Exp Mol Pathol* 80: 192-196.

Leinonen, M., Nieminen, P., Kotaniemi-Talonen, L., Malila, N., Tarkkanen, J., Laurila, P. & Anttila, A. (2009).

Age-specific evaluation of primary human papillomavirus screening vs conventional cytology in a randomized setting. *J Natl Cancer Inst* 2; 101(23): 1612-1623.

Levin, C.E., Sellors, J., Shi, J.F., Ma, L., Qiao, Y.L., Ortendahl, J., O'Shea, M.K. & Goldie, S.J. (2010). Cost-effectiveness analysis of cervical cancer prevention based on a rapid human papillomavirus screening test in a high-risk region of China. *Int J Cancer* 1; 127(6): 1404-1411.Lichtig, H., Algrisi, M., Botzer, L.E., Abadi, T., Verbitzky, Y., Jackman, A., Tommasino, M., Zehbe I. & Sherman, L. (2006). HPV16 E6 natural variants exhibit different activities in functional assays relevant to the carcinogenic potential of E6. *Virology* 350: 216-219.

Li, J., Zhang, Z., Bidder, M., Funk, M.C., Nguyen, L., Goodfellow, P.J. & Rader, J.S. (2005). IGSF4 promoter methylation and expression silencing in human cervical cancer. *Gynecol Oncol* 96: 150-158.

Lilli, F.B.(2005). Determination of human papillomavirus (HPV) load and type in high-grade cervical lesions surgically resected from HIV-infected women during follow-up of HPV infection. *Clin Infect Dis* 40, 451-457.

Longatto-Filho A, Schmitt FC. (2007). Gynecological cytology: too old to be a pop star but too young to die. *Diagn Cytopathol* 35(10): 672-673.

Luzzatto, L., van Haaften, C., Boon, M.E. (20049. Proliferation patterns of cervical cells as visualized in Leiden liquid cytology slides. *Diagn Cytopathol* 31(1): 5-9.

Meisels, A. & Fortin R. (1976). Condylomatous lesions of the cervix and vagina. I. Cytologic patterns. *Acta Cytol* 20(6): 505-509.

Mendez, F., Munoz, N., Posso, H., Molano, M., Moreno, V., van den Brule, A.J., Ronderos, M., Meijer, C. & Munoz, A. (2005). Cervical co-infection with human papillomavirus (HPV) types and possible implications for the prevention of cervical cancer by HPV vaccines. *J Infect Dis* 192: 1158–1165.

Mendoza-Lorenzo, P., Maldonado, R., Pacheco, R., Mendez, A., Pina-Sanchez, P. & Rangel, A. (2007). An oligoarray for the detection of human papillomavirus type 16 variants. *Int J Gynecol Cancer* 17: 1083–1091.

Molden, T., Nygård, J.F., Kraus, I., Karlsen, F., Nygård, M., Skare, G.B., Skomedal, H., Thoresen, S.Ø. & Hagmar, B. (2005). Predicting CIN2+ when detecting HPV mRNA and DNA by PreTect HPV-proofer and consensus PCR: A 2-year follow-up of women with ASCUS or LSIL Pap smear. *Int J Cancer* 10: 973-977.

Monsonego, J., Bohbot, J.M., Pollini, G., Krawec, C., Vincent, C., Merignargues, I., Haroun, F., Sednaoui, P., Monfort, L., Dachez, R. & Syrjänen, K. (2005). Performance of the Roche AMPLICOR human papillomavirus (HPV) test in prediction of cervical intraepithelial neoplasia (CIN) in women with abnormal PAP smear. *Gynecol Oncol* 99(1): 160-168.

Monsonego, J., Hudgens, M.G., Zerat, L., Zerat, J.C., Syrjänen, K,. Halfon, P., Ruiz, F. & Smith J. (2011). Evaluation of oncogenic human papillomavirus RNA and DNA tests with liquid-based cytology in primary cervical cancer screening: The FASE study. *J Cancer* 129(3): 691-701.

Munoz, N., Bosch, F.X., de Sanjose, S., Herrero, R., Castellsague, X. & Shah, K.V. (2003). Epidemiologic classification of human papillomavirus types associated with cervical cancer. *N Engl J Med* 348: 518-527.

Munoz, N., Mendez,F., Posso, H., Molano, M., Van den Brule, A., Ronderos, M., Meijer, C. & Munoz, A., for the Instituto National de Cancerologia HPV Study Group. (2004). Incidence, duration and determinants of cervical human papillomavirus infection in a cohort of Colombian women with normal cytological results. *J Infect Dis* 190: 234-242.

Muñoz, N., Castellsague, X., de Gonzale, A.B. & Gissman, L. (2006). Chapter I: HPV in the etiology of human cancer. *Vaccine* 24(3): S1-S7.

Nam, K., Chung, S., Kim, J., Jeon, S. & Bae, D. (2009). Factors associated with HPV persistence after conization in patients with negative margins. *J Gynecol Oncol* ;20(2): 91-915.

Nakagawa, S., Yoshikawa, H., Yasugi, T., Kimura, M., Kawana, K., Matsumoto, K., Yamada, M., Onda, T. & Taketani, Y. (2000). Ubiquitous presence of E6 and E7 transcrips in human papillomavirus-positive cervical carcinoma regardless of its type. *J Med Virol* 62: 251-258.

Nance, K.V. (2007). Evolution of Pap testing at a community hospital - a ten years experience. *Diagnostic Cytopathology* 35: 148-153.

National Cancer Institute Workshop. (1989). The 1988 Bethesda System for reporting cervical/vaginal cytological diagnoses. *JAMA* 18; 262(7): 931-934.

Naucler, P., Ryd, W., Törnberg, S., Strand, A., Wadell, G., Elfgren, K., Rådberg, T., Strander, B., Johansson, B., Forslund, O., Hansson, B.G., Rylander, E. & Dillner, J. (2007). Human papillomavirus and Papanicolaou tests to screen for cervical cancer. *N Engl J Med* 18; 357(16): 1589-1597.

Naucler, P., Ryd, W., Törnberg, S., Strand, A., Wadell, G., Elfgren, K., Rådberg, T,. Strander, B., Forslund, O., Hansson, B.G., Hagmar, B., Johansson, B., Rylander, E. & Dillner, J. (2009). Efficacy of HPV DNA testing with cytology triage and/or repeat HPV DNA testing in primary cervical cancer screening. *J Natl Cancer Inst.* 101: 88-99.

Ogilvie, G.S., Patrick, D.M., Schulzer, M., Sellors, J.W., Petric, M., Chambers, K., White, R. & FitzGerald, J.M. (2005). Diagnostic accuracy of self collected vaginal specimens for human papillomavirus compared to clinician collected human papillomavirus specimens: a meta-analysis. *Sex Transm Infect* 81(3): 207-212.

Rowson, K.E. & Mahy, B.W. (1967). Human papova (wart) virus. *Bacteriol Rev* 31(2): 110-131.

Pagliusi, S.R. & Garland, S.M. (2007). International standard reagents for HPV detection. *Dis Markers* 23(4): 283-296

Papillo, J.L, St John, T.L. & Leiman, G. (2008). Effectiveness of the ThinPrep Imaging System: clinical experience in a low risk screening population. *Diagnostic Cytopathology* 36: 155-160.

Parkin, D.M., Bray, F., Ferlay, J. & Pisani, P. (2005) Global cancer statistics, 2002. *CA Cancer J Clin* 55: 74-108.

Perrons, C., Jelley, R., Kleter, B., Quint, W. & Brink, N. (2005). Detection of persistent high risk human papillomavirus infection with Hybrid Capture II and specific SPF10/LiPA. *J Clin Virol* 32: 278-285.

Pfister H, Gissmann L, zur Hausen H. (1977). Partial characterization of the proteins of human papilloma viruses (HPV) 1-3. *Virology* 83(1): 131-137.

Poljak, M., Ostrbenk, A., Seme, K., Ucakar, V., Hillemanns, P., Bokal, E.V., Jancar, N. & Klavs, I. (2011). Comparison of clinical and analytical performance of the Abbott Realtime High Risk HPV test to the performance of hybrid capture 2 in population-based cervical cancer screening. *J Clin Microbiol* 49(5): 1721-1729.

Psyrri, A. & Di Maio, D. (2008). Human papillomavirus in cervical and headand neck cancer. *Nature Clin Prac Oncol* 5: 24-31.

Rebolj, M., Bonde, J., Njor, S.H. & Lynge, E. (2011). Human papillomavirus testing in primary cervical screening and the cut-off level for hybrid capture 2 tests: systematic review. BMJ 23; 342:350.

Rodriguez, A.C., Shiffman, M., Herrero, R., Wacholder, S., Hidesteim, A., Castle, P.E., Solomon, D. & Burk, R. (2008). Rapid clearance of human papillomavirus and implications for clinical focus on persistent infections. *J Natl Cancer Inst* 100: 513-517.

Ronco, G., Giorgi-Rossi, P., Carozzi, F., Confortini, M., Dalla Palma, P., Del Mistro, A., Gillio-Tos, A., Minucci, D., Naldoni, C., Rizzolo, R., Schincaglia, P., Volante, R., Zappa, M., Zorzi, M., Cuzick, J. & Segnan, N. (2008). New Technologies for Cervical Cancer Screening Working Group. Results at recruitment from a randomized controlled trial comparing human papillomavirus testing alone with conventional cytology as the primary cervical cancer screening test. J *Natl Cancer Inst* 2; 100(7): 492-501.

Sahebali, S., Depuydt, C.E., Segers, K., Vareecken, A.J., Van Marck, E. & Bogers, J.J. (2003). Ki-67 immunocytochemistry in liquid based cervical cytology: useful as an adjunctive tool? *J Clin Pathol* 56: 681-686.

Wentzensen, N. & von knebel Doeberitz, M. (2007). Biomarkers in cervical cancer screening. *Dis Markers* 23, 315-330.

Sanchez, G.I., Kleter, B., Gheit, T., van Doorn, L.J., de Koning, M.N., de Sanjosé, S., Alemany, L., Bosch, X.F., Tommasino, M., Muñoz, N. & Quint, W.G. (2011). Clinical evaluation of polymerase chain reaction reverse hybridization assay for detection and identification of human papillomavirus type 16 variants. *J Clin Virol* 51(3): 165-169.

Sarian, L.O., Derchain, S.F., Naud, P., Roteli-Martinsm C., Longatto-Filho, A., Tatti, S., Branca, M., Erzen, M., Serpa-Hammes, L., Matos, J., Gontijo, R., Bragança, J.F., Lima, T.P., Maeda, M.Y., Lörincz, A., Dores, G.B., Costa, S., Syrjänen, S.& Syrjänen, K. (2005). Evaluation of visual inspection with acetic acid (VIA), Lugol's iodine (VILI), cervical cytology and HPV testing as cervical screening tools in Latin America. *J Med Screen* 12(3): 142-149.

Sasieni, P.D., Cuzick, J. & Lynch-Framery, E. (1996). Estimating the efficacy of screening by auditing smear histories of women with and without cervical cancer. *Br J Cancer* 73: 1001-1005.

Saunier, M., Monnier-Benoit, S. & Mauny, F. (2008). HPV16 DNA load and physical state allow the identification of HPV16 infected women with high-grade lesions or cervical carcinoma. *J Clin Microbiol* 17: 22-30.

Schmitt, M., Bravo, I.G., Snijders, P.J., Gissmann, L., Pawlita, M. & Waterboer, T. (2006). Bead-based multiplex genotyping of human papillomaviruses. *J Clin Microbiol* 44: 504–512.

Schmitt, M., Dondog, B., Waterboer, T., Pawlita, M., Tommasino, M. & Gheit, T. (2010). Abundance of Multiple High-Risk Human Papillomavirus (HPV) Infections Found in Cervical Cells Analyzed by Use of an Ultrasensitive HPV Genotyping Assay. *J Clin Microbiol* 48(1): 143–149.

Schwarz, E., Freese, U.K., Gissmann, L., Mayer, W., Roggenbuck, B., Stremlau, A. & zur Hausen, H. (1985). Structure and transcription of human papillomavirus sequences in cervical carcinoma cells. *Nature* 314(6006): 111-114.

Shah, K.V., Solomon, L., Daniel, R., Cohn, S. & Vlahov, D. (1997). Comparison of PCR and hybrid capture methods for detection of human papillomavirus in injection drug-using women at high risk of human immunodeficiency virus infection. *J Clin Microbiol* 35: 517–519.

Sichero, L., Ferreira, S., Trottier, H., Duarte-Franco, E., Ferenczy, A. & Franco, E.L. (2007). High grade cervical lesions are caused preferentially by non-European variants of HPVs 16 and 18. *Int J Cancer* 120: 1763–1768.

Scott, M., Nakagawa, M. & Moscicki, A. (2001). Cell-mediated immune response to human papillomavirus infection. *Clin Diagn Lab Immunol* 8: 209-213.

Seedlacek, T.V. (1999). Advances in the diagnosis and treatment of human papillomavirus infections. *Clin Obstet Gynecol* 42: 206-220.

Skomedal, H., Kraus, I., Silva, I., Molden, T., Hovland, S., Morland, G., Morland, E. & Karlsen, F. (2006). Direct Detection of Cervical Carcinogenesis through mRNA, in *Emerging issues on HPV infections:from science to practice*, Joseph Monsonego Editor, pp 82-102 Paris.

Schmidt, D., Bergeron, C., Denton, K.J. & Ridder, R. (2011). p16/Ki-67 dual stain cytology in the triage of ASCUS and LSIL Papanicolaou cytology. *Cancer Cytopathol* 25; 119(3): 158-166.

Wise-Draper, T.M. & Wells, S.I. (2008). Papillomavirus E6 and E7 proteins and their cellular targets. *Front Biosci* 1: 1003-1017.

Smith, J.S., Lindsay, L., Hoots, B., Keys, J., Franceschi, S. & Winer, R. (2007). Human papillomavirus type distribution in invasive cervical cancer and high-grade cervical lesions: A meta-analysis update. *Int J Cancer* 121: 621-632.

Solomon, D., Schiffman, M.H. & Tarone, R. (2001). Comparison of three management strategies for patients with atypical squamous cells of undetermined significance: baseline results from a randomized trial. *J Natl Cancer Inst* 93: 293-297.

Solomon, D. Chapter 14: role of triage testing in cervical cancer screening. (2003). *J Natl Cancer Inst Monogr* 31: 97-106.

Solomon, D. (2003). Role of triage testing in cervical cancer screening. J Natl Cancer Inst Monogr: 97-101

zur Hausen, H. (2002). Papillomaviruses and cancer: from basic studies to clinical application. *Nat Rev Cancer* 2(5): 342-350.

Stanley, M., Lowy, D.R. & Frazer, I. (2006). Chapter 12: Prophylactic HPV vaccines: underlying mechanisms. *Vaccine* 24: S106-S113.

Stoler, M.H. & Schiffman, M. (2001). Interobserver reproducibility of cervical cytologic and histologic interpretations: realistic estimates from the ASCUS-LSIL Triage Study. *JAMA* 285: 1500-1505.

Stoler, M.H. (2004). The pathology of cervical neoplasia, in: *Cervical cancer: from etiology to prevention*, Rohan TE, Shah KW Editors, pp. 1-50.Jemal, A, Siegel, R, Xu, J & Ward, E. (2010). Cancer statistics, 2010. CA Cancer J Clin 60: 277-300.

Snijders, P.J., Steenbergen, R D., Heideman, D.A. & Meijer, C.J. (2006) HPV-mediated cervical carcinogenesis: concepts and clinical implications. *J Pathol* 208: 152-164.

Stoykova, B., Kuzmanov, G. & Dowie, R. (2008). Putting National Institute for Health and Clinical Excellence guidance into practice: a cost minimization model of a national roll-out of liquid based cytology in England. *Int J Technol Assess Health Care* 24(4): 391-398.

Tang, S.M., Tao, J.P., McCoy J. & Zheng, Z.M. (2006). The E7 oncoprotein is translated from spliced E6*I transcripts in high-risk human papillomavirus type 16- or type 18-positive cervical cancer cell lines via translation reinitiation. *J Virol* 80: 4249-4251.

Tsoumpou, I,, Arbyn, M. & Kyrgiou, M. (2009). p16^{INK4a} immunostaining in cytological and histological specimens from the uterine cervix: a systematic review and meta-analysis. *Cancer Treatment Rev* 35: 210–220.

Wentzenses, N., Bergeron, C., Cas, F., Eschenbach, D., Vinokurova, S. & von Knebel, D.M. (2005). Evalutation of a nuclear score for p16 INK4astained cervical squamous cells in liquid-based cytology samples. *Cancer* 105: 461-467.

Tsu, V. & Levin, C.E. (2008). Making the case for cervical cancer prevention: what about equity? *Reprod Health Matters* 16: 104-112.

van den Brule, A.J., Pol, R., Fransen-Daalmeijer, N., Schouls, L.M., Meijer, C.J. & Snijders, P.J. (2002). GP5+/6+ PCR followed by reverse line blot analysis enables rapid and high-throughput identification of human papillomavirus genotypes. *J Clin Microbiol* 40: 779–787.

Varnai, A.D., Bollmann, M., Bankfalvi, A., Speich, N., Schmitt, C., Griefingholt, H., Kovács, K., Klozoris, C. & Bollmann, R. (2008). Predictive testing of early cervical pre-cancer by detecting human papillomavirus E6/E7 mRNA in cervical cytologies up to high-grade squamous intraepithelial lesions: diagnostic and prognostic implications. *Oncol Report* 19: 457-465.

Welters, M.J., Kenter, G.G., Piersma, S.J., Vloon, A.P., Löwik, M.J., Berends-van der Meer, D.M., Drijfhout, J.W., Valentijn, A.R., Wafelman, A.R., Oostendorp, J., Fleuren, G.J., Offringa, R., Melief, C.J. & van der Burg, S.H. (2008). Induction of Tumor-Specific CD4+ and CD8+ T-Cell Immunity in Cervical Cancer Patients by a Human Papillomavirus Type 16 E6 and E7 Long Peptides Vaccine. *Clin Cancer Res* 14: 178-187.

Wentzensen, N., Vinokurova, S. & von Knebel, D.M. (2004). Systematic review of genomic integration sites of human papillomavirus genomes in epithelial dysplasia and invasive cancer in the female lower genital tract. *Cancer Res* 64: 3878-3884.

Wright, T.C. Jr, Cox, J.T, Massad, L.S., Twiggs, L.B. & Wilkinson, E.J. (2002). ASCCP-Sponsored Consensus Conference 2001 Consensus Guidelines for the management of women with cervical cytological abnormalities. *JAMA* 24;287(16): 2120-2129.

Xi, L.F., Hughes, J.P., Castle, P.E., Edelstein, Z.R., Wang, C., Galloway, D.A., Koutsky, L.A., Kiviat ,N.B. & Schiffman, M. (2011). Viral load in the natural history of human papillomavirus type 16 infection: a nested case-control study. *J Infect Dis* 15; 203(10): 1425-1433.

Xiang, L., Yang, H., Li, J., Wu, X. & Zhou, X. (2011). Different amplification patterns of the human telomerase RNA gene in invasive cervical carcinomas and cervical intraepithelial neoplasia grade III. *Diagn Cytopathol* 4, in press.

Yang YX, Yang AH, Yang ZJ, Wang ZR, Xia XH. (2006). Involvement of tumor suppressor in lung cancer 1 gene expression in cervical carcinogenesis. *Int J Gynecol Cancer* ;16(5): 1868-1872.

Zappacosta R. & Rosini S. (2008). Cervical Cancer Screening: From Molecular Basis to Diagnostic Practice, Going Through New Technologies. *Technol in Cancer Res and Treat* 7(3): 161-174.

Zappacosta, R., Caraceni, D., Ciccocioppo, L., Ottaviantonio, M., Conti, F., Andreozzi, S., Petrucci, F. & Rosini S. (2010). Is HPV-DNA testing a useful tool in predicting low-grade squamous intraepithelial lesion outcome? A retrospective longitudinal study. *Int J Immunopathol Pharmacol* 23(1): 317-326.

Zielinski, G.D., Bais, A.G., Helmerorst, T.J., Verheijen, R.H., De Shipper, F.A. & Snijders, P.J. (2004). HPV testing and monitoring of women after treatment of CIN3: review of the literature and meta-analysis. *Obstet Gynecol Surv* 59: 543-553.

zur Hausen, H.(2002). Papillomaviruses and cancer: from basic studies to clinical application. *Nat Rev Cancer* 2: 342-350.

9

Molecular Diagnosis of Human Papillomavirus

I. Dutra[1,3], I. Foroni[1,3], A.R. Couto[1,3], M. Lima[2,3] and J. Bruges-Armas[1,3]
[1] *Serviço Especializado de Epidemiologia e Biologia Molecular, Hospital de Santo Espírito de Angra do Heroísmo*
[2] *Grupo de Epidemiologia e Genética Humana do Departamento de Biologia da Universidade dos Açores*
[3] *Genetics and Arthritis Research Group (GARG), Institute for Molecular and Cell Biology (IBMC), University of Porto*
Portugal

1. Introduction

The Papillomaviruses are small double-stranded DNA viruses that infect squamous epithelia. They display absolute species-specificity: human papillomavirus (HPV) only infect humans, rabbit papillomaviruses only infect rabbits and so forth. They are also exquisitely tissue tropic, undergoing a complete infectious cycle only in fully differentiating squamous epithelium (Stanley, 2010). Nearly 100 HPVs were described based on the isolation of complete genomes (de Villiers et al., 2004). The circular genome, whose size is close to 8.0 kilobases (kb), is enclosed in a protein shell made from the major (L1) and minor (L2) capsid proteins resulting in virions of approximately 55nm in diameter. It can be divided into 3 domains: a noncoding upstream regulatory region (URR), an early region with 6 genes (E6, E7, E1, E2, E4 and E5), and a late region encoding two genes (L1 and L2). The early genes are involved in DNA replication, transcriptional regulation and cellular transformation. The late genes encode capsid proteins and facilitate the entry of viral DNA into the cell (Tjalma et al., 2005). Approximately 35 HPV types are known to infect the human genital mucosa. They can be grouped as "high risk" (HR) or "low risk" (LR) based on their epidemiologic association with cancer. HR types such as HPV16 and HPV18 are associated with low and high-grade intraephitelial lesions and invasive cancer. The LR types such as HPV6 and HPV11 are associated with genital warts or condyloma acuminate, recurrent respiratory papillomatosis, and low-grade cervical intraepithelial lesions (LSIL) (Trottier and Franco, 2006). The recognition that infection with HPV is essential for the development of cervical cancer led to the development of cervical cancer prevention strategies which incorporate HPV testing.

There are a variety of HPV tests in use worldwide and several of these may be adequate to use for cervical cancer screening and HPV vaccination. An ideal assay should have (Organization, 2009):

1. good sensitivity and specificity as evaluated in internal proficiency testing;
2. ease of transfer to laboratories with varying levels of experience and resources;
3. affordable cost, to allow use in low-resource settings.

It is important that quality assurance programs are established, both in HPV serology and DNA typing, in order to evaluate laboratory performance as well as assay characteristics. The WHO global reference laboratory recommends proficiency panels composed of a series of validated samples, traceable to International Standards, sent to unknown challenges to HPV LabNet members. Results allow an evaluation of individual laboratory performances and an evaluation of whether assays platforms used by multiple laboratories are robust in terms of the generation of acceptable results. HPV cannot be easily propagated by standard in vitro culture systems, and in malignant tissue there are little or no infectious HPV particles (Organization, 2009). Other classical direct virological diagnosis techniques, such as electron microscopy and immunohistochemistry, lack the sensitivity and specificity for the routine detection of HPV (Poljak and Kocjan, 2010). For these reasons, the preferred assay formats are based on the detection of HPV nucleic acids.

Molecular methods for HPV DNA detection can be grouped in two main categories: those that rely on signal amplification to detect the targets, and those that rely on target amplification; most of them are based on polymerase chain reaction (PCR). Results of HPV detection are strongly influenced by the technique, and comparison between assays is not always possible. This is why all HPV testing steps need careful standardization including sample collection, extraction and testing. Stability during transport and storage is very important for a good quality DNA. The viral nucleic acid must be preserved to avoid false negative results caused by degradation by endogenous endonucleases. To assess the integrity of genomic DNA in the specimen and its stability for molecular techniques it is crucial to use internal controls such as β-globin. There are several commercially available kits (PreservCyt, Cytyc Corp.) for sample transportation that adequately preserve nucleic acids for molecular diagnosis even after long periods of ambient temperature storage (Molijn et al., 2005, Chan et al., 2006). The choice of which DNA extraction method to use depends on the quality of the clinical material and the diagnostic test that will be executed.

In this chapter, the paramount methods for screening and typing high risk HPV types will be described (Table 2). In particular, we describe molecular methods for the identification of HPVs based on signal amplified hybridization, polymerase chain reaction (PCR), DNA sequencing, type-specific probes, reverse line-blot hybridization, *in situ* hybridization, southern blot hybridization and immunological techniques, including ELISA and western-blot. In addition, we give examples of commercially available kits, for each assay, and point out advantages and limitations of its use.

2. Signal amplified hybridization assays

Hybrid Capture to HPV detection was first introduced by Digene Corporation (Gaithesburg, MD,USA) in 1995. This assay is a non radioactive amplification method, based on the hybridization of the target HPV-DNA to labeled RNA probes in solution. It captures the resulting hybrids detecting them by a specific monoclonal antibody and a chemiluminescent substrate, providing a semi-quantitative measurement of HPV-DNA. The second generation of hybrid capture assay - hc2 - uses microtiter plate instead of tubes for the detection of 13 high-risk HPV types: 16, 18, 31, 33, 35, 39, 45, 51, 52, 56, 58, 59 and 68, on liquid-based cervical specimens (Clavel et al., 1999). Specimens containing the target DNA hybridize with a specific HPV RNA probe cocktail. The resultant RNA:DNA hybrids are captured onto the surface of a microplate well coated with antibodies specific for RNA:DNA hybrids, and detected with a chemiluminiscent substrate. Several alkaline phosphatase molecules are conjugated to each antibody. Multiple conjugated antibodies bind to each captured hybrid resulting in substantial signal amplification. As the substrate is cleaved by the bound alkaline phosphatase, light is emitted being measured as relative light units (RLUs) on a luminometer (Figure 1). The intensity of the light emitted denotes the presence or absence of target DNA in the specimen. An RLU measurement equal to or greater than the Cutoff Value (CO) indicates the presence of high risk HPV DNA sequences in the specimen, whereas an RLU measurement lesst han the CO indicates the absence of the specific high risk HPV DNA sequences tested or HPV DNA levels below the detection limit of the assay (Digene, 2004). This assay has an excellent sensitivity (93% according to referral Kaiser Study population) since it can detect HPV16 DNA of a concentration down to 1pg/ml. It is considered the most reliable signal amplified hybridization assay and is a CE-IVD test. On the other hand, it does not detect all high risk HPV types or very low levels of infection. Cross hybridizations with low risk types 6 and 11 may happen (Castle et al., 2002, Seme et al., 2006). Despite the negative aspects, it is still the gold standard technique for HPV detection, highly recommended for comparative evaluations. The hc2 assay has been used in the majority of key randomized controlled and other clinical trials that have proved the clinical value of HPV testing (Cox, 2009, Meijer et al., 2009). For this reason it has been recommended that new HPV assays should show that they possess similar characteristics as hc2 in the process of clinical validation of the test, before it can be used for cervical cancer screening purposes (Meijer et al., 2009).

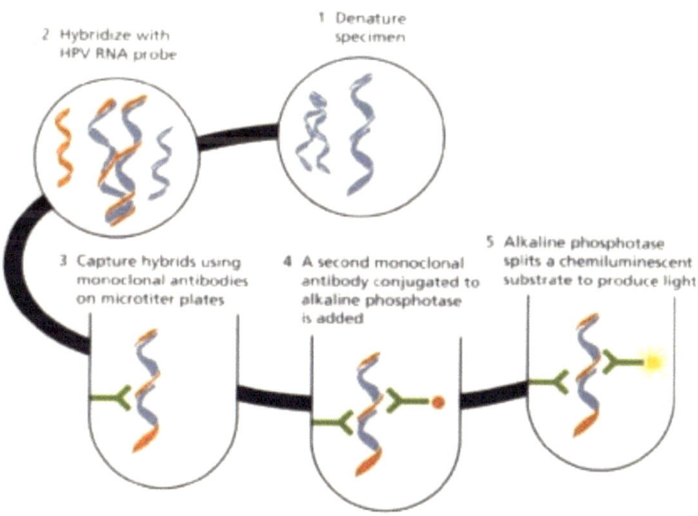

Fig. 1. Hybrid Capture2 test principle, adapted from www.papillomavirus.cz/eng/diagnosis_kits_hybrid.html

The Cervista™ is another FDA approved qualitative test that detects the DNA from 14 high risk HPV types: 16, 18, 31, 33, 35, 39, 45, 51, 52, 56, 58, 59, 66 and 68. The detection of DNA from targeted HPV types, with similar characteristics, is performed with three different probe mixtures. It uses the Invader® chemistry, a signal amplification method for the detection of specific nucleic acid sequences. This method uses two types of isothermal reactions: a primary reaction that occurs on the targeted DNA sequence and a secondary reaction that produces a fluorescent signal. In the primary reaction, two types of sequence specific oligonucleotides - a probe oligonucleotide and an Invader oligonucleotide - bind to the DNA target sequence. When these oligonucleotides overlap by at least one base pair on the target sequence, an invasive structure forms that acts as a substrate for the Cleavase® enzyme. The enzyme cleaves the 5′ portion (flap) of the probe at the position of the overlap. The probes are present in large molar excess and cycle rapidly on and off the target sequence so that many cleaved 5′ flaps are generated per target sequence. The cleaved flaps then bind to a universal hairpin fluorescence resonance energy transfer (FRET) oligonucleotide creating another invasive structure that the Cleavase enzyme recognizes as a substrate. The enzyme cleaves the FRET oligonucleotides between the fluorophore and quencher and produces a fluorescence signal as the cleaved flaps cycle on and off. For each copy of target, the combined primary and secondary reactions result in 10^6 - 10^7 fold signal amplification per hour. The flap sequences and FRET oligonucleotides are universal since they are not complementary to the targeted sequence (Technologies, 2009). Oligonucleotides that bind to the human histone 2 gene (*HIST2H2BE*) are also present in all three oligonucleotides mixtures. This serves as an internal control, producing a semi-quantitative signal from cellular DNA present in the sample (Day et al., 2009). The Cervista™ HPV 16/18 uses de same chemistry for the identification of the two most highly oncogenic and persistent HPV types. It does not allow the exact determination of HPV type(s) present in the clinical specimen, but rather express the result as negative or positive (Day et al., 2009, Poljak and Kocjan, 2010). Sensitivity of the Cervista HPV HR test for detection of ≥CIN2 among women with ASCUS cytology was 92.8% (84.1-96.9) and the negative predictive value (NPV) was 99.1% (98.1-99.6). Sensitivity for detection of ≥CIN3 among women with ASCUS cytology was 100% (85.1-100) and the NPV was 100% (99.4-100). HPV 16/18 genotyping test sensitivity of ≥CIN2 was 68.8 (56.6-78.8) and NPV was 96.0% (93.9-97.4). HPV 16/18 genotyping test sensitivity of ≥CIN3 was 77.3 (56.6-89.9) and NPV was 99.0% (97.7-99.6)(Einsteina et al., 2010). The reproducibility, tested at three different testing centers, resulted in an overall inter-run reproducibility agreement of 98.8% [1-sided 95% Confidence Lower Limit = 96.9%] and an overall inter-site reproducibility agreement of 98.7% [1-sided 95% Confidence Lower Limit = 97.9%] (Day et al., 2009). The Cervista HPV HR test showed no cross-reactivity with DNA from seven non-oncogenic HPV types or 17 different infectious agents at up to 10 copies per reaction (Day et al., 2009). This assay uses standard laboratory equipment and instrumentation, such as thermal cyclers and fluorescence plate readers reducing the need for additional equipment. It has technology proficiency, due to common reaction conditions for all DNA targets, and the simple analysis yields objective results producing straightforward interpretation. It should be used in conjunction with clinical information derived from other diagnostics and screening tests, physical examinations, and full medical history in accordance with appropriate patient management procedures (Day et al., 2009). The limitations of Cervista includes: 1) Cervista HPV HR only detects 14 high-risk HPV types and the Cervista 16/18 only detects 2 high risk types; 2) the Cervista HPV HR test shows cross-reactivity to two HPV types of unknown risk - HPV types 67 and 70 - while the Cervista 16/18 test shows cross-reactivity to high levels of high risk HPV 31 (an HPV16 positive result was observed with 10^7 copies/reaction of HPV31); 3) very low levels of infection may cause false negative results; 4) false-negatives can also take place with cervical specimens contaminated with high-levels of contraceptive jelly and/or anti-fungal creams, when DNA was isolated with the Genfind™ DNA extraction kit; 5) the Cervista HPV HR and 16/18 have been validated only for use with cervical cytology specimens collected in Preserv Cyt® solution using a Rovers Cervex® Brush, Wallach Papette® or endocervical Brush/Spatula; 6) performance of Cervista HPV HR and HPV 16/18 were established exclusively using DNA extracted with the Genfind™ DNA extraction kit and using cervical cytology PreserveCyt® specimen processed on the ThinPrep 2000 processor; 7) the performance of the Cervista HPV HR and HPV 16/18 test has not been established for HPV vaccinated individuals (Technologies, 2009).

AMPLICOR HPV is a CE-IVD PCR based test launched in 2003, by Roche, in America, and in 2004 in Europe. It is capable of detecting 13 HR HPV types with simultaneous assessment of the presence of the human β-globin gene as a positive control. It expresses the result of the test HR HPV in either negative or positive. The method involves the isolation of nucleic acids, PCR amplification, hybridization and absorbance detection. It makes use of a pool of PCR primers designed to amplify HPV DNA from 13 high risk genotypes: 16, 18, 31, 33, 35, 39, 45, 51, 52, 56, 58, 59 and 68. Capture probe sequences are located in polymorphic regions of L1 bound by these primers. One additional primer set is used to amplify the human β-globin gene to provide control for cell adequacy, extraction and amplification. After PCR amplification, the HPV amplicon and the β-globin amplicon are hybridized to the olinucleotide probles bound to the well of the microwell plate. This hybridization of amplicon to the probes increases the overall specificity of the test. Following the hybridization reaction the plate is washed to remove unbound material and avidin-horseradish peroxidase conjugate binds to the biotin-labeled amplicon hybridized to the oligonucleotide probes bound to the microwell plate. The absorbance of the reaction mixture is measured at 450nm (Monsonego et al., 2005, van Ham et al., 2005). This test has shown high analytical sensitivity with an specificity (Poljak et al., 2005) and overall specificity of 96.5% and sensitivity of 96.1% (Sun et al., 2005). It is comparable to hc2 assay in detecting high grade CIN among women examined for abnormal PAP test. This test sensitivity in detecting both CIN1 and CIN2-3 is practically identical with the sensitivity of colposcopy (with minor abnormality cutoff) but, such as hc2, AMPLICOR assay cannot compete with the specificity of cervical (LBC) cytology (Monsonego et al., 2005). The current version of Amplicor is not well suited for high throughput testing since it includes many manual steps. The recommended extraction of DNA using the AmpliLute liquid media extraction kit is especially time-consuming, labor intensive and prone to potential cross-contamination, especially when large numbers of samples are being processed. AMPLICOR HPV test does not detect HPV 26, 53, 66, 73 and 82, HPV types that have been classified as probably high risk types (26, 53, 66) or high risk (73 and 82) types in a large epidemiological study (Munoz et al., 2003). Although this test is sensitive, specific, feasible, and easy to handle in routine it does not provide specific genotype information.

A new rapid screening test - careHPV (QIAGEN, Gaithersburg, MD, USA) - based on the simplified hc2 technology - has been developed to detect 14 high-risk types of carcinogenic human Papillomavirus: 16, 18, 31, 33, 35, 39, 45, 51, 52, 56, 58, 59, 66 and 68, in about 2.5 h (Qiao et al., 2008). This test is very promising as a primary "screen and treat strategy"due to the ability to obtain accurate HPV results in a few hours. This strategy is especially important for remote and low resource regions of the world where follow-up is difficult (Qiagen, 2009). The advantages of the use of this test are: 1) it can be run in any setting (no special needs of humidity, temperature, mains electricity or water are required) by a healthcare worker with minimum laboratory training; 2) cervical samples can be collected by a healthcare worker or can be self-collected by the patient herself; 3) the results are easily interpreted and are available in approximately 3 hours (Qiagen, 2009). Limitations include the low throughput with only 24-90 specimens processed manually. However, it is very promising for developing countries HPV screening strategies such as China (Levin et al., 2010, Canfell et al., 2011, Shi et al., 2011) and Thailand (Trope et al., 2009). A cross sectional study assessed the clinical accuracy of careHPV, comparing it with the hc2, in two county hospitals in rural China. A sensitivity and specificity for CIN2+ of 90.0 and 84.2% while standard hc2 parameters were 97.1 and 85.6%, respectively (Qiao et al., 2008).

3. Polymerase chain reaction (PCR) assays

The polymerase chain reaction (PCR) is a molecular technique capable of amplifying selectively a particular DNA sequence several million-fold. It consists of repeated cycles of heating and cooling in which a heat stable enzyme (Taq polymerase) uses a denatured double strand DNA to synthesize new molecules of DNA. The starting point for DNA synthesis are the primers (forward and reverse), short strands of nucleic acid, which selectively recognise flanking regions of the DNA template. The sensitivity of this methodology is about 10-100 HPV viral genomes in a background of 100ng cellular DNA (Zaravinos et al., 2009). The sensitivity and specificity of PCR-based methods vary, depending on several aspects such as: DNA extraction procedures, site and type of clinical sample, sample transport and storage, primer sets, size of the PCR product, reaction conditions and performance of the DNA polymerase used in the reaction and ability to detect multiple types (Garland and Tabrizi, 2006).

3.1 Type-specific and consensus primer PCR methods

HPV detection by PCR can be performed using either type-specific primers, which amplify a single HPV genotype, or consensus/general primers, which are usually directed to a highly conserved region of the L1 gene. Type-specific primers are designed to amplify exclusively a single HPV genotype and in order to detect the presence of HPV-DNA in a single sample, multiple type-specific PCR reactions must be performed separately (Molijn et al., 2005). The use of multiple type-specific PCR reactions has the disadvantages of being labor-intensive, costly, time consuming and requiring the evaluation of the type-specificity of each PCR primer set (Molijn et al., 2005, Zaravinos et al., 2009).

The use of consensus primers (Table 1) is more convenient because they can amplify a broad-spectrum of HPV genotypes. Most laboratories use consensus primers targeting the L1 region, since it is the most conserved part of the genome, referring to the assay as L1 consensus PCR. Amplification of each of the primer sets will result in different size amplicons and consequently can result in a variation in sensitivity for detection of certain HPV types, particularly when samples contain multiple genotypes (Garland and Tabrizi, 2006). There are numerous L1 consensus PCR primers that can be used. The first was described in 1989 by Manos and colleagues (Manos et al., 1989). This assay is a set of degenerated primers, MY09/MY11, designed with the intent of amplifying in a single reaction all the included genotypes. It generates a 450pb amplicon ready for typing determination by subsequent molecular techniques such as restriction fragment length polymorphism and DNA sequencing (Manos et al., 1989). At the time that MY09/11 was described, only 5 of the 20 or more known HPV genotype sequences had been reported: HPV 6, 11, 16, 18, and 33 and the primer set was not entirely homologous even among these 5 genotypes. The intertypic sequence variation was compensated by introducing one or more degeneracies at the priming sites, resulting in a mixture of 24 unique oligonucleotide sequences (Gravitt et al., 2000). The disadvantage of this design is that the synthesis of oligonucleotides containing degeneracies is not highly reproducible and results in high batch-to-batch variation (Molijn et al., 2005). The degenerate MY09/11 primers were afterwards replaced by a set of 18 defined primers, PGMY09/11, to improve specificity and sensitivity. This amplification system combines a number of distinct forward and reverse primers, aimed at the same position of the viral genome. They do not contain random degeneracy but may contain inosine, which matches any nucleotide. Gravitt (Gravitt et al., 2000) and colleagues grouped the virus types by sequence homology in each of the two primer binding regions: a set of 5 upstream oligonucleotides comprising the PGMY11 primer pool and a set of 13 downstream oligonucleotides comprising the PGMY09 (Gravitt et al., 2000) primer set. Using a defined mixture of non-degenerate primers has the advantages that the oligonucleotides can be synthesized with high reproducibility and PCR is performed at optimal annealing temperatures (Molijn et al., 2005).

Other example of consensus primers is the GP5/6, incorporating one forward and one reverse primer aimed at short regions of homology conserved amongst HPV types 1a, 6, 8, 11, 13, 16, 18, 30, 31, 32 and 33 (Snijders et al., 1990). To improve efficiency, part of these sequences were used to elongate GP5 and GP6 at their 3′ ends to generate the primers GP5+/6+ (de Roda Husman et al., 1995). The GP5+/6+ primer set generates a 160pb amplicon and reveales an improved HPV detection, reflected by a 10 to 100 fold higher sensitivity, compared with the GP5/6. The mismatching between the primers and the non complementary HPV types (it was only 100% complementary to just a few HPV genotypes) is overcome by setting a low annealing temperature at the PCR reaction (Zaravinos et al., 2009). Qu and colleagues (Qu et al., 1997) compared the MY09/11 and GP5+/6+ primer sets in a group of cervicovaginal samples and concluded that despite good agreement in the detection of HPV DNA -positive and -negative status, there is a significant difference in the detection of multiple types within samples. The MY-PCR primer set was more robust than the GP+-PCR method. The second was relatively inefficient in the amplification of HPV types 53 and 61 compared with the MY-PCR, which was inefficient in the amplification of HPV35. Chan and colleagues (Chan et al., 2006) compared the 3 methods: PGMY09/11, MY09/11, GP5+/6+ in 2006 and concluded that PGMY09/11 showed higher sensitivity with a positive rate of 95.8% compared to 84.2% of the MY09/11 and GP5+/6+ methods. Regarding samples with multiple infection, PGMY09/11 primer set detected most of them (9/11, 81.8%), MY09/11 detected 2/11 (18.2%), whereas GP5+/6+ failed to detect any of these.

General primers in the E1 region have also been described, and several other broad-spectrum PCR primers were reported, but have not been extensively used in clinical situations (Molijn et al., 2005) and therefore will not be mentioned in this chapter.

Primer	Sequence (5′-3′)[a]	Amplimer length (bp)	Target[b]
MY09/11	(MY09)CGT CCM ARR GGA WAC TGA TC (MY11)GCM CAG GGW CAT AAY AAT GG	450	L1
PGMY09/ 11	(PGMY11)A GCA CAG GGA CAT AAC AAT GG (PGMY11B)GCG CAG GGC CAC AAT AAT GG (PGMY11C)GCA CAG GGA CAT AAT AAT GG (PGMY11D)GCC CAG GGC CAC AAC AAT GG (PGMY11E)GCT CAG GGT TTA AAC AAT GG (PGMY09F)CGT CCC AAA GGA AAC TGA TC (PGMY09G)CGA CCT AAA GGA AAC TGA TC (PGMY09H)CGT CCA AAA GGA AAC TGA TC (PGMY09I*a*)G CCA AGG GGA AAC TGA TC (PGMY09J)CGT CCC AAA GGA TAC TGA TC (PGMY09K)CGT CCA AGG GGA TAC TGA TC (PGMY09L)CGA CCT AAA GGG AAT TGA TC (PGMY09M)CGA CCT AGT GGA AAT TGA TC (PGMY09N)CGA CCA AGG GGA TAT TGA TC (PGMY09P*a*)G CCC AAC GGA AAC TGA TC (PGMY09Q)CGA CCC AAG GGA AAC TGG TC (PGMY09R)CGT CCT AAA GGA AAC TGG TC (HMB01*b*) GCG ACC CAA TGC AAA TTG GT	450	L1
GP5/6	(GP5)TTT GTT ACT GTG GTA GAT AC (GP6) TGA TTT ACA GTT TAT TTT TC	140-150	L1
GP5+/6+	(GP5+)TTT GTT ACT GTG GTA GAT ACT AC (GP6+)GAA AAA TAA ACT GTA AAT CAT ATT C	160	L1

[a] M, A1C; R, A1G; S, G1C; W, A1T; Y, C1T.

[b] L1, HPV late structural protein 1.

Table 1. Specifications of oligonucleotides used as primers for general HPV detection by PCR

3.2 Polymerase chain reaction-restriction fragment length polymorphisms assays (PCR-RFLP)

PCR-RFLP assay is an alternative technique developed to identify and characterize species detecting variations at the DNA sequence level. It involves the digestion of the PCR product with specific restriction endonucleases to generate DNA profiles. Appropriate software such as Webcutter v2.0 (http://rna.lundberg.gu.se/cutter2/) is used in order to find the most suitable restriction site. The restriction enzymes will generate several fragments of variable lengths which can be resolved by gel electrophoresis, producing DNA fingerprinting patterns (Kado et al., 2001). This method depends on the availability of restriction enzymes capable of detecting specific mutations. In addition to several in-house genotyping protocols based on PCR-RFLP, there is one commercially available kit. The BIOTYPAP kit (Biotools,

Nave, Spain) allows the detection and identification of 31 HPV types: 6, 11, 13, 16, 18, 30-35, 39, 40, 42-44, 51-54, 56-59, 61, 62, 64 and 66-69, and one subtype (subHPV-44 or subHPV-55). The kit consists of a multiplex amplification reaction, using two pairs of primers. One pair of primers (Pair1- GEN1 and GEN2) hybridizes with sequences common to all tested HPV genotypes (L1 and L2 genes), and therefore, indicates HPV presence. The second pair of primers (Pair 2 - ONC1 and ONC2) hybridizes with specific sequences for oncogenic HPV genotypes (E6 and E7 genes). The first pair of primers renders a band of approximately 450 bp, while Pair 2 renders a product of approximately 250 bp. Amplification products are then subjected to a restriction fragment analysis, on which different restriction patterns will indicate presence of a given HPV genotype (Figure 2) (BIOTYPAP Kit, 2009). Mammas and colleagues (Mammas et al., 2010) used the kit for genotyping of HPV in four children with respiratory papillomatosis. The use of PCR-RFLP has been shown to be useful in the identification of multiple HPV infections as well as the detection of novel HPV types (Kay et al., 2002).

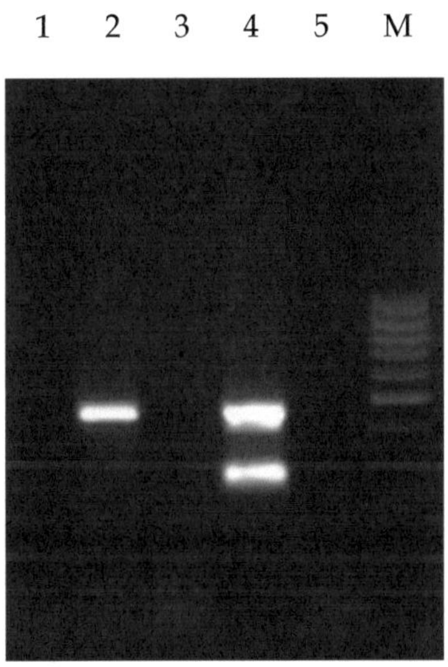

Fig. 2. Detection of HPV with BIOTYPAP Kit. Lane 1 and Lane 3: samples from healthy patients; Lane 2: patient infected with a generic HPV; Lane 4: patient infected with an oncogenic HPV; Lane 5: negative control; M: 100 bp Ladder, adapted from (BIOTYPAP Kit, 2009).

3.3 Polymerase chain reaction-restriction fragment mass polymorphism assay (PCR-RFMP)

The PCR-RFMP assay is based on PCR amplification, restriction enzyme digestion, and analysis by MALDI-TOF mass spectrometry. The precise sizing of oligonucleotides after genotype-specific base variation is detected by fragment scission using type IIS restriction enzymes (Lee et al., 2011). The use of a type IIS restriction enzyme makes the RFMP assay sequence independent and applicable to a wide variety of HPV genotypes, because these enzymes have cleavage sites at a fixed distance from their recognition sites. It is a simple and rapid protocol (4-4,5 h) and accurately detects and identifies at least 74 different HPV genotypes (Hong et al., 2008). When Lee (Lee et al., 2011) and colleagues compared the assay with the well established automated direct sequencing, the PCR-RFMP had a higher analytical sensitivity - 92% and 84% respectively.

3.4 Real-time polymerase chain reaction based assays (rtq-PCR)

Real-time PCR reaction, also called quantitative real time PCR, is a technique capable of amplifying and simultaneously quantifying the target DNA molecules. At each PCR cycle it is possible to measure the amount of amplified product. The detection is performed using non-specific fluorescent dyes that intercalate with any double-stranded DNA or using sequence-specific DNA probes. The reaction is performed in a Real-time PCR thermocycler. After each cycle, to estimate the DNA concentration, the fluorescence is measured with a detector and is compared with a control used as reference. Given its capacity to detect the presence and abundance of a specific DNA sequence, rtq-PCR techniques have been developed to quantify HPV-DNA in clinical samples. Type-specific probes can be combined with fluorescence probes although multiplexing several type-specific primers within one reaction is technically difficult. Consensus primers are used in this technique but are less amenable to quantification than a type-specific system (Molijn et al., 2005). This methodology has the following advantages: 1) it is capable of detecting the viral load; 2) the reaction can be performed on multiplex, with the use of different fluorochromes which emit fluorescence as the PCR reaction proceeds; 3) using a 7-log dynamic range to extrapolate viral load/concentration in the standard curve, it is possible to detect nucleic acids at very small concentrations which would not be detectable by conventional PCR; 4) it is extremely reproducible, rapid and pertinent in a clinical setting (Zaravinos et al., 2009).

Novel RT-PCR methods have been released and are capable of being used as high-throughput screening tools. The GenoID (GenoID Ltd., Budapest, Hungary) is a molecular beacon-based one-step multiplex real-time PCR system which detects 15 high-risk HPV types: 16, 18, 26, 31, 33, 35, 39, 45, 51, 52, 56, 58, 59, 66 and 68) and 5 low-risk HPV types: 6, 11, 42, 43 and 44. The optimized PCR reaction mixture contains 16 forward, 16 reverse primers and 20 type-specific molecular beacon probes targeted to a special sequence of the L1 gene, where a highly variable sequence is flanked by two conserved sequences. Molecular beacons detecting high-risk types are 5-FAM-3-DABCYL-labeled, molecular beacons for low-risk detection are 5-TET-3-DABCYL-labelled, while the internal control added before sample DNA extraction is detected by a 5-FAMTexasRed-3-DABCYL wavelength-shifting molecular beacon. Accordingly, fluorescent data for HPV detection are collected at 530 nm for high-risk types, 560 nm in case of low-risk types and the reaction internal control is detected at 610 nm on a Roche LightCycler 2.0 instrument (Takacs et al., 2008). The sensitivity for detected types varies between 22 and 700 copies/reaction; the assay shows some cross-reactions, however without comprising the overall clinical applicability of the system.

The Abbott Real Time High Risk HPV test (Abbott Molecular Inc., Des Plaines, IL, USA) is performed on the *m*2000rt real-time PCR instrument (Abbott Molecular) and is designed to individually genotype HPV16 and HPV18 and detect other 12 HPVs: 31, 33, 35, 39, 45, 51, 52, 56, 58, 59, 66 and 68 using a modified GP5+/6+ primer mix consisting of three forward and two reverse primers. The assay uses four channels for detecting fluorescent probes: one for detecting the internal control (human beta-globin), a second one for detecting HPV16, a third one for detecting HPV-18, and a fourth one for detecting the remaining 12 hr-HPV genotypes. The assay turnaround time is 6 to 8 hours for 96 samples and depends on the method used for DNA extraction. The fully automated high throughput *m2000sp* instrument (Abbott Molecular Inc.) or smaller *m24sp* instrument (Abbott Molecular Inc.) can be used for DNA extraction, or alternatively DNA can be prepared manually (Poljak et al., 2009). Halfon and colleagues (Halfon et al., 2010b) evaluated the clinical performance of the Abbott Real time HR HPV test, in comparison with biopsy, hybrid capture II and Linear Array, for detection of high-grade disease (CIN2+) in women with abnormal cytology who referred to undergo colposcopic evaluation. All tests had high sensitivity in detecting CIN2+ lesions: Abbott RT HR HPV had 90%, LA had 92% and HCII had 95% and similar specificities: 50%, 47% and 50% for Abbott RT HR HPV, LA, HCII respectively. The authors concluded that the Abbott RT HR HPV assay is good and closely correlated with the other two assays with the advantages of automation and ability to identify HPV16 and HPV18. Another study compared the performance of Abbott RT HR HPV test with that of Hybrid Capture II in 250 liquid-based cervical cytology samples diagnosed with ASCUS, collected from Asian Screening Population. The two tests showed high concordance (absolute agreement: 90%; 95% CI = 0.726–0.874). For detecting cases with underlying HSIL/CIN2+, both tests achieved 100% sensitivity and 100% NPV but Abbott provided higher specificity (20.83% vs 12.50%). The RT-PCR assay is found to provide enhanced sensitivity and specificity for triage of ASCUS (Wong et al., 2011). This assay is also a reliable, sensitive and specific diagnostic tool for the detection and partial genotyping of targeted HPV genotypes in formalin-fixation and subsequent paraffin/paraplast embedding cervical cancer tissue specimens (Kocjan et al., 2011).

The cobas 4800 HPV Test (Roche Molecular Diagnostics, Pleasanton, CA, USA) is a real-time PCR assay for the detection of 14 high-risk HPV types in a single analysis in patient specimens. The test specifically identifies HPV16 and HPV18 while concurrently detecting the rest of the high risk types: 31, 33, 35, 39, 45, 51, 52, 56, 58, 59, 66 and 68. The cobas 4800 System consists of the cobas x 480 instrument for fully automated sample preparation directly from primary sample tubes and the cobas z 480 analyser for real-time PCR based amplification and detection. The cobas x 480 instrument is an automated multi-channel pipetting instrument used to extract, purify, and prepare target nucleic acid for subsequent PCR testing on the cobas z 480 analyser. After completion of sample preparation the cobas x 480 instrument automatically sets up the PCR in a microwell plate. The microwell plate with the PCR-ready samples is then manually unloaded, sealed, and transferred to the cobas z 480 analyser for amplification and detection using real-time PCR (Figure 3) (cobas 4800, 2010). When Castle and colleagues (Castle et al., 2009) described the cobas 4800 HPV DNA Test and compared its performance with the LA test, the percentage of total agreement was 94.7% (95%CI, 92,5%-96%5%), in 531 tested samples. A study enrolling 47,208 women from 61 clinical centers across USA (ATHENA study) evaluated the clinical performance of the cobas 4800 HPV DNA test. The clinical validation of the assay was achieved by determining its performance characteristics for the detection of CIN2+ or worse and CIN3 or worse and by comparing with hc2 test. Sensitivy rates for CIN 2 and CIN 3 were 90% (95%CI, 81.5%-94.8%) and 93,5% (95%CI, 82.5%-97.8%), respectively. The specificity for high grade disease detected by cobas 4800 HPV Test was also comparable with hc2: 70.5% (95%CI, 68.1%-72.7%) vs 71.1% (95%CI, 68.8%-73.4%), respectively. The main advantage of the assay over hc2 is that it provides information on HPV16 and HPV18 separately (Stoler et al., 2011).

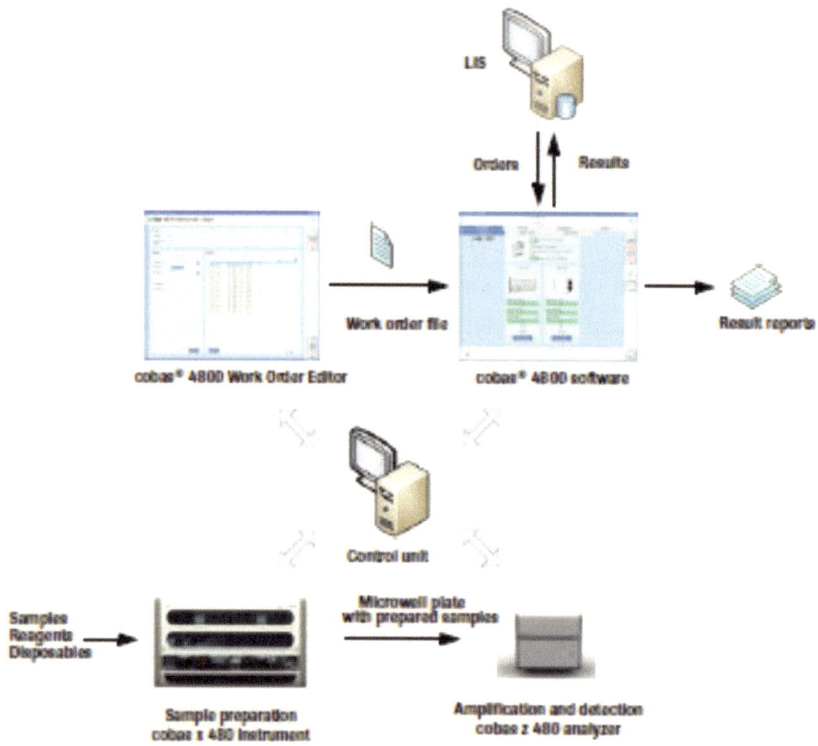

Fig. 3. cobas 4800 HPV Test system overview, adapted from (cobas 4800, 2010)

3.5 Reverse-transcription polymerase chain reaction assays (RT-PCR)

Although the majority of HPV detection strategies are DNA based, it is possible to look for specific HPV viral RNA by incorporating a reverse transcriptase (RT) step before PCR amplification (Molijn et al., 2005). Reverse transcriptase is a DNA polymerase enzyme that transcribes single-stranded RNA into double-stranded DNA. In RT-PCR a specific mRNA is first 'reverse transcribed' into its DNA complement (cDNA) and then amplified using traditional PCR or rtq-PCR methods. The most relevant transcripts for diagnostic purposes are those encoding viral oncoproteins E6 and E7. The detection of viral mRNA can be done by reverse transcriptase PCR or by nucleic acid sequence-based amplification (NASBA) (Poljak and Kocjan, 2010).

The Pretect HPV-Proofer (HPV-Proofer; NorChip, Klokkarstua, Norway) is based on real-time multiplex NASBA and has the advantage of detection type-specific E6/E7 mRNA from the carcinogenic HPV types: 16, 18, 31, 33, and 45. Two primer and probe-sets are included in each reaction vessel. This assay can therefore be used in monitoring a persistent viral infection. Also, it is possible to detect the transforming potential of the infection, due to the oncogenic capacity of E6/E7 genes (Molden et al., 2007). The protocol of this assay is based on isothermal RNA amplification, accomplished by the simultaneous enzymatic activity of avian myeloblastosis virus (AMV) reverse transcriptase, T7 RNA polymerase, and RNase H. For detection, two different types of probes are used, an ECL probe and a molecular beacon probe direct against E6/E7 mRNA (Figure 4). As performance control, to avoid false negatives due to degradation of nucleic acid, a primer set and probe directed against the human U1 small nuclear ribonucleoprotein-specific A protein (U1A mRNA) is included. Two differently labeled molecular beacon probes are used in each multiplex reaction. Fluorescein (FAM) is used as a fluorophore for the detection of HPV16, 31 and 33; Texas Red (TxR) is used for the detection of U1A, HPV 18 and 45. All the molecular beacons contain the non-fluorescent quencher Dabsyl CPG (1-dimethoxytrityloxy-3-[*O*-(N-4′-sulfonyl-4-(dimethylamino)-azobenzene)-3-aminopropyl]-propyl-2-*O*-succinoyl-long chain alkylamino-CPG) (Kraus et al., 2004, Molden et al., 2007). The performance of HPV-Proofer requires standard laboratory equipment, the lambda FL600 fluorescence reader- NASBA platform (Bio-Tek, Wnooski, VT, USA) and PreTect Analysis software (NorChip) for analysis of the experimental data. The analytical sensitivity of the assay is less than 10 SiHA cells, equivalent to 20 copies of HPV16 and less than 1 HeLa cell equivalent to 25 copies of HPV18 (Lie et al., 2005). All studies that have compared HPV-Proofer with hc2 or different in-house or commercial PCR-based HPV DNA assays, showed that HPV-Proofer has a lower clinical sensitivity for the detection of CIN2+ lesions than DNA-based assays, but a significantly higher clinical specificity (Kraus et al., 2004, Lie et al., 2005, Molden et al., 2007, Szarewski et al., 2008).

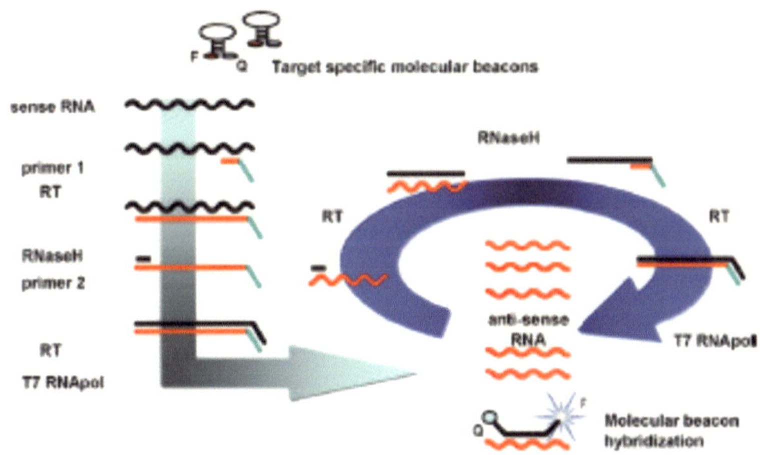

Fig. 4. Schematic presentation of NASBA including molecular beacon detection, adapted from (Molden et al., 2007)

The NucliSENS EasyQ HPV v1 (NucliSENS; bioMÉRIEUX) is a real-time nucleic acid amplification and multiplex detection assay for the qualitative determination of E6/E7 mRNAs of the HPVs 16, 18, 31, 33 and 45. The assay utilizes the nucleic acid sequence-based amplification (NASBA) technology, detecting both viral and bacterial nucleic acids. NucliSENS EasyQ HPV version 1 was launched in 2007 and was based on the original PreTect Proofer assay, except for the NucliSENS hardware platform and the software for NASBA measurements and data analysis (NucliSENS Director software). The latest NucliSENS EasyQ HPV assay version 1 has recently been improved in the following ways:

taking into account the RNA nature of the HPV-specific targets, the five positive controls for the different subtypes and the U1A internal control were changed from single stranded DNA to RNA; also, in order to facilitate handling and to increase reproducibility of the assay, the positive controls are no longer provided in liquid phase but in freeze-dried accuspheres; aiming to improve and harmonize the sensitivity for the five HPV types covered by the assay, the concentrations of the primers and beacons for HPV16 and the U1A internal control were re-adjusted; the extraction protocol on NucliSENS EasyMAG® system was optimized; the HPV assay protocols were updated and the NucliSENtral ™ HPV software V1.1 introduced to further improve the convenience of operator use for results reporting (Jeantet et al., 2009). The calculated analytical sensitivity ranges from $2.3x10^2$ to $3.0x10^4$ copies/mL, showing the highest sensitivity for HPV45 and the lowest for HPV31 (Jeantet et al., 2009). Halfon and colleagues (Halfon et al., 2010a) compared this mRNA assay with the hc2 assay in a population of atypical cells of undetermined significance/low-grade squamous intraepithelial lesion/high-grade squamous intraepithelial lesion (ASCUS/LSIL/HSIL) patients. The clinical sensitivity of NucliSENS EasyQ HPV was 63% for the detection of CIN2+ or HSIL, significantly higher than the sensitivity of hc2 and LA (49% and 45%, respectively). The sensitivity of the assay is significantly lower than that of hc2 and LA (76% vs 95% ans 76% vs 92% respectively).

The APTIMA HPV Assay (Gen-Probe Incorporated, San Diego, CA) is a multiplex nucleic acid test that detects HPV E6/E7 mRNA from 14 high-risk HPV types: 16, 18, 31, 33, 35, 39, 45, 51, 52, 56, 58, 59, 66 and 68. The assay provides a qualitative result (positive/negative) for the presence/absence of these high-risk HPV types, but does not determine the specific HPV type present in the specimen. The APTIMA HPV Assay involves three main steps, which take place in a single tube: capture of the target mRNA using HPV-specific capture oligomers and magnetic microparticles; target mRNA amplification using transcription-mediated amplification, and detect the amplification products (amplicons) using the Hybridization Protection Assay (Dockter et al., 2009a). An internal control transcript is added to each reaction to verify the performance of each step of the assay: capture, amplification and detection. One positive calibrator and one negative calibrator are used to determine the validity of the run and to establish the assay cutoff values for the internal control and analyse signals. A positive control and a negative control are also processed as separate samples and used to determine run validity. The assay can be performed on the semi-automated Direct TubeSampling (DTS) systems, or on the fully automated TIGRIS DTS system (Gen-Probe Incorporated, San Diego, CA). The throughput is approximately 180 specimens for 1 operator in about 5 to 6 hours for the DTS systems and approximately 1000 specimens in about 14 hours for the TIGRIS DTS system (Dockter et al., 2009a). The analytical sensitivity of the assay in the semi-automated DTS systems was between 38 and 488 HPV mRNA copies and in fully automated TIGRIS DTS system was between 17 and 275 HPV mRNA copies. The overall analytical specificity of the assay was equal to or greater than 99% in both systems. Dockter and colleagues (Dockter et al., 2009b) evaluated APTIMA HPV Assay performance for detection of high risk HPV and high-grade cervical intraepithelial neoplasia (CIN) compared to hc2. The mRNA based assay was found to be highly sensitive and specific for the detection of high-risk HPV in clinical samples, with a sensitivity of 92% and a specificity of 98%. The results obtained in the DTS and TIGRIS DTS systems were equivalent. Another study compared the sensitivity and specificity of several tests, including APTIMA HPV Assay, for the detection of high-grade CIN in a population referred to colposcopy because of abnormal cytology (Szarewski et al., 2008). Four adjuvant tests had sensitivities greater than 95% for high-grade disease (CIN2+ and CIN3+ respectively): Amplicor (98.9% and 99.5%), Hybrid Capture II (99.6% and 99.5%), Linear Array (98.2% and 99.0%) and APTIMA (95.2% and 97.4%). Of these, APTIMA showed the highest specificity (42.2% and 38.8%).

4. Sequencing reaction (GP6+) – big dye terminator cycle sequencing kit

As previously mentioned, sequencing methods of PCR products are also now available for high throughput allowing its application to routine clinical analysis (Ekstrom et al., 2011). Nested PCR amplification of a conserved region of the HPV *L1* gene, with the consensus GP5+/GP6+ primers, followed by genotyping with direct DNA sequencing (BigDye Terminators, Applied Biosystems) and alignment of the hypervariable region of the L1 gene against known HPV genotype sequences, stored in the GenBank database, usually determines the genotype of the HPV isolates detected (Molijn et al., 2005). LoTemp™ HiFi® DNA polymerase has shown to be 10 times more efficient, than other Taq DNA polymerases, in amplifying HPV plasmid DNA by MY09/MY11 PCR and about 100 to 1000 times more efficient when the first amplification was followed by a GP5+/GP6+ nested PCR in tandem (Lee et al., 2007). The nested PCR technology described by Molijn *et al.* proved to be a sensitive method for the detection of 1-10 copies of purified genomic DNA of HPV types 16, 18 or 6B. However, 10^4 - 10^5 copies of genomic DNA were needed as PCR templates for UV visualization of a positive primer amplicon after electrophoresis. Reproducibility of this nested PCR assay was confirmed (Molijn et al., 2005).The exploitation of this method allows the identification of new HPV types given that it is not intended for the identification of specific types. Sequencing protocols, in particular the requirement for template purification, are too labor-intensive for routine applications. In the presence of samples infected with more than one genotype of HPV are unsuitable for HPV determination. Sequences which represent a minority species, in the total of the PCR product, may remain undetected underestimating the prevalence of infections with multiple HPV genotypes. After detecting a sample with multiple HPV infection the genotype can be deduced by two methods: 1) database homology search (BLAST) and 2) phylogenetic analyses (Kleter et al., 1999). In any case, it is time consuming and not totally reliable. Thus, this method is not readily adapted to routine diagnostic labs.

5. Type-specific probe assays

5.1 DNA Microarray genotyping assays

The DNA microarray system has been largely used in HPV typing (Jacobs et al., 1997). A DNA microarray is a collection of microscopic DNA probes attached to a solid surface by a covalent bond. Each probe contains picomoles of a specific DNA sequence like a short section of a gene. The cDNA targets are fluorescently labelled and under high-stringency conditions hybridize with the probes on the surface of a chip. In each spot the fluorescent light is detected by excitation with monochromatic light and transformed in image by software. This technology can screen a high number of markers per individual and it is particularly suited for strategy using large populations. An example of this methodology is HPVDNAChip (Biomedlab, Seoul, South Korea) which contains 22 type-specific probes, allowing identification of 15 high-risk types: 16, 18, 31, 33, 35, 39, 45, 51, 52, 56, 58, 59, 66, 68, 69 and 7 low-risk types: 6, 11, 34, 40, 42, 43 and 44. In summary, target HPV DNA is amplified by PCR with hpv1/hpv2 primers and labeled utilizing Cy5-dCTP or Cy5-dUTP, with primers and conditions described by manufacturer. Secondly, the PCR product is hybridized onto the chip and, after washing, the hybridized signals are visualized with a DNA chip scanner (Seo et al., 2006). The HPVDNAChip test was successfully implemented in a population based study in Korea with 2.470 women (Hwang et al., 2004) and in a study that compared the performance of four HPV genotyping assays on a panel of 824 samples; the analytical sensitivity of the test was around 80% and specificity for the individual HPV types was above 94% (Klug et al., 2008).

The GG HPVCHIP (GoodGene, Seoul, South Korea) allows the identification of 42 alpha-HPV types; 15 high-risk types: 16, 18, 31, 33, 35, 39, 45, 51, 52, 56, 58, 59, 68, 69 and 70; Three probable high-risk types: 26, 53 and 66; 20 low-risk types:6, 7, 10, 11, 27, 32, 40, 42, 44, 54, 55, 57, 61, 62, 72, 73, 91, CP8304/81, and MM7/83, MM8/84; and four undetermined-risk types: 30, 34, 67 and MM4/82. The DNA chips collect multiple oligonucleotide probes of the 42 HPV types and human β-globin gene. The DNA is amplified with Cy5-labelled primer for E6, E7 and L1 gene and the produced amplicons are applied onto the DNA chip, followed by hybridization and the genotypes of HPV within sample are identified by a fluorescent scanner (Kim et al., 2006). The performance of the GG DNACHIP was compared with PCR sequencing on 100 cervical cancer specimens and both methods detected 98% (98/100) high-risk types of the samples tested (Kim et al., 2006).

The HPV GenoArray Test Kit (GenoArray, HybriBio Limited, Hong Kong) uses both DNA amplification and Hybrio's proprietary flowthrough hybridization technique to simultaneously identify 21 alpha-HPV types: 6, 11, 16, 18, 31, 33, 35, 39, 42-45, 51-53, 56, 58, 59, 66, 68 and 81. The test employs a macroarray format with a nylon membrane onto which HPV genotype-specific oligonucleotides probes have been immobilized (Grisaru et al., 2008). Liu and colleagues (Liu et al., 2010) compared the HPV GenoArray test with Linear Array, revealing concordant or compatible results for 97,5% of the samples and discordant results for only eight samples (2,5%). The assay appears to be highly sensitive and specific for the genotyping of HPV and has the advantage that specifically detects HPV52, which overcomes a limitation of the Linear Array.

Less frequent in peer-reviewed literature are the kits GeneTrack HPV DNA Chip (GeneTrack, Genomic Tree, Daejeon, South Korea) and GeneSQUARE HPV Microarray (Kurabo Industries, Osaka, Japan). The first identifies 28 HPV types: 6, 11, 16, 18, 31, 33, 35, 39, 40, 42-45, 51, 52, 54, 56, 58, 59, 62, 66-72 and consists in the amplification of a 450 bp region of the L1 gene using MY09/11/HMB01 primers and of an internal control (portion of the human interferon-2 gene). To determine the HPV genotype, the amplicons are hybridized on a DNA chip with eight microarrays chambers, each containing a duplicate of the 28 type-specific probes and a replicate of a human cellular target-specific probe (Oh et al., 2004, Poljak and Kocjan, 2010). The GeneSQUARE HPV is a microarray system in development that utilizes a multiplex PCR to amplify and identify 23 alpha-HPVs: 6, 11, 16, 18, 30, 31, 33-35, 39, 40, 42, 45, 51-54, 56, 58, 59, 61, 66 and 68. Type-specific primer pairs are used in the assay and the upstream primer in each pair is labeled with biotin at the 5'end. After hybridization, the microarray is washed, dried and scanned (Figure 5) (Ermel et al., 2010, Matsushita et al., 2011). Ermel and colleagues (Ermel et al., 2010) compared the hc2,

Linear Array and GeneSQUARE methods and the sample proportion agreement was very good, particularly between Linear Array and GeneSQUARE.

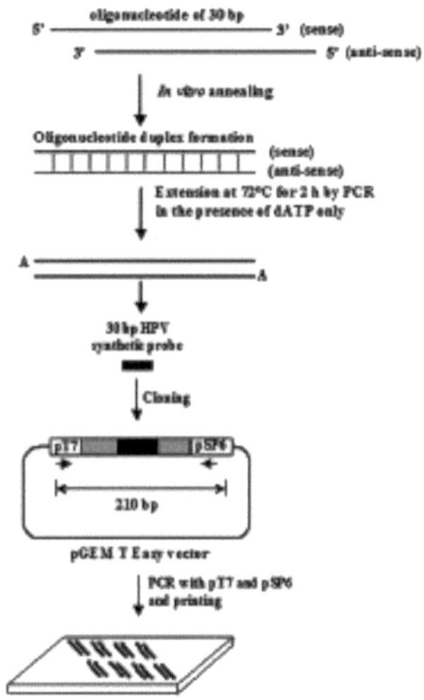

Fig. 5. Protocol for HPV-specific probe synthesis by oligonucleotide shuffling used in GeneTrack, adapted from (Oh et al., 2004)

The Infiniti HPV assays (AutoGenomics, Carlsbad, CA, USA) are commercially available genotyping platforms for HPV genotyping that uses multiplex PCR, followed by automated processing for primer extension, hybridization and detection (Erali et al., 2009). It groups three assays: Infiniti HPV Genotyping Assay, Infiniti HPV-HR Quad assay and Infiniti HPV-Quad Assay. The Infiniti HPV-Quad assay targets the E1 gene of the HPV genome and identifies five individual HPV types: 16, 18, 31, 33, and 45, five combinations of HPV types: 35/68, 39/56, 58/52, 59/51, 6/11 and a β-globin internal control. When Erali and colleagues (Erali et al., 2009) compared this assay with Hybrid Capture II, the overall concordance of positive and negative results was 83% among the 197 specimens tested.

The PANArray HPV Genotyping Chip (PANArray, PANAGENE, Daejeon, Korea) uses peptide nucleic acid probes for the identification of 31 HPV types: 6, 11, 16, 18, 26, 31-35, 39, 40, 42-45, 51-54, 56, 58, 59, 62, 66, 68-70, 73, 81, 83 and one subtytpe, subHPV-44 or HPV-55. MY09/11 PCR products nested with GP5+/biotinylated-GP6+ primers are used for the genotyping (Poljak and Kocjan, 2010). A study comparing the genotyping results of PANArray to sequencing with MY09/11 PCR products showed excellent agreement except for samples reflecting multiple infections (Choi et al., 2009).

Another illustration of this methodology is Clart HPV 2 assay (Genomica, Madrid, Spain), developed for the detection and genotyping of 35 HPV types: 6, 11, 16, 18, 26, 31, 33, 35, 39,

40, 42, 43, 44, 45, 51, 52, 53, 54, 56, 58, 59, 61, 62, 66, 68, 70, 71, 72, 73, 81, 82, 83, 84, 85 and 89. It uses biotinylated primers that amplify a 450bp fragment within L1 region. Co-amplification of an 892 bp region of the CFTR gene and 1,202 bp fragment of a transformed plasmid provides a control to ensure DNA extraction and PCR efficiency (Pista et al., 2011). The performance of Clart HPV 2 requires standard laboratory equipment and the Clinical Arrays Processor (Genomica) for fully automated microarray processing and genotyping analysis (Poljak and Kocjan, 2010). A comparative evaluation of Clart HPV 2 with Hybrid Capture 2 Test on samples with cervical intraepithelial neoplasia grade 2 or worse showed a clinical sensitivity of 96.9% and specificity of 71.9% (Pista et al., 2011). When Galan-Sanchez and colleagues (Galan-Sanchez and Rodriguez-Iglesias, 2009) compared INNO-LIPA HPV Genotyping v2, Linear Arrays HPV Genotyping Test and Clart HPV 2 the results were absolutely concordant in 31 samples, compatible (some but not all genotypes) in 44 samples and discordant in only 3 samples; concluding that all the 3 methods are highly comparable and suitable for clinical and epidemiological studies. The advantages of this methodology, made a successful use in large-population-based study in Spain, where 2362 women from three different regions were investigated (Gomez-Roman et al., 2009).

The PapilloCheck HPV-Screening Test (Greiner Bio-One GmbH, Frickenhausen, Germany) is one of the two most frequently used PCR-microarrays-based assays (Poljak and Kocjan, 2010). It is a PCR-based test using a consensus primer set targeting the E1 HPV gene. HPV oligoprobes immobilized on a DNA chip allow for the identification of 24 HPV types: 6, 11, 16, 18, 31, 33, 35, 39, 40, 42-45, 51-53, 56, 58, 59, 66, 68, 70, 73 and 82. Each PapilloCheck chip contains 12 wells defined by elevated rims, each of which contains one PapilloCheck array with 28 probes, each in 5 replicate spots (Dalstein et al., 2009). This test utilizes the amplification of 350 pb HPV DNA fragment as a new consensus primer set: each reverse primer was extended at 5′ end with a universal tag. Additionally, a region within the human ADAT1 gene is simultaneously amplified using fluorescent-labeled primers with Cy5-dUTP. The amplicons hybridize to HPV specific oligoprobes immobilized on the DNA chip the readings are performed on a CheckScanner instrument (Dalstein et al., 2009). Several comparative evaluations of PapilloCheck with other HPV assays have been published (Halfon et al., 2010c, Hesselink et al., 2010, Iftner et al., 2010, Schopp et al., 2010, Kitchener et al., 2011). This genotyping test was compared with SPF10PCRLiPav and PGMY09/11 on Hybrid Capture2 pretested samples (Schopp et al., 2010). From results of 826 cervical samples, the PapilloCheck found 100% sensitivity in HPV types 53, 56 and 33. The lowest detection rate was observed for type 35 (72,2%) and the detection rates for the identification of high-grade intraephitelial neoplasia (CIN2+) ranged from 93,7% (PGMY09/11 PCR) to 98,4% (PapilloCheck, SPF10 PCR, HC2), leading to the conclusion that the PapilloCheck gives comparable results on established PCR methods (Schopp et al., 2010). Halfon and colleagues (Halfon et al., 2010c) compared PapilloCheck, Linear Array and hc2 in 239 women referred for colposcopy and histology, concluding that all tests showed a good sensitivity (greater than 90%) without statistically relevant differences between them.

The application of microarray technology as a diagnostic toll shows great advantages, since microarray can discriminate HPV genotypes and identify multiple infections (Kim et al., 2003). Ideally, a larger number of HPV type-specific probes could be spotted on a chip, augmenting the quantity of HPVs genotyped by assay. Unfortunately this method requires the presence of expensive equipment and therefore is not suitable for all the laboratories.

5.2 Suspension array genotyping assays (HPV-SA)

The HPV-SA provides a rapid and cost-effective method to simultaneously detect different HPV genotypes. This technology uses microspheres as array elements that carry appropriate receptor molecules such as DNA oligonucleotide probes, antibodies, or other proteins. Microspheres are readily suspendable in solution and possess distinct optical properties. Each bead can easily be differentiated based on variations and intensity of colour. The most common detection systems are light scatter or fluorescence from an internal dye. The Luminex xMAP system is a flexible analyzer based on the principle of flow cytometry. It incorporates a proprietary process to internally dye polystyrene beads with two spectrally distinct fluorochromes. Each bead set is usually coupled to a single oligonucleotide probe specific for one HPV type. Genotyping is done by reverse hybridization using biotinylated PCR amplicons. After denaturing and hybridization of target HPV sequences to the bead-bound probes, labeling of the hybridized biotinylated amplicons is done using R-phycoerythrin-labelled streptavidin, serving as a reporter fluorophore. The bead sets are then read and analysed on a Luminex analyser (Poljak and Kocjan, 2010).

There are several in-house genotyping protocols based on xMAP technology. Jiang and colleagues (Jiang et al., 2006) developed a rapid high-throughput DNA suspension assay, capable of simultaneously typing 26 HPVs: 6, 11, 16, 18, 26, 31, 33-35, 39, 40, 42-45, 51-54, 56, 58, 59, 66, 68, 73 and 82. The HPV-SA consists of 26 different microsphere sets with spectral addresses. Each microsphere set shows an HPV type-specific probe on its surface, and they can be combined allowing up to 26 different HPV targets to be measured simultaneously in a single reaction vessel (Figure 6). Another in-house SA protocol was developed by Oh and colleagues (Oh et al., 2007) combining PCR amplification with Luminex hybridization. The use of HPV type-specific probes and YBT L1/GP6-1 primers detects HPVs 6, 16, 18, 31, 35, 42, 51, 52, 55, 56, 58, 59, 66, 67 and 68. The authors compared the SA to the established HPV DNA microarray chip for PCR products derived from 53 clinical samples. The evaluation showed excellent agreement as the SA was a very sensitive and reproducible technique for simultaneously genotyping of all clinically relevant genital HPV types (Oh et al., 2007).

In addition, at least two commercial assays based on this technology are available at present. The Multiplex HPV Genotyping kit v1.0 (Progen/Multimetrix, Heidelberg, Germany) is a research use only (RUO) assay that allows detection and identification of 24 HPV types: 6, 11, 16, 18, 26, 31, 33, 35, 39, 42-45, 51-53, 56, 58, 59, 66, 68, 70, 73 and 82. The sample is subjected to PCR amplification, using sets of biotinylated primers contained in the kit. The amplicons are added to bead mix, containing 26 distinct bead populations coupled to 24 HPV, one β-globin and one hybridization control specific oligonucleotide probe. The β-globin control serves as quality control for genomic DNA in the PCR. After thermal denaturing and hybridization of target sequences to the bead-bound probes, labeling of the hybridized biotinylated PCR products is achieved by R-phycoerythrin labeled streptavidin. Schmitt and colleagues (Schmitt et al., 2006) compared the performance of Multiplex Human

Papillomavirus Genotyping assay to an estabilished reverse line blot assay on GP5+/6+ PCR products derived from 94 clinical samples. The evaluation showed an excellent agreement but also a higher sensitivity of the Multiplex assay.

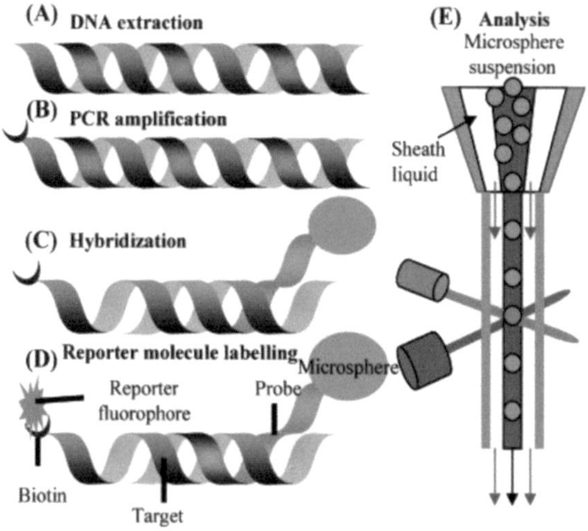

Fig. 6. Schematic representation of the HPV-SA. After HPV DNA extraction (A), the template was amplified with the MY09/11 primer set (B). PCR products are transferred to a PCR tube containing the 26-plex HPV-SA and hybridized (C). After washing, the hybridized microspheres were incubated with streptavidin-R-phycoerythrin at room temperature for 30 min (D). Finally, the mixture is analysed on the Luminex100 analyser (E), adapted from (Jiang et al., 2006).

The digene HPV genotyping LQ Test RUO (Digene LQ Test; Qiagen) uses multiplex, bead-based xMAP technology and an automated, high-throughput read-out by either the LiquidChip 200 workstation (Qiagen, Hilden, Germany) or Luminex 100 IS System (Luminex Corporation, Austin, TX, USA). The test was developed for identification of 18 high-risk HPVs: 16, 18, 26, 31, 33, 35, 39, 45, 51-53, 56, 58, 59, 66, 68, 73 and 82 using GP5+/6+ PCR products. Read-out of this assay is expressed as the medium fluorescent intensity of the reporter fluorescence for each genotype (Geraets et al., 2009b). When compared with in-house GP5+/6+, the assay demonstrated high agreement for overall detection and type-specific identification (Geraets et al., 2009b).

6. Reverse line-blot hybridization-based HPV genotyping assays

It is the most common method used for HPV genotyping nowadays. In these types of assays a fragment of the HPV genome is first amplified by PCR, using biotinylated HPV-specific primers, and the resulting amplicons are then denatured and hybridized with HPV-specific oligonucleotide probes immobilized as parallel lines on nylon or a nitrocellulose membrane strip. After hybridization, streptavidin-conjugated alkaline phosphatase or horseradish peroxidase is added, which binds to any biotinilated hybrid formerly produced (Figure 7). Incubation with chromogenic substrates yields a colored precipitate at the probe positions where hybridization occurs. The genotyping strip is then visually interpreted by comparison with the test reference guide for each of the targeted HPV types. The principle of INNO-

LiPA HPV Genotyping assay is based on the amplification of a 65bp region of the HPV *L1* gene, using biotinylated SPF10 primers, followed by the hybridization of the resulting amplicons with HPV specific oligonucleotide probes immobilized on a nitrocellulose strip. This is one of the most widely used HPV genotyping kits and there are several versions developed of which the first version, the INNO-LiPA$_{25}$ HPV genotyping V1.0 (Labo Biomedical Products, Rijswick, The Netherlands) allowed the identification of 26 HPVs: 6, 11, 16, 18, 31, 33, 34, 35, 39, 40, 42,43, 44, 45, 51, 52, 53, 54, 56, 58, 59, 66, 68, 70, 73 and 74 (Kleter et al., 1999). More recent versions of this assay, the INNO-LiPA HPV Genotyping v2 and INNO-LiPA HPV Genotyping CE Assays (Innogenetics) allowed the identification of 24 and 17 individual types, respectively. The latest version, INNO-LiPA HPV Genotyping *Extra*, allows the simultaneous identification of 28 different HPV types: 6, 11, 16, 18, 26, 31, 33, 35, 39, 40, 43, 44, 45, 51, 52, 53, 54, 56, 58, 59, 66, 68, 69/71, 70, 73, 74 and 82. The former assay contains an additional primer pair, in the amplification mix, for the amplification of the *HLA-DPB1* gene to check for PCR inhibition, sample quality and DNA extraction, as well as an anticontamination system based on uracil-N-glycosylase (Poljak and Kocjan, 2010). Several evaluation studies have been performed in recent years. A recent study compared real-time multiplex HPV PCR assays with INNO-LiPA Genotyping *Extra* suggesting increased sensitivity of DNA HPV detection by type-specific multiplex HPV PCR assays (Else et al., 2011). Another interesting and important assessment was the comparative evaluation of different extraction methods for genotyping with INNO-LiPA and Linear array genotyping tests. This study suggests that the use of consistent protocols for DNA purification is a priority to guarantee intra-assay reproducibility over time (Dona et al., 2011). INNO-LiPA HPV Genotyping *Extra* is also recommended for the use with paraffin-embedded tissue. After comparison with Linear Array HPV Genotyping Test the INNO-LiPA genotyping *Extra* revealed greater sensitivity for HPV genotyping from archival tissue (Tan et al., 2010). INNO-LiPA *Extra* has a sensitivity of 20-70 viral copies per assay (estimated for HPV-16, 18, 31, 45 and 52) (Seme et al., 2009).

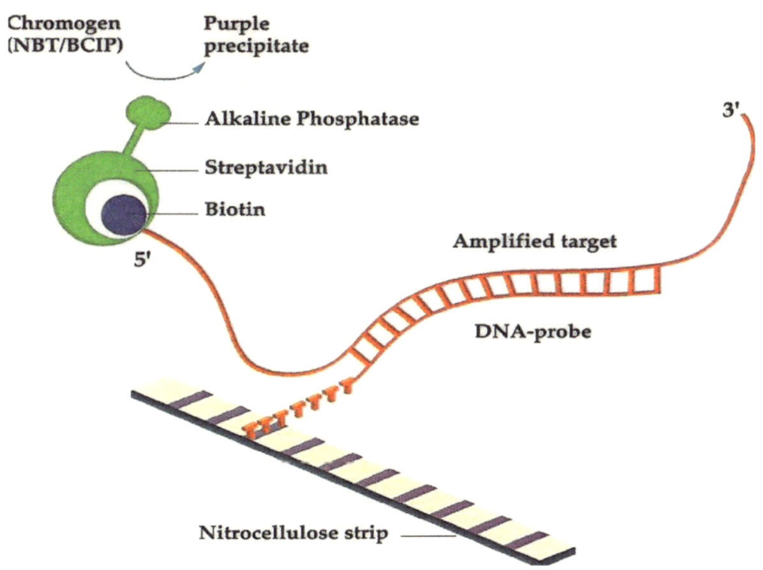

Fig. 7. INNO-LiPA HPV Genotyping test principle, adapted from INNO-LiPA brochure.

As with INNO-LiPA, Linear Array HPV Genotyping assay is based on the amplification of a region of the HPV *L1* gene (450 bp). This genotyping test also amplifies a 268bp region of the human β-globin gene, using biotinylated primer sets PGM09/PGMY11 and PC04/GH20, respectively. Subsequent hybridization of the resulting amplicons is made onto a single-typing nylon strip coated with HPV type specific and β-globin specific oligonucleotide probes. This test is one of the most commonly used HPV genotyping assays which combines PCR amplification and reverse line-blot hybridization for the identification of 36 HPV types: 6, 11, 16, 18, 26, 31, 33, 35, 39, 40, 42, 44, 45, 51, 52, 53, 54, 56, 58, 59, 61, 62, 64, 66, 67, 68, 69, 70, 71, 72, 73, 81, 82, 83, 84 and 89 and one subtype (subHPV-82 or IS39) (Poljak and Kocjan, 2010). It is registered for use in the European Union (CE-IVD) but not available for use in the United States. Numerous comparative evaluations of Linear Array with other HPV genotyping assays have been performed. All studies reported high concordance amongst hybridization genotyping methods and suitability for clinical and epidemiological studies (Galan-Sanchez and Rodriguez-Iglesias, 2009). Linear Array has revealed good correlation and perfect agreement with hc2, with high sensitivity; 100% detection of cervical intraepithelial neoplasia (CIN) III was shown by both Linear array and hc2 (Paolini et al., 2011). Comparison of this genotyping assay with real-time multiplex HPV PCR assays, holding as constant the DNA extraction method (Qiagen Spin blood kit), revealed that multiplex PCR assays detect more HPV-positive specimens for the 14 HPV types common to both than Linear Array HPV genotyping assay. Type-specific agreements between the assays were good but were often driven by negative agreement in HPV types with low prevalence, as evidenced by reduced proportions of positive agreement. An alternate DNA extraction technique (Qiagen MinElute kit) impacted subsequent HPV detection in both the multiplex PCR and Linear Array (Roberts et al., 2011). A comparative evaluation with INNO-LiPA has shown high concordance amongst both methods; however, when comparing individual HPV types, Linear Array was able to detect significantly more HPV-16, 18, 39, 40, 42, 54, 58, 59, 66, 70 and 68/73, and fewer HPV-11, 31 and 52 than INNO-LiPA (Castle et al., 2008). Furthermore, INNO-LiPA was able to detect more multiple HPV infections and a greater number of HPV types per multiple infection (Castle et al., 2008). Linear array has shown a sensitivity of 98.2% and a specificity of 32.8% for the detection of CIN II+ lesions (Szarewski et al., 2008).

The Digene HPV Genotyping RH Test RUO is a reverse line-blot assay designed for the detection and identification of 18 HPV types: 16, 18, 26, 31, 33, 35, 39, 45, 51, 52, 53, 56, 58, 59, 66, 68, 73 and 82. As the previous genotyping tests it is based on the PCR amplification of a 150bp region of the HPV *L1* gene using biotinylated GP5+ and GP6+ primers, followed by the hybridization of the resulting amplicons onto a single-typing nitrocellulose strip containing 18 HPV type-specific probe lines (Geraets et al., 2009a). Digene HPV genotyping RH Test RUO was compared to INNO-LiPA genotyping test *Extra* showing comparable genotyping results. However, INNO-LiPA identified significantly more samples with multiple HPV types (Seme et al., 2009). Another evaluation study compared the Digene genotyping RH test with the in-house Reverse Line Blot (RLB) genotyping assay. Both genotyping assays demonstrated high concordance, in 493 HC2-positive samples, for overall HR HPV detection and type-specific identification of the 18 HR types. The Digene RH Test revealed positivity for one or more HR HPV type(s) in 86.6% of the HC2-positive women, and negativity was confirmed in 97.9% of the HC2-negative women. The Digene HPV

Genotyping RH Test revealed a high genotyping agreement with the established RLB assay on GP5+/6+ amplimers (Geraets et al., 2009a). It was reported recently another study encompassing the Digene HPV Genotyping RH test. The objective was to test whether the RH Test and LQ Test (XMap based) can be used as an universal hrHPV genotyping test. Self-collected 416 cervico-vaginal specimens from an epidemiologic study were analyzed with Amplicor. The amplimers obtained were also tested with the RH Test and LQ Test for identification of 18 HPV types, including the 13 hrHPVs targeted by Amplicor. 197 specimens were positive by Amplicor, in which the RH Test and LQ Test identified one of the 13 hrHPVs in 94.4% and 98.0%, respectively. In 219 specimens remaining negative by Amplicor, the RH Test and LQ Test, performed on the Amplicor amplification products, still detected one of the 13 hrHPVs in 3.7% and 5.5% respectively, and include identification of HPV53, 66, and 82. Overall, the RH and LQ Tests demonstrated high concordance with Amplicor for hrHPV detection (κ=0.908 and κ=0.923, respectively). The authors suggest that the digene HPV Genotyping RH and LQ Tests can be directly used for amplimers generated by the Amplicor HPV Test (Geraets et al., 2011). The latest version of Digene RH test (v1.0) includes an additional primer pair for human β-globin gene amplification, serving as an internal control for PCR inhibition and adequate sample taking and DNA purification (Poljak and Kocjan, 2010).

The EasyChip HPB Blot kit (HPV Blot kit; King Car, Taiwan) is a reverse dot-blot assay designed for the identification, in the latest version, of 39 types of HPV: 6, 11, 16, 18, 26, 31, 32, 33, 35, 37, 39, 42, 43, 44, 45, 51, 52, 53, 54, 55, 56, 58, 59, 61, 62, 66, 67, 68, 69, 70, 72, 74, 82, CP8061, CP8304, L1AE5, MM4, MM7 and MM8. The biotinylated PCR amplicons of several HPV general primer sets or their combinations can be used for genotyping, including MY11/MY09, PGMY11/PGMY09, GP5+/GP6+, MY11/GP6+, MY11/GP6+ nested with GP5+/GP6+ and SPF1/GP6+. The latest version of this kit provides two standardized PCR amplification mixes: in the first, a modificed MY11/GP6+ primers set is used to amplify a 190bp region of the HPV *L1* gene; in the second, the quality of extracted DNA is validated by amplification of a 136bp region of the human *GAPDH* gene. The resulting amplicons from an individual DNA sample are genotyped together on a single-typing nylon membrane containing the 39 HPV type-specific and one GAPDH-specific oligonucleotide probe marked in duplicate (Poljak and Kocjan, 2010). The evaluation of the sensitivity, specificity, reliability and reproducibility of the EasyChip HPV blot for HPV genotyping was performed in two studies. In the first, type-specific sensitivity and specificity for the 39 types of HPV were examined. The operating environment, reliability, reproducibility and blot interpretation were assessed by a quality assurance system. Each batch experiment contained samples from 89 cervical specimens and 7 extrinsic controls. Caski, HeLa and Jurkat cells, male human blood cell DNA and sterile water were used to assess reliability. Furthermore, pairs of sibling controls were used to assess reproducibility. The overall sensitivity of HPV detection was 1-50 copies of HPV genome equivalent. There was no cross-reactivity with amplicons of other HPV genotypes. One hundred batch experiments demonstrated that the reliability was excellent. The intra-batch and inter-batch reproducibility was 98 and 97%, respectively. The authors concluded that the EasyChip HPV blot is a highly sensitive, reliable and reproducible tool for detection and identification of HPV genotypes (Lin et al., 2007). The second study compared the efficacy of HPV detection and typing with a general PCR-based genotyping array with EasyChip HPV Blot.

The concordance of the two tests in determining HPV positivity was 96.8% (419/433), with a Cohen's kappa=0.93 (95% CI: 0.90-0.97) and McNemar's test of P=1.0, which indicates excellent agreement. The overall concordance of the two tests in the identification of type-specific HPV was 91.0%. Sensitivity (90-100%), specificity (99.2-100%), and accuracy (98.6-100%) rates of HPV Blot against the gold standard were satisfactory for HPV-16, 18, 58, 33, 52, 39, 45, 31, 51, 70 while HPV-71 (63.6%) had suboptimal sensitivity. The authors conclude that the modified MY11/GP6+ PCR-based HPV Blot assay is accurate and sensitive for detection and genotyping of HPV in cervical swab samples (Lin et al., 2008).

M&D REBA HPV-ID® is a molecular diagnostic kit for genotyping HPV; it detects 15 high-risk genotypes:16, 18, 31, 33, 35, 39, 45, 51, 52, 56, 58, 59, 68, 53, 66 and 10 low-risk genotypes: 6, 11, 42, 43, 44, 70, 72, 81, 84, 87 , simultaneously. Genetic target of REBA HPV-ID® is the HPV *L1* gene, which is expressed at the late stage of infection cycles in the host cells. The kit is based on one-step nested PCR with biotinylated MY09/11 and GP5+/6+ primers and subsequent genotyping of the resulting amplicons with a single typing strip containing 23 HPV type-specific probes and one HPVV universal probe. There are no evaluation studies about this kit in peer-reviewed literature (**Inc**, **M&D**, Poljak and Kocjan, 2010).

The reverse hybridization methodology uses standard laboratory equipment and the methodology is both reproducible and rapid. The price per sample can limit its use.

7. *In situ* hybridization assays (ISH)

In situ hybridization allows the detection of intact viral DNA directly in tissues sections or cell preparations (*in situ*). The method is based on the recognition and following bond of the labelled probe with the complementary viral target. The sample is fixed in fixative solution in order to preserve the tissue morphology and to prevent loss of genetic material (Carlson and Hu). The result of the hybridization reaction is evaluated microscopically and the appearance of a specific precipitate is indicative of infection (Huang et al., 1998, Poljak and Kocjan, 2010). Generally the assay is based on four steps: tissue fixation, permeabilization of tissue samples, hybridization of the sample with probes, and detection of the HPV positive cells. Critical points for a successful ISH test are the hybridization and post-hybridization treatment. Hybridization is performed by incubating the fixed tissue with the solution containing the hybridization probe and washing the tissue to remove the unbound probes. During these steps, many parameters play a crucial role. Different lengths of probes and different labelling conditions are an example (Montgomery, 2002). The ISH probe cocktails available in the market for HPV detection are several. The latest generation probes utilize stacked antibodies to enhance the sensitivities and probes containing viral genomic DNA in double strand form (INFORM HPV III test). The target of the probes can be the viral DNA and mRNA sequences or viral mRNA transcript in human cells. ISH assay showed a low sensitivity (50%) but a significantly higher specificity (Caussy et al., 1988). The values can vary, depending on the commercially method utilized.

INFORM HPV III test (Ventana, Tucson, AZ, USA) represents the last generation commercial kit for detecting HPV DNA in cytological and histological specimens. It utilizes stacked antibodies to enhance the sensitivity of the technique (Poljak and Kocjan, 2010). The antibody stacks consist of a primary antibody that binds the dinitro-phenol hapten linked to the probe, a secondary antibody, a biotinylated tertiary antibody, and a streptavidin-alkaline phosphatase conjugate that generate the final colour precipitates. Several are the probe cocktails available for low and high HPV risk detection. The probe B and C target 12 HPVs: 16, 18, 31, 33, 35, 39, 45, 51, 52, 56, 58, and 66.

GenPoint HPV Biotinylated DNA probe is the last generation ISH kit using the GenPoint Tyramide Signal Amplification System (Dako) (Glostrup, Denmark). It can be used in both cytological and histological specimens. The probe is biotin-labeled and consists of a viral genomic double-stranded DNA of 500 bp (Gebeyehu et al., 1987). Biotin can be detected by using enzyme conjugates of streptavidin to produce covalent bounds with tyramide substrates and chromogenic indicator dye diaminobenzidine (DAB) (Bobrow et al., 1989). DAB is oxidized by peroxidase enzymes to produce a dark brown precipitate that can be visualized on Dako Hybridizer and Autostainer Plus (Poljak and Kocjan, 2010). The probe cocktail recognises 13 HPVs: 16, 18, 31, 33, 35, 39, 45, 51, 52, 56, 58, 59, and 68. In a comparative study of INFORM III, GenPoint, and HPV PCR evaluated on 58 tissue specimens, GenPoint showed the same specificity (100%) then INFORM III but lower sensitivity (Kong et al., 2007).

Zyto*Fast* HPV Probes (ZytoVision, Bremerhaven, Germany) are specific probes for the detection of viral DNA and mRNA of E6, E7, and L1 proteins. It can be used in both cytological and histological specimens. The probes are biotin or digoxigenin labelled and consist of HPV-type-specific oligonucleotides (Poljak and Kocjan, 2010). The target is indirectly detected using an antidigoxigenin or antibiotin enzyme conjugated antibody. The use of a chromogenic substrate leads to the formation of a colour precipitate that is visualised by light microscopy. The ZytoFast HPV Kit is designed for the detection of low risk HPV types 6 and 11 and high risk types 16, 18, 31, and 33.

HPV OncoTect Test Kit (OncoTect; IncellDx, El Camino Real Menlo Park, CA, USA; Invirion Diagnostics, Oak Brook, IL, USA) measures the number of transforming cells and the quantity of E6, E7 mRNA in each intact human cell. The kit works as indicator of disease activity. The percentage of tested cells that overexpress the viral mRNAs provides a specific indication about the risk of an HPV infection can turn into cervical cancer (IncellDx, 2010)(IncellDx, 2010)(IncellDx, 2010)(IncellDx, 2010)(IncellDx, 2010, Bhat et al., 2007). Generally, HPV OncoTect Test is used in parallel with other HPV protocols (Poljak and Kocjan, 2010). The sensitivity and the specificity of the test are high (83.3% and 91.3% respectively) and is significantly increased (Narimatsu and Patterson, 2005). It is possible to detect 95% of infected cells in moderate dysplasia (HPV OncoTect™, 2010, Liu et al., 2007).

The advantages and disadvantages of this technique depends on the methodologies and the kind of probe used (Feldman et al., 1997): double stranded DNA probes are easy to use but need reannealing during the hybridization (decreasing the probe availability); single stranded DNA probes does not need probe denaturation and no reannealing during hybridization but it is technically complex. RNA probes have high specific activity, no probe denaturation needed, no reannealing, but less tissue penetration. Finally, oligonucleotide probes have stable good tissue penetration (small size), no self-hybridization, but lower specific activity, so less sensitive, less stable hybrids, and access to DNA synthesizer needed. The ISH based tests for HPV detection are insufficiently clinically validated. They are not used in routine screening because the methodology is too laborious and not sufficiently sensible (Poljak and Kocjan, 2010).

Test name	Test principle	Nucleic acid target	Types		Performance	
			Detected	Genotyped	Sensitivity	Specificity
hc2	Signal amplified hybr.	DNA	HPVs16, 18, 31, 33, 35, 39, 45, 51, 52, 56, 58, 59 and 68.	-	93%	
Cervista™	Signal amplified hybr.	DNA	HPVs16, 18, 31, 33, 35, 39, 45, 51, 52, 56, 58, 59, 66 and 68.	-	92,8%	
Amplicor	Signal amplified hybr.	DNA	HPVs16, 18, 31, 33, 35, 39, 45, 51, 52, 56, 58, 59 and 68.	-	96,1%	96,5%
careHPV	Signal amplified hybr.	DNA	HPVs16, 18, 31, 33, 35, 39, 45, 51, 52, 56, 58, 59, 66 and 68.	-	90,0%	84,2%
GenoID	rtq-PCR	DNA	HPVs16, 18, 26, 31, 33, 35, 39, 45, 51, 52, 56, 58, 59, 66, 68, 6, 11, 42, 43 and 44.	-		
Abbott Real Time HR HPV test	rtq-PCR	DNA	HPVs31, 33, 35, 39, 45, 51, 52, 56, 58, 59, 66 and 68.	HPV16 and HPV18.	90,0%	50%
Cobas4800	rtq-PCR	DNA	HPVs31, 33, 35, 39, 45, 51, 52, 56, 58, 59, 66 and 68.	HPV16 and HPV18.	90,0%	70,5%
Pretect HPV-Proofer	RT-PCR	mRNA	HPVs16, 18, 31, 33 and 45.	-	78,1%	75,5%
NucliSENS EasyQ HPV v1	RT-PCR	mRNA	HPVs16, 18, 31, 33 and 45.	-	63%	
APTIMA HPV Assay	RT-PCR	mRNA	HPVs16, 18, 31, 33, 35, 39, 45, 51, 52, 56, 58, 59, 66 and 68.	-	92%	98%

Test name	Test principle	Nucleic acid target	Types		Performance	
			Detected	**Genotyped**	**Sensitivity**	**Specificity**
HPVDNA chip	DNA Microarray	DNA	-	HPVs16, 18, 31, 33, 35, 39, 45, 51, 52, 56, 58, 59, 66, 68, 69, 6, 11, 34, 40, 42, 43 and 44.	80%	94%
GG HPVCHIP	DNA Microarray	DNA	-	HPVs16, 18, 31, 33, 35, 39, 45, 51, 52, 56, 58, 59, 68, 69, 70, 26, 53, 66, 6, 7, 10, 11, 27, 32, 40, 42, 44, 54, 55, 57, 61, 62, 72, 73, 91, CP8304/81, MM7/83, MM8/84, 30, 34, 67 and MM4/82.		
HPV GenoArray Test Kit	DNA Microarray	DNA		HPVs6, 11, 16, 18, 31, 33, 35, 39, 42-45, 51-53, 56, 58, 59, 66, 68 and 81.		
GeneTrack HPV DNA Chip	DNA Microarray	DNA		HPVs6, 11, 16, 18, 31, 33, 35, 39, 40, 42-45, 51, 52, 54, 56, 58, 59, 62 and 66-72.		
Clart HPV2	DNA Microarray	DNA	-	HPVs6, 11, 16, 18, 26,	96,9%	71,9%

Test name	Test principle	Nucleic acid target	Types		Performance	
			Detected	Genotyped	Sensitivity	Specificity
				31, 33, 35, 39, 40, 42, 43, 44, 45, 51, 52, 53, 54, 56, 58, 59, 61, 62, 66, 68, 70, 71, 72, 73, 81, 82, 83, 84, 85 and 89.		
Multiplex HPV genotyping kit v1.0	Suspension array	DNA	-	HPVs6, 11, 16, 18, 26, 31, 33, 35, 39, 42-45, 51-53, 56, 58, 59, 66, 68, 70, 73 and 82.		
digene HPV genotyping LQ Test	Suspension array	DNA	-	HPVs16, 18, 26, 31, 33, 35, 39, 45, 51-53, 56, 58, 59, 66, 68, 73 and 82.		
INNO-LiPA v2	Reverse line-blot	DNA	-	HPVs6, 11, 16, 18, 26, 31, 33, 35, 39, 40, 43, 44, 45, 51, 52, 53, 54, 56, 58, 59, 66, 68, 69/71, 70, 73, 74 and 82.		
Linear Array HPV	Reverse line-blot	DNA	-	HPVs6, 11, 16, 18, 26, 31, 33, 35, 39, 40, 42, 44, 45, 51,	98,2%	32,8%

Test name	Test principle	Nucleic acid target	Types		Performance	
			Detected	Genotyped	Sensitivity	Specificity
				52, 53, 54, 56, 58, 59, 61, 62, 64, 66, 67, 68, 69, 70, 71, 72, 73, 81, 82, 83, 84 and 89.		
Digene HPV Genotyping	Reverse line-blot	DNA	-	HPVs16, 18, 26, 31, 33, 35, 39, 45, 51, 52, 53, 56, 58, 59, 66, 68, 73 and 82.		
EasyChip HPB Blot	Reverse line-blot	DNA	-	HPVs6, 11, 16, 18, 26, 31, 32, 33, 35, 37, 39, 42, 43, 44, 45, 51, 52, 53, 54, 55, 56, 58, 59, 61, 62, 66, 67, 68, 69, 70, 72, 74, 82, CP8061, CP8304, L1AE5, MM4, MM7 and MM8.	90,0%	99,2%
INFORM HPV III	*In situ* hybridization	DNA	HPVs16, 18, 31, 33, 35, 39, 45, 51, 52, 56, 58 and 66.	-	~50%	
GenPoint HPV Biotinylated DNA	*In situ* hybridization	DNA	HPVs16, 18, 31, 33, 35, 39, 45, 51, 52, 56, 58, 59 and 68.	-	-	100%

Table 2. Most important commercially available assays for HPV detection and/or genotyping.

8. Southern blot hybridization assays

Southern blot hybridization was the first assay used to detect integrated HPV (Cooper et al., 1991) and is generally used to classify new viral types (Lorincz, 1996). In Southern blot hybridization, the genome is extracted and the DNA chain is broken using restriction enzymes. The products are integrated into a gel and separated by electrophoresis. The fragments are denatured in situ, transferred to a nitrocellulose membrane, and hybridized with cloned HPV genomic probes. The probes are then labelled, often using radioisotopes. The detection of the labelled DNA hybrids is visualized by autoradiography. The sensitivity and the specificity of the assay are high, ranging between 70% and 80% the first and 90% the second (Caussy et al., 1988).There are no commercial kits available; the method is entirely laboratory-based, with existing reagents and methodologies. Despite high sensibility, specificity and application to cells and biopsies, Southern Blot is not suitable for routine application: it is time consuming, labourious, expensive and requires large amount of purifying DNA and radio labeled probes.

9. Immunological techniques

9.1 Enzyme-linked immunosorbent (ELISA) assays

ELISA, also known as an enzyme immunoassay (EIA), is a technique used to detect the presence of antigens or antibodies in wide variety biological samples. The basic steps of this technique are the immobilization of the antigen and its detection by a labeled antibody. The immobilization can be accomplished by direct adsorption to the assay plate or indirectly via a capture antibody that has been already attached to the solid phase. The detection can be performed either directly by a labeled primary antibody or indirectly by a labeled secondary antibody. The labeled antibody reacts with a colourless substrate to produce a coloured product. The most widely used ELISA methods for detecting antigens is the Sandwich system (Figure 8) (Baker et al., 2009) . In this format, the antigen is sandwiched between two similar or different antibodies: a capture antibody, already bond to the solid phase, and an enzyme-conjugated secondary antibody.The enzyme reacted with the substrate producing a colour reaction which can be observed visually or measured with a spectrophotometer. The enzyme activity is directly proportional with the amount of the test antigen. Sandwich ELISA is especially used when the concentration of antigens is low or in presence of contaminating protein, as its sensitivity is 2-5 times more than other Elisa assays (Baker et al., 2009). The assay is very specific and simple (Biosupply, 2010, Chung et al., 2010) and there is no need to purify the antigen prior to use. On the other hand, only monoclonal antibodies can be used as matched pairs. They detect different epitopes on the antigen without impeding each other's binding (Biosupply, 2010).

To detect specific antibodies, the most widely used ELISA systems are the "indirect" and "competitive" systems (Figure 8). In the indirect system the antigen is directly adsorbed onto a solid phase and the primary and the conjugate antibodies are added to the plate successively. The intensity of the colour development between substrate-conjugate enzyme indicates the amount of antigen present. In the indirect ELISA there are many binding sites for the antibody, consequently more enzyme can be detected. A large variety of enzyme-linked secondary antibodies are commercially available. The method is sensitive and versatile. The same enzyme-linked secondary antibody can detect many primary antibodies in one species. A non-specific signal might occur if cross-reactivity happens with the secondary antibody and an extra incubation step is required in the procedure. "Competitive" system is useful for identification and quantification of either antigen or antibody. The antigen is first incubated in presence of the unlabeled antibody, forming antigen-antibody complex, and after add to an antigen-coated plate. The production of colour elicited by antibody-antigen-substrate complex will be inversely proportional to the amount of antigen in the sample. In competitive ELISA, the secondary antibody competes with the sample antigen which is associated with the primary antibody. The more antigen in the sample the less labelled antibody is retained in the plate and the weaker the signal. It is possible to use impure samples (Biomaterials, 2007)(Biomaterials, 2007)(Biomaterials, 2007)(Biomaterials, 2007) and the assay is precise, rapid, accurate, and reproducible (Zhou et al., 2002). The use of monoclonal antibodies is not so adequate because they are more difficult to find and cost more. The sensitivity and specificity are lower than the sandwich assay (Chung et al., 2010).

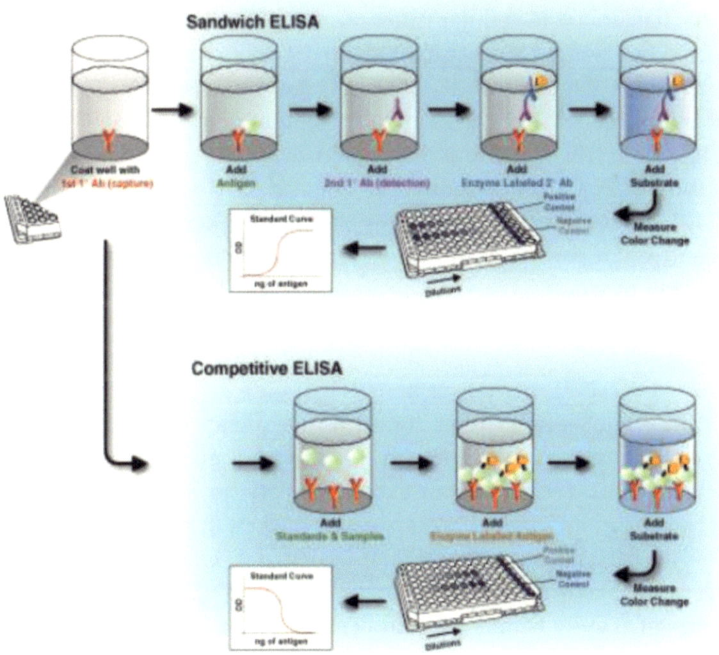

Fig. 8. Schematic representation of Sandwich and competitive ELISA.

The ELISA methodology is widely used to detect HPV antigens (Gutierrez-Xicotencatl et al., 2009). Several works are focused on antibodies against the viral HPV16L1 capsid protein and the viral HPV16E6 and HPV16E7 oncoproteins. L1 is the major capsid protein and it represents 80%-90% of the total viral proteins(Favre et al., 1975). The most of the antibody-mediated immune responses are directed against L1 antigen (Carter et al., 2000, Rocha-Zavaleta et al., 2003). A high frequency of anti-16L1 antibodies was found in patients with high-risk HPV-associated LSIL and with cervical cancer. While a low antibody response was found from women without evidence of HPV infection and with low-risk HPV-associated LSIL (Cason et al., 1992, Ghosh et al., 1993, Di Lonardo et al., 1994, Rocha-Zavaleta et al., 2004, Leon et al., 2009). Furthermore, it is possible to discriminate between high-risk HPV and low-risk HPV types by using the epitopes of the L1 capsid protein. The viral oncogenes E6 and E7 are associated with cancer; they modify the cell cycle in order to favour the viral genome replication and consequent late gene expression (Munger and Howley, 2002). Most HPV-positive cancer cells maintain the expression of E6 and E7 (Baker et al., 1987, Shirasawa et al., 1987). A higher HPV16E6 and HPV16E7 seropositivity was observed in patients with cervical cancer compared to healthy or with subjects displaying early lesions (Kanda et al., 1992, Ghosh et al., 1993, Viscidi et al., 1993, Di Lonardo et al., 1994, Dillner et al., 1994, Fujii et al., 1995, Fisher et al., 1996). Hence, E6 and E7 oncoproteins might be used to monitor infected woman at the very late stage of the infection.

Several studies were focused on biomarker identification for early stages of cervical cancer in order to perform an early diagnosis of woman at risk of infection. For this reason the detection of viral HPV16E2, HPV16E4, and HPV16E5 proteins were studied. The expression of the HPVE4 protein is linked to cellular differentiation status (Breitburd et al., 1987, Chow et al., 1987a, Chow et al., 1987b, Doorbar et al., 1989, Palefsky et al., 1991) playing important role in the viral life cycle (Doorbar et al., 1986, Jareborg and Burnett, 1991). HPVE2 is the first protein to be expressed. High E2 levels repress expression of the E6 and E7 oncoproteins. When the HPV genome is integrated in its host, E2 function are disrupted, preventing repression of E6/E7 (Munger and Howley, 2002). In relation to the expression of HPV16E2 and HPV16E4 there are conflicting opinions. Some authors found elevated responses for E2 antigen in patients with cervical cancer. Others reported anti-E2 antibodies in normal subjects and in women with CIN lesions (Dillner, 1990, Dillner et al., 1994, Veress et al., 1994, Marais et al., 1997). A higher E4 seropositivity was observed in pre-cancerous and cancerous lesions as well as in healthy individuals (Jochmus-Kudielka et al., 1989, Crum et al., 1990, Kochel et al., 1991, Snyder et al., 1991, Kanda et al., 1992, Dillner et al., 1994, Muller et al., 1995), while other studies found a frequency of E4 antibodies in cancer patients higher than in normal subjects (Suchankova et al., 1991, Ghosh et al., 1993, Gaarenstroom et al., 1994). Moreover, an expression of the E4 protein was observed in patients with high-risk and low-risk HPV-associated but not in patients with cervical cancer (Crum et al., 1990, Vazquez-Corzo et al., 2003). HPV16E5 is a weakly oncogenic protein which potentiates the transforming activity of E7(Bouvard et al., 1994, Valle and Banks, 1995), but its biological activity is mostly unknown. Chang et. al (Chang et al., 2001) studied the HPV-16 E5 protein and found its expression in the lower third of the epithelium in LSIL.

ELISA assays are quick, convenient, and very accurate. The method can achieve high sensitivities and specificities, favorably comparable with other radioimmunoassay (Moore et al., 1999, Leng et al., 2008). It can be performed in a small laboratory and it has the advantage of automation and multiplexing (Leng et al., 2008, Adler et al., 2009). Moreover, ELISA assays need small volume of blood and do not use radioisotopes or a costly radiation system. It is suitable for large numbers of specimens. False positive results might happen if the blocking solution is ineffective and the enzyme/substrate reaction is short term and needs a rapid reading. It is a time-consuming methodology (>1.5h), uses refrigerated reagents and probe design is difficult, but many kits are available.Considering PCR as a reference, ELISA methods are less sensitive than PCR (81.8%, 53%, 72.2% vs. 100%) but more specific (100%, 99%, 92.2% vs. 78%) for invasive cervical cancer (Meschede et al., 1998, Lack et al., 2005, Zaghloul, 2011) .

9.2 Detection of HPV antibodies - western blot

Western blot (alternatively, protein immunoblot) is an analytical technique used to identify proteins based on their ability to bind a specific antibody. The analysis can detect the target from a mixture of a great number of proteins from tissue homogenate or extract. It uses gel electrophoresis to separate native or denatured proteins by the length of the polypeptide or by the 3-D structure of the protein (Towbin et al., 1979). The proteins are transferred to a membrane made of nitrocellulose or polyvinylidene difluoride (PVDF) to make the proteins accessible to antibody detection (Khan et al., 2005). The membrane is "probed" for the protein of interest with a modified antibody which is linked to a reporter enzyme. When the enzyme is exposed to an appropriate substrate drives a colorimetric reaction (Renart et al., 1979).

Several works based on Western Blot technique have studied the high correlation between the oncogene proteins and cervical cancer (Jochmus-Kudielka et al., 1989, Kochel et al., 1991, Suchankova et al., 1991, Fujii et al., 1995) and the possible role of the protein E4 in cancer disease (Jochmus-Kudielka et al., 1989, Ghosh et al., 1993, Pedroza-Saavedra et al., 2000, Middleton et al., 2003) but the results were controversial. The sensitivity of the Western blot assay is 67%. The specificity increases to 78%(Pedroza-Saavedra et al., 2000).

There are kits based on detection of antigens using horseradish peroxidase (HRP) conjugated antibodies and the chemiluminescent substrate luminol. Chemiluminescent system detects the protein target using the light produced by the catalysis of an enzyme substrate. It is rapid and allows accurate identification of samples. With this assay it is possible to detect the target protein from a mixture of antigens (Molijn et al., 2005); it is, nevertheless, expensive, demanding and complex and it is impossible to analyze a large number of samples simultaneously (Molijn et al., 2005).

10. Conclusions

There are two major purposes for the use of molecular HPV diagnosis. The first is to identify women at cervical cancer risk; these can be detected through community-based screening programs or through clinical counseling. In this scenario, the use of a highly sensitive assay will overestimate some HPV infections that would be cleared by the immune system in less than 24 months (Moscicki, 2007). If a less sensitive or even a quantitative assay is chosen, the efficacy in identifying women at risk of progression might be more effective. The other purpose includes vaccination trials, epidemiological and natural history studies (Molijn et al., 2005). In this case, contrarily to the clinical application, a highly sensitive and reproducible assay is required, and it should include the broadest spectrum of HPV types.

The ideal HPV testing for both goals should be a single assay with adjustable cut-off for detection, linked to a genotyping method (Molijn et al., 2005). Unfortunately, such method does not exist and combined detection systems have to be used. The molecular assays are the gold standard for HPV testing and there are specific characteristics that positively distinguish each method. For instance, the extremely high sensitivity and specificity of PCR assays and the need of only small amounts of DNA template, makes it the support of several other high-quality assays. Within the signal amplification assays, hc2 is considered the most reliable assay and is a CE-IVD test. On the other hand, Southern blot technique is more expensive, requires large amount of purifying DNA and it is difficult to apply in routine practice due to time consumption; *in situ* hybridization is not as sensitive as the PCR and hc2 methods. The sampling and HPV DNA detection assays bearing different sensitivity and specificity, as shown above, are the most accountable aspects for the heterogeneity of the results. To overcome such problems, a combined detection system, to detect the presence of the HPV, and an antibody profile against different viral antigens, to stage the infection, will improve the signaling of persistent infections and prevent cervical cancer.

11. References

Adler M, Schulz S, Spengler M (2009) Cytokine Quantification in Drug Development: A comparison of sensitive immunoassay platforms. . (Biotech., C., ed).

Baker CC, Phelps WC, Lindgren V, Braun MJ, Gonda MA, Howley PM (1987) Structural and transcriptional analysis of human papillomavirus type 16 sequences in cervical carcinoma cell lines. J Virol 61:962-971.

Baker GB, Dunn S, Lajtha A, Holt A (2009) Handbook of neurochemistry and molecular biology. .

Biomaterials A (2007) APC Biomaterials, LLC - Frequently Asked Questions. Biosupply (2010) Introduction to Antibodies - Enzyme-Linked Immunosorbent Assay (ELISA). BIOTYPAP Kit (2009) BIOTYPAP Kit - Kit for Papillomavirus (HPV) DNA detection and typing in human clinical samples. (BIOTOOLS, B. M. L., S.A., ed).

Bobrow MN, Harris TD, Shaughnessy KJ, Litt GJ (1989) Catalyzed reporter deposition, a novel method of signal amplification. Application to immunoassays. J Immunol Methods 125:279-285.

Bouvard V, Matlashewski G, Gu ZM, Storey A, Banks L (1994) The human papillomavirus type 16 E5 gene cooperates with the E7 gene to stimulate proliferation of primary cells and increases viral gene expression. Virology 203:73-80.

Breitburd F, Croissant O, Orth G (1987) Expression of human papillomavirus type 1 E4 gene products in warts.

Canfell K, Shi JF, Lew JB, Walker R, Zhao FH, Simonella L, Chen JF, Legood R, Smith MA, Nickson C, Qiao YL (2011) Prevention of cervical cancer in rural China: evaluation of HPV vaccination and primary HPV screening strategies. Vaccine 29:2487-2494.

Carlson C, Hu Z Optimizing In Situ Hybridization Protocols.

Carter JJ, Koutsky LA, Hughes JP, Lee SK, Kuypers J, Kiviat N, Galloway DA (2000) Comparison of human papillomavirus types 16, 18, and 6 capsid antibody responses following incident infection. J Infect Dis 181:1911-1919.

Cason J, Kambo PK, Best JM, McCance DJ (1992) Detection of antibodies to a linear epitope on the major coat protein (L1) of human papillomavirus type-16 (HPV-16) in sera from patients with cervical intraepithelial neoplasia and children. Int J Cancer 50:349-355.

Castle PE, Porras C, Quint WG, Rodriguez AC, Schiffman M, Gravitt PE, Gonzalez P, Katki HA, Silva S, Freer E, Van Doorn LJ, Jimenez S, Herrero R, Hildesheim A (2008)

Comparison of two PCR-based human papillomavirus genotyping methods. J Clin Microbiol 46:3437-3445.

Castle PE, Sadorra M, Lau T, Aldrich C, Garcia FA, Kornegay J (2009) Evaluation of a prototype real-time PCR assay for carcinogenic human papillomavirus (HPV) detection and simultaneous HPV genotype 16 (HPV16) and HPV18 genotyping. J Clin Microbiol 47:3344-3347.

Castle PE, Schiffman M, Burk RD, Wacholder S, Hildesheim A, Herrero R, Bratti MC, Sherman ME, Lorincz A (2002) Restricted cross-reactivity of hybrid capture 2 with nononcogenic human papillomavirus types. Cancer Epidemiol Biomarkers Prev 11:1394-1399.

Caussy D, Orr W, Daya AD, Roth P, Reeves W, Rawls W (1988) Evaluation of methods for detecting human papillomavirus deoxyribonucleotide sequences in clinical specimens. J Clin Microbiol 26:236-243.

Chan PK, Cheung TH, Tam AO, Lo KW, Yim SF, Yu MM, To KF, Wong YF, Cheung JL, Chan DP, Hui M, Ip M (2006) Biases in human papillomavirus genotype prevalence assessment associated with commonly used consensus primers. Int J Cancer 118:243-245.

Chang JL, Tsao YP, Liu DW, Huang SJ, Lee WH, Chen SL (2001) The expression of HPV-16 E5 protein in squamous neoplastic changes in the uterine cervix. J Biomed Sci 8:206-213.

Choi JJ, Kim C, Park H (2009) Peptide nucleic acid-based array for detecting and genotyping human papillomaviruses. J Clin Microbiol 47:1785-1790.

Chow LT, Nasseri M, Wolinsky SM, Broker TR (1987a) Human papillomavirus types 6 and 11 mRNAs from genital condylomata acuminata. J Virol 61:2581-2588.

Chow LT, Reilly SS, Broker TR, Taichman LB (1987b) Identification and mapping of human papillomavirus type 1 RNA transcripts recovered from plantar warts and infected epithelial cell cultures. J Virol 61:1913-1918.

Chung MK, Riby J, Li H, Iavarone AT, Williams ER, Zheng Y, Rappaport SM (2010) A sandwich enzyme-linked immunosorbent assay for adducts of polycyclic aromatic hydrocarbons with human serum albumin. Anal Biochem 400:123-129.

Clavel C, Masure M, Bory JP, Putaud I, Mangeonjean C, Lorenzato M, Gabriel R, Quereux C, Birembaut P (1999) Hybrid Capture II-based human papillomavirus detection, a sensitive test to detect in routine high-grade cervical lesions: a preliminary study on 1518 women. Br J Cancer 80:1306-1311. cobas 4800 (2010) cobas 4800 System (LTD, R. D., ed).

Cooper K, Herrington CS, Stickland JE, Evans MF, McGee JO (1991) Episomal and integrated human papillomavirus in cervical neoplasia shown by non-isotopic in situ hybridisation. J Clin Pathol 44:990-996.

Cox JT (2009) History of the use of HPV testing in cervical screening and in the management of abnormal cervical screening results. J Clin Virol 45 Suppl 1:S3-S12.

Crum CP, Barber S, Symbula M, Snyder K, Saleh AM, Roche JK (1990) Coexpression of the human papillomavirus type 16 E4 and L1 open reading frames in early cervical neoplasia. Virology 178:238-246.

Dalstein V, Merlin S, Bali C, Saunier M, Dachez R, Ronsin C (2009) Analytical evaluation of the PapilloCheck test, a new commercial DNA chip for detection and genotyping of human papillomavirus. J Virol Methods 156:77-83.

Day SP, Hudson A, Mast A, Sander T, Curtis M, Olson S, Chehak L, Quigley N, Ledford J, Yen-Lieberman B, Kohn D, Quigley DI, Olson M (2009) Analytical performance of

the Investigational Use Only Cervista HPV HR test as determined by a multi-center study. J Clin Virol 45 Suppl 1:S63-72.
de Roda Husman AM, Walboomers JM, van den Brule AJ, Meijer CJ, Snijders PJ (1995) The use of general primers GP5 and GP6 elongated at their 3' ends with adjacent highly conserved sequences improves human papillomavirus detection by PCR. J Gen Virol 76:1057-1062.
de Villiers EM, Fauquet C, Broker TR, Bernard HU, zur Hausen H (2004) Classification of papillomaviruses. Virology 324:17-27.
Di Lonardo A, Campo MS, Venuti A, Marcante ML (1994) Brief report: antibody response to E6, E7, and L1 proteins of human papillomavirus 16 in an Italian population. J Med Virol 43:357-361.
Digene (2004) Hybrid capture 2 high-risk HPV DNA test - an in vitro nucleic acid hybridization assay with signal amplification using microplate chemiluminiscence for the qualitative detection of human papillomavirus (HPV) types 16, 18, 31, 33, 35, 39, 45, 51, 52, 56, 58, 59 and 68 in cervical specimens. . Product insert 1-22.
Dillner J (1990) Mapping of linear epitopes of human papillomavirus type 16: the E1, E2, E4, E5, E6 and E7 open reading frames. Int J Cancer 46:703-711.
Dillner J, Lenner P, Lehtinen M, Eklund C, Heino P, Wiklund F, Hallmans G, Stendahl U (1994) A population-based seroepidemiological study of cervical cancer. Cancer Res 54:134-141.
Dockter J, Schroder A, Eaton B, Wang A, Sikhamsay N, Morales L, Giachetti C (2009a) Analytical characterization of the APTIMA HPV Assay. J Clin Virol 45 Suppl 1:S39-47.
Dockter J, Schroder A, Hill C, Guzenski L, Monsonego J, Giachetti C (2009b) Clinical performance of the APTIMA HPV Assay for the detection of high-risk HPV and high-grade cervical lesions. J Clin Virol 45 Suppl 1:S55-61.
Dona MG, Benevolo M, Pimpinelli F, Battista M, Rollo F, Stivali F, Moscarelli A, Giuliani M, Di Carlo A, Vocaturo A (2011) Comparative evaluation of different DNA extraction methods for HPV genotyping by linear array and INNO-LiPA. J Med Virol 83:1042-1047.
Doorbar J, Campbell D, Grand RJ, Gallimore PH (1986) Identification of the human papilloma virus-1a E4 gene products. EMBO J 5:355-362.
Doorbar J, Coneron I, Gallimore PH (1989) Sequence divergence yet conserved physical characteristics among the E4 proteins of cutaneous human papillomaviruses. Virology 172:51-62.
Einsteina MH, Martensb MG, Garciac FAR, Ferrisd DG, Mitchellc AL, P. S, Daye SP, Olsone MC (2010) Clinical validation of the Cervista® HPV HR and 16/18 genotyping tests for use in women with ASC-US cytology. Gynecologic Oncology 118:116-122
Ekstrom J, Bzhalava D, Svenback D, Forslund O, Dillner J (2011) High throughput sequencing reveals diversity of human papillomaviruses in cutaneous lesions. Int J Cancer.
Else EA, Swoyer R, Zhang Y, Taddeo FJ, Bryan JT, Lawson J, Van Hyfte I, Roberts CC (2011) Comparison of real-time multiplex human papillomavirus (HPV) PCR assays with INNO-LiPA HPV genotyping extra assay. J Clin Microbiol 49:1907-1912.
Erali M, Pattison DC, Wittwer CT, Petti CA (2009) Human papillomavirus genotyping using an automated film-based chip array. J Mol Diagn 11:439-445.
Ermel A, Qadadri B, Morishita A, Miyagawa I, Yamazaki G, Weaver B, Tu W, Tong Y, Randolph M, Cramer H, Brown D (2010) Human papillomavirus detection and typing in thin prep cervical cytologic specimens comparing the Digene Hybrid

Capture II Assay, the Roche Linear Array HPV Genotyping Assay, and the Kurabo GeneSquare Microarray Assay. J Virol Methods 169:154-161.

Favre M, Orth G, Croissant O, Yaniv M (1975) Human papillomavirus DNA: physical map. Proc Natl Acad Sci U S A 72:4810-4814.

Feldman RS, Meyer JS, Quenzer LF (1997) Principles of Neuropsychopharmacology. .

Fisher SG, Benitez-Bribiesca L, Nindl I, Stockfleth E, Muller M, Wolf H, Perez-Garcia F, Guzman-Gaona J, Gutierrez-Delgado F, Irvin W, Gissmann L (1996) The association of human papillomavirus type 16 E6 and E7 antibodies with stage of cervical cancer. Gynecol Oncol 61:73-78.

Fujii T, Matsushima Y, Yajima M, Sugimura T, Terada M (1995) Serum antibody against unfused recombinant E7 protein of human papillomavirus type 16 in cervical cancer patients. Jpn J Cancer Res 86:28-34.

Gaarenstroom KN, Kenter GG, Bonfrer JM, Korse CM, Gallee MP, Hart AA, Muller M, Trimbos JB, Helmerhorst TJ (1994) Prognostic significance of serum antibodies to human papillomavirus-16 E4 and E7 peptides in cervical cancer. Cancer 74:2307-2313.

Galan-Sanchez F, Rodriguez-Iglesias MA (2009) Comparison of human papillomavirus genotyping using commercial assays based on PCR and reverse hybridization methods. APMIS 117:708-715.

Garland SM, Tabrizi S (2006) Methods for HPV Detection: Polymerase Chain Reaction Assays. Monsonego J (ed): Emerging Issues on HPV Infections:From Science to Practice Basel, Karger 63-72.

Gebeyehu G, Rao PY, SooChan P, Simms DA, Klevan L (1987) Novel biotinylated nucleotide--analogs for labeling and colorimetric detection of DNA. Nucleic Acids Res 15:4513-4534.

Geraets DT, Heideman DA, de Koning MN, Snijders PJ, Meijer CJ, van Doorn LJ, Quint WG (2009a) High genotyping concordance between the digene HPV Genotyping RH Test and the Reverse Line Blot genotyping assay on GP5+/6+-PCR products. J Clin Virol 46 Suppl 3:S16-20.

Geraets DT, Heideman DA, de Koning MN, Snijders PJ, van Alewijk DC, Meijer CJ, van Doorn LJ, Quint WG (2009b) High-throughput genotyping of high-risk HPV by the digene HPV Genotyping LQ Test using GP5+/6+-PCR and xMAP technology. J Clin Virol 46 Suppl 3:S21-26.

Geraets DT, Lenselink CH, Bekkers RL, van Doorn LJ, Quint WG, Melchers WJ (2011) Universal human papillomavirus genotyping by the digene HPV Genotyping RH and LQ Tests. J Clin Virol 50:276-280.

Ghosh AK, Smith NK, Stacey SN, Glew SS, Connor ME, Arrand JR, Stern PL (1993) Serological response to HPV 16 in cervical dysplasia and neoplasia: correlation of antibodies to E6 with cervical cancer. Int J Cancer 53:591-596.

Gomez-Roman JJ, Echevarria C, Salas S, Gonzalez-Moran MA, Perez-Mies B, Garcia-Higuera I, Nicolas Martinez M, Val-Bernal JF (2009) A type-specific study of human papillomavirus prevalence in cervicovaginal samples in three different Spanish regions. APMIS 117:22-27.

Gravitt PE, Peyton CL, T.Q. A, Wheeler CM, Coutlée F, Hildesheim A, Schiffman MH, Scott DR, Apple RJ (2000) Improved amplification of genital human papillomaviruses. J Clin Microbiol 38:357-361.

Grisaru D, Avidor B, Niv J, Marmor S, Almog B, Leibowitz C, Graidy M, Giladi M (2008) Pilot study of prevalence of high-risk human papillomavirus genotypes in Israeli Jewish women referred for colposcopic examination. J Clin Microbiol 46:1602-1605.

Gutierrez-Xicotencatl L, Plett-Torres T, Madrid-Gonzalez CL, Madrid-Marina V (2009) Molecular diagnosis of human papillomavirus in the development of cervical cancer. Salud Publica Mex 51 Suppl 3:S479-488.

Halfon P, Benmoura D, Agostini A, Khiri H, Martineau A, Penaranda G, Blanc B (2010a) Relevance of HPV mRNA detection in a population of ASCUS plus women using the NucliSENS EasyQ HPV assay. J Clin Virol 47:177-181.

Halfon P, Benmoura D, Agostini A, Khiri H, Penaranda G, Martineau A, Blanc B (2010b) Evaluation of the clinical performance of the Abbott RealTime High-Risk HPV for carcinogenic HPV detection. J Clin Virol 48:246-250.

Halfon P, Benmoura D, Khiri H, Penaranda G, Blanc B, Riggio D, Sandri MT (2010c) Comparison of the clinical performance of carcinogenic HPV typing of the Linear Array and Papillocheck HPV-screening assay. J Clin Virol 47:38-42.

Hesselink AT, Heideman DA, Berkhof J, Topal F, Pol RP, Meijer CJ, Snijders PJ (2010) Comparison of the clinical performance of PapilloCheck human papillomavirus detection with that of the GP5+/6+-PCR-enzyme immunoassay in population-based cervical screening. J Clin Microbiol 48:797-801.

Hong SP, Shin SK, Lee EH, Kim EO, Ji SI, Chung HJ, Park SN, Yoo W, Folk WR, Kim SO (2008) High-resolution human papillomavirus genotyping by MALDI-TOF mass spectrometry. Nat Protoc 3:1476-1484.

HPV OncoTect™ E, E7 mRNA Kit. (2010) HPV OncoTect Brochure.

Huang CC, Qiu JT, Kashima ML, Kurman RJ, Wu TC (1998) Generation of type-specific probes for the detection of single-copy human papillomavirus by a novel in situ hybridization method. Mod Pathol 11:971-977.

Hwang HS, Park M, Lee SY, Kwon KH, Pang MG (2004) Distribution and prevalence of human papillomavirus genotypes in routine pap smear of 2,470 korean women determined by DNA chip. Cancer Epidemiol Biomarkers Prev 13:2153-2156.

Iftner T, Eberle S, Iftner A, Holz B, Banik N, Quint W, Straube AN (2010) Prevalence of low-risk and high-risk types of human papillomavirus and other risk factors for HPV infection in Germany within different age groups in women up to 30 years of age: an epidemiological observational study. J Med Virol 82:1928-1939.

Inc MD REBA HPV-ID. http://mndkoreacokr/img/Product%20information/REBA%20HPV-IDpdf.

IncellDx I (2010) IncellDx Announces a Supply Agreement with Accuri to Offer Complete Solution for Cervical Cancer Screening.

Jacobs MV, Snijders PJ, van den Brule AJ, Helmerhorst TJ, Meijer CJ, Walboomers JM (1997) A general primer GP5+/GP6(+)-mediated PCR-enzyme immunoassay method for rapid detection of 14 high-risk and 6 low-risk human papillomavirus genotypes in cervical scrapings. J Clin Microbiol 35:791-795.

Jareborg N, Burnett S (1991) Immunofluorescent detection of bovine papillomavirus E4 antigen in the cytoplasm of cells permissive in vitro for viral DNA amplification. J Gen Virol 72 (Pt 9):2269-2274.

Jeantet D, Schwarzmann F, Tromp J, Melchers WJ, van der Wurff AA, Oosterlaken T, Jacobs M, Troesch A (2009) NucliSENS EasyQ HPV v1 test - Testing for oncogenic activity of human papillomaviruses. J Clin Virol 45 Suppl 1:S29-37.

Jiang HL, Zhu HH, Zhou LF, Chen F, Chen Z (2006) Genotyping of human papillomavirus in cervical lesions by L1 consensus PCR and the Luminex xMAP system. J Med Microbiol 55:715-720.

Jochmus-Kudielka I, Schneider A, Braun R, Kimmig R, Koldovsky U, Schneweis KE, Seedorf K, Gissmann L (1989) Antibodies against the human papillomavirus type 16 early

proteins in human sera: correlation of anti-E7 reactivity with cervical cancer. J Natl Cancer Inst 81:1698-1704.
Kado S, Kawamata Y, Shino Y, Kasai T, Kubota K, Iwasaki H, Fukazawa I, Takano H, Nunoyama T, Mitsuhashi A, Sekiya S, Shirasawa H (2001) Detection of human papillomaviruses in cervical neoplasias using multiple sets of generic polymerase chain reaction primers. Gynecol Oncol 81:47-52.
Kanda T, Onda T, Zanma S, Yasugi T, Furuno A, Watanabe S, Kawana T, Sugase M, Ueda K, Sonoda T, et al. (1992) Independent association of antibodies against human papillomavirus type 16 E1/E4 and E7 proteins with cervical cancer. Virology 190:724-732.
Kay P, Meehan K, Williamson AL (2002) The use of nested polymerase chain reaction and restriction fragment length polymorphism for the detection and typing of mucosal human papillomaviruses in samples containing low copy numbers of viral DNA. J Virol Methods 105:159-170.
Khan MJ, Castle PE, Lorincz AT, Wacholder S, Sherman M, Scott DR, Rush BB, Glass AG, Schiffman M (2005) The elevated 10-year risk of cervical precancer and cancer in women with human papillomavirus (HPV) type 16 or 18 and the possible utility of type-specific HPV testing in clinical practice. J Natl Cancer Inst 97:1072-1079.
Kim CJ, Jeong JK, Park M, Park TS, Park TC, Namkoong SE, Park JS (2003) HPV oligonucleotide microarray-based detection of HPV genotypes in cervical neoplastic lesions. Gynecol Oncol 89:210-217.
Kim KH, Yoon MS, Na YJ, Park CS, Oh MR, Moon WC (2006) Development and evaluation of a highly sensitive human papillomavirus genotyping DNA chip. Gynecol Oncol 100:38-43.
Kitchener HC, Gilham C, Sargent A, Bailey A, Albrow R, Roberts C, Desai M, Mather J, Turner A, Moss S, Peto J (2011) A comparison of HPV DNA testing and liquid based cytology over three rounds of primary cervical screening: extended follow up in the ARTISTIC trial. Eur J Cancer 47:864-871.
Kleter B, van Doorn LJ, Schrauwen L, Molijn A, Sastrowijoto S, ter Schegget J, Lindeman J, ter Harmsel B, Burger M, Quint W (1999) Development and clinical evaluation of a highly sensitive PCR-reverse hybridization line probe assay for detection and identification of anogenital human papillomavirus. J Clin Microbiol 37:2508-2517.
Klug SJ, Molijn A, Schopp B, Holz B, Iftner A, Quint W, P JFS, Petry KU, Kruger Kjaer S, Munk C, Iftner T (2008) Comparison of the performance of different HPV genotyping methods for detecting genital HPV types. J Med Virol 80:1264-1274.
Kochel HG, Monazahian M, Sievert K, Hohne M, Thomssen C, Teichmann A, Arendt P, Thomssen R (1991) Occurrence of antibodies to L1, L2, E4 and E7 gene products of human papillomavirus types 6b, 16 and 18 among cervical cancer patients and controls. Int J Cancer 48:682-688.
Kocjan BJ, Seme K, Poljak M (2011) Comparison of the Abbott RealTime High Risk HPV test and INNO-LiPA HPV Genotyping Extra test for the detection of human papillomaviruses in formalin-fixed, paraffin-embedded cervical cancer specimens. J Virol Methods.
Kong CS, Balzer BL, Troxell ML, Patterson BK, Longacre TA (2007) p16INK4A immunohistochemistry is superior to HPV in situ hybridization for the detection of high-risk HPV in atypical squamous metaplasia. Am J Surg Pathol 31:33-43.
Kraus I, Molden T, Erno LE, Skomedal H, Karlsen F, Hagmar B (2004) Human papillomavirus oncogenic expression in the dysplastic portio; an investigation of biopsies from 190 cervical cones. Br J Cancer 90:1407-1413.

Lack N, West B, Jeffries D, Ekpo G, Morison L, Soutter WP, Walraven G, Boryseiwicz L (2005) Comparison of non-invasive sampling methods for detection of HPV in rural African women. Sex Transm Infect 81:239-241.
Lee JK, Hong YJ, Um TH, Lee EH, Chi HS, Koh JS, Yim HW, Cha YJ (2011) Detection and identification of human papillomavirus using a PCR-restriction fragment mass polymorphism assay. Mol Med Report
Lee SH, Vigliotti VS, Vigliotti JS, Pappu S (2007) Routine human papillomavirus genotyping by DNA sequencing in community hospital laboratories. Infect Agent Cancer 2:11.
Leng SX, McElhaney JE, Walston JD, Xie D, Fedarko NS, Kuchel GA (2008) ELISA and multiplex technologies for cytokine measurement in inflammation and aging research. J Gerontol A Biol Sci Med Sci 63:879-884.
Leon S, Sanchez R, Patarroyo MA, Camargo M, Mejia A, Urquiza M, Patarroyo ME (2009) Prevalence of HPV-DNA and anti-HPV antibodies in women from Girardot, Colombia. Sex Transm Dis 36:290-296.
Levin CE, Sellors J, Shi JF, Ma L, Qiao YL, Ortendahl J, O'Shea MK, Goldie SJ (2010) Cost-effectiveness analysis of cervical cancer prevention based on a rapid human papillomavirus screening test in a high-risk region of China. Int J Cancer 127:1404-1411.
Lie AK, Risberg B, Borge B, Sandstad B, Delabie J, Rimala R, Onsrud M, Thoresen S (2005) DNA- versus RNA-based methods for human papillomavirus detection in cervical neoplasia. Gynecol Oncol 97:908-915.
Lin CY, Chao A, Yang YC, Chou HH, Ho CM, Lin RW, Chang TC, Chiou JY, Chao FY, Wang KL, Chien TY, Hsueh S, Huang CC, Chen CJ, Lai CH (2008) Human papillomavirus typing with a polymerase chain reaction-based genotyping array compared with type-specific PCR. J Clin Virol 42:361-367.
Lin CY, Chen HC, Lin RW, You SL, You CM, Chuang LC, Pan MH, Lee MH, Chou YC, Chen CJ (2007) Quality assurance of genotyping array for detection and typing of human papillomavirus. J Virol Methods 140:1-9.
Liu SS, Leung RC, Chan KK, Cheung AN, Ngan HY (2010) Evaluation of a newly developed GenoArray human papillomavirus (HPV) genotyping assay and comparison with the Roche Linear Array HPV genotyping assay. J Clin Microbiol 48:758-764.
Lorincz AT (1996) Molecular methods for the detection of human papillomavirus infection. Obstet Gynecol Clin North Am 23:707-730.
M&D REBA HPV-ID. http://mndkoreacokr/img/Product%20information/REBA%20HPV-IDpdf.
Mammas IN, Sourvinos G, Vakonaki E, Giamarelou P, Michael C, Spandidos DA (2010) Novel human papilloma virus (HPV) genotypes in children with recurrent respiratory papillomatosis. Eur J Pediatr 169:1017-1021.
Manos MM, Ting Y, Wright DK, Lewis AJ, Broker TR, Wolinsky SM (1989) Use of polymerase chain reaction amplification for the detection of genital papillomaviruses. Cancer Cells 7:209-214.
Marais D, Rose RC, Williamson AL (1997) Age distribution of antibodies to human papillomavirus in children, women with cervical intraepithelial neoplasia and blood donors from South Africa. J Med Virol 51:126-131.
Matsushita K, Sasagawa T, Miyashita M, Ishizaki A, Morishita A, Hosaka N, Saikawa K, Hoshina S, Bi X, Ichimura H (2011) Oral and cervical human papillomavirus infection among female sex workers in Japan. Jpn J Infect Dis 64:34-39.
Meijer CJ, Berkhof J, Castle PE, Hesselink AT, Franco EL, Ronco G, Arbyn M, Bosch FX, Cuzick J, Dillner J, Heideman DA, Snijders PJ (2009) Guidelines for human

papillomavirus DNA test requirements for primary cervical cancer screening in women 30 years and older. Int J Cancer 124:516-520.
Meschede W, Zumbach K, Braspenning J, Scheffner M, Benitez-Bribiesca L, Luande J, Gissmann L, Pawlita M (1998) Antibodies against early proteins of human papillomaviruses as diagnostic markers for invasive cervical cancer. J Clin Microbiol 36:475-480.
Middleton K, Peh W, Southern S, Griffin H, Sotlar K, Nakahara T, El-Sherif A, Morris L, Seth R, Hibma M, Jenkins D, Lambert P, Coleman N, Doorbar J (2003) Organization of human papillomavirus productive cycle during neoplastic progression provides a basis for selection of diagnostic markers. J Virol 77:10186-10201.
Molden T, Kraus I, Skomedal H, Nordstrom T, Karlsen F (2007) PreTect HPV-Proofer: real-time detection and typing of E6/E7 mRNA from carcinogenic human papillomaviruses. J Virol Methods 142:204-212.
Molijn A, Kleter B, Quint W, van Doorn LJ (2005) Molecular diagnosis of human papillomavirus (HPV) infections. J Clin Virol 32 Suppl 1:S43-51.
Monsonego J, Bohbot JM, Pollini G, Krawec C, Vincent C, Merignargues I, Haroun F, Sednaoui P, Monfort L, Dachez R, Syrjanen K (2005) Performance of the Roche AMPLICOR human papillomavirus (HPV) test in prediction of cervical intraepithelial neoplasia (CIN) in women with abnormal PAP smear. Gynecol Oncol 99:160-168.
Montgomery SM (2002) In situ Hybridization. .
Moore KA, Werner C, Zannelli RM, Levine B, Smith ML (1999) Screening postmortem blood and tissues for nine classes [correction of cases] of drugs of abuse using automated microplate immunoassay. Forensic Sci Int 106:93-102.
Moscicki AB (2007) HPV infections in adolescents. Dis Markers 23:229-234.
Muller M, Viscidi RP, Ulken V, Bavinck JN, Hill PM, Fisher SG, Reid R, Munoz N, Schneider A, Shah KV, et al. (1995) Antibodies to the E4, E6, and E7 proteins of human papillomavirus (HPV) type 16 in patients with HPV-associated diseases and in the normal population. J Invest Dermatol 104:138-141.
Munger K, Howley PM (2002) Human papillomavirus immortalization and transformation functions. Virus Res 89:213-228.
Munoz N, Bosch FX, de Sanjose S, Herrero R, Castellsague X, Shah KV, Snijders PJ, Meijer CJ (2003) Epidemiologic classification of human papillomavirus types associated with cervical cancer. N Engl J Med 348:518-527.
Narimatsu R, Patterson BK (2005) High-throughput cervical cancer screening using intracellular human papillomavirus E6 and E7 mRNA quantification by flow cytometry. Am J Clin Pathol 123:716-723.
Oh TJ, Kim CJ, Woo SK, Kim TS, Jeong DJ, Kim MS, Lee S, Cho HS, An S (2004) Development and clinical evaluation of a highly sensitive DNA microarray for detection and genotyping of human papillomaviruses. J Clin Microbiol 42:3272-3280.
Oh Y, Bae SM, Kim YW, Choi HS, Nam GH, Han SJ, Park CH, Cho Y, Han BD, Ahn WS (2007) Polymerase chain reaction-based fluorescent Luminex assay to detect the presence of human papillomavirus types. Cancer Sci 98:549-554.
Organization WH (2009) Human papillomavirus laboratory manual, First edition.
Palefsky JM, Winkler B, Rabanus JP, Clark C, Chan S, Nizet V, Schoolnik GK (1991) Characterization of in vivo expression of the human papillomavirus type 16 E4 protein in cervical biopsy tissues. J Clin Invest 87:2132-2141.

Paolini F, Rollo F, Brandi R, Benevolo M, Mariani L, Cercato MC, Vocaturo A, Venuti A (2011) High risk human papillomavirus genotyping in clinical samples: evaluation of different commercial tests. Int J Immunopathol Pharmacol 24:127-138.

Pedroza-Saavedra A, Cruz A, Esquivel F, De La Torre F, Berumen J, Gariglio P, Gutierrez L (2000) High prevalence of serum antibodies to Ras and type 16 E4 proteins of human papillomavirus in patients with precancerous lesions of the uterine cervix. Arch Virol 145:603-623.

Pista A, Verdasca N, Oliveira A (2011) Clinical performance of the CLART human papillomavirus 2 assay compared with the hybrid capture 2 test. J Med Virol 83:272-276.

Poljak M, Fujs K, Seme K, Kocjan BJ, Vrtacnik-Bokal E (2005) Retrospective and prospective evaluation of the Amplicor HPV test for detection of 13 high-risk human papillomavirus genotypes on 862 clinical samples. Acta Dermatovenerol Alp Panonica Adriat 14:147-152.

Poljak M, Kocjan BJ (2010) Commercially available assays for multiplex detection of alpha human papillomaviruses. Expert Rev Anti Infect Ther 8:1139-1162.

Poljak M, Kovanda A, Kocjan BJ, Seme K, Jancar N, Vrtacnik-Bokal E (2009) The Abbott RealTime High Risk HPV test: comparative evaluation of analytical specificity and clinical sensitivity for cervical carcinoma and CIN 3 lesions with the Hybrid Capture 2 HPV DNA test. Acta Dermatovenerol Alp Panonica Adriat 18:94-103.

Qiagen (2009) The CareHPV Test. Qiagen 4.

Qiao YL, Sellors JW, Eder PS, Bao YP, Lim JM, Zhao FH, Weigl B, Zhang WH, Peck RB, Li L, Chen F, Pan QJ, Lorincz AT (2008) A new HPV-DNA test for cervical-cancer screening in developing regions: a cross-sectional study of clinical accuracy in rural China. Lancet Oncol 9:929-936.

Qu W, Jiang G, Cruz Y, Chang CJ, Ho GY, Klein RS, Burk RD (1997) PCR detection of human papillomavirus: comparison between MY09/MY11 and GP5+/GP6+ primer systems. J Clin Microbiol 35:1304-1310.

Renart J, Reiser J, Stark GR (1979) Transfer of proteins from gels to diazobenzyloxymethyl-paper and detection with antisera: a method for studying antibody specificity and antigen structure. Proc Natl Acad Sci U S A 76:3116-3120.

Roberts CC, Swoyer R, Bryan JT, Taddeo FJ (2011) Comparison of real-time multiplex human papillomavirus (HPV) PCR assays with the linear array HPV genotyping PCR assay and influence of DNA extraction method on HPV detection. J Clin Microbiol 49:1899-1906.

Rocha-Zavaleta L, Ambrosio JP, Mora-Garcia Mde L, Cruz-Talonia F, Hernandez-Montes J, Weiss-Steider B, Ortiz-Navarrete V, Monroy-Garcia A (2004) Detection of antibodies against a human papillomavirus (HPV) type 16 peptide that differentiate high-risk from low-risk HPV-associated low-grade squamous intraepithelial lesions. J Gen Virol 85:2643-2650.

Rocha-Zavaleta L, Pereira-Suarez AL, Yescas G, Cruz-Mimiaga RM, Garcia-Carranca A, Cruz-Talonia F (2003) Mucosal IgG and IgA responses to human papillomavirus type 16 capsid proteins in HPV16-infected women without visible pathology. Viral Immunol 16:159-168.

Schmitt M, Bravo IG, Snijders PJ, Gissmann L, Pawlita M, Waterboer T (2006) Bead-based multiplex genotyping of human papillomaviruses. J Clin Microbiol 44:504-512.

Schopp B, Holz B, Zago M, Stubenrauch F, Petry KU, Kjaer SK, Iftner T (2010) Evaluation of the performance of the novel PapilloCheck HPV genotyping test by comparison with two other genotyping systems and the HC2 test. J Med Virol 82:605-615.

Seme K, Fujs K, Kocjan BJ, Poljak M (2006) Resolving repeatedly borderline results of Hybrid Capture 2 HPV DNA Test using polymerase chain reaction and genotyping. J Virol Methods 134:252-256.

Seme K, Lepej SZ, Lunar MM, Iscic-Bes J, Planinic A, Kocjan BJ, Vince A, Poljak M (2009) Digene HPV Genotyping RH Test RUO: comparative evaluation with INNO-LiPA HPV Genotyping Extra Test for detection of 18 high-risk and probable high-risk human papillomavirus genotypes. J Clin Virol 46:176-179.

Seo SS, Song YS, Kim JW, Park NH, Kang SB, Lee HP (2006) Good correlation of HPV DNA test between self-collected vaginal and clinician-collected cervical samples by the oligonucleotide microarray. Gynecol Oncol 102:67-73.

Shi JF, Canfell K, Lew JB, Zhao FH, Legood R, Ning Y, Simonella L, Ma L, Kang YJ, Zhang YZ, Smith MA, Chen JF, Feng XX, Qiao YL (2011) Evaluation of primary HPV-DNA testing in relation to visual inspection methods for cervical cancer screening in rural China: an epidemiologic and cost-effectiveness modelling study. BMC Cancer 11:239.

Shirasawa H, Tomita Y, Sekiya S, Takamizawa H, Simizu B (1987) Integration and transcription of human papillomavirus type 16 and 18 sequences in cell lines derived from cervical carcinomas. J Gen Virol 68 (Pt 2):583-591.

Snijders PJ, van den Brule AJ, Schrijnemakers HF, Snow G, Meijer CJ, Walboomers JM (1990) The use of general primers in the polymerase chain reaction permits the detection of a broad spectrum of human papillomavirus genotypes. J Gen Virol 71:173-181.

Snyder KA, Barber SR, Symbula M, Taylor PT, Crum CP, Roche JK (1991) Binding by immunoglobulin to the HPV-16-derived proteins L1 and E4 in cervical secretions of women with HPV-related cervical disease. Cancer Res 51:4423-4429.

Stanley M (2010) Pathology and epidemiology of HPV infection in females. Gynecol Oncol 117:S5-10.

Stoler MH, Wright TC, Jr., Sharma A, Apple R, Gutekunst K, Wright TL (2011) High-risk human papillomavirus testing in women with ASC-US cytology: results from the ATHENA HPV study. Am J Clin Pathol 135:468-475.

Suchankova A, Ritterova L, Krcmar M, Krchnak V, Vagner J, Jochmus I, Gissmann L, Kanka J, Vonka V (1991) Comparison of ELISA and western blotting for human papillomavirus type 16 E7 antibody determination. J Gen Virol 72 (Pt 10):2577-2581.

Sun R, Kornegay J, Ahmad A, Current R, Ding K, Joshi S, Kosarikov D, Kotadia R, Rudra N, Young T, Yu K (2005) Evaluation of the Roche AMPLICOR® Human Papillomavirus (HPV) Test. Poster.

Szarewski A, Ambroisine L, Cadman L, Austin J, Ho L, Terry G, Liddle S, Dina R, McCarthy J, Buckley H, Bergeron C, Soutter P, Lyons D, Cuzick J (2008) Comparison of predictors for high-grade cervical intraepithelial neoplasia in women with abnormal smears. Cancer Epidemiol Biomarkers Prev 17:3033-3042.

Takacs T, Jeney C, Kovacs L, Mozes J, Benczik M, Sebe A (2008) Molecular beacon-based real-time PCR method for detection of 15 high-risk and 5 low-risk HPV types. J Virol Methods 149:153-162.

Tan SE, Garland SM, Rumbold AR, Tabrizi SN (2010) Human papillomavirus genotyping using archival vulval dysplastic or neoplastic biopsy tissues: comparison between the INNO-LiPA and linear array assays. J Clin Microbiol 48:1458-1460.

Technologies TW (2009) Cervista™ HPV HR test - Manual. In vitro diagnostic medical device 5,6.

Tjalma WA, Van Waes TR, Van den Eeden LE, Bogers JJ (2005) Role of human papillomavirus in the carcinogenesis of squamous cell carcinoma and adenocarcinoma of the cervix. Best Pract Res Clin Obstet Gynaecol 19:469-483.

Towbin H, Staehelin T, Gordon J (1979) Electrophoretic transfer of proteins from polyacrylamide gels to nitrocellulose sheets: procedure and some applications. Proc Natl Acad Sci U S A 76:4350-4354.

Trope LA, Chumworathayi B, Blumenthal PD (2009) Preventing cervical cancer: stakeholder attitudes toward CareHPV-focused screening programs in Roi-et Province, Thailand. Int J Gynecol Cancer 19:1432-1438.

Trottier H, Franco EL (2006) The epidemiology of genital human papillomavirus infection. Vaccine 24:1-15.

Valle GF, Banks L (1995) The human papillomavirus (HPV)-6 and HPV-16 E5 proteins co-operate with HPV-16 E7 in the transformation of primary rodent cells. J Gen Virol 76 (Pt 5):1239-1245.

van Ham MA, Bakkers JM, Harbers GK, Quint WG, Massuger LF, Melchers WJ (2005) comparison of two commercial assays for detection of human papillomavirus (HPV) in cervical scrape specimens: validation of the Roche AMPLICOR HPV test as a means to screen for HPV genotypes associated with a higher risk of cervical disorders. J Clin Microbiol 43:2662-2667.

Vazquez-Corzo S, Trejo-Becerril C, Cruz-Valdez A, Hernandez-Nevarez P, Esquivel-Guadarrama R, Gutierrez-Xicotencatl Mde L (2003) [Association between presence of anti-Ras and anti-VPH16 E4/E7 antibodies and cervical intraepithelial lesions]. Salud Publica Mex 45:335-345.

Veress G, Konya J, Csiky-Meszaros T, Czegledy J, Gergely L (1994) Human papillomavirus DNA and anti-HPV secretory IgA antibodies in cytologically normal cervical specimens. J Med Virol 43:201-207.

Viscidi RP, Sun Y, Tsuzaki B, Bosch FX, Munoz N, Shah KV (1993) Serologic response in human papillomavirus-associated invasive cervical cancer. Int J Cancer 55:780-784.

Wong OG, Lo CK, Szeto E, Cheung AN (2011) Efficacy of Abbott RealTime High Risk HPV test in evaluation of atypical squamous cells of undetermined significance from an Asian screening population. J Clin Virol 51:136-138.

Zaghloul MZ (2011) Human bocavirus (HBoV) in children with respiratory tract infection by enzyme linked immunosorbent assay (ELISA) and qualitative polymerase chain reaction (PCR). Virol J 8:239.

Zaravinos A, Mammas IN, Sourvinos G, Spandidos DA (2009) Molecular detection methods of human papillomavirus (HPV). Int J Biol Markers 24:215-222.

Zhou YM, Liu GD, Wu ZY, Shen GL, Yu RQ (2002) An amperometric immunosensor based on a conducting immunocomposite electrode for the determination of Schistosoma japonicum antigen. Anal Sci 18:155-159.

Part 3

Recent Advances in Fundamental Human Papillomavirus Research

10

Molecular Bases of Human Papillomavirus Pathogenesis in the Development of Cervical Cancer

Adolfo Pedroza-Saavedra[1], Tanya Plett-Torres[1], Lilia Chihu-Amparán[1], Minerva Maldonado-Gama[1], Ana M. González-Jaimes[1], Fernando Esquivel-Guadarrama[2] and Lourdes Gutiérrez-Xicotencatl[1]

[1]*Department of Epidemiological Interactions, Center of Research on Infectious Diseases, National Institute of Public Health.*
[2]*Faculty of Medicine, Autonomous University of Morelos State.*
[1,2]*Cuernavaca, Morelos, Mexico*

1. Introduction

Human papillomavirus (HPV) is a DNA virus which belongs to the newly named *Papillomaviridae* family (de Villiers et al., 2004). The papillomaviruses induce a variety of proliferative lesions in the skin and internal mucosa. Nearly half of the over 200 types of HPVs can infect the genital mucosa, producing benign epithelial lesions. However, a subset of these viruses is found in over 90% of malignant carcinomas of the genital tract, the majority of which contain the HPV16 and 18 types considered to be of "High Risk" (HR), as they help the progression into cervical cancer (Lorincz et al., 1992; Shah & Buscema, 1988).

The mechanisms through which HPVs induce cell transformation have been intensively investigated in the last few years. The most abundant viral transcripts in tumor and tumor cell lines are produced from the *E6* and *E7* Open Reading Frames (ORFs) that are known to be oncogenic. These two genes from HPV are necessary and sufficient to induce HPV-mediated transformation of murine cells (Yasumoto et al., 1986), transform human fibroblasts (Pirisi et al., 1987), and in cooperation with *ras* are capable of transforming baby rat kidney cells (Phelps et al., 1988) and primary human keratinocytes (Yoshida et al., 2008). The best evidence for the role of E6 and E7 proteins in malignancy comes from biochemical studies. E6 and E7 oncoproteins from the HR-HPV types have the ability to alter pathways involved in cell cycle control, interacting with and neutralizing the regulatory function of primarily two suppressor proteins, p53 and pRb respectively (Dyson et al., 1992; Werness et al., 1990). These effects produce genetic instability and accumulation of mutations that might contribute to the oncogenic process. Besides, several other target proteins for E6 and E7 oncoproteins have been identified and probably those interactions also promote cellular transformation. The latest oncogene identified from HPV was the *E5* from HPV16. The E5 oncoprotein showed to be capable of increasing the half-life of Epidermal Growth Factor

(EGF) and Platelet-Derived Growth Factor (PDGF) receptors (Leechanachai et al., 1992). Contrary to *E6* and *E7*, the *E5* oncogene is lost in the late stages of cervical cancer due to viral integration to the cellular genome. However, the close association with growth factor receptors could suggest that E5 has a key role in viral life cycle and may have an important function in the early development of the neoplasia.

The oncogenes mentioned above codify for oncoproteins that have developed a plethora of strategies resulting in the alteration of cell cycle and apoptosis control by targeting the same or different cellular pathways, favoring viral persistence and leading to a strong synergism in promoting cellular transformation. Several studies have been performed to elucidate the mechanisms through which these HPV oncogenes allow the cellular transformation and the generation of the cervical cancer. Recently, the development of genomic and proteomic techniques has promoted the research of cervical cancer progression due to HPV infection, allowing the identification of protein interaction networks and the discovery of biomarkers useful for diagnostic and therapeutic systems.

2. Organization and classification of human papillomaviruses

HPV is a non enveloped DNA virus with icosahedral capsid that surrounds one copy of circular double stranded DNA close to 8 kb long. HPV genome codes for eight proteins classified as early (E) and late (L) proteins expressed from polycistronic mRNA by a positive DNA strand. Between E and L coding sequences is a Long Control Region (LCR) that has low conservation among members of the *Papillomaviridae* family. This region promotes and enhances the viral gene expression and it does not include ORFs (de Villiers et al., 2004; Syrjänen & Syrjänen, 1999). The HPVs maintain high fidelity of their genome as they use the host cell proofreading polymerases, generating mutations at similar rates as the host DNA genome. HPVs involve different genotypes, defined as a complete cloned genome whose *L1* ORF most conserved segment has a DNA sequence at least 10% different from any other HPV type (Bernard, 2005; de Villiers et al., 2004; Myers et al., 1996). HPV subtypes may be found (differences between 2-10% of homology) like HPV55 that is a subtype of HPV44. The HPV variants are defined as those that show differences of less than 2% of homology in nucleotide sequence in the coding regions and 5% in the non-coding regions from the original isolate (prototype) (Bernard et al., 1994; Bernard, 2005; de Villiers et al., 2004). Now at days, more than 200 suggested types have been detected and 100 types have been completely sequenced, all of them registered at the German Cancer Research Center in Heidelberg, Germany (Bernard, 2005; de Villiers et al., 2004).

All HPV types are epitheliotropic and may be found in mucous tissue and/or in skin (de Villiers, 1989; Myers et al., 1996). Recently, the new taxonomy of papillomaviruses grouped them in 16 higher-order cluster groups (super-groups or major branches) named *genus* which share from 23 to 43% of identity. The genera are identified by Greek letters (alpha to pi) and divided in lower-order clusters named *species* that share 60-70% of identity within a genus and 71-89% within a species (de Villiers et al., 2004). Species are identified by numbers and group HPV types with common phylogenetical, biological and pathological properties (Bernard, 2005; de Villiers et al., 2004). HPVs are classified into five genera (alpha, beta, gamma, mu and nu) (Bernard et al., 2010). The alpha-papillomavirus genus contains all the clinically important HPVs associated with mucosal and genital lesions. While, the beta-papillomavirus genus includes all cutaneous HPV types involved in *Epidermodysplasia verruciformis* or skin cancer in immunosupressed subjects, the gamma-papillomavirus genus includes cutaneous HPV types distinguished by intracytoplasmic inclusion bodies in histological tests (Bernard, 2005; de Villiers, 1989; de Villiers et al., 2004).

There are a limited number of variants for each HPV type, some of which are highly divergent, especially those taken from ethnic groups that evolved without geographical contact. Thus, it seems that each HPV type was not transferred from other species, has been with the human race since its origins, evolved together and spread as human ethnic groups arose and populated the world (Bernard, 2005). The HPV16 variants can be divided into six geographically clustered phylogenetic groups, the European (E), African 1 and 2 (Af1 and Af2, respectively), Asian (As), Asian-American (AA) and North American (NA) (Yamada et al., 1997). Clinically speaking, there is an interesting concern on the biological activity of HPV variants because some of them are more frequently detected (94%) in high-grade cervical lesions than the HPV16 prototype (6%) (Zehbe et al., 1998) and being associated to the development of cervical lesions grade 2-3 (Xi et al., 2002). However, more epidemiological and laboratory studies need to be performed to confirm these observations. Bravo and Alonso suggested an alternative classification system based on the nucleotide sequence of the *E1* and *E2* ORFs. Also, they proposed that concatenated E1-E2 proteins sequences can be incorporated as a suitable evolutionary standard for *Papillomaviridae* classification (Bravo & Alonso, 2007). Due to the increasing number of new sequences of Papillomaviruses (PVs), Bernard and coworkers proposed the expansion of the family *Papillomaviridae.* To accomplish this, the names of genera were extended to the end of the Greek alphabet (from *Alphapapillomavirus* to *Omegapapillomavirus*), followed by the prefix "*Dyo*" (i.e., "a second time"), omitting the designation from *Dyoalphapapillomavirus* to *Dyogammapapillomavirus* because the *Alpha, Beta* and *Gamma* genera include the most common and medically important HPVs. Also, they named the rest of PVs genera waiting for classification as *Rho* to *Omega*, assigning the terms "*Dyodelta*-PVs", "*Dyoepsilon*-PVs" and so on, for the new PV genus (Bernard et al., 2010).

Phylogenetical analysis of the *E5*, *E6* and *E7* gene sequences have revealed that only *E6* and *E7* genes from the alpha genus are highly conserved (>75% and >65% homology, respectively). However, when only the HR-HPV types of the alpha genus are considered the homologies go up to 80% for *E6* and up to 70% for *E7* sequences. The less conserved viral sequences from the alpha genus are those from the *E5* gene, since the homology in this genus is only of 25% and 40% when only the HR-HPV types are considered. Few years ago, Bravo and Alonso (2004) described the evolutionary characteristics of the E5 proteins and compared them with the E6 and E7 oncogenic proteins and with the structural proteins L1 and L2. They showed that there is a clear pattern of divergence from late to early genes at the protein level, which increased in the progression $L1 < L2 < E6 \approx E7 < E5$. Among the E5 proteins from the alpha genus it was clear that there was not an evident sequence similarity and that the evolutionary divergence between present proteins rises to 80% (Bravo & Alonso, 2004). The few common characteristics for the alpha genus E5 proteins are the high hydrophobicity, the high Ile+Leu+Val content and the presence of transmembranal regions. Taking into consideration these characteristics of the E5 protein, Bravo and Alonso (2004) identified 4 groups of E5 proteins in the alpha genus (E5α, E5β, E5γ and E5δ) and proposed that besides of the phylogenetic characteristics, the chemical part of the proteins have to be taken into consideration to have a more specific classification, as it has been suggested that the protein chemistry is an important restriction for protein evolution (Babbit & Gerlt, 1997).

On the other hand, Wang and coworkers (2010) showed that the Canine Papillomavirus type 2 (CPV2) encodes an E7 protein that has Ser substituted for Cys at the LXCXE motif, important in the E7 proteins from the alpha genus, to bind and degrade the pRb protein. This mutation in the CVP2 E7 protein abrogates pRb binding at this site; however a new domain with a binding site for pRb was identified at the C-terminal region of canine E7, and was able to degrade the pRb protein. At the same time, these researchers demonstrated that the HPV4 E7 protein also binds pRb in a similar way as CPV2 E7 protein and by screening of HPV genome sequences identified that the LXSXE motif of the CPV2 E7 protein was also present in the gamma HPV genus (Wang et al., 2010).

Altogether these data show that phylogenetic sequence analysis is important to trace the papillomaviruses evolution and define ancestors, but also showed that when chemical and biological characteristics of the oncogenic HPV proteins are integrated into the analysis, there is a better classification of HPVs within the genus, as subgroups were identified. However, more work needs to be done before this type of integrative analysis can be used to give some light between clinical manifestations and the development of cancer associated to HPV.

3. Viral cycle and HPV integration into the genome of host cell

During HPV infection, the different viral proteins are expressed sequentially (Middleton et al., 2003; Peh et al., 2002). The HPV infection starts in the basal cell layer of the cervix since these cells express the specific receptors for viral entry and also because are the only cells in the squamous epithelium capable of dividing. Molecules like heparan sulfate and glycosaminoglycans seem to mediate the attachment of the virions via interaction of the major capsid protein, L1, to the basal membrane of human keratinocytes. The internalization of some HPV types is a slow process mediated by clathrin-coated vesicles, or the caveolae-dependent route (Bousarghin et al., 2003; Horvath et al., 2010). Once the virus has penetrated the cell, disassembly of HPV particles occurs in cytoplasmic vesicles, followed by the delivery of the viral DNA into the nucleus mediated by L2 (Day et al., 2004). After infection, HPV genomes are established as autonomous replicating extra-chromosomal elements or episomes and start a low expression level of the *E6* and *E7* genes (Middleton et al., 2003; Moody & Laimins, 2010). The *E6* and *E7* gene expression is achieved by cellular transcription factors that interact with the LCR, a region where the E2 protein interacts to repress or to activate viral transcription. The promoter region from HPVs contains TATA boxes for binding cellular transcriptional factors like TFIID and an epithelial cell-specific enhancer, which holds binding sites for transcription factors like Sp-1 and AP-1, among others (Butz & Hoppe-Seyler, 1993; Doorbar, 2005; Middleton et al., 2003; Tan et al., 1994). The expression of E6 leads mainly to the ubiquitin-dependent proteolysis of p53 (Farthing & Vousden, 1994; Münger et al., 1992; Rapp & Chen, 1998), preventing cell growth inhibition in both undifferentiated and differentiated cells (Moody & Laimins, 2010) and the E7 expression to the liberation of the transcription factor E2F by sequestration of pRb (Münger et al., 1992), effects that promote cellular proliferation and genome instability throughout the infected tissue.

While the basal HPV infected cell migrates to upper layers and differentiates, the viral cycle continues with the E1, E2, E4 and E5 protein expression and viral DNA replication (Doorbar, 2005; Longworth & Laimins, 2004; Middleton et al., 2003; Peh et al., 2002). First, the E1 protein hexamerizes to recruit the cellular DNA polymerase and replication accessory proteins, while it displaces Histone H1 and functions as a helicase/ATPase to start the viral genome replication (Hughes & Romanos, 1993; Lambert, 1991; Swindle & Engler, 1998). It has been observed that the E1 and E2 expression is auto-regulated and activated by replication. The E2 protein modulates E1 expression and E6 splicing differentially regulates E1 and E2 expression (Hubert & Laimins, 2002). Once the viral replication has finished, E2 levels raise and repress the E6 and E7 expression by binding to the HPV early promoter as a dimmer and promoting the liberation of cellular transcriptional activator factors (Tan et al., 1994).

On the other hand, the E4 protein is translated from a spliced E1^E4 transcript to form a fusion protein that contains the first 5 amino acids (aa) from the E1 protein and the E4 ORF. In warts, E4 exists as multiple species that are formed from a combination of progressive proteolysis of the N-terminal residues, oligomerization, and phosphorylation. The species resulting from proteolysis are the 17 kDa species in the parabasal cell layer of epithelium and this is coincident with viral genome amplification. The E4 16, 11 and 10 kDa species are accumulated in superficial keratinocytes, where capsid proteins expression and assembly occurs (Doorbar et al., 1988; Middleton et al., 2003). It is known that E4 binds to zinc, cytoskeleton and cytokeratins (Roberts et al., 1994; Wang et al., 2004). Therefore, it is suggested that E4 may alter the normal keratinization process to benefit the viral cycle progress and generate a cytoskeleton collapse (Gaillard et al., 1992) inducing apoptosis through alteration of mitochondrial function (Raj et al., 2004) and favoring the viral particle liberation (Gaillard et al., 1992). However, in natural infections only a limited amount of keratin collapse has been observed (Doorbar et al., 1996). The E4 protein sequesters the CDK1/Cyc B1 complex (CDK, Cyclin dependent kinase and Cyc, Cyclin) onto the cytokeratin network, preventing their nuclear accumulation and therefore inducing inhibition of the G2/M transition of the cell cycle (Davy et al., 2002; Nakahara et al., 2002) and allowing viral and genomic DNA replication. The HPV16 E4 coding region possesses a splicing enhancer element required for the early viral mRNA splicing (Rush et al., 2005), especially for the expression of late viral transcripts of E1^E2, E1, E4 and E5, thus regulating the viral DNA amplification (Wilson et al., 2005).

Other protein suggested to be expressed at the same time as E4 is E5, both of which may contribute to viral genome amplification (Doorbar, 2006; Syrjänen & Syrjänen, 1999). A polycistronic mRNA containing the E5 sequence is the most abundant transcript in HPV positive cervical carcinomas *in situ* (Stoler et al., 1992). E5 transcripts expression is very low in undifferentiated cells (Reagan & Laimins, 2008). The E5 mRNA and protein are mainly present in the lower third of the epithelium of Low Grade Squamous Intraepithelial Lesions (LSILs), and might contribute to neoplastic proliferation during the early stages of infection (Chang et al., 2001; Stoler et al., 1992), or to be essential for malignant transformation (Stoppler et al., 1996). The gene encoding the viral E5 protein is frequently disrupted or lost when viral DNA is integrated into human genome (Pater & Pater, 1985). Even though, E5 protein expression pattern in cervical epithelia has not been accomplished yet, it has been observed that E5 function is needed to maintain the cell proliferation stimuli driven by the

EGF Receptor (EGFR) signaling pathway at this stage (Syrjänen & Syrjänen, 1999). In this way, the E5 function complements the E7 and E6 functions, to generate and maintain the transformed phenotype (Stöppler et al., 1996).

A special characteristic of the viral cycle is that the last stages take place in terminally differentiated keratinocytes (Schiller et al., 2010). In this stage, viral particles are generated when the expression of capsid proteins (L1 and L2) starts by a promoter localized in the late region of the HPV genome. The L1 and L2 proteins polymerize into icosahedral capsids in a thermodynamic stable and spontaneous process that involves the binding of the HPV DNA to the N-terminal sequence of the L2 protein (Hagensee et al., 1993; Zhou et al., 1994). During their formation, HPV capsids require maturation (formation of intermolecular disulfide bonds in L1), event that leads to stability and virions liberation in the external surface of the squamous epithelium by cellular death (Buck et al., 2005; Syrjänen & Syrjänen, 1999). Up to now, it is still unknown if encapsidation of the viral genome takes place during or after capsid assembly (Conway & Meyers, 2009; Holmgren et al., 2005), but it has been suggested that L2 uses E2 to recruit the viral genome to the site of virion assembly (Holmgren et al., 2005).

During HPV productive infections that lead to cervical lesions, the viral genome is episomal with a great copy number that depends on differentiated cells. Throughout the HPV persistent infection, there is a gradual deregulation in the expression of E6 and E7 proteins that may lead to the development of low-grade cervical lesions, where one third of the epithelium is formed by E6/E7 expressing basal cells. The progression from High Grade Squamous Intraepithelial Lesions (HSILs) to cancer usually occurs in lesions that contain integrated copies of the viral genome. This event leads to an abortive infection (Farthing & Vousden, 1994; Münger et al., 2004; Peitsaro et al., 2002) and cells cannot longer produce new viral particles (Matlashewski, 2006). It has been observed that the viral integration occurs mainly between *E1-E2* ORFs, event that produces the loss of *E2* and *E4* genes expression. Thus, the loss of *E2* and *E4* genes generates a down-replication of the viral genome, G2 arrest, and E6 and E7 over-expression (Jeon & Lambert, 1995; Wilson et al., 2005). Thus, the integration of the HPV DNA in the host genome represents an important event in cervical carcinogenesis (Pett & Coleman, 2007), as this may cause cellular immortalization (Band et al., 1990; Jeon & Lambert, 1995; Münger et al., 1992; zur Hausen, 2000), reduction of cellular differentiation, cellular dysplasia and TNF-α non-responder cells (TNF, Tumor Necrosis Factor) (Syrjänen & Syrjänen, 1999; zur Hausen, 2000).

Besides increasing the transcript stability and protein expression of the viral E6 and E7 oncoproteins, integration of the viral genome may cause chromosomal rearrangements (Jeon & Lambert, 1995) and influences cancer progression through interaction with hTERT, p53 and pRB (Raibould et al., 2011). The integration of HPV sequences in the host genome occurs randomly, although in invasive genital carcinomas or cervical cancer-derived cell lines, HPV genome has been found frequently integrated near fragile sites, like translocation breakpoints (Koopman et al., 1999; Mammas et al., 2008), or modifying proto-oncogenes sequences either by rearrangement or amplification as has been observed for *myc* genes (Ocadiz et al., 1987; Sastre-Garau et al., 2000). Disruption or deregulation of defined critical cellular gene functions by insertional mutagenesis of HPV genome fragments has been hypothesized as the major promoting factor in the pathogenesis of HPV-associated cancers (Wentzensen et al., 2004). Further investigation on early integration events needs to be done to describe the mechanism by which viral infection is aborted and cell transformation is generated.

4. Role and function of HPV oncoproteins

4.1 E5 oncoprotein

4.1.1 E5 biochemical properties

The E5 oncoproteins are small highly hydrophobic proteins important in the carcinogenic process and recently have been identified as potential oncogenes, although their role is not well understood (Bouvard et al., 1994). The E5 proteins from both animal and human sources can transform mammalian cells with different degrees of efficiency (Bouvard et al., 1994; Horwitz et al., 1989; Straight et al., 1993). Both BPV-1 (bovine papillomavirus) and HPV E5 proteins are transmembrane proteins localized in Golgi and endosomes, but they have also been found in plasmatic membrane and endoplasmic reticulum (ER) (Cartin & Alonso, 2003; Conrad et al., 1993; Disbrow et al., 2005; Lewis et al., 2008). The E5 oncoprotein from HPV16 has 83 aa residues with an estimated molecular weight of 10 kDa. The E5 protein presents three transmembranal helices and short hydrophilic regions at the C- and N-terminus (Alonso & Reed, 2002; Ullman et al., 1994; Yang et al., 2003), being the first hydrophobic region important for cellular localization of E5 (Fig. 1) (Cortese et al., 2010; Lewis et al., 2008). In HaCat cells (immortalized human keratinocytes) this region confers anchorage-independent growth and is associated with the capacity of these cells to invade extracellular matrix in organotypic "*raft*" assays (Barbaresi et al., 2010; Lewis et al., 2008). It has been demonstrated that E5 proteins contribute to cellular transformation by increasing the mitogenic signal from growth factor receptors to the nucleus (Leechanachai et al., 1992).

4.1.2 E5 functional properties

A proposed mechanism for E5 transforming activity is through increasing the half-life of the tyrosine kinase-containing growth factor receptors like EGFR, the phosphorylation state of this receptor or both (Genther-Williams et al., 2005; Straight et al., 1993, 1995; Tomakidi et al., 2000). It has been also proposed that HPV E5 proteins interact with the 16 kDa subunit of the protonic ATPase, inhibiting the acidification of endosomes and retarding the receptor degradation (Andresson et al., 1995; Briggs et al., 2001; Conrad et al., 1993; Straight et al., 1995). At the same time, E5 induces a number of functional effects like causing alkalinization of endocellular pH, tyrosinase activation, melanin deposition and modulation of sensitivity to dopamine mimetic drugs as it has been shown in melanocytes that express E5 from HPV16 (Di Domenico et al., 2009). The second and third transmembranal domains cooperate to bind the protonic ATPase-16 kDa subunit (Adam et al., 2000; Rodriguez et al., 2000). However, some contradictory studies indicate that E5 proteins bind, but do not disturb the activity of the vacuolar protonic ATPase (Adam et al., 2000; Ashby et al., 2001; Rodriguez et al., 2000), and it has been shown that the final effect is due to a perturbation of the endocytic trafficking (S.L. Chen et al., 1996c). In contrast, it has been demonstrated that HPV16 E5 stimulates the EGFR-mediated signal transduction by inhibiting the interaction with c-Cbl and decreasing the receptor degradation pathway (B. Zhang et al., 2005a) (Fig. 2). Recently, it was shown that HPV16 E5 down-modulates the KGFR/FGFR2b (keratinocyte growth factor receptor) by interference of the endocytic receptor pathway and perturbing the differentiation process (Belleudi et al., 2011).

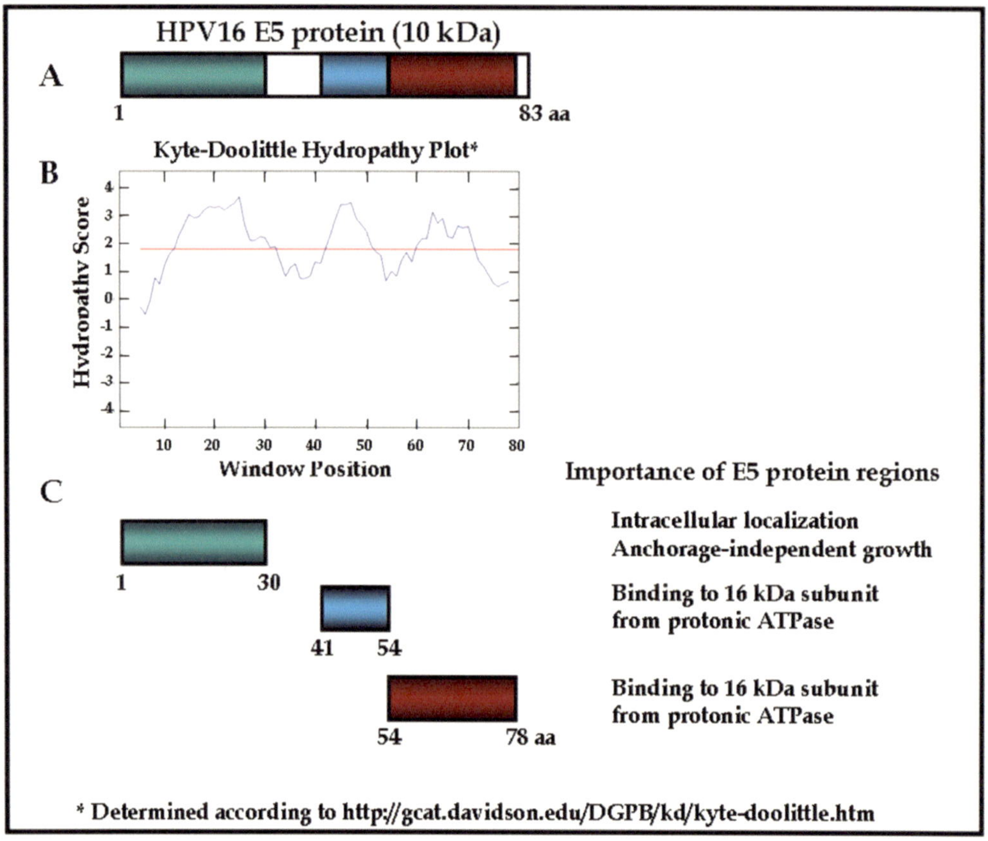

Fig. 1. Biochemical characteristics of the HPV16 E5 oncoprotein. (**A**) The E5 protein with 83 amino acid residues has an estimated molecular weight of 10 kDa. (**B**) E5 is divided in three hydrophobic regions as estimated by the Kyte-Doolittle Hydropathy Plot. (**C**) The first region (aa 1-30) is important for membrane localization and for anchorage-independent growth. The second (aa 41-54) and third (aa 54-78) hydrophobic regions contain the domains for binding to the protonic ATPase-16 kDa subunit.

The expression of E5 protein has been associated with the expression of other members of the EGFR family (i.e. ErbB1, ErbB4) as well as the activity of ErbB2 (Crusius et al., 1998) and components of the EGF signaling pathway, like MAPKs (ERK1/2) (Crusius et al., 1997; S.H. Kim et al., 2006). The activation of members of the MAPK pathway may lead to regulation of other set of genes implicated in growth, as was observed that HPV16 E5 favors the over-expression of transcriptional factors such as c-Fos and c-Jun that form the AP-1 complex (S.L. Chen et al., 1995, 1996a, 1996b), and stimulates transcription of genes involved in cell growth. During the cell cycle the E5 proteins from HPV11 and 16 have shown to be able to modulate cell proliferation, due to repression of $p21^{Waf1}$ gene expression through *c-jun* activation (Tsao et al., 1996). In addition, our laboratory has identified that HPV16 E5 increases the down-regulation of $p27^{Kip1}$ CDK inhibitor in an EGFR dependent pathway, allowing the cells to stay for longer time into the cell cycle due to an increment in the S-phase (Pedroza-Saavedra et al., 2010) (Fig. 2). Also, HPV16 E5 is able to activate other type of transcriptional factors like NF-κB and leading to COX-2 expression (S.H. Kim et al., 2009)

(Fig. 2). More recently, it has been suggested that HPV16 E5 protein can act independently of the EGFR through the PLCγ1 (Crusius et al., 1999) and on MAPKs (ERK1/2 and p38) activities, when the cells are placed under stress conditions (Crusius et al., 2000). On the other hand, E5 is also able to induce the expression of other type of receptors like the EP4 subtype of prostaglandin E2 receptor, which increases the colony-forming efficiency and the Vascular Endothelial Growth Factor (VEGF) secretion in cervical cancer cells, both of which are required for tumor growth, angiogenesis and metastasis (Oh et al., 2009).

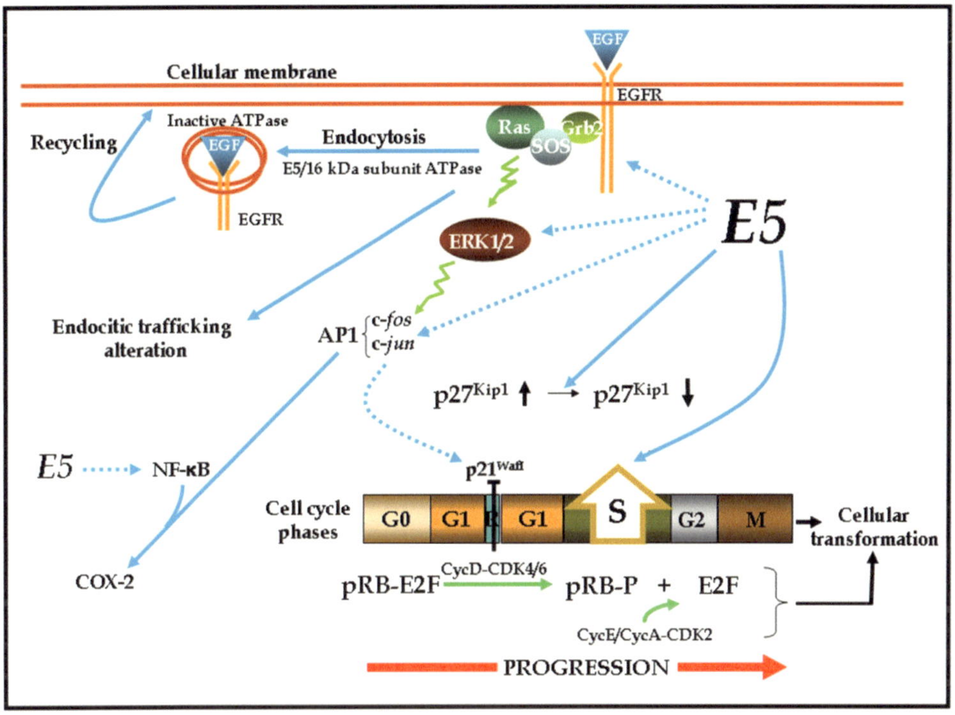

Fig. 2. Important functions of HPV16 E5 in the cell. E5 can modify the half-life of the EGFR through binding with the protonic ATPase-16 kDa subunit, avoiding acidification of endosomes and favoring the recycling of receptors and perturbing the endocytic trafficking. E5 targets molecular components of the MAPKs cascade that have incidence on the progression of the cell cycle. E5 decreases the level of the CDK inhibitor $p21^{Waf1}$ and modulates $p27^{Kip1}$ protein levels allowing deregulation of the cell cycle, by increasing the S-phase of the cell cycle and promoting cellular transformation.

Other important activity observed for E5 proteins is the ability to keep the major histocompatibility complex (MHC) class I in Golgi, preventing its transport to the cell surface. In the case of HPV16 E5, this blockage is rescued by treatment with interferon. Unlike BPV E5, HPV16 E5 does not affect the synthesis of HLA class I heavy chains, but rather interferes with the transporter associated with antigen processing (TAP). The absence of cell surface HLA class I molecules in E5 expressing cells may allow the HPV to establish an infection by avoiding immune clearance of virus-infected cells by CTLs (Araibi et al., 2004; Ashrafi et al., 2005; Marchetti et al., 2002, 2006). In this context, Gill and coworkers (1998) observed that women with increasingly severe HPV16-associated lesions have decreasing T cell HPV16 E5-specific proliferative responses. At the same time, HPV16 E5 impairs TRAIL- and FasL-mediated apoptosis in HaCat cells possibly as a mechanism to escape immune surveillance that otherwise would be likely to detect infected cells at an early stage in the viral life cycle (Kabsch et al., 2004).

Finally, the close association of E5 with growth factors and their receptors, and the fact that the *E5* ORF is lost in cervical carcinoma cells, suggest that E5 may play a critical role in the genesis of cervical cancer as an initiator of the transformation process, as it has been shown to happen with the Ras oncoprotein in colorectal cancer (Gryfe et al., 1997; Takami et al., 1995). Additionally, these findings support the idea that the E5 protein could be an early predictor marker of cervical cancer (Gill et al., 1998; Hsieh et al., 2000; Kell et al., 1994).

4.2 E6 oncoprotein

4.2.1 E6 biochemical properties

E6 proteins from HPVs comprise molecules between 151 and 158 amino acids that are usually localized within the cell nucleus (Nomine et al., 2006; Rapp & Chen, 1998). It has been difficult to study E6 proteins because they are expressed at very low levels in HPV infected cells and are difficult to purify in a stable folded form as they tend to aggregate in complexes of misfolded molecules when over-expressed in bacteria (Nominé et al., 2001; Ristriani et al., 2002).

In general, the E6 proteins contain two Cys-Xaa_2-Cys-$Xaa_{29\text{-}30}$-Cys-Xaa_2-Cys zinc binding domains located at the N- and C-terminal parts of the molecule. These domains are novel types of zinc-binding structures characterized by αβαβ secondary structures separated by 29 to 30 residues (Ullman et al., 1996). The E6 C-terminal domain is a DNA binding site that consists of 3-stranded β-sheet (S1, S2 and S3) with two short helices (H1 and H2) packed on one of its sides, a peripheric zinc binding site that protrudes away from the β sheet and that involves the long loop (L2) connecting H1 and H2 with a short C-terminal helix (H3). E6 has a main hydrophobic core (conserved among HPVs) between the β-sheet and helices H1 and H2, that it is not exposed to water in the full-length E6 protein. This part of the E6 protein has a mostly positive charge potential, except for a neutral area at the top of H1 and H2 corresponding to the hydrophobic patch. Conserved amino acids are on the surface of the N- and C-terminal zinc binding motifs of E6 protein in all HPV species. Some may participate in generic functions shared by all HPVs E6 proteins like trans-activation, transformation, and protein-protein interactions, while others may have a structural role. In this sense, it seems that specific amino acids located at the hydrophilic sites in high- and low-risk HPVs, allow certain physicochemical characteristics which confer them the ability to recognize different subsets of cellular molecules. An example is the C-terminal region from HPV16 E6, which displays a strong positive charge at the nucleic acid binding site and the highest surface potential (Nominé et al., 2006).

The HPV16 E6 full-length protein is composed of 151 amino acids (Rapp & Chen, 1998), with a calculated molecular weight of 18 kDa and with a bimodal half-life in SiHa cells of 30 min and 4 h that seem to be related to E6 interactions with target proteins (Androphy et al., 1987). HPV16 E6 protein C-terminal region has an IEP of 10.6 (IEP, Isoelectric Point) and it is the part of the molecule necessary for binding to p53, while the N-terminal region contains the binding site for E6AP (Lxxϕ Lsh motif) important for p53 degradation (Howie et al., 2009;

Thomas et al., 1999). These LxxϕLsh motifs (where xx is a dipeptide and one of the residues is Asp, Glu, Asn or Gln; ϕ is a hydrophobic residue; s is a small amino acid; h is an amino acid capable of accepting hydrogen bonds) are Leucine-rich amphipathic helices and binding through these motifs is a conserved property of the E6 proteins from HPVs from the alpha genus. In this sense, the minimal segment still functional for p53 degradation comprises residues 1-142 and coordinates with two Zn^{+2} ions (Beerheide et al., 1999; Lipari et al., 2001) by means of conserved cysteine residues 30, 33, 63 and 66 at the N-terminal and residues 103, 106, 136 and 139 at the C-terminal (Nominé et al., 2001), where the loss of the Zn^{+2} at the C-terminal domain leads to loss of tertiary structure and protein aggregation (Y. Liu et al., 2009). Other proteins like E6AP, E6BP, IRF3, Paxilin and MCM7 are also able to bind E6 through these LxxϕLsh motifs, interaction that appears to regulate the activity of different subset of proteins (J.J. Chen et al., 1998; Elston et al., 1998; Tong & Howley, 1997).

Besides, the E6 proteins from oncogenic HPV types have a motif designated XT/SXV at their C-terminal motifs that mediates binding to specific domains known as PDZ (Howie et al., 2009). The PDZ domains are approximately 90 amino acid stretches. The PDZ proteins known to bind E6 are hDlg1 and 4, tumor suppressor proteins (Kiyono et al., 1997; S.S. Lee et al., 1997), MAGI-1, -2 and -3, Membrane Associated Guanylate kinase homolog proteins (Thomas et al., 2001), MUPP-1 a multi PDZ protein (S.S. Lee et al., 2000), hScrib (Nakagawa & Huibregtse 2000) and PTPN3, both tyrosine phosphatase proteins (Jing et al., 2007). These proteins bind to E6 by the PDZ domain (aa 141-151) (Pim et al., 2009; Storrs & Silverstein, 2007; Y. Zhang et al., 2007), acting as an adaptor to link the ubiquitin ligase to the target for ubiquitination by means of its C-terminal region (Pim et al., 2009). Moreover, differences in binding PDZs by different HPV E6 proteins have been associated with the pathogenicity of HPV types as a single amino acid substitution in this binding motif among HR-HPV E6 proteins has a profound effect upon its binding to PDZ bearing target proteins (Thomas et al., 2001).

E6 protein may be found full length and C-terminally truncated (E6*) expressed from a subset of spliced transcripts, differing in number depending on the HPV type (HPV16 E6 presents 4 species, while HPV18 E6 only one). The E6* protein of HPV18 has the first 44 amino acids of the full-length protein and thereafter is composed by 13 unique amino acids derived from E6 intronic sequences. One of these sequences results in an E6* protein of 7 kDa able to bind to E6AP, but not p53. This interference with the p53-mediated E6 degradation by E6* re-activates the p53-dependent growth arrest and apoptotic functions (Pim et al., 2009). In this sense, the presence of E6 over E6* may lead to aggressive cancers as E6* is present at low levels in Asian-American HPV16 variant, the one detected in the most aggressive cancers, and at high levels in African variant, together with higher levels of p53 (Filippova et al., 2009).

4.2.2 E6 functional properties

The HR-HPV E6 proteins are distributed in the cytoplasm and the nucleus, and its expression leads to the transformation of NIH3T3 cells as well as the immortalization of human mammary epithelial cells (Holt et al., 1996). The first function associated to E6 protein was its anti-apoptotic activity due to the ability to mediate the p53 degradation through the E6/E6AP complex, allowing the regulation of expression of proteins controlling the cell cycle, being the most important the CDK inhibitor $p21^{Waf1}$ (Cooper et al., 2003). The p73 protein, homologue in structure and function to p53, also binds to E6 but its degradation is not promoted by the oncoprotein (Das et al., 2003). However, in HPV18 transformed cells there is an abrogation of p53 degradation due to the Pitx2a protein that binds to E6 and interferes with the E6/E6AP complex, leading to the accumulation of functional p53 protein (Wei, 2005). In this case, the anti-apoptotic effect of E6 is carried out through the interference of the p53/PUMA/Bax cascade (M. Vogt et al., 2006).

On the other hand, E6 is able to transactivate the survivin promoter and along with E7, transactivate the c-IAP-2 promoter and confer resistance to apoptosis (Yuan et al., 2005). Isoforms of E6 regulate the extrinsic apoptosis in a concentration-dependent manner. When low levels of large (E6) and short E6 (E6*) proteins are expressed, the cells become resistant to TNF. On the other hand, with moderate and high levels of expression, there is a sensitization to TNF aided by the E6 protein ability to form complexes with each other. In this sense, the cellular response to TNF depends on the ratio of the two E6 isoforms, being high levels of large E6 responsible for the low response to TNF and E6* reverting the E6 effect (Filippova et al., 2009). The resistance to TNF-mediated apoptosis is related to high levels of E6 and low levels of E6*. Other ways by which E6 protein regulates cell death pathways is by inhibiting the transactivation action of IRF3 (Ronco et al., 1998) and by inhibiting TLR9 transcription generating functional loss of TLR9-regulated pathways (Hasan et al., 2007).

In contrast, the capacity of E6/E6AP-mediated p53 degradation favors the accumulation of genetic alterations. A possible explanation is that E6 alters molecules implicated in DNA-repairing such as degradation of MGMT (Srivenugopal & Ali-Osman, 2002) and MCM7 proteins, producing chromosomal abnormalities (Kühne & Banks, 1998; Kukimoto et al., 1998). Also E6 from the HR-HPVs increases cellular telomerase activity via transcriptional activation of the telomerase catalytic subunit, hTERT (X. Liu et al., 2005) and degradation of the telomerase inhibitor NFX1-91 (Gewin et al., 2004), events that lead to reconstitution of telomerase activity allowing the immortalization process in the cells (J.P. Liu, 1999; Longworth & Laimins, 2004).

Recent studies have demonstrated that HR-HPV E6 proteins have a PDZ-binding motif, which probably mediates the disruption of signal transduction where PDZ proteins are implicated (Watson et al., 2003). It has been reported that E6 binds PDZ proteins and promotes their ubiquitination and further degradation as observed for hDlg (Grm & Banks, 2004), MUPP-1 (S.S. Lee et al., 2000; Massimi et al., 2004), h-SCRIB (Thomas et al., 2005), MAGI-1, -2 and -3 (Thomas et al., 2001, 2002). The MAGUK family protein MAGI-2 interacts with PTEN tumor suppressor (Wu et al., 2000), which inactivates IP_3. Thus, PKB remains activated promoting cell survival and proliferation. Additionally, HPV E6 oncoprotein has been linked to the MAPK signaling pathway by increasing the levels of MAPK1/2, MEK 1/2, and BRaf specially the E6 variant in amino acid 83, promoting cell proliferation by another pathway (Chakrabarti et al., 2004).

Other molecules that bind E6 proteins (in some cases with its concomitant degradation) are the Rap GTPase-activating protein E6TP1 (Gao et al., 1999; L. Singh et al., 2003), the CDK inhibitor $p16^{INK4a}$ (Malanchi et al., 2004), the regulator of insulin signaling pathway tuberin (Lu et al., 2004), the regulator TRIP-Br1 for the E2F/DP1/pRb complex during cell-cycle (Gupta et al., 2003), the extracellular matrix Ca^{+2}-binding protein fibulin-1 (Du et al., 2002) and the putative Ca^{+2} binding protein E6BP (J.J. Chen et al., 1995). Viral oncoproteins induce mislocation of select PDZ proteins allowing disruption of tight junctions and cause polarity defects in epithelial cells. The development of human cancers is frequently associated with a failure of epithelial cells to form tight junctions and to establish proper apicobasal polarity and this is probably another pathway that E6 follows to disrupt the cellular system (Latorre et al., 2005). On the other hand, E6 interacts and promotes the degradation of NHERF-1, a PDZ domain containing protein leading to the activation of the PI3K/AKT signaling pathway (Accardi et al., 2011), and promoting cellular proliferation also by this mechanism. Furthermore, E6 protein participates in the up-regulation of SGLT1 promoting the glucose intake in tumor cells (Leiprecht et al., 2011).

4.3 E7 oncoprotein

4.3.1 E7 biochemical properties

The nucleotide sequence of *E7* oncogenes are highly conserved among different HPV types. The *E7* ORF encodes for a small acidic phosphoprotein of 98 amino acids. The predicted molecular weight of this E7 protein is 11 kDa and 14 kDa when phosphorylated *in vitro*, characteristics that are observed in the E7 protein from HPV16 (Armstrong & Roman, 1993). However, the electrophoretic mobility of HPV16 E7 protein observed when analyzed by SDS-PAGE is approximately 17 kDa and this molecular weight is not affected by *in vitro* phosphorylation by CKII (Armstrong & Roman, 1992; Gage et al., 1990). Heck and coworkers (1992) showed that the anomalous behavior of the HPV16 E7 protein resides within the amino-terminal residues that confer a net negative charge to the protein.

The E7 proteins of different HPV types are highly similar among them and share 3 regions of homology with the Adenovirus E1A protein and with the SV40 large T antigen (Fig. 3) (Barbosa et al., 1990; Brokaw et al., 1994). The amino-terminal portion of E7 protein contains the CR1 (Consensus Region 1) between amino acids 1-20 important for DNA synthesis and cellular transformation (Gulliver et al., 1997). The CR2 (aa 21-43) contains the binding site for pRb (aa 21-26), the phosphorylation sites for CKII (aa 31 and 32) and the site for binding the cyclin A-E2F complex (Barbosa et al., 1990; Gulliver et al., 1997; Münger et al., 1989). Although the C-terminal region of the HPV16 E7 (aa 44-98) does not contain an extensive amino acid homology with the CR3 of E1A, it consists of a metal binding domain composed of two CXXC motifs separated by 29 amino acids (Fig. 3) (Brokaw et al., 1994; Phelps et al., 1988). The E7 proteins from HPV16 and 18 are able to bind Zn^{+2} with the CXXC motifs, sites that are important for dimerization and intracellular stabilization of the molecule (Clemmens et al., 1995). This region also contains a low affinity pRb binding site and is involved in the disruption of the E2F/pRb1 complex (Braspenning et al., 1998).

Different molecular weights for E7 have been reported and suggested that the negative charge and the N-terminal region of the protein are related to these changes. Pulse-chase experiments by Smotkin and Wettstein (1987) with HPV16 were unable to detect changes in the E7 protein mobility in SDS-PAGE, suggesting that no other modifications were present. However, other groups have reported the presence of two E7 species in HPV6, 16 and 18 (Gage et al., 1990; Greenfield et al., 1991; Sato et al., 1990; Selvey et al., 1994), but neither the origin or the biological significance have been explained. The presence of phosphorylated species of E7 can explain some of the different molecular weights, although treatment of E7 protein with alkaline phosphatase suggests the presence of other posttranslational modifications (Selvey et al., 1994). Differences in cellular localization also exist for the E7 protein, some groups have reported this protein as cytoplasmic, but others have found it in nucleus (Kanda et al., 1991; Sato et al., 1990; Selvey et al., 1994).

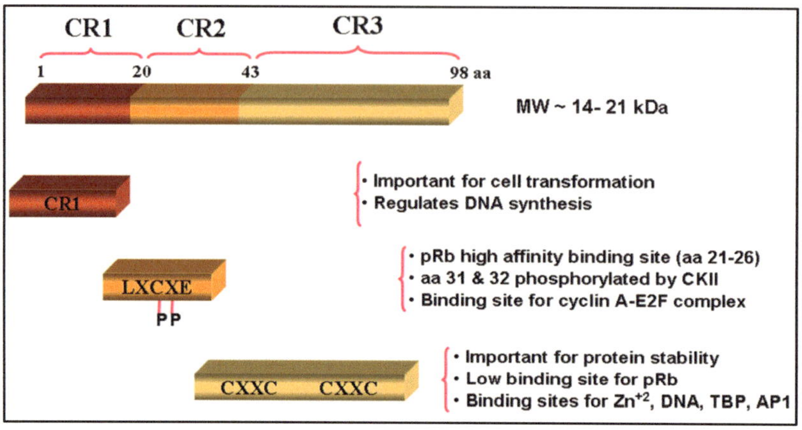

Fig. 3. Biochemical characteristics of HPV16 E7 protein. The HPV16 E7 protein has been reported with different eletrophoretical molecular weights (from 14-21 kDa), differences that have been partially explained by the net negative charge of the protein. E7 shares 3 homology regions with the Adenovirus E1A protein and with the SV40 large T antigen denoted as CR1, 2 and 3. Mutational analysis of the E7 protein has shown that CR1 is important for cellular transformation; CR2 contains the high affinity binding site (LXCXE) for pRb and the phosphorylation sites for CKII (aa 31 and 32); CR3 contains two binding motifs (CXXC) for Zn^{+2} important for the protein stability and DNA binding.

The HPV16 E7 is able to translocate through the nuclear pores via a non-classical Ran-dependent pathway, independent of the main cytosolic Kap beta import receptors (Angeline et al., 2003), and it possesses two NLSs and one NES domains to shuttle between nucleus and cytoplasm (Knapp et al., 2009). Recently, our group identified 3 isoforms of E7 from HPV16 present in CasKi cells, E7a1 (17.5 kDa and IEP of 4.68), E7a (17 kDa and IEP of 6.18) and E7b (16 kDa and IEP of 6.96). The processing of the E7 protein was followed up by pulse-chase experiments and found that the first isoform synthesized was a 17 kDa protein and after approximately 1 h, it was processed to a faster moving band of 16 kDa with a short half-life (Valdovinos-Torres et al., 2008). A broad phosphorylated band of a calculated molecular weight of 17.5 kDa was also identified, and this could be the 17 kDa protein that due to the change in charge because phosphorylation is retarded in the SDS-PAGE. However, the lower molecular weight band of 16 kDa could not be explained by phosphorylation and it is suggested that an unidentified posttranslational modification could exist and generated the E7b isoform (Valdovinos-Torres et al., 2008). Until now, the only posttranslational modification identified for E7 has been the phosphorylation. However, immunofluorescence experiments in our laboratory have shown that a fraction of E7 is present in ER and Golgi apparatus (Fig. 4 and Valdovinos-Torres et al., 2008). This suggests that during the processing and transit of E7 through the different cell compartments, the protein could be posttranslationally modified.

According with the amino acid sequence of the HPV16 E7 protein, it contains putative posttranslational modification sites such as the Asp 29 that can be glycosylated, or modified by sulphation at Tyr 23 and 26, and phosphorylated in four other residues apart from the already known Ser residues 31 and 32. Until now, it is unknown if all these posttranslational modifications apply to E7 protein, but some of them could explain the different molecular weights found and their presence in different cell compartments.

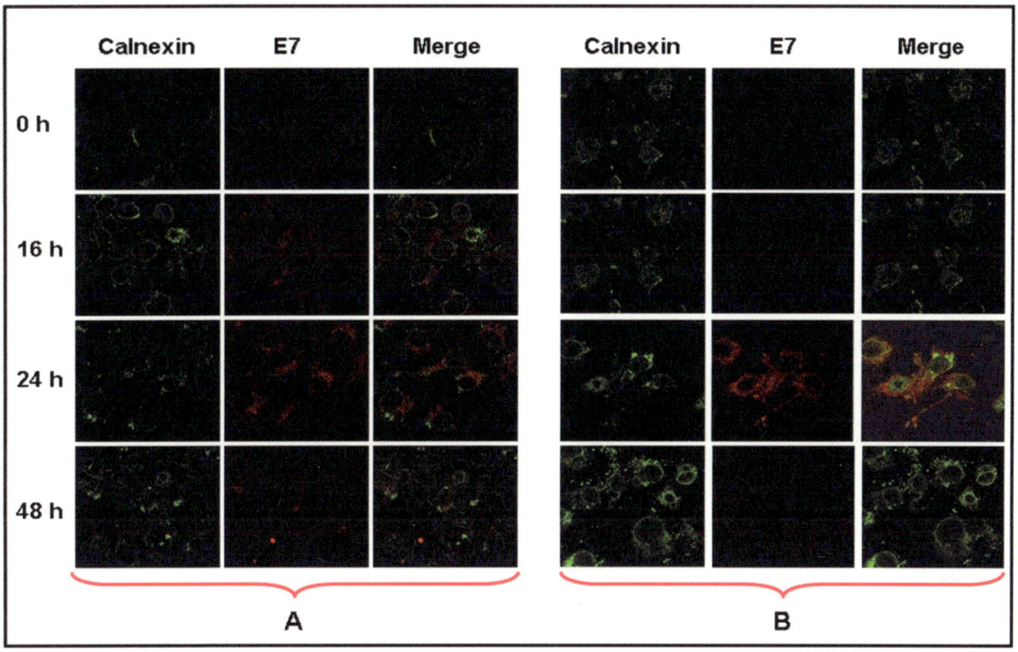

Fig. 4. Immunolocalization of HPV16 E7 protein. Cos-7 cells were transiently transfected with the pcDNA-E7 plasmid and chased for different times (0, 16, 24 and 48 h). Cells were fixed (4% p-formaldehyde) and permeabilized with 0.2% saponine. Cell preparations were tested with different anti-E7 antibodies produced in our laboratory (Valdovinos-Torres et al., 2008). **(A)** Cells were tested with D11 anti-E7 monoclonal antibody and with anti-calnexin polyclonal antibody as marker for ER. **(B)** Cells were tested with B4 anti-E7 monoclonal antibody and calnexin as in **A**. Secondary fluorescent antibodies were anti-rabbit IgG conjugated with Alexa 488 (green) or anti-mouse IgG conjugated with Alexa 594 (red). Images were taken at a magnification of 1000X using Confocal Microscope. The results showed that E7 protein is recognized by different antibodies in different cell compartments as the B4 monoclonal antibody recognized the E7 protein at the ER (co-localized with calnexin), while the D11 monoclonal antibody recognized a different isoform of E7 as no co-localization with calnexin was observed.

4.3.2 E7 functional properties

The E7 proteins are the major oncoproteins of HPVs that do not have known intrinsic enzymatic activities. Expression of HR-HPVs *E6* and *E7* genes in primary human keratinocytes is necessary for immortalization (Hawley-Nelson et al., 1989; Münger et al., 1989). The HPV16 *E7* gene encodes a multifunctional oncoprotein that can subvert multiple cellular regulatory pathways. Studies on mucosal HPV types showed that E7 deregulates the cell cycle mainly by binding to and promoting degradation of the tumor suppressor pRb protein (Caldeira et al., 2005; Collins et al., 2005), resulting in the dissociation of pRb from E2F transcription factors and the premature cell progression into the S-phase of the cell cycle. This activity is mediated by the LXCXE motif and the CR3 zinc binding domain of the E7 protein (Singh et al., 2005). However, E7 from HR-HPVs can also bind E2F1 and activates

E2F1-driven transcription independent of pRb (Hwang et al., 2002). It has been postulated that E7 binds and activates µ-calpain (Darnell et al., 2007) to target pRb, that in turn is poliubiquitinated by cullin 2 (Huh et al., 2007) and degraded by the 26S proteasome through the interaction of E7 with the subunit 4 of the proteasome (Berezutskaya & Bagchi, 1997). In a similar way, E7 affects the pRb-related pocket proteins p107, p130 (Davies et al., 1993; B. Zhang et al., 2006) and the retinoblastoma protein associated factor p600 (Huh et al., 2005). However, cells try to defend themselves from the HPV infection through the expression or activation of molecules such as the transglutaminase 2 that inhibits pRb binding to HPV18 E7, by incorporating polyamine (J.H. Jeon et al., 2003) and PAI-2, and regulating ARF protein expression, which in turn protects pRb from the accelerated degradation mediated by E7 (Darnell et al., 2003). At the same time, the E7 oncoprotein is able to modulate the G2/M phase of the cell cycle by regulating the kinase of the histone H1 through a complex with the p107 protein, effect that allows progression of the viral cycle (Davies et al., 1993). It has also been shown that HPV16 E7 associates mainly with the cyclin A-E2F complex, or to cyclin E retaining their CDK2-associated kinase activity (Ghittoni et al., 2010; He et al., 2003). On the contrary, E7 inhibits the activity of CDK inhibitors $p21^{Waf1}$ (Funk et al., 1997; Jones et al., 1997), $p27^{Kip1}$ (Zerfass et al., 1996) and indirectly the $p16^{INK4a}$ (Giarrè et al., 2001). The regulation of all these cell cycle proteins by E7 may allow the activation of a subset of substrates important for the completion of the viral life cycle.

Apart from the already described E7-protein interactions, there are other groups of E7-target proteins that allow the modification of several different pathways such as metabolism, metastasis, transcription, apoptosis among others, and these subsets of E7-target proteins have been summarized in Table 1.

Finally, E7 has evolved to escape the immune-response by interfering with cytokines signaling pathways: abrogates the immune surveillance by binding to IRF-1 and preventing activation of the INFα and β promoters (Barnard & McMillan, 1999; Park et al., 2000), as well as represses the TGF-β2 promoter by releasing E2F from pRb (Lee et al., 2002b; Murvai et al., 2004). The cytotoxic response against HPV is also evaded by E7 through the down-regulation of TAP1, a key protein for peptide transportation from cytosol into the ER, reducing MHC I-dependent antigen presentation, impairing in this way a specific CTL response (Vambutas et al., 2001).

Cellular differentiation–dependent HPV life cycle has been difficult to study due to the lack of an *in vitro* culture system to differentiate epithelial cells efficiently. The recently development of xenographs and raft cultures have allowed the replication of HPV under *in vitro* conditions (Chow & Broker, 1997). And now, it is important that the activity of the oncogenic viral proteins be examined in their proper physiological contexts with complete viral genomes rather than relying on over-expression assays in different cell types.

5. Proteomics and genomics in the study of HPV

Recent advances in proteomics and genomics have allowed the study of modifications of profiles of cellular proteins and gene transcripts involved in a particular phenomenon compared to a normal status. In this way, Lee and coworkers (2004) identified a group of modulators regulated by *E7* oncogene using proteomics and genomics technology. By using MALDI-TOF MS, 47 spots were identified in a HPV-negative cervical cancer cell line (C33A) stably transfected with HPV16 E7. Proteins like disulfide isomerase A3, integrase interactor 1 protein, glutathione S-transferase P and *vav* proto-oncogene were down-regulated, whereas HSP60, Ku70 binding protein, 26S proteosome subunit were up-regulated. In the genomic approach using DNA microarrays the researchers showed that IL-12Rβ, cytochrome c and TNF II were induced by *E7* oncogene (K.A. Lee et al., 2004).

Activity Pathways subgroups	Proteins Modulated by HPV E7	References
1) Metabolism-related	Pyruvate kinase α-glucosidase	Zwerschke et al.,1999, 2000
2) Metastasis suppressors	Nm23-H1 Nm23-H2	Mileo et al., 2006
3) Transcription factors	TBP TAF-110 AP-1 family factors MPP2 SMAD3 MYC p48 from ISGF3 complex	Massimi et al., 1996 Mazzarelli et al., 1995 Antinore et al., 1996 Lüscher-Firzlaff et al., 1999 D.K. Lee et al., 2002b Y.W. Wang et al., 2007 Barnard & McMillan, 1999
4) Transcriptional coactivators	pCAF acetyltransferase FHL2 Skip IRF1 SRC-1 p300 TAF9	Avvakumov et al., 2003 Campo-Fernández et al., 2007 Prathapam et al., 2001 Park et al., 2000 Baldwin et al., 2006 Bernat et al., 2003 Enzenauer et al., 1998
5) Transcriptional repressors	E2F6	McLaughlin-Drubin et al., 2008
6) DNA modifying enzymes	DNMT1 BRG-1 from SW1/SNF complex	Burgers et al., 2007 D. Lee et al., 2002a
7) Histone-related	Mi2β from NURD complex	Brehm et al., 1999
8) Tumor suppressor	BRCA1 hTid1-TNF-α modulator	Y. Zhang et al., 2005b Schilling et al., 1998
9) Senescence regulators	DEK PML	Wise-Draper et al., 2005 Bischof et al., 2005
10) Anti-apoptotic	Mcl-1	Y.W. Cheng et al., 2008
11) Pro-apoptotic	PP2A Siva-1 IGFBP-3	Pim et al., 2005 Severino et al., 2007 Mannhardt et al., 2000
12) Miscellaneous	TAP-1 γ-tubulin IkB kinase complex F-actin	Vambutas et al., 2001 Nguyen et al., 2007 Spitkovsky et al., 2002 Rey et al., 2000

Table 1. Subsets of E7-target proteins according to activity pathways.

On the other hand, Yim and coworkers (2004b) analyzed the genomic and proteomic expression patterns in 2 different HPV16 E6 transfected human carcinoma cell lines. They reported that among 1024 known genes and expressed sequence tags (ESTs) tested by cDNA microarray and by performing two dimensional gel electrophoresis and MALDI-TOF-MS, the authors found that only the genes and proteins of CDK5, Bak, and I-TRAF matched in both systems, the cDNA microarray and the proteomics. In addition, proteomic profiling of altered proteins by anti-cancer drugs on cervical cancer cells may contribute to provide the fundamental resources for investigation of disease-specific target proteins, elucidation of the novel mechanisms of action and development of new drugs (Yim & Park, 2006) as it has been analyzed with the 5-fluorouracil (5FU) drug (Yim et al., 2004a).

Other study with a genomic approach carried on by Garner-Hamrick and coworkers (2004), analyzed the mRNA from primary human keratinocytes infected with retroviruses that expressed the HPV18 *E6* and *E7* genes and used to generate probes for querying Affymetrix U95A microarrays, which contain >12,500 human gene sequences. The results showed that HPV18 *E6/E7* expression significantly altered the expression of 1,381 genes. A large increase of transcripts associated with DNA and RNA metabolism was observed, with major increases noted for transcription factors, splicing factors and DNA replication elements, among others. Multiple genes associated with protein translation were down-regulated. In addition, major alterations were found in transcripts associated with the cell cycle and cell differentiation.

This review does not include an exhaustive search of all gene transcripts or proteins which expression pattern is altered in each report. In Tables 2 and 3 were summarized only those important genes or proteins that were strongly associated to the phenomenon studied.

HPV Gene	Research Focused on	Concluding Remarks	Refe-rence
		HPV16	
E6/E7	Anti-tumor immunity	Down-regulated: MCP-1, osteopontin and midkine.	Smahel et al., 2005b
E6/E7	Chromosome alterations	HPV16-negative tumors had loss at 18q12.1–23 but gain in HPV16-positive tumors.	Smeets et al., 2006
E6/E7	Chromosome amplifications	Duplication of chromosome 5q and 20q and macrodeletions in chromosomes 6q and 20q.	Ramirez et al., 2004
E6, E7	Chromosome amplifications	Genes (DNA metabolism) up-regulated: 6 in chromosome 20q and 25 in chromosome 5.	Klingelhutz et al., 2005
E6/E7	Differenti-ation	Blocked or delayed differentiation. Alteration in TGFβ expression /TGFβ inducible genes.	Nees et al., 2000
E6/E7	Differenti-ation	Altered expression of 80 cellular genes: INF-responsive genes, NF-kB stimulated genes, cell cycle progression and DNA synthesis.	Nees et al., 2001

HPV Gene	Research Focused on	Concluding Remarks	Refe-rence
E7	Effect of E7 on p53 stability	E7 can modulate normal turnover of p53. No transcriptional consequences on p53 targets.	Eichten et al., 2002
E6/E7	Episome integration	53 genes up-regulated: IFN modulators, EGFR, cytoskeleton proteins, and 32 genes down-regulated during episomal integration.	Alazawi et al., 2002
E6/E7	Episome loss and integration	Activation of antiviral response genes MX1, MX2, OAS1, TRIM22, GIP3 and IRF7.	Pett et al., 2006
E6	Gene expression	Up- or down-regulated genes: 85 in RKO and 70 in A549 cells. Genes and proteins matched: CDK5, Bak and I-TRAF.	Yim et al., 2004b
E6/E7	Gene expression	Expression of 13 genes from HPV16-positive cell lines is down-regulated.	Ruutu et al., 2005
E7	Host cell effectors interaction	E7 interacts with Siva-1 factor.	Severino et al., 2007
E6/E7	Immorta-lization	Over-expression of IGFBP-3 is a late event after E6/E7 expression in the infected cells.	Berger et al., 2002
E6/E7	Immorta-lization and progression	HPV immortalized EGFR null cells have elevated levels of mRNAs of $p21^{Waf1}$ and insulin-like growth factor-binding protein-2 (IGFBP2).	Woodworth et al., 2000
E7	Immuno-surveillance	Induction of IL12Rβ1, cytochrome c and TNFR type II.	K.A. Lee et al., 2004
E6, E7	miRNA in carcinoma	Up-regulation of miR-363 and down-regulation of miR-181a, mR-218, and miR-29a.	Wald et al., 2011
E6/E7	Oncogenicity and metastases	Down-regulation of CKIs (p57 and p16) and up-regulation of S100 proteins (A6, A10) might be involved in the increase of oncogenicity.	Smahel et al., 2005a
E6/E7, E7	Regulation of cellular genes	54 up- or down-regulated genes involved in DNA damage, differentiation, signal transduction, immune response, cell-cycle.	Duffy et al., 2003
E7	Senescence	Associated genes: BRAK, DOC1 and IGFBP-3 but down-regulated in immortalization.	Schwarze et al., 2002
E6/E7	Tumor angiogenesis	Down-regulation thrombospondin-1, maspin and up-regulation of IL-8 and VEGF.	Toussaint et al., 2004
		HPV 18	
E6	Effects of E6 gene knockdown	359 genes up- or down-regulated. Cell cycle: p21; apoptosis: CASP4, CASP6, IGFBP3; ubiquitin proteolysis pathway: UBE3A; differentiation: KRT4, KRT6E, KRT18; anti-oncogenes RECK, VEL.	Min et al., 2009

HPV Gene	Research Focused on	Concluding Remarks	Reference
E6/E7	E2-induced senescence	E2 induces senescence by up-regulating 10 genes (p21) and down-regulating 24.	Wells et al., 2003
E6/E7	Gene expression	Affects DNA synthesis genes: MCM, cdc6, cdc7, PCNA. Regulators: cdk 1-2, CycB, Wee1, CycE. Centrosome abnormalities: Bub1, TTK.	Garner et al., 2004

Table 2. Genomics in HPV research.

HPV Protein	Research Focused on	Concluding Remarks	Reference
		HPV 16	
E6	Chemotherapeutic agents sensitization	Cdc2 is the most dramatically up-regulated protein.	Z.G. Liu et al., 2007
E5	Early cervical cancer markers related to E5	Both EGFR and TfR assays detected HSIL with very high accuracy (100% and 96.3%, respectively).	Keesee et al., 2002
E6/E7****	Expression levels for protein features	This large-scale analysis provides a framework for understanding the cooperation between oncoproteins in HPV-driven carcinogenesis.	Merkley et al., 2009
E5 */**	Expression of membrane proteins	Decreased amount of calnexin and increased hsp70 expression, both associated to MHC-I processing.	Leykauf et al., 2004
E5/E6/E7	HPV proteins immunogenicity	E7 proteins of HR-HPV types are more reactive in cancer patients and discriminating between cancer and HSIL or LSIL patients.	Luevano et al., 2010
E7 */***	Immunosurveillance	36 proteins down-regulated and 11 up-regulated including Ku-70 binding protein involved in DNA metabolism and hsp60 KD protein 1.	K.A. Lee et al., 2004
E6 */***	Protein expression	In RKO and A539 cells: 26 up- and down-regulated proteins. Only three proteins matched with its corresponding gene: CDK5, Bak and I-TRAF.	Yim et al., 2004b
E7*/***	Proteins modulated by E7	Two down-regulated proteins: actin and leukocyte elastase inhibitor and 26 proteins up-regulated, amongst these: catalase and peroxiredoxin.	K.A. Lee et al., 2005
E6/E7 */***	Proteins modulated by E6, E7 or E6/E7	Annexin III, gp96, transaldolase 1, elongation factor 1, proteasome 26S were up-regulated and have been confirmed at the transcriptional level.	Ciotti et al., 2009

HPV Protein	Research Focused on	Concluding Remarks	Reference
E7 */***	Resistance to oxidative stress-induced apoptosis	E7 induces higher resistance to ROS-induced cell injury, probably via the modulation anti-oxidant enzymes, including catalase and peroxiredoxin.	Shim et al., 2005
		HPV 18	
E6/E7 */***	Anti-cancer effect of 5-fluorouracil treatment	22 proteins up-regulated (CIDE-B, caspase-3, caspase-8, Apo-1/CD95 (Fas) and 12 proteins down-regulated (BUB3, c-myc protein, src substrate cortactin, transforming protein p21A, among others).	Yim & Park 2006; Yim et al., 2004a
E6/E7 */***	Anti-cancer effect of paclitaxel treatment	Paclitaxel showed anti- proliferative activity through the (DR)-mediated apoptotic pathway with TRAIL-dependent caspase-8 activation and the mitochondrial-mediated pathway with down-regulation of bcl-2 by cytochrome c release.	K.H. Lee et al., 2005; Yim & Park 2006

Used systems: * 2-DE: two-dimensional electrophoresis; ** nanoESI-MS: nanoelectrospray ionization mass spectrometry; *** MALDI-TOF-MS: matrix-assisted laser desorption/ionization time of flight mass spectrometry; ****2D-DIGE: two-dimensional difference gel electrophoresis.

Table 3. Proteomics in HPV research.

Working with genomics and proteomics is a great challenge as the following issues must be overcome: 1) The use of a standard genomic chip or an appropriate cell line has not been achieved, leading to results not easily comparable between different laboratories; 2) Many genes can be down-regulated or up-regulated during transcriptional profile analysis of a particular phenomenon, but this may not correspond necessarily at all with the proteomic profile; 3) Only a lesser number of proteins actually are modified as consequence of an alteration in the expression of the related gene; 4) Changes in gene expression may predict changes in protein expression, but not necessarily changes in functionality that in most cases is related to protein posttranslational modifications; 5) There are many human genes in data banks that codify for hypothetical proteins which activity or function are not yet known. Therefore, the expression of selected genes needs to be confirmed by means of other kind of procedures like real-time RT-PCR and the corresponding protein analysis by Western blot or in functional assays. In this regard, only two reports showed that some of the proteins studied with altered gene expression matched with the altered protein expression levels (Ciotti et al., 2009; Yim et al., 2004b). More remains to be done in genomics and proteomics, because once all the proteins modified in their expression have been characterized, the researchers need to investigate the way by which the proteins interact with each other, the sequence in which those interactions take place, and finally to establish the mechanism through which cervical cancer develops. This information is of great value when anti-cancer drugs are assayed to attack tumor cells, because the identification of the cellular targets of the drug will help to design better molecules to induce specific malignant cell death. In the case of HPV, these studies are focused on the research of the proteins or genes that are altered by the presence of HR-HPV in the cell. In this sense, the identification of a biomarker to design chips would be useful in high-throughput screening test for uterine cervical cancer (Kim et al., 2006; Steinau et al., 2005), early diagnosis and prediction of response to therapy.

6. Conclusions

Intense work has been done to elucidate the molecular mechanisms through which the HPV E5, E6 and E7 oncoproteins generate cellular transformation. At the same time, it has became clear that the HPV oncoproteins use and modify different signal pathways, specially those related to cell growth, differentiation and apoptosis. The study of the transformation process associated to HPV has given some light about target proteins and disturbed mechanisms that could be considered for the design of drugs, which in the future would be specifically generated for the treatment of HPV associated cancers.

Early detection remains one of the most important issues in cervical cancer research. Therefore, intensive screening to search for biomarkers (genes and/or proteins) particularly sensitive to differences between early and late stage cancer patients is the main target of the new technology. The development of the genomics and proteomics in cervical cancer associated to HPV infection will help in the identification of most accurate biomarkers for an automated early detection of this kind of cancer, as this approach allows the correlation of changes in host gene expression with the biological functions of viral genes. Although proteomics and genomics have simplified the analysis of a great quantity of genes or proteins that are modulated by the presence of HPV oncoproteins in a cell, a major concern has always existed as to whether the discovered biomarkers and the derived multivariate models are truly associated with the disease process. There is still much to do regarding to how these genes or its codified proteins are interconnected and which of them are actually important to the carcinogenic process.

7. References

Accardi, R., Rubino, R., Scalise, M., Gheit, T., Shahzad, N., Thomas, M., Banks. L., Indiveri, C., Sylla, B.S., Cardone, R.A., Reshkin, S.J. & Tommasino, M. (2011). E6 and E7 from human papillomavirus type 16 cooperate to target the PDZ protein Na/H exchange regulatory factor-1. *J Virol*. Vol. 85, No. 16, pp. (8208-8216).

Adam, J.L., Briggs, M.W. & McCance, D.J. (2000). A mutagenic analysis of the E5 protein of human papillomavirus type 16 reveals that E5 binding to the vacuolar H+-ATPase is not sufficient for biological activity, using mammalian and yeast expression systems. *Virol*. Vol. 272, No. 2, pp. (315-325).

Alazawi, W., Pett, M., Arch, B., Scott, L., Freeman, T., Stanley, M.A. & Coleman, N. (2002). Changes in cervical keratinocyte gene expression associated with integration of human papillomavirus 16. *Cancer Res*. Vol. 62, No. 23, pp. (6959-6965).

Alonso, A. & Reed, J. (2002). Modelling of the human papillomavirus type 16 E5 protein. *Biochim Biophys Acta*. Vol. 1601, No. 1, pp. (9-18).

Andresson, T., Sparkowski, J., Goldstein, D.J. & Schlegel, R. (1995). Vacuolar H(+)-ATPase mutants transform cells and define a binding site for the papillomavirus E5 oncoprotein. *J Biol Chem*. Vol. 270, No. 12, pp. (6830-6837).

Androphy, E.J., Hubbert, N.L., Schiller, J.T. & Lowy, D.R. (1987). Identification of the HPV-16 E6 protein from transformed mouse cells and human cervical carcinoma cell lines. *EMBO J*. Vol. 6, No. 4, pp. (989-992).

Angeline, M., Merle, E. & Moroianu, J. (2003). The E7 oncoprotein of high-risk human papillomavirus type 16 enters the nucleus via a nonclassical Ran-dependent pathway. *Virol*. Vol. 317, No. 1, pp. (13-23).

Antinore, M.J., Birrer, M.J., Patel, D., Nader, L. & McCance, D.J. (1996). The human papillomavirus type 16 E7 gene product interacts with and trans-activates the AP1 family of transcription factors. *EMBO J*. Vol. 15, No. 8, pp. (1950-1960).

Araibi, E.H., Marchetti, B., Ashrafi, G.H. & Campo, M.S. (2004). Downregulation of major histocompatibility complex class I in bovine papillomas. *J Gen Virol*. Vol. 85, No. 10, pp. (2809-2814).

Armstrong, D.J. & Roman, A. (1992). Mutagenesis of human papillomavirus types 6 and 16 E7 open reading frames alters the electrophoretic mobility of the expressed proteins. *J Gen Virol*. Vol. 73, No. 5, pp. (1275-1279).

Armstrong, D.J. & Roman, A. (1993). The anomalous electrophoretic behavior of the human papillomavirus type 16 E7 protein is due to the high content of acidic amino acid residues. *Biochem Biophys Res Commun*. Vol. 192, No. 3, pp. (1380-1387).

Ashby, A.D., Meagher, L., Campo, M.S. & Finbow, M.E. (2001). E5 transforming proteins of papillomaviruses do not disturb the activity of the vacuolar H(+)-ATPase. *J Gen Virol*. Vol. 82, No. 10, pp. (2353-2362).

Ashrafi, G.H., Haghshenas, M.R., Marchetti, B., O'Brien, P.M. & Campo, M.S. (2005). E5 protein of human papillomavirus type 16 selectively downregulates surface HLA class I. *Int J Cancer*. Vol. 113, No. 2, pp. (276-283).

Avvakumov, N., Torchia, J. & Mymryk, J.S. (2003). Interaction of the HPV E7 proteins with the pCAF acetyltransferase. *Oncogene*.Vol. 22, No. 25, pp. (3833-3841).

Babbitt, P.C. & Gerlt, J.A. (1997). Understanding enzyme superfamilies. Chemistry As the fundamental determinant in the evolution of new catalytic activities. J Biol Chem. Vol. 272, No. 49 pp. (30591-30594).

Baldwin, A., Huh, K.W. & Münger, K. (2006). Human papillomavirus E7 oncoprotein dysregulates steroid receptor coactivator 1 localization and function. *J Virol*. Vol. 80, No. 13, pp. (6669-6677).

Band, V., Zajchowski, D., Kulesa, V. & Sager, R. (1990). Human Papillomavirus DNAs immortalize normal human mammary epithelial cells and reduce their growth factor requirements. *Proc Natl Acad Sci USA*. Vol. 87, No. 1, pp. (463-467).

Barbaresi, S., Cortese, M.S., Quinn, J., Ashrafi, G.H., Graham, S.V. & Campo, M.S. (2010). Effects of human papillomavirus type 16 E5 deletion mutants on epithelial morphology: functional characterization of each transmembrane domain. *J Gen Virol*. Vol. 91, No. 2, pp. (521-530).

Barbosa, M.S., Edmonds, C., Fisher, C., Schiller, J.T., Lowy, D.R. & Vousden, K.H. (1990). The region of the HPV E7 oncoprotein homologous to adenovirus E1a and SV40 large T antigen contains separate domains for Rb binding and casein kinase II phosphorylation. *EMBO J*. Vol. 9, No. 1, pp. (153-160).

Barnard, P. & McMillan, N.A. (1999). The human papillomavirus E7 oncoprotein abrogates signaling mediated by interferon-alpha. *Virol.* Vol. 259, No. 2, pp. (305-313).

Beerheide, W., Bernard, H.U., Tan, Y.J., Ganesan, A., Rice, W.G. & Ting, A.E. (1999). Potential drugs against cervical cancer: zinc-ejecting inhibitors of the human papillomavirus type 16 E6 oncoprotein. *J Natl Cancer Inst.* Vol. 91, No. 14, pp. (1211-1220).

Belleudi, F., Leone, L, Purpura, V., Cannella, F., Scrofani, C. & Torrisi, M.R. (2011). HPV16 E5 affects the KGFR/FGFR2b-mediated epithelial growth through alteration of the receptor expression, signaling and endocytic traffic. *Oncogene.* May 30. [Epub ahead of print].

Berezutskaya, E. & Bagchi, S. (1997). The human papillomavirus E7 oncoprotein functionally interacts with the S4 subunit of the 26 S proteasome. *J Biol Chem.* Vol. 272, No. 48, pp. (30135-30140).

Berger, A.J., Baege, A., Guillemette, T., Deeds, J., Meyer, R., Disbrow, G., Schlegel, R. & Schlegel, R. (2002). Insulin-like growth factor-binding protein 3 expression increases during immortalization of cervical keratinocytes by human papillomavirus type 16 E6 and E7 proteins. *Am J Pathol.* Vol. 161, No. 2, pp. (603-610).

Bernard, H.U., Chan, S.Y. & Delius, H. (1994). Evolution of papillomaviruses. *Curr Top Microbiol Immunol.* Vol. 186, pp. (33-53).

Bernard, H.U. (2005). The clinical importance of the nomenclature, evolution and taxonomy of human Papillomaviruses. *J Clin Virol.* Vol. 32, S1, pp. (S1-S6).

Bernard, H.U., Burk, R.D., Chen, Z., van Doorslaer, K., zur Hausen, H. & de Villiers, E.M. (2010). Classification of papillomaviruses (PVs) based on 189 PV types and proposal of taxonomic amendments. *Virol.* Vol. 401, No. 1, pp. (70-79).

Bernat, A., Avvakumov, N., Mymryk, J.S. & Banks, L. (2003). Interaction between the HPV E7 oncoprotein and the transcriptional coactivator p300. *Oncogene.* Vol. 22, No. 39, pp. (7871-7881).

Bischof, O., Nacerddine, K. & Dejean, A. (2005). Human papillomavirus oncoprotein E7 targets the promyelocytic leukemia protein and circumvents cellular senescence via the Rb and p53 tumor suppressor pathways. *Mol Cell Biol.* Vol. 25, No. 3, pp. (1013-1024).

Bousarghin, L., Touze, A., Sizaret, P.Y. & Coursaget P. (2003). Human Papillomavirus types 16, 31 and 58 use different endocytosis pathways to enter cells. *J Virol.* Vol. 77, No. 6, pp. (3846-3850).

Bouvard, V., Matlashewski, G., Gu, Z-M., Storey, A. & Banks L. (1994). The human papillomavirus type 16 E5 gene cooperates with the E7 gene to stimulate proliferation of primary cells and increases viral gene expression. *Virol.* Vol. 203, No. 1, pp. (73-80).

Braspenning, J., Marchini, A., Albarani, V., Levy, L., Ciccolin, F., Cremonesi, C., Ralston, R., Gissmann, L., Tommasino, M. (1998). The CXXC Zn binding motifs of the human papillomavirus type 16 E7 oncoprotein are not required for its *in vitro* transforming activity in rodent cells. *Oncogene.* Vol. 16, No. 8, pp. (1085-1089).

Bravo, I.G. & Alonso, A. (2004). Mucosal human papillomaviruses encode four different E5 proteins whose chemistry and phylogeny correlate with malignant or benign growth. J Virol. Vol. 78, No. 24, pp. (13613-13626).

Bravo, I.G. & Alonso, A. (2007). Phylogeny and evolution of papillomaviruses based on the E1 and E2 proteins. *Virus Genes*. Vol. 34, No. 3, pp. (249-262).

Brehm, A., Nielsen, S.J., Miska, E.A., McCance, D.J., Reid, J.L., Bannister, A.J. & Kouzarides, T. (1999). The E7 oncoprotein associates with Mi2 and histone deacetylase activity to promote cell growth. *EMBO J*. Vol. 18, No. 9, pp. (2449-2458).

Briggs, M.W., Adam, J.L. & McCance, D.J. (2001). The human papillomavirus type 16 E5 protein alters vacuolar H(+)-ATPase function and stability in *Saccharomyces cerevisiae*. *Virol*. Vol. 280, No. 2, pp. (169-175).

Brokaw, J.L., Yee, C.L. & Münger, K. (1994). A mutational analysis of the amino terminal domain of the human papillomavirus type 16 E7 oncoprotein. *Virol*. Vol. 205, No. 2, pp. (603-607).

Buck, C.B., Thompson, C.D., Pang, Y.Y.S., Lowy, D.R. & Schiller, J.T. (2005). Maturation of Papillomavirus capsids. *J Virol*. Vol. 79, No. 5, pp. (2839-2846).

Burgers, W.A., Blanchon, L., Pradhan, S., de Launoit, Y., Kouzarides, T. & Fuks, F. (2007). Viral oncoproteins target the DNA methyltransferases. *Oncogene*. Vol. 26, No. 11, pp. (1650-1655).

Butz, K. & Hoppe-Seyler, F. (1993). Transcriptional control of Human Papillomavirus (HPV) oncogene expression: composition of the HPV type 18 upstream regulatory region. *J Virol*. Vol. 67, No. 11, pp. (6476-6486).

Caldeira, S., Dong, W. & Tommasino, M. (2005). Analysis of E7/Rb associations. *Methods Mol Med*. Vol. 119, pp. (363-379).

Campo-Fernández, B., Morandell, D., Santer, F.R., Zwerschke, W. & Jansen-Dürr, P. (2007). Identification of the FHL2 transcriptional coactivator as a new functional target of the E7 oncoprotein of human papillomavirus type 16. *J Virol*. Vol. 81, No. 2, pp. (1027-1032).

Cartin, W. & Alonso, A. (2003). The human papillomavirus HPV2a E5 protein localizes to the Golgi apparatus and modulates signal transduction. *Virol*. Vol. 314, No, 2, pp. (572-579).

Chakrabarti, O., Veeraraghavalu, K., Tergaonkar, V., Liu, Y., Androphy, E.J., Stanley, M.A. & Krishna, S. (2004). Human Papillomavirus type 16 E6 amino acid 83 variants enhance E6-medated MAPK signaling and differentially regulate tumorigenesis by Notch signaling and oncogenic Ras. *J Virol*. Vol. 78, No. 11, pp. (5934-5945).

Chang, J.L., Tsao, Y.P., Liu, D.W., Huang, S.J., Lee, W.H. & Chen, S.L. (2001). The expression of HPV-16 E5 protein in squamous neoplastic changes in the uterine cervix. *J Biomed Sci*. Vol. 8, No. 2, pp. (206–213).

Chen, J.J., Reid, C.E., Band, V. & Androphy, E.J. (1995). Interaction of papillomavirus E6 oncoproteins with a putative calcium-binding protein. *Science*. Vol. 269, No. 5223, pp. (529-531).

Chen, J.J., Hong, Y., Rustamzadeh, E., Baleja, J.D. & Androphy, E.J. (1998). Identification of an alpha helical motif sufficient for association with papillomavirus E6. *J Biol Chem*. Vol. 273, No. 22, pp. (13537–13544).

Chen, S.L., Tsao, Y.P., Yang, C.M., Lin, Y.K., Huang, C.H. & Kuo, S.W. (1995). Differential induction and regulation of the c-*jun*, *junB*, *junD* and c-*fos* by human papillomavirus type 11 E5a oncoprotein. *J Gen Virol*. Vol. 76, No. 11, pp. (2653-2659).

Chen, S.L., Huang, C.H., Tsai, T.C., Lu, K.Y. & Tsao, Y.P. (1996a). The regulation mechanism of c-*jun* and *junB* by human papillomavirus type 16 E5 oncoprotein. *Arch Virol*. Vol. 141, No. 5, pp. (791-800).

Chen, S.L., Lin, Y.K., Li, L.Y., Tsao, Y.P., Lo, H.Y., Wang, W.B. & Tsai, T.C. (1996b). E5 proteins of human papillomavirus types 11 and 16 transactivate the c-*fos* promoter through the NF1 binding element. *J Virol*. Vol. 70, No. 12, pp. (8558-8563).

Chen, S.L., Tsai, T.Z., Han, C.P. & Tsao, Y.P. (1996c). Mutational analysis of human papillomavirus type 11 E5a oncoprotein. *J Virol*. Vol. 70, No. 6, pp. (3502-3508).

Cheng, Y.W., Lee, H., Shiau, M.Y., Wu, T.C., Huang, T.T. & Chang, Y.H. (2008). Human papillomavirus type 16/18 upregulates the expression of interleukin-6 and antiapoptotic Mcl-1in non-small cell lung cancer. *Clin Cancer Res*. Vol. 14, No. 15, pp. (4705–4712).

Chow, L.T. & Broker, T.R. (1997). In vitro experimental systems for HPV: epithelial raft cultures for investigations of viral reproduction and pathogenesis and for genetic analyses of viral proteins and regulatory sequences. *Clin Dermatol*. Vol. 15, No. 2, PP. (217-227).

Ciotti, M., Marzano, V., Giuliani, L., Nuccetelli, M., D'Aguanno, S., Azzimonti, B., Bernardini, S., Perno, C.F., Urbani, A., Favalli, C. & Federici, G. (2009). Proteomic investigation in A549 lung cell line stably infected by HPV16E6/E7 oncogenes. *Respiration*. Vol. 77, No. 4, pp. (427-439).

Clemmens, K.E., Brent, R., Gyiuris, J. & Münger, K. (1995). Dimerization of the human papillomavirus E7 oncoprotein *in vivo*. *Virol*. Vol. 214, pp. (289-293).

Collins, A.S., Nakahara, T., Do, A. & Lambert, P.F. (2005). Interactions with pocket proteins contribute to the role of human papilomavirus type 16 E7 in the papillomavirus life cycle. *J Virol*. Vol. 79, No. 23, pp. (14769-14780).

Conrad, M., Bubb, V.J., & Schlegel, R. (1993). The human papillomavirus type 6 and 16 E5 proteins are membrane-associated proteins which associate with the 16-kilodalton pore-forming protein. *J Virol*. Vol. 67, No. 10, pp. (6170-6178).

Conway, M.J. & Meyers, C. (2009). Replication and assembly of human papillomaviruses. *J Dent Res*. Vol. 88, No. 4, pp. (307-317).

Cooper, B., Schneider, S., Bohl, J., Jiang, Y., Beaudet, A. & Vande Pol, S. (2003). Requirement of E6AP and the features of human papillomavirus E6 necessary to support degradation of p53. *Virol*. Vol. 306, No. 1, pp. (87-99).

Cortese, M.S., Ashrafi, G.H. & Campo, M.S. (2010). All 4 di-leucine motifs in the first hydrophobic domain of the E5 oncoprotein of human papillomavirus type 16 are essential for surface MHC class I downregulation activity and E5 endomembrane localization. *Int J Cancer*. Vol. 126, No. 7, pp. (1675–1682).

Crusius, K., Auvinen, E. & Alonso, A. (1997). Enhancement of EGF- and PMA-mediated MAP kinase activation in cells expressing the human papillomavirus type 16 E5 protein. *Oncogene*. Vol. 15, No. 12, pp. (1437-1444).

Crusius, K., Auvinen, E., Steuer, B., Gaissert, H. & Alonso, A. (1998). The human papillomavirus type 16 E5-protein modulates ligand-dependent activation of the EGF receptor family in the human epithelial cell line HaCaT. *Exp Cell Res*. Vol. 241, No. 1, pp. (76-83).

Crusius, K., Kaszkin, M., Kinzel, V. & Alonso, A. (1999). The human papillomavirus type 16 E5 protein modulates phospholipase C-gamma-1 activity and phosphatidyl inositol turnover in mouse fibroblasts. *Oncogene*. Vol. 18, No, 48, pp. (6714-6718).

Crusius, K., Rodriguez, I. & Alonso, A. (2000). The human papillomavirus type 16 E5 protein modulates ERK1/2 and p38 MAP kinase activation by an EGFR-independent process in stressed human keratinocytes. *Virus Genes*. Vol. 20, No. 1, pp. (65-69).

Darnell, G.A., Antalis, T.M., Johnstone, R.W., Stringer, B.W., Ogbourne, S.M., Harrich, D. & Suhrbier, A. (2003). Inhibition of retinoblastoma protein degradation by interaction with the serpin plasminogen activator inhibitor 2 via a novel consensus motif. *Mol Cell Biol*. Vol. 23, No. 18, pp. (6520-6532).

Darnell, G.A., Schroder, W.A., Antalis, T.M., Lambley, E., Major, L., Gardner, J., Birrell, G., Cid-Arregui, A. & Suhrbier, A. (2007). Human papillomavirus E7 requires the protease calpain to degrade the retinoblastoma protein. *J Biol Chem*. Vol. 282, No. 52, pp. (37492-37500).

Das, S., El-Deiry, W.S. & Somasundaram, K. (2003). Efficient growth inhibition of HPV 16 E6-expressing cells by an adenovirus-expressing p53 homologue p73beta. *Oncogene*. Vol. 22, No. 52, pp. (8394-8402).

Davies, R., Hicks, R., Crook, T., Morris, J. & Vousden, K. (1993). Human papillomavirus type 16 E7 associates with a histone H1 kinase and with p107 through sequences necessary for transformation. *J Virol*. Vol. 67, No. 5, pp. (2521-2528).

Davy, C.E., Jackson, D.J., Wang, Q., Raj, K., Masterson, P.J., Fenner, N.F., Southern, S., Cuthill, S., Millar, J.B. & Doorbar, J. (2002). Identification of a G(2) arrest domain in the E1^E4 protein of human papillomavirus type 16. *J Virol*. Vol. 76, No. 19, pp. (9806–9818).

Day, P.M., Baker, C.C., Lowy, D.R., & Schiller, J.T. (2004). Establishment of papillomavirus infection is enhanced by promyelocytic leukemia protein (PML) expression. *Proc Natl Acad Sci USA*. Vol. 101, No. 39, pp. (14252-14257).

de Villiers, EM. (1989). Minireview: Heterogeneity of the Human Papillomavirus group. *J Virol*. Vol. 63, No. 11, pp. (4898-4903).

de Villiers, E.M., Fauquet, C., Broker, T.R., Bernard, H.U. & zur Hausen, H. (2004). Classification of Papillomaviruses. *Virol*. Vol. 324, No. 1, pp. (17-27).

Di Domenico, F., Foppoli, C., Blarzino, C., Perluigi, M., Paolini, F., Morici, S., Coccia, R., Cini, C. & De Marco, F. (2009). Expression of Human papillomavirus type 16 E5 protein in amelanotic melanoma cells regulates endo-cellular pH and restores tyrosinase activity. *J Exp Clin Cancer Res*. Vol. 28, No. 1, pp. (4).

Disbrow, G.L., Hanover, J.A. & Schlegel, R. (2005). Endoplasmic reticulum-localized human papillomavirus type 16 E5 protein alters endosomal pH but not trans-Golgi pH. *J Virol*. Vol. 79, No. 9, pp. (5839-5846).

Doorbar, J., Evans, H.S., Coneron, I., Crawford, L.V. & Gallimore, P.H. (1988). Analysis of HPV-1 E4 gene expression using epitope-defined antibodies. *EMBO J*. Vol. 7, No. 3, pp. (825-833).

Doorbar, J., Medcalf, E. & Napthine, S. (1996). Analysis of HPV1 E4 complexes and their association with keratins *in vivo*. *Virol*. Vol. 218, No. 1, pp. (114–126).

Doorbar, J. (2005). The papillomavirus life cycle. *J Clin Virol*. Vol. 32, Suppl 1, pp. (S7-S15).

Doorbar, J. (2006). Molecular biology of human papillomavirus infection and cervical cancer. *Clin Sci*. Vol. 110, No. 5, pp. (525-541).

Du, M., Fan, X., Hong, E. & Chen, J.J. (2002). Interaction of oncogenic papillomavirus E6 proteins with fibulin-1. *Biochem Biophys Res Commun*. Vol. 296, No. 4, pp. (962-969).

Duffy, C.L., Phillips, S.L. & Klingelhutz, A.J. (2003). Microarray analysis identifies differentiation-associated genes regulated by human papillomavirus type 16 E6. *Virol*. Vol. 314, No. 1, pp. (196-205).

Dyson, N., Guida, P., Munger, K. & Harlow, E. (1992). Homologous sequences in adenovirus E1A and human papillomavirus E7 proteins mediate interaction with the same set of cellular proteins. *J Virol*. Vol. 66, No. 12, pp. (6893-6902).

Eichten, A., Westfall, M., Pietenpol, J.A. & Munger, K. (2002). Stabilization and functional impairment of the tumor suppressor p53 by the human papillomavirus type 16 E7 oncoprotein. *Virol*. Vol. 295, No. 1, pp. (74-85).

Elston, R.C., Napthine, S. & Doorbar, J. (1998). The identification of a conserved binding motif within human papillomavirus type 16 E6 binding peptides, E6AP and E6BP. *J Gen Virol*. Vol. 79, No. 2, pp. (371-374).

Enzenauer, C., Mengus, G., Lavigne, A., Davidson, I., Pfister, H. & May, M. (1998). Interaction of human papillomavirus 8 regulatory proteins E2, E6 and E7 with components of the TFIID complex. *Intervirology*. Vol. 41, No. 2-3, pp. (80-90).

Farthing, A.J. & Vousden, K.H. (1994). Functions of Human Papillomavirus E6 and E7 oncoproteins. *Trends Microbiol*.Vol. 2, No. 5, pp. (170-173).

Filippova, M., Filippov, V.A., Kagoda, M., Garnett, T., Fodor, N. & Duerksen-Hughes, J. (2009). Complexes of human papillomavirus type 16 E6 proteins form pseudo-death-inducing signaling complex structures during Tumor Necrosis Factor-Mediated Apoptosis. *J Virol*. Vol. 83, No. 1, pp. (210-227).

Funk, J.O., Waga, S., Harry, J.B., Espling, E., Stillman, B. & Galloway, D.A. (1997). Inhibition of CDK activity and PCNA-dependent DNA replication by p21 is blocked by interaction with the HPV-16 E7 oncoprotein. *Genes Dev*. Vol. 11, No. 16, pp. (2090-2100).

Gage, J.R., Meyers, C. & Wettstein, F.O. (1990). The E7 proteins of the nononcogenic human papillomavirus type 6b (HPV-6b) and of the oncogenic HPV-16 differ in retinoblastoma protein binding and other properties. *J Virol*. Vol. 64, No. 2, pp. (723-730).

Gaillard-R, C., Breitburd, F. & Orth, G. (1992). Human Papillomavirus type 1 E4 N-terminal ends have distinct cellular localizations when transiently expressed *in vitro*. *J Virol*. Vol. 66, No. 2, pp. (816-823).

Gao, Q., Srinivasan, S., Boyer, S,N., Wazer, D.E. & Band, V. (1999). The E6 oncoproteins of high-risk papillomaviruses bind to a novel putative GAP protein, E6TP1, and target it for degradation. *Mol Cell Biol*. Vol. 19, No. 1, pp. (733-744).

Garner-Hamrick, P.A., Fostel, J.M., Chien, W.M., Banerjee, N.S., Chow, L.T., Broker, T.R. & Fisher, C. (2004). Global effects of human papillomavirus type 18 E6/E7 in an organotypic keratinocyte culture system. *J Virol*. Vol. 78, No. 17, pp. (9041-9050).

Genther-Williams, S.M., Disbrow, G.L., Schlegel, R., Lee, D., Threadgill, D.W. & Lambert, P.F. (2005). Requirement of epidermal growth factor receptor for hyperplasia induced by E5, a high-risk human papillomavirus oncogene. *Cancer Res*. Vol. 65, No. 15, pp. (6534-6542).

Gewin, L., Myers, H., Kiyono, T. & Galloway, D.A. (2004). Identification of a novel telomerase repressor that interacts with the human papillomavirus type-16 E6/E6-AP complex. *Genes Dev*. Vol. 18, No. 18, pp. (2269-2282).

Ghittoni, R., Accardi, R., Hasan, U., Gheit, T., Sylla, B. & Tommasino, M. (2010). The biological properties of E6 and E7 oncoproteins from human papillomaviruses. *Virus Genes*. Vol. 40, No. 1, pp. (1-13).

Giarrè, M., Caldeira, S., Malanchi, I., Ciccolini, F., Leão, M.J. & Tommasino, M. (2001). Induction of pRb degradation by the human papillomavirus type 16 E7 protein is essential to efficiently overcome p16INK4a-imposed G1 cell cycle Arrest. *J Virol*. Vol. 75, No. 10, pp. (4705-4712).

Gill, D.K., Bible, J.M., Biswas, C., Kell, B., Best, J.M., Punchard, N.A. & Cason, J. (1998). Proliferative T-cell responses to human papillomavirus type 16 E5 are decreased amongst women with high-grade neoplasia. *J Gen Virol*. Vol. 79, No. 8, pp. (1971-1976).

Greenfield, I., Nickerson, J., Penman, S. & Stanley, M. (1991). Human papillomavirus 16 E7 protein is associated with the nuclear matrix. *Proc Natl Acad Sci USA*. Vol. 88, No. 24, pp. (11217-11221).

Grm, H.S. & Banks, L. (2004). Degradation of hDlg and MAGIs by human papillomavirus E6 is E6-AP-independent. *J Gen Virol*. Vol. 85, No. 10, pp. (2815-2819).

Gryfe, R., Swallow, C., Bapat, B., Redston, M., Gallinger, S. & Couture, J. (1997). Molecular biology of colorectal cancer. *Curr Probl Cancer*. Vol. 21, No. 5, pp. (233-300).

Gulliver, G.A., Herber, R.L., Liem, A. & Lambert, P.F. (1997). Both conserved region 1 (CR1) and CR2 of the human papillomavirus type 16 E7 oncogene are required for induction of epidermal hyperplasia and tumor formation in transgenic mice. *J Virol*. Vol. 71, No. 8, pp. (5905-5914).

Gupta, S., Takhar, P.P., Degenkolbe, R., Koh, C.H., Zimmermann, H., Yang, C.M., Guan Sim, K., Hsu, S.I. & Bernard, H.U. (2003). The human papillomavirus type 11 and 16 E6 proteins modulate the cell-cycle regulator and transcription cofactor TRIP-Br1. *Virol*. Vol. 317, No. 1, pp. (155-164).

Hagensee, M.E., Yaegashi, N. & Galloway, D.A. (1993). Self-assembly of human papillomavirus type 1 capsids by expression of the L1 protein alone or by coexpression of the L1 and L2 capsid proteins. *J Virol*. Vol. 67, No. 1, pp. (315-322).

Hasan, U.A., Bates, E., Takeshita, F., Biliato, A., Accardi, R., Bouvard, V., Mansour, M., Vincent, I., Gissmann, L., Iftner, T., Sideri, M., Stubenrauch, F. & Tommasino, M. (2007). TLR9 expression and function is abolished by the cervical cancer-associated human papillomavirus type 16. *J Immunol*. Vol. 178, No. 5, pp. (3186-3197).

Hawley-Nelson, P., Vousden, K.H., Hubbert, N.L., Lowy, D.R. & Schiller, J.T. (1989). HPV16 E6 and E7 proteins cooperate to immortalize human foreskin keratinocytes. *EMBO J*. Vol. 8, No. 12, pp. (3905-3910).

He, W., Staples, D., Smith, C. & Fisher, C. (2003). Direct activation of cyclin-dependent kinase 2 by human papillomavirus E7. *J Virol*. Vol. 77, No. 19, pp. (10566-10574).

Heck, D.V., Yee, C.L., Howley, P.M. & Münger, K. (1992). Efficiency of binding the retinoblastoma protein correlates with the transforming capacity of the E7 oncoproteins of the human papillomaviruses. *Proc Natl Acad Sci USA*. Vol. 89, No. 10, pp. (4442-4446).

Holmgren, S.C., Patterson, N.A., Ozbun, M.A. & Lambert, P.F. (2005). The minor capsid protein L2 contributes to two steps in the human papillomavirus type 31 life cycle. *J Virol.* Vol. 79, No. 7, pp. (3938-3948).

Holt, S., Gollahon, L., Willingham, T., Barbosa, M. & Shay, J. (1996). p53 levels in human mammary epithelial cells expressing wild-type and mutant human papillomavirus type 16 (HPV-16) E6 proteins. *Int J Oncol.* Vol. 8, No. 2, pp. (263-270).

Horvath, C.A.J., Boulet, G.A.V., Renoux, V.M., Delvenne, P.O. & Bogers, J.P.J. (2010). Mechanisms of cell entry by human papillomaviruses: an overview. *Virol J.* Vol. 7, No. 1, pp. 11.

Horwitz, B.H., Settleman, J., Prakash, S.S. & DiMaio, D. (1989). Structure, activity, and regulation of the bovine papillomavirus *E5* gene and its transforming protein product. *Curr Top Microbiol Immunol.*Vol. 144, pp. (143-151).

Howie, H.L., Katzenellenbogen, R.A. & Galloway, D.A. (2009). Papillomavirus E6 proteins. *Virol.* Vol. 384, No. 2, pp. (324-334).

Hsieh, C.H., Tsao, Y.P., Wang, C.H., Han, C.P., Chang, J.L., Lee, J.Y. & Chen, S.L. (2000). Sequence variants and functional analysis of human papillomavirus type 16 *E5* gene in clinical specimens. *Arch Virol.* Vol. 145, No. 11, pp. (2273-2284).

Hubert, W.G. & Laimins, L.A. (2002). Human Papillomavirus Type 31 Replication Modes during the Early Phases of the Viral Life Cycle Depend on Transcriptional and Posttranscriptional Regulation of E1 and E2 Expression. *J Virol.* Vol. 76, No. 5, pp. (2263-2273).

Hughes, F.J. & Romanos, M.A. (1993). E1 protein of Human Papillomavirus is a DNA helicase/ATPase. *Nucl Acids Res.* Vol. 21, No. 25, pp. (5817-5823).

Huh, K.W., DeMasi, J., Ogawa, H., Nakatani, Y., Howley, P.M. & Munger, K. (2005). Association of the human papillomavirus type 16 E7 oncoprotein with the 600-kDa retinoblastoma protein-associated factor, p600. *Proc Natl Acad Sci USA.* Vol. 102, No. 32, pp. (11492-11507).

Huh, K., Zhou, X., Hayakawa, H., Cho, J.Y., Libermann, T.A., Jin, J., Harper, J.W. & Munger, K. (2007). Human papillomavirus type 16 E7 oncoprotein associates with the cullin 2 ubiquitin ligase complex, which contributes to degradation of the retinoblastoma tumor suppressor. *J Virol.* Vol. 81, No. 18, pp. (9737-9747).

Hwang, S.G., Lee, D., Kim, J., Seo, T. & Choe, J. (2002). Human papillomavirus type 16 E7 binds to E2F1 and activates E2F1-driven transcription in a retinoblastoma protein-independent manner. *J Biol Chem.* Vol. 277, No. 4, pp. (2923-2930).

Jeon, J.H., Choi, K.H., Cho, S.Y., Kim, C.W., Shin, D.M., Kwon, J.C., Song, K.Y., Park, S.C. & Kim, I.G. (2003). Transglutaminase 2 inhibits Rb binding of human papillomavirus E7 by incorporating polyamine. *EMBO J.* Vol. 22, No. 19, pp. (5273-5282).

Jeon, S. & Lambert, P.F. (1995). Integration of Human Papillomavirus type 16 DNA into the human genome leads to increased stability of E6 and E7 mRNAs: Implications for cervical carcinogenesis. *Proc Natl Acad Sci USA.* Vol. 92, No. 5, pp. (1654-1658).

Jing, M., Bohl, J., Brimer, N., Kinter, M. & Vande Pol, S.B. (2007). Degradation of tyrosine phosphatase PTPN3 (PTPH1) by association with oncogenic human papillomavirus E6 proteins. *J Virol.* Vol. 81, No. 5, pp. (2231-2239).

Jones, D.L., Alani, R.M. & Munger, K. (1997). The human papillomavirus E7 oncoprotein can uncouple cellular differentiation and proliferation in human keratinocytes by abrogating p21Cip1-mediated inhibition of cdk2. *Genes Dev*. Vol. 11, No. 16, pp. (2101-2111).

Kabsch, K., Mossadegh, N., Kohl, A., Komposch, G., Schenkel, J., Alonso, A. & Tomakidi, P. (2004). The HPV-16 E5 protein inhibits TRAIL- and FasL-mediated apoptosis in human keratinocyte raft cultures. *Intervirology*. Vol. 47, No. 1, pp. (48-56).

Kanda, A., Zanma, S., Watanabe, S., Furuno, A. & Yoshiike, K. (1991). Two Inmunodominant regions of the human papillomavirus type 16 E7 protein are masked in the nuclei of monkey COS-1 cells. *Virol*. Vol. 182, pp. (723-731).

Keesee, S.K., Domanik, R. & Patterson, B. (2002). Fully automated proteomic detection of cervical dysplasia. *Anal Quant Cytol Histol*. Vol. 24, No. 3, pp. (137-146).

Kell, B., Jewers, R.J., Cason, J., Pakarian, F., Kaye, J.N. & Best, J.M. (1994). Detection of E5 oncoprotein in human papillomavirus type 16-positive cervical scrapes using antibodies raised to synthetic peptides. *J Gen Virol*. Vol. 75, No. 9, pp. (2451-2456).

Kim, K.H., Yoon, M.S., Na, Y.J., Park, C.S., Oh, M.R. & Moon, W.C. (2006). Development and evaluation of a highly sensitive human papillomavirus genotyping DNA chip. *Gynecol Oncol*. Vol. 100, No. 1, pp. (38-43).

Kim, S.H., Juhnn, Y.S., Kang, S., Park, S.W., Sung, M.W., Bang, Y.J. & Song, Y.S. (2006). Human papillomavirus 16 E5 up-regulates the expression of vascular endothelial growth factor through the activation of epidermal growth factor receptor, MEK/ERK1,2 and PI3K/Akt. *Cell Mol Life Sci*. Vol. 63, No. 7-8, pp. (930-938).

Kim, S.H., Oh, J.M., No, J.H., Bang, Y.J., Juhnn, Y.S. & Song, Y.S. (2009). Involvement of NF-kappaB and AP-1 in COX-2 upregulation by human papilomavirus 16 E5 oncoprotein. *Carcinogenesis*. Vol. 30, No. 5, pp. (753-757).

Kiyono, T., Hiraiwa, A., Fujita, M., Hayashi, Y., Akiyama, T. & Ishibashi, M. (1997). Binding of high-risk human papillomavirus E6 oncoproteins to the human homologue of the Drosophila discs large tumor suppressor protein. *Proc Natl Acad Sci USA*. Vol. 94, No. 21, pp. (11612–11616).

Klingelhutz, A.J., Qian, Q., Phillips, S.L., Gourronc, F.A., Darbro, B.W. & Patil, S.R. (2005). Amplification of the chromosome 20q region is associated with expression of HPV-16 E7 in human airway and anogenital epithelial cells. *Virol*. Vol. 340, No. 2, pp. (237-244).

Knapp, A.A., McManus, P.M., Bockstall, K. & Moroianu, J. (2009). Identification of the nuclear localization and export signals of high risk HPV16 E7 oncoprotein. *Virol*. Vol. 383, No. 1, pp. (60-68).

Koopman, L.A., Szuhai, K., van Eendenburg, J.D.H., Bezrookove, V., Kenter, G.G., Schuuring, E., Tanke, H. & Fleuren, G.J. (1999). Recurrent integration of Human Papillomaviruses 16, 45 and 67 near translocation breakpoints in new cervical cancer cell lines. *Cancer Res*. Vol. 59, No. 21, pp. (5615-5624).

Kühne, C. & Banks, L. (1998). E3-ubiquitin ligase/E6-AP links multicopy maintenance protein 7 to the ubiquitination pathway by a novel motif, the L2G box. *J Biol Chem*. Vol. 273, No. 51, pp. (34302-34309).

Kukimoto, I., Aihara, S., Yoshiike, K. & Kanda, T. (1998). Human papillomavirus oncoprotein E6 binds to the C-terminal region of human minichromosome maintenance 7 protein. *Biochem Biophys Res Commun*. Vol. 249, No. 1, pp. (258-262).

Lambert, P. (1991). Papillomavirus DNA replication. *J Virol*. Vol. 65, No. 7, pp. (3417-3420).

Latorre, I.J., Roh, M.H., Frese, K.K., Weiss, R.S., Margolis, B. & Javier, R.T. (2005). Viral oncoprotein-induced mislocalization of select PDZ proteins disrupts tight junctions and causes polarity defects in epithelial cells. *J Cell Sci*. Vol. 118, No. 18, pp. (4283-4293).

Lee, D., Lim, C., Seo, T., Kwon, H., Min, H. & Choe, J. (2002a). The viral oncogene human papillomavirus E7 deregulates transcriptional silencing by Brm-related gene 1 via molecular interactions. *J Biol Chem*. Vol. 277, No. 50, pp. (48842-48848).

Lee, D.K., Kim, B.C., Kim, I.Y., Cho, E.A., Satterwhite, D.J. & Kim, S.J. (2002b). The human papilloma virus E7 oncoprotein inhibits transforming growth factor-beta signaling by blocking binding of the Smad complex to its target sequence. *J Biol Chem*. Vol. 277, No. 41, pp. (38557-38564).

Lee, K.A., Shim, J.K., Kho, C.W., Park, S.G., Park, B.C., Kim, J.W., Lim, J.S., Choe, Y.K., Paik, S.G. & Yoon, D.Y. (2004). Protein profiling and identification of modulators regulated by E7 oncogene in the C33A cell line by proteomics and genomics. *Proteomics*. Vol. 4, No. 3, pp. (839-848).

Lee, K.A., Kang, J.W., Shim, J.H., Kho, C.W., Park, S.G., Lee, H.G., Paik, S.G., Lim, J.S. & Yoon, D.Y. (2005) Protein profiling and identification of modulators regulated by human papillomavirus 16 E7 oncogene in HaCaT keratinocytes by proteomics. *Gynecol Oncol*. Vol. 99, No. 1, pp. (142-152).

Lee, K.H., Yim, E.K., Kim, C.J., Namkoong, S.E., Um, S.J. & Park, J.S. (2005). Proteomic analysis of anti-cancer effects by paclitaxel treatment in cervical cancer cells. *Gynecol Oncol*.Vol. 98, No. 1, pp. (45-53).

Lee, S.S., Weiss, R.S. & Javier, R.T. (1997). Binding of human virus oncoproteins to hDlg/SAP97, a mammalian homolog of the Drosophila discs large tumor suppressor protein. *Proc Natl Acad Sci USA*. Vol. 94, No. 13, pp. (6670-6675).

Lee, S.S., Glaunsinger, B., Mantovani, F., Banks, L. & Javier, R.T. (2000). Multi-PDZ domain protein MUPP1 is a cellular target for both adenovirus E4-ORF1 and high-risk papillomavirus type 18 E6 oncoproteins. *J Virol*. Vol. 74, No. 20, pp. (9680-9693).

Leechanachai, P., Banks, L., Moreau, F. & Matlashewski, G. (1992). The E5 gene from human papillomavirus type 16 is an oncogene which enhances growth factor-mediated signal transduction to the nucleus. *Oncogene*. Vol. 7, No. 1, pp. (19-25).

Leiprecht, N., Munoz, C., Alesutan, I., Siraskar, G., Sopjani, M., Föller, M., Stubenrauch, F., Iftner, T. & Lang, F. (2011). Regulation of Na(+)-coupled glucose carrier SGLT1 by human papillomavirus 18 E6 protein. *Biochem Biophys Res Commun*. Vol. 404, No. 2, pp. (695-700).

Lewis, C., Baro, M.F., Marques, M., Grüner, M., Alonso, A. & Bravo, I.G. (2008). The first hydrophobic region of the HPV16 E5 protein determines protein cellular location and facilitates anchorage-independent growth. *Virol J*. Vol. 5, No. 1, pp. (30).

Leykauf, K., Salek, M., Schluter, H., Lehmann, W.D. & Alonso, A. (2004). Identification of membrane proteins differentially expressed in human papillomavirus type 16 E5-transfected human keratinocytes by nanoelectrospray ionization mass spectrometry. *J Gen Virol*. Vol. 85, No. 6, pp. (1427-1431).

Lipari, F., McGibbon, G.A., Wardrop, E. & Cordingley, M.G. (2001). Purification and biophysical characterization of a minimal functional domain and of an N-terminal Zn+2-binding fragment from the human papillomavirus type 16 E6 protein. *Biochemistry*. Vol. 40, No. 5, pp. (1196-1204).

Liu, J.P. (1999). Studies of the molecular mechanisms in the regulation of telomerase activity. *FASEB J*. Vol. 13, No. 15, pp. (2091-2104).

Liu, X., Yuan, H., Fu, B., Disbrow, G.L., Apolinario, T., Tomaic, V., Kelley, M.L., Baker, C.C., Huibregtse, J. & Schlegel, R. (2005). The E6AP ubiquitin ligase is required for transactivation of the hTERT promoter by the human papillomavirus E6 oncoprotein. *J Biol Chem*. Vol. 280, No. 11, pp. (10807-10816).

Liu, Y., Cherry, J.J., Dineen, J.V., Androphy, E.J. & Baleja, J.D. (2009) Determinants of stability for the E6 protein of papillomavirus type 16. *J Mol Biol*. Vol. 386, No. 4, pp. (1123-1137).

Liu, Z.G., Zhao, L.N., Liu, Y.W., Li, T.T., Fan, D.M. & Chen, J.J. (2007). Activation of Cdc2 contributes to apoptosis in HPV E6 expressing human keratinocytes in response to therapeutic agents. *J Mol Biol*. Vol. 374, No. 2, pp. (334-345).

Longworth, M.S. & Laimins, L.A. (2004). Pathogenesis of Human Papillomaviruses in differentiating epithelia. *Microbiol Mol Biol Rev*. Vol. 68, No. 2, pp. (362-372).

Lorincz, A.T., Reid, R., Jenson, A.B., Greenberg, M.D., Lancaster, W. & Kurman, R.J. (1992). Human papillomavirus infection of the cervix: relative risk associations of 15 common anogenital types *Obstet Gynecol*. Vol. 79, No. 3, pp. (328-337).

Lu, Z., Hu, X., Li, Y., Zheng, L., Zhou, Y., Jiang, H., Ning, T., Basang, Z., Zhang, C. & Ke, Y. (2004). Human papillomavirus 16 E6 oncoprotein interferences with insulin signaling pathway by binding to tuberin. *J Biol Chem*. Vol. 279, No. 34, pp. (35664-35670).

Luevano, M., Bernard, H.U., Barrera-Saldaña, H.A., Trevino, V., Garcia-Carranca, A., Villa, L.L., Monk, B.J., Tan, X., Davies, D.H., Felgner, P.L. & Kalantari, M. (2010). High-throughput profiling of the humoral immune responses against thirteen human papillomavirus types by proteome microarrays. *Virol*. Vol. 405, No. 1, pp. (31-40).

Lüscher-Firzlaff, J.M., Westendorf, J.M., Zwicker, J., Burkhardt, H., Henriksson, M., Müller, R., Pirollet, F. & Lüscher, B. (1999). Interaction of the fork head domain transcription factor MPP2 with the human papilloma virus 16 E7 protein: enhancement of transformation and transactivation. *Oncogene*. Vol. 18, No. 41, pp. (5620-5630).

Malanchi, I., Accardi, R., Diehl, F., Smet, A., Androphy, E., Hoheisel, J. & Tommasino, M. (2004). Human Papillomavirus Type 16 E6 Promotes Retinoblastoma Protein Phosphorylation and Cell Cycle Progression. *J Virol*. Vol. 78, No. 4, pp. (13769-13778).

Mammas, I.N., Sourvinos, G., Giannoudis, A. & Spandidos, D.A. (2008). Human papillomavirus (HPV) and host cellular interactions. *Pathol Oncol Res*. Vol. 14, No. 4, pp. (345-354).

Mannhardt, B., Weinzimer, S.A., Wagner, M., Fiedler, M., Cohen, P., Jansen-Durr, P. & Zwerschke, W. (2000). Human papillomavirus type 16 E7 oncoprotein binds and inactivates growth-inhibitory insulin-like growth factor binding protein 3. *Mol Cell Biol*. Vol. 20, No. 17, pp. (6483-6495).

Marchetti, B., Ashrafi, G.H., Tsirimonaki, E., O'Brien, P.M. & Campo, M.S. (2002). The bovine papillomavirus oncoprotein E5 retains MHC class I molecules in the Golgi apparatus and prevents their transport to the cell surface. *Oncogene*. Vol. 21, No. 51, pp. (7808-7816).

Marchetti, B., Ashrafi, G.H., Dornan, E.S., Araibi, E.H., Ellis, S.A. & Campo, M.S. (2006). The E5 protein of BPV-4 interacts with the heavy chain of MHC class I and irreversibly retains the MHC complex in the Golgi apparatus. *Oncogene*. Vol. 25, No. 15, pp. (2254-2263).

Massimi, P., Pim, D., Storey, A. & Banks, L. (1996). HPV-16 E7 and adenovirus E1a complex formation with TATA box binding protein is enhanced by casein kinase II phosphorylation. *Oncogene*. Vol. 12, No. 11, pp. (2325-2330).

Massimi, P., Gammoh, N., Thomas, M. & Banks, L. (2004). HPV E6 specifically targets different cellular pools of its PDZ domain-containing tumour suppressor substrates for proteasome-mediated degradation. *Oncogene*. Vol. 23, No. 49, pp. (8033-8039).

Matlashewski, G. (2006) Chapter 11: Papillomaviruses, In: *Fundamentals of Molecular Virology*, Nicholas H. Acheson, pp. (114-122), John Wiley and Sons Ltd, ISBN 9780471351511, USA.

Mazzarelli, J.M., Atkins, G.B., Geisberg, J.V. & Ricciardi, R.P. (1995). The viral oncoproteins Ad5 E1A, HPV16 E7 and SV40 TAg bind a common region of the TBP-associated factor-110. *Oncogene*. Vol. 11, No. 9, pp. (1859-1864).

McLaughlin-Drubin, M.E., Huh, K.W. & Münger, K. (2008). Human papillomavirus type 16 E7 oncoprotein associates with E2F6. *J Virol*. Vol. 82, No. 17, pp. (8695-8705).

Merkley, M.A., Hildebrandt, E., Podolsky, R.H., Arnouk, H., Ferris, D.G., Dynan, W.S. & Stöppler, H. (2009). Large-scale analysis of protein expression changes in human keratinocytes immortalized by human papilloma virus type 16 *E6* and *E7* oncogenes. *Proteome Sci*. Vol. 7, No. 1, pp. (29).

Middleton, K., Peh, W.L., Southern, S., Griffin, H., Sotlar, K., Nakahara, T., El-Sherif, A., Morris, L., Seth, R., Hibma, M., Jenkins, D., Lambert, P., Coleman, N. & Doorbar, J. (2003). Organization of human papillomavirus productive cycle during neoplastic progression provides a basis for selection of diagnostic markers. *J Virol*. Vol. 77, No. 19, pp. (10186-10201).

Mileo, A.M., Piombino, E., Severino, A., Tritarelli, A., Paggi, M.G. & Lombardi, D. (2006). Multiple interference of the human papillomavirus-16 E7 oncoprotein with the functional role of the metastasis suppressor Nm23-H1 protein. *J Bioenerg Biomembr*. Vol. 38, No. 3-4, pp. (215-225).

Min, W., Wen-li, M., Zhao-hui, S., Ling, L., Bao, Z. & Wen-ling, Z. (2009). Microarray analysis identifies differentially expressed genes induced by human papillomavirus type 18 E6 silencing RNA. *Int J Gynecol Cancer*. Vol. 19, No. 4, pp. (547-563).

Moody, C.A. & Laimins, L.A. (2010). Human papillomavirus oncoproteins: pathways to transformation. *Nat Rev Cancer*. Vol. 10, No. 8, pp. (550-560).

Münger, K., Phelps, W.C., Bubb, V., Howley, P.M. & Schlegel, R. (1989). The E6 and E7 genes of the human papillomavirus type 16 together are necessary and sufficient for transformation of primary human keratinocytes. *J Virol*. Vol. 63, No. 10, pp. (4417-4421).

Münger, K., Scheffner, M., Huibregste, J.M. & Howley, P.M. (1992). Interactions of the HPV E6 and E7 oncoproteins with tumour suppressor gene products. *Cancer Surv*. Vol. 12, pp. (197-217).

Münger, K., Baldwin, A., Edwards, K.M., Hayakawa, H., Nguyen, C.L., Owens, M., Grace, M. & Huh, K. (2004). Mechanisms of human papillomavirus-induced oncogenesis. *J Virol.* Vol. 78, No. 21, pp. (11451-11460).

Murvai, M., Borbely, A.A., Konya, J., Gergely, L. & Veress, G. (2004). Effect of human papillomavirus type 16 E6 and E7 oncogenes on the activity of the transforming growth factor-beta2 (TGF-beta2) promoter. *Arch Virol.* Vol. 149, No. 12, pp. (2379-2392).

Myers, G., Lu, H., Calef, C. & Leitner. T. (1996). Heterogeneity of Papillomaviruses. *Sem Cancer Biol.* Vol. 7, No. 6, pp. (349-358).

Nakahara, T., Nishimura, A., Tanaka, M., Ueno, T., Ishimoto, A. & Sakai, H. (2002). Modulation of the cell division cycle by human papillomavirus type 18 E4. *J Virol.* Vol. 76, No. 21, pp. (10914-10920).

Nakagawa, S. & Huibregtse, J.M. (2000). Human scribble (Vartul) is targeted for ubiquitin-mediated degradation by the high-risk papillomavirus E6 proteins and the E6AP ubiquitin-protein ligase. *Mol Cell Biol.* Vol. 20, No. 21, pp. (8244-8253).

Nees, M., Geoghegan, J.M., Munson, P., Prabhu, V., Liu, Y., Androphy, E. & Woodworth, C.D. (2000). Human papillomavirus type 16 E6 and E7 proteins inhibit differentiation-dependent expression of transforming growth factor-beta2 in cervical keratinocytes. *Cancer Res.* Vol. 60, No. 15, pp. (4289-4298).

Nees, M., Geoghegan, J.M., Hyman, T., Frank, S., Miller, L. & Woodworth, C.D. (2001). Papillomavirus type 16 oncogenes downregulate expression of interferon-responsive genes and upregulate proliferation-associated and NF-kappaB-responsive genes in cervical keratinocytes. *J Virol.* Vol. 75, No. 9, pp. (4283-4296).

Nguyen, C.L., Eichwald, C., Nibert, M.L. & Münger, K. (2007). Human papillomavirus type 16 E7 oncoprotein associates with the centrosomal component gamma-tubulin. *J Virol.* Vol. 81, No. 24, pp. (13533-13543).

Nominé, Y., Ristriani, T., Laurent, C., Lefèvre, J.F., Weiss, E., & Travé, G. (2001). Formation of soluble inclusion bodies by HPV E6 oncoprotein fused to Maltose-binding protein. *Protein Expr Purif.* Vol. 23, No. 1, pp. (22–32).

Nominé, Y., Masson, M., Charbonnier, S., Zanier, K., Ristriani, T., Deryckère, F., Sibler, A.P., Desplancq, D., Atkinson, R.A., Weiss, E., Orfanoudakis, G., Kieffer, B. & Travé, G. (2006). Structural and functional analysis of E6 oncoprotein: insights in the molecular pathways of human papillomavirus mediated pathogenesis. *Mol Cell.* Vol. 21, No. 5, pp. (665–678).

Ocadiz, R., Sauceda, R., Cruz, M., Graef, A.M. & Gariglio, P. (1987). High correlation between molecular alterations of the *c-myc* oncogene and carcinoma of the uterine cervix. *Cancer Res.* Vol. 47, No. 15, pp. (4173-4177).

Oh, J.M., Kim, S.H., Lee, Y.I., Seo, M., Kim, S.Y., Song, Y.S., Kim, W.H. & Juhnn, Y.S. (2009). Human papillomavirus E5 protein induces expression of the EP4 subtype of prostaglandin E2 receptor in cyclic AMP response element-dependent pathways in cervical cancer cells. *Carcinogenesis.* Vol. 30, No. 1, pp. (141-149).

Park, J.S., Kim, E.J., Kwon, H.J., Hwang, E.S., Namkoong, S.E. & Um, S.J. (2000). Inactivation of interferon regulatory factor-1 tumor suppressor protein by HPV E7 oncoprotein. Implication for the E7-mediated immune evasion mechanism in cervical carcinogenesis. *J Biol Chem.* Vol. 275, No. 10, pp. (6764-6769).

Pater, M.M. & Pater, A. (1985). Human papillomavirus types 16 and 18 sequences in carcinoma cell lines of the cervix. *Virol.* Vol. 145, No. 2, pp. (313-318).

Pedroza-Saavedra, A., Lam, E.W., Esquivel-Guadarrama, F. & Gutierrez-Xicotencatl, L. (2010). The human papillomavirus type 16 E5 oncoprotein synergizes with EGF-receptor signaling to enhance cell cycle progression and the down-regulation of p27(Kip1). *Virol.* Vol. 400, No. 1, pp. (44-52).

Peh, L.W., Middleton, K., Christensen, N., Nicholls, P., Egawa, K., Soltar, K., Brandsma, J., Percival, A., Lewis, J., Liu, J.W. & Doorbar, J. (2002). Life cycle heterogeneity in animal models of human papillomavirus-associated disease. *J Virol.* Vol. 76, No. 20, pp. (10401-10416).

Peitsaro, P., Johansson, B. & Syrjänen, S. (2002). Integrated human Papillomavirus type 16 is frequently found in cervical cancer precursors as demonstrated by a novel quantitative Real-time PCR technique. *J Clin Microbiol.* Vol. 40, No. 3, pp. (886-891).

Pett, M.R., Herdman, M.T., Palmer, R.D., Yeo, G.S., Shivji, M.K., Stanley, M.A. & Coleman, N. (2006). Selection of cervical keratinocytes containing integrated HPV16 associates with episome loss and an endogenous antiviral response. *Proc Natl Acad Sci USA.* Vol. 103, No. 10, pp. (3822-3827).

Pett, M. & Coleman, N. (2007) Integration of high-risk human papillomavirus: a key event in cervical carcinogenesis? *J Pathol.* Vol. 212, No. 4, pp. (356-367).

Phelps, W.C., Yee, C.L., Münger, K. & Howley, P.M. (1988). The human papillomavirus type 16 E7 gene encodes transactivation and transformation functions similar to those of adenovirus E1A. *Cell.* Vol. 53, No. 4, pp. (539-547).

Pim, D., Massimi, P., Dilworth, S.M. & Banks, L. (2005). Activation of the protein kinase B pathway by the HPV-16 E7 oncoprotein occurs through a mechanism involving interaction with PP2A. *Oncogene.* Vol. 24, No. 53, pp. (7830-7838).

Pim, D., Tomaic, V. & Banks, L. (2009). The human papillomavirus (HPV) E6* proteins from high-risk, mucosal HPVs can direct degradation of cellular proteins in the absence of full-length E6 protein. *J Virol.* Vol. 83, No. 19, pp. (9863-9874).

Pirisi, L., Yasumoto, S., Feller, M., Doniger, J. & DiPaolo, J.A. (1987). Transformation of human fibroblasts and keratinocytes with human papillomavirus type 16 DNA. *J Virol.* Vol. 61, No. 4, pp. (1061-1066).

Prathapam, T., Kühne, C. & Banks, L. (2001). The HPV-16 E7 oncoprotein binds Skip and suppresses its transcriptional activity. *Oncogene.* Vol. 20, No. 52, pp. (7677-7685).

Raibould, R., Fiander, A. & Hibbitts S. (2011). Human Papillomavirus Integration and its Role in Cervical Malignant Progression. *Open Clin Canc J.* Vol. 5, pp. (1-7).

Raj, K., Berguerand, S., Southern, S., Doorbar, J. & Beard, P. (2004). E1 empty set E4 protein of human papillomavirus type 16 associates with mitochondria. *J Virol.* Vol. 78, No. 13, pp. (7199-7207).

Ramirez, R.D., Sheridan, S., Girard, L., Sato, M., Kim, Y., Pollack, J., Peyton, M., Zou, Y., Kurie, J.M., Dimaio, J.M., Milchgrub, S., Smith, A.L., Souza, R.F., Gilbey, L., Zhang, X., Gandia, K., Vaughan, M.B., Wright, W.E., Gazdar, A.F., Shay, J.W. & Minna, J.D. (2004). Immortalization of human bronchial epithelial cells in the absence of viral oncoproteins. *Cancer Res.* Vol. 64, No. 24, pp. (9027-9034).

Rapp, L. & Chen, J.J. (1998). The Papillomavirus E6 proteins. *Biochem Biophys Acta.*Vol. 1378, No. 1, pp. (F1-F9).

Reagan, J.A. & Laimins, L.A. (2008). Bap31 Is a Novel Target of the Human Papillomavirus E5 Protein. *J Virol.* Vol. 82, No. 20, pp. (10042-10051).

Rey, O., Lee, S., Baluda, M.A., Swee, J., Ackerson, B., Chiu, R. & Park, N.H. (2000). The E7 oncoprotein of human papillomavirus type 16 interacts with F-actin *in vitro* and *in vivo*. *Virol.* Vol. 268, No. 2, pp. (372-381).

Ristriani, T., Nominé, Y., Laurent, C., Weiss, E. & Travé, G. (2002). Protein mutagenesis with monodispersity-based quality probing: selective inactivation of p53 degradation and DNA-binding properties of HPV E6 oncoprotein. *Protein Expr Purif.* Vol. 26, No. 3, pp. (357–367).

Roberts, S., Ashmole, I., Gibson, L.J., Rookes, S.M., Barton, G.J. & Gallimore, P.H. (1994). Mutational analysis of Human Papillomavirus E4 proteins: Identification of structural features important in the formation of cytoplasmic E4/ cytokeratin networks in epithelial cells. *J Virol.* Vol. 68, No. 10, pp. (6432-6445).

Rodriguez, M.I., Finbow, M.E. & Alonso, A. (2000). Binding of human papillomavirus 16 E5 to the 16 kDa subunit c (proteolipid) of the vacuolar H+-ATPase can be dissociated from the E5-mediated epidermal growth factor receptor overactivation. *Oncogene.* Vol. 19, No. 33, pp. (3727-3732).

Ronco, L.V., Karpova, A.Y., Vidal, M. & Howley, P.M. (1998). Human papillomavirus 16 E6 oncoprotein binds to interferon regulatory factor-3 and inhibits its transcriptional activity. *Genes Dev.* Vol. 12, No. 13, pp. (2061-2072).

Rush, M., Zhao, X. & Scwartz, S. (2005). A splicing enhancer in the E4 coding region of Human Papillomavirus type 16 is required for early mRNA splicing and polyadenylation as well as inhibition of premature late gene expression. *J Virol.* Vol. 79, No. 18, pp. (12002-12015).

Ruutu, M., Johansson, B., Grenman, R. & Syrjanen, S. (2005). Two different global gene expression profiles in cancer cell lines established from etiologically different oral carcinomas. *Oncol Rep.* Vol. 14, No. 6, pp. (1511-1517).

Sastre-Garau, X., Favre, M., Coutrier, J. & Orth, G. (2000) Distinct patterns of alteration of *myc* genes associated with integration of Human papillomavirus type 16 or type 45 DNA in two genital tumours. *J Gen Virol.* Vol. 81, No. 8, pp. (1983-1993).

Sato, H., Watanabe, S., Furuno, A. & Yoshiike, K. (1990). Human papillomavirus type 16 E7 protein expressed in *Escherichia coli* and monkey COS-1 cells: immunoflorescence detection of the nuclear E7 protein. *Virol.* Vol. 170, No. 1, pp. (311-315).

Schiller, J.T. Day, P.M. & Kines, R.C. (2010). Current understanding of the mechanism of HPV infection. *Gynecol Oncol.* Vol. 118, Suppl. 1, pp. (S12-S17).

Schilling, B., De-Medina, T., Syken, J., Vidal, M., & Munger, K. (1998). A novel human DnaJ protein, hTid-1, a homolog of the Drosophila tumor suppressor protein Tid56, can interact with the human papillomavirus type 16 E7 oncoprotein. *Virol.* Vol. 247, No. 1, pp. (74-85).

Schwarze, S.R., DePrimo, S.E., Grabert, L.M., Fu, V.X., Brooks, J.D. & Jarrard, D.F. (2002). Novel pathways associated with bypassing cellular senescence in human prostate epithelial cells. *J Biol Chem.* Vol. 277, No. 17, pp. (14877-14883).

Selvey, L.A., Dunn, L.A., Tindle, R.W., Park, D.S. & Frazer, I.H. (1994). Human papillomavirus (HPV) type 18 E7 protein is a short-lived steroid-inducible phosphoprotein in HPV-transformed cell lines. *J Gen. Virol.* Vol. 75, No. 7, pp. (1647-1653).

Severino, A., Abbruzzese, C., Manente, L., Valderas, A.A., Mattarocci, S., Federico, A., Starace, G., Chersi, A., Mileo, A.M. & Paggi, M.G. (2007). Human papillomavirus-16 E7 interacts with Siva-1 and modulates apoptosis in HaCaT human immortalized keratinocytes. *J Cell Physiol.* Vol. 212, No. 1, pp. (118-125).
Shah, K.V. & Buscema, J. (1988). Genital warts, papillomaviruses, and genital malignancies. *Annu Rev Med.* Vol. 39, pp. (371-379).
Shim, J.H., Cho, K.J., Lee, K.A., Kim, S.H., Myung, P.K., Choe, Y.K. & Yoon, D.Y. (2005). E7-expressing HaCaT keratinocyte cells are resistant to oxidative stress-induced cell death via the induction of catalase. *Proteomics.* Vol. 5, No. 8, pp. (2112-2122).
Singh, L., Gao, Q., Kumar, A., Gotoh, T., Wazer, D.E., Band, H., Feig, L.A. & Band, V. (2003). The high-risk human papillomavirus type 16 E6 counters the GAP function of E6TP1 toward small Rap G proteins. *J Virol.* Vol. 77, No. 2, pp. (1614-1620).
Singh, M., Krajewski, M., Mikolajka, A. & Holak, T.A. (2005). Molecular determinants for the complex formation between the retinoblastoma protein and LXCXE sequences. *J Biol Chem.* Vol. 280, No. 45, pp. (37868-37876).
Smahel, M., Smahelova, J., Tejklova, P., Tachezy, R. & Jelinek, F. (2005a). Analysis of tumor progression by transcriptional profiling of mouse MK16 cell lines transformed with human papillomavirus type 16 E6 and E7 oncogenes and activated H-ras. *Oncol Rep.* Vol. 14, No. 6, pp. (1665-1674).
Smahel, M., Smahelova, J., Tejklova, P., Tachezy, R. & Marinov, I. (2005b). Characterization of cell lines derived from tumors induced by TC-1 cells in mice preimmunized against HPV16 E7 oncoprotein. *Int J Oncol.* Vol. 27, No. 3, pp. (731-742).
Smeets, S.J., Braakhuis, B.J., Abbas, S., Snijders, P.J., Ylstra, B., van de Wiel, M.A., Meijer, G.A., Leemans, C.R. & Brakenhoff, R.H. (2006). Genome-wide DNA copy number alterations in head and neck squamous cell carcinomas with or without oncogene-expressing human papillomavirus. *Oncogene.* Vol. 25, No. 17, pp. (2558-2564).
Smotkin, D. & Wettstein, F.O. (1987). The major human papillomavirus protein in cervical cancers is a cytoplasmic phosphoprotein. *J Virol.* Vol. 61, No. 5, pp. (1686-1689).
Spitkovsky, D., Hehner, S.P., Hofmann, T.G., Möller, A. & Schmitz, M.L. (2002). The human papillomavirus oncoprotein E7 attenuates NF-kappa B activation by targeting the Ikappa B kinase complex. *J Biol Chem.* Vol. 277, No. 28, pp. (25576-25582).
Srivenugopal, K.S. & Ali-Osman, F. (2002). The DNA repair protein, O(6)-methylguanine-DNA methyltransferase is a proteolytic target for the E6 human papillomavirus oncoprotein. *Oncogene.* Vol. 21, No. 38, pp. (5940-5945).
Steinau, M., Lee, D.R., Rajeevan, M.S., Vernon, S.D., Ruffin, M.T. & Unger, E.R. (2005). Gene expression profile of cervical tissue compared to exfoliated cells: impact on biomarker discovery. *BMC Genomics.* Vol. 6, pp. (64-71).
Stoler, M.H., Rhodes, C.R., Whitbeck, A., Wolinsky, S.M., Chow, L.T. & Broker, T.R. (1992). Human papillomavirus type 16 and 18 gene expression in cervical neoplasias. *Hum Pathol.* Vol. 23, No. 2, pp. (117-128).
Stöppler, M.C., Straight, S.W., Tsao, G., Schlegel, R., McCance, D.J. (1996). The E5 gene of HPV-16 enhances keratinocyte immortalization by full-length DNA. *Virol.* Vol. 223, No. 1, pp. (251-254).
Storrs, C.H. & Silverstein, S.J. (2007). PATJ, a tight junction-associated PDZ protein, is a novel degradation target of high-risk human papillomavirus E6 and the alternatively spliced isoform 18 E6. *J Virol.* Vol. 81, No. 8, pp. (4080-4090).

Straight, S.W., Hinkle, P.M., Jewers, R.J. & McCance, D.J. (1993). The E5 oncoprotein of human papillomavirus type 16 transforms fibroblasts and effects the downregulation of the epidermal growth factor receptor in keratinocytes. *J Virol.* Vol. 67, No. 8, pp. (4521-4532).

Straight, S.W., Herman, B. & McCance, D.J. (1995). The E5 oncoprotein of human papillomavirus type 16 inhibits the acidification of endosomes in human keratinocytes. *J Virol.* Vol. 69, No. 5, pp. (3185-3192).

Swindle, C.S. & Engler, J.A. (1998). Association of the Human Papillomavirus type 11 E1 protein with Histone H1. *J Virol.* Vol. 72, No. 3, pp. (1994-2001).

Syrjänen, S.M. & Syrjänen, J.K. (1999). New concepts on the role of Human Papillomavirus in cell cycle regulation. *Ann Med.* Vol. 31, No. 3, pp. (175-187).

Takami, K., Yana, I., Kurahashi, H. & Nishisho, I. (1995). Multistep carcinogenesis in colorectal cancers.Southeast Asian. *J Trop Med Public Health.* Vol. 26, Suppl 1, pp. (190-196).

Tan, S-H., Leong, L.E.C., Walker, P.A. & Bernard, H.U. (1994). The Human Papillomavirus type 16 E2 transcription factor binds with a low cooperativity to two flanking sires and represses the E6 promoter through displacement of Sp1 and TFIID. *J Virol.* Vol. 68, No. 10, pp. (6411-6420).

Thomas, M., Pim, D. & Banks, L. (1999). The role of the E6-p53 interaction in the molecular pathogenesis of HPV. *Oncogene.* Vol. 18, No. 53, pp. (7690 -7700).

Thomas, M., Glaunsinger, B., Pim, D., Javier, R. & Banks, L. (2001). HPV E6 and MAGUK protein interactions: determination of the molecular basis for specific protein recognition and degradation. *Oncogene.* Vol. 20, No. 39, pp. (5431-5439).

Thomas, M., Laura, R., Hepner, K., Guccione, E., Sawyers, C., Lasky, L. & Banks, L. (2002). Oncogenic human papillomavirus E6 proteins target the MAGI-2 and MAGI-3 proteins for degradation. *Oncogene.* Vol. 21, No. 33, pp. (5088-5096).

Thomas, M., Massimi, P., Navarro, C., Borg, J.P. & Banks, L. (2005). The hScrib/Dlg apico-basal control complex is differentially targeted by HPV-16 and HPV-18 E6 proteins. *Oncogene.* Vol. 24, No. 41, pp. (6222-6230).

Tomakidi, P., Cheng, H., Kohl, A., Komposch, G. & Alonso, A. (2000). Modulation of the epidermal growth factor receptor by the human papilomavirus type 16 E5 protein in raft cultures of human keratinocytes. *Eur J Cell Biol.* Vol. 79, No. 6, pp. (407-412).

Tong, X. & Howley, P.M. (1997). The bovine papillomavirus E6 oncoprotein interacts with paxillin and disrupts the actin cytoskeleton. *Proc Natl Acad Sci USA.* Vol. 94, No. 9, pp. (4412-4417).

Toussaint-Smith, E., Donner, D.B. & Roman, A. (2004). Expression of human papillomavirus type 16 E6 and E7 oncoproteins in primary foreskin keratinocytes is sufficient to alter the expression of angiogenic factors. *Oncogene.* Vol. 23, No. 17, pp. (2988-2995).

Tsao, Y.P., Li, L.Y., Tsai, T.C. & Chen, S.L. (1996). Human papillomavirus type 11 and 16 E5 represses p21(WafI/SdiI/CipI) gene expression in fibroblasts and keratinocytes. *J Virol.* Vol. 70, No. 11, pp. (7535-7539).

Ullman, C.G., Haris, P.I., Kell, B., Cason, J., Jewers, R.J., Best, J.M., Emery, V.C. & Perkins, S.J. (1994). Hypothetical structure of the membrane-associated E5 oncoprotein of human papillomavirus type 16. *Biochem Soc Trans.* Vol. 22, No. 4, pp. (439S).

Ullman, C.G., Haris, P.I., Galloway, D.A., Emery, V.C. & Perkins, S.J. (1996). Predicted alpha-helix/beta-sheet secondary structures for the zinc-binding motifs of human papillomavirus E7 and E6 proteins by consensus prediction averaging and spectroscopic studies of E7. *Biochem J*. Vol. 319, No. 1, pp. (229-239).

Valdovinos-Torres, H., Orozco-Morales, M., Pedroza-Saavedra, A., Padilla-Noriega, L., Esquivel-Guadarrama, F. & Gutierrez-Xicotencatl, L. (2008). Different Isoforms of HPV-16 E7 Protein are Present in Cytoplasm and Nucleus. *Open Virol J*. Vol. 2, pp. (15-23).

Vambutas, A., DeVoti, J., Pinn, W., Steinberg, B.M. & Bonagura, V.R. (2001). Interaction of human papillomavirus type 11 E7 protein with TAP-1 results in the reduction of ATP-dependent peptide transport. *Clin Immunol*. Vol. 101, No. 1, pp. (94-99).

Vogt, M., Butz, K., Dymalla, S., Semzow, J. & Hoppe-Seyler, F. (2006). Inhibition of Bax activity is crucial for the antiapoptotic function of the human papillomavirus E6 oncoprotein. *Oncogene*. Vol. 25, No. 29, pp. (4009-4015).

Wald, A.I., Hoskins, E.E., Wells, S.I., Ferris, R.L. & Khan, S.A. (2011). Alteration of microRNA profiles in squamous cell carcinoma of the head and neck cell lines by human papillomavirus. *Head Neck*. Vol. 33, No. 4, pp. (504-512).

Wang, Q., Grifin, H., Sotherd, S., Jackson, D., Martin, A., McIntosh, P., Davy, C., Masterson, P.J., Walker, P.A., Laskey, P., Oary, M.B. & Doorbar, J. (2004). Functional analysis of the human papillomavirus type 16 E1^E4 protein provides a mechanism for *in vitro* and *in vivo* keratin filament reorganization. *J Virol*. Vol. 78, No. 2, pp. (821-833).

Wang, Y.W., Chang, H.S., Lin, C.H. & Yu, W.C. (2007). HPV-18 E7 conjugates to c-Myc and mediates its transcriptional activity. *Int J Biochem Cell Biol*. Vol. 39, No. 2, pp. (402-412).

Wang, J., Zhou, D., Prabhu, A., Schlegel, R. & Yuan, H. (2010). The canine papillomavirus and gamma HPV E7 proteins use an alternative domain to bind and destabilize the retinoblastoma protein. *PLoS Pathog*. Vol. 6, No. 9, pp. (e1001089).

Watson, R.A., Thomas, M., Banks, L. & Roberts, S. (2003). Activity of the human papillomavirus E6 PDZ-binding motif correlates with an enhanced morphological transformation of immortalized human keratinocytes. *J Cell Sci*. Vol. 116, No. 24, pp. (4925-4934).

Wei, Q. (2005). Pitx2a binds to human papillomavirus type 18 E6 protein and inhibits E6-mediated P53 degradation in HeLa cells. *J Biol Chem*. Vol. 280, No. 56, pp. (37790-37797).

Wells, S.I., Aronow, B.J., Wise, T.M., Williams, S.S., Couget, J.A. & Howley, P.M. (2003). Transcriptome signature of irreversible senescence in human papillomavirus-positive cervical cancer cells. *Proc Natl Acad Sci USA*. Vol. 100, No. 12, pp. (7093-7098).

Wentzensen, N., Vinokurova, S. & von Knebel Doeberitz, M. (2004). Systematic review of genomic integration sites of human papillomavirus genomes in epithelial dysplasia and invasive cancer of the female lower genital tract. *Cancer Res*. Vol. 64, No. 11, pp. (3878-3884).

Werness, B.A., Levine, A.J. & Howley, P.M. (1990). Association of the human papillomavirus types 16 and 18 E6 proteins with p53. *Science*. Vol. 248, No. 4951, pp. (76-79).

Wilson, R., Fhrmann, F. & Laimins, L.A. (2005). Role of the E1^E4 protein in the differentiation-dependent life cycle of Human Papillomavirus type 31. *J Virol*. Vol. 79, No. 11, pp. (6732-6740).

Wise-Draper, T.M., Allen, H.V., Thobe, M.N., Jones, E.E., Habash, K.B., Munger, K. & Wells, S.I. (2005). The human DEK proto-oncogene is a senescence inhibitor and an upregulated target of high-risk human papillomavirus E7. *J Virol*. Vol. 79, No. 22, pp. (14309-14317).

Woodworth, C.D., Gaiotti, D., Michael, E., Hansen, L. & Nees, M. (2000). Targeted disruption of the epidermal growth factor receptor inhibits development of papillomas and carcinomas from human papillomavirus-immortalized keratinocytes. *Cancer Res*. Vol. 60, No. 16, pp. (4397-4402).

Wu, X., Hepner, K., Castelino-Prabhu, S., Do, D., Kaye, M.B., Yuan, X.J., Wood, J., Ross, C., Sawyers, C.L. & Whang, Y.E. (2000). Evidence for regulation of the PTEN tumor suppressor by a membrane-localized multi-PDZ domain containing scaffold protein MAGI-2. *Proc Natl Acad Sci USA*. Vol. 97, No. 8, pp. (4233-4238).

Xi, L.F., Carter, J.J., Galloway, D.A., Kuypers, J., Hughes, J.P., Lee, S.K., Adam, D.E., Kiviat, N.B. & Koutsky, L.A. (2002). Acquisition and Natural History of Human Papillomavirus Type 16 Variant Infection among a Cohort of Female University Students1. *Cancer Epidemiol Biomarkers Preven*. Vol. 11, No. 4, pp. (343–351).

Yamada, T., Manos, M., Peto, J., Greer, C.E., Muñoz, N., Bosch, F.X. & Wheeler, C.M. (1997). Human Papillomavirus Type 16 Sequence Variation in Cervical Cancers: a Worldwide Perspective. *J Virol*. Vol. 71, No. 3, pp. (2463–2472).

Yang, D.H., Wildeman, A.G. & Sharom, F.J. (2003). Overexpression, purification, and structural analysis of the hydrophobic E5 protein from human papillomavirus type 16. *Protein Expr Purif*. Vol. 30, No. 1, pp. (1-10).

Yasumoto, S., Burkhardt, A.L., Doniger, J. & DiPaolo, J.A. (1986). Human papillomavirus type 16 DNA-induced malignant transformation of NIH 3T3 cells. *J Virol*. Vol. 57, No. 2, pp. (572-577).

Yim, E.K., Lee, K.H., Bae, J.S., Namkoong, S.E., Um, S.J. & Park, J.S. (2004a). Proteomic analysis of antiproliferative effects by treatment of 5-fluorouracil in cervical cancer cells. *DNA Cell Biol*. Vol. 23, No. 11, pp. (769-776).

Yim, E.K., Meoyng, J., Namakoong, S.E., Um, S.J. & Park, J.S. (2004b). Genomic and proteomic expression patterns in HPV-16 E6 gene transfected stable human carcinoma cell lines. *DNA Cell Biol*. Vol. 23, No.12, pp. (826-835).

Yim, E.K. & Park, J.S. (2006). Role of proteomics in translational research in cervical cancer. *Expert Rev Proteomics*. Vol. 3, No. 1, pp. (21-36).

Yoshida, S., Kajitani, N., Satsuka, A., Nakamura, H. & Sakai, H. (2008). Ras modifies proliferation and invasiveness of cells expressing human papillomavirus oncoproteins. *J Virol*. Vol. 82, No. 17, pp. (8820-8827).

Yuan, H., Fu, F., Zhuo, J., Wang, W., Nishitani, J., An, D.S., Chen, I.S. & Liu, X. (2005). Human papillomavirus type 16 E6 and E7 oncoproteins upregulate c-IAP2 gene expression and confer resistance to apoptosis. *Oncogene*. Vol. 24, No. 32, pp. (5069-5078).

Zehbe, I., Wilander, E., Delius, H. & Tommasino, M. (1998). Human Papillomavirus 16 E6 variants are more prevalent in invasive carcinoma than the prototype. *Cancer Res*. Vol. 58, No. 4, pp. (829-833).

Zerfass-Thome, K., Zwerschke, W., Mannhardt, B., Tindle, R., Botz, J.W. & Jansen-Durr, P. (1996). Inactivation of the cdk inhibitor p27KIP1 by the human papillomavirus type 16 E7 oncoprotein. *Oncogene*. Vol. 13, No. 11, pp. (2323-2330).

Zhang, B., Srirangam, A., Potter, D.A. & Roman, A. (2005a). HPV16 E5 protein disrupts the c-Cbl-EGFR interaction and EGFR ubiquitination in human foreskin keratinocytes. *Oncogene*. Vol. 24, No. 15, pp. (2585-2588).

Zhang, B., Chen, W. & Roman, A. (2006). The E7 proteins of low- and high-risk human papillomaviruses share the ability to target the pRB family member p130 for degradation. *Proc Natl Acad Sci USA*. Vol. 103, No. 2, pp. (437-442).

Zhang, Y., Fan, S., Meng, Q., Ma, Y., Katiyar, P., Schlegel, R. & Rosen, E.M. (2005b). BRCA1 interaction with human papillomavirus oncoproteins. *J Biol Chem*. Vol. 280, No. 39, pp. (33165-33177).

Zhang, Y., Dasgupta, J., Ma, R.Z., Banks, L., Thomas, M. & Chen, X.S. (2007). Structures of a human papillomavirus (HPV) E6 polypeptide bound to MAGUK proteins: mechanisms of targeting tumor suppressors by a high-risk HPV oncoprotein. *J Virol*. Vol. 81, No. 7, pp. (3618-3626).

Zhou, X., Sun, X.Y., Louis, K. & Frazer, I.H. (1994). Interaction of Human papillomavirus (HPV) type 16 capsid proteins with HPV DNA requires an intact L2 N-terminal sequence. *J Virol*. Vol. 68, No. 2, pp. (619-625).

zur Hausen, H. (2000). Papillomaviruses in human cancers. In: *Infectious causes of cancer: Targets for intervention*, JJ Goedert, pp. (245-261), Humana Press, ISBN 9780896037724, USA.

Zwerschke, W., Mazurek, S., Massimi, P., Banks, L., Eigenbrodt, E. & ansen-Dürr, P. (1999). Modulation of type M2 pyruvate kinase activity by the human papillomavirus type 16 E7 oncoprotein. *Proc Natl Acad Sci USA*. Vol. 96, No. 4, pp. (1291-1296).

Zwerschke, W., Mannhardt, B., Massimi, P., Nauenburg, S., Pim, D., Nickel, W., Banks, L., Reuser, A.J. & Jansen-Dürr, P. (2000). Allosteric activation of acid alpha-glucosidase by the human papillomavirus E7 protein. *J Biol Chem*. Vol. 275, No. 13, pp. (9534-9541).

11

The Interaction between Human Papillomavirus Proteins and Cytoskeletal Filaments

Zehra Safi Oz
Zonguldak Karaelmas University, Department of Medical Biology
Turkey

1. Introduction

Cancer is a disease in which uncontrolled cell division begins, cell integrity and transmission collapse. Cervical cancer is the second most common cancer among women worldwide. The oncogenic human papillomavirus (HPV) types are the most significant risk factors in its aetiology. HPV causes deformation of genomic integrity, control of cell cycle, cell adhesion and apoptosis by suppressing tumor suppressor genes and interacting with cellular proteins via various proteins on carcinogenesis process. While doing all these functions, HPV undoubtedly interacts with the members of cytoskeleton which enable cellular motility and integrity. This causes deformation of intercellular junction and tissue integrity. Formation of "koilos" which is created by HPV in cells and has an important place in the diagnosis of virus in gynecologic and non-gynecologic samples can be thought as the result of interaction of HPV-cytoskeleton. In this chapter the relation between HPV proteins and members of cytoskeleton will be studied through tumor suppressor genes. First of all HPV genomic structure and HPV proteins will be mentioned generally, then cytoskeleton and its members will be explained together with HPV proteins which they are in interaction with.

2. HPV genomic structure and function

Human papillomaviruses (HPVs) are small, nonenveloped, icosahedral, double-stranded circular DNA viruses belong to the *Papovaviridae* family. HPVs specifically infect keratinized stratified epithelia. The circular DNA approximetely 8,000 bp in size, contained within a spherical protein capsid, composed of 72 capsomers. The viral capsid has developed to complete several roles that are crucial to establish viral infection. The HPV genome is enclosed by an icosahedral capsid (T=7) of 55 nm in diameter composed by two structural proteins, the major protein L1 and the minor capsid protein L2 (Horvath et al., 2010; Howley 1996; Longworth & Laimins, 2004; Prétet et al., 2007). To date, over 100 different viral types have been recognized and new types are regularly added to this list. These viruses can be classified into mucosal and cutaneous subtypes. Within each of these HPV groups, individual viruses are designated high risk or low risk according to their oncologic potential: high risk viruses such as HPV16,18 are frequently found in carcinomas. Low-risk types are responsible for benign lesions or condylomas (Blachon & Demeret, 2003, Howley 1996; Longworth & Laimins, 2004; Mu¨nger et al,, 2004, Prétet et al., 2007).

HPV types belong to four of those genera, i.e., Alphapapillomavirus, Gammapapillomavirus, Mupapillomavirus and Nupapillomavirus have been associated with cutaneous warts, especially foot and hand warts (Koning et al., 2011). Genitally transmitted HPV types are contained within genus Alfapapillomavirus and viruses from this group, such as HPV 6 and 11, are major sexually transmitted pathogens (Brentijens et al., 2002; de Villiers et al., 2004, Myers et al., 1994 as cited in Doorbar, 2005). These viruses are associated with benign papillomas. Contrary, the high-risk viruses from supergroup A, such as HPV16 and 18, cause mucosal lesions that can progress in some individuals to high-grade neoplasia and cancer (Bosch et al., 2002; Walboomers et al., 1999 as cited in Doorbar, 2005). The second major group of human papillomaviruses (also known as Beta papillomaviruses) are contained within supergroup B such as HPV5. This virus causes inapparent or latent infections in the general population (de Villiers et al., 2004; Myers et al., 1994; Ramoz et al., 2002, as cited in Doorbar 2005). The third major group of human papillomaviruses (also known as Gammapapillomaviruses) are gamma papillomaviruses such as HPV4. This virus cause cutaneous warts in the general population that can superficially resemble those caused by supergroup A papillomaviruses such as HPV2. The remaining group of HPVs are contained within supergroup E (also classified as Mu and Nu-papillomaviruses (de Villiers et al., 2004, Myers et al., 1994 as cited in Doorbar, 2005). Only three human members from this group are known, and all cause cutaneous papillomas in the general population. HPV1 is the most well studied member of this group, and like HPV2 in supergroup A, causes verrucas and palmar warts (Doorbar, 2005).

The HPV genome includes several open reading frames (late and early gene regions and the non-coding long control region (LCR) that encode proteins involved in viral DNA replication (E1 and E2), viral gene expression regulation (E2), virus assembly (E4) and the immortalisation and transformation of infected epithelial cells (E5, E6 and E7; high-risk HPV only). These proteins play a role in genome organization, regulation of gene expression, and cellular transport. HPV proteins and their functions were documented in Table 1. The open reading frames L1 and L2 encode the two capsid proteins (Howley 1996; Prétet et al., 2007). These proteins are expressed in the upper layers of infected tissue (Ozbun & Meyers, 1998, as cited in Doorbar, 2005). HPVs L1 and L2 capsid proteins form the structure of the virion and facilitate viral DNA packaging and maturation.

The papillomavirus E1 and E2 proteins play significant roles in viral genome replication. (Munger et al., 2004). The E1 protein also exhibits DNA helicase/ATPase activity (Hughes & Romanos 1993, Longworth & Laimins, 2004). E1 proteins bind to specific DNA elements in the viral origin of replication and assemble into hexameric helicases with the assist of a second viral protein, E2 (Wilson et al., 2002). The viral E2 protein is also crucial for the viral origin of replication (Dao et al., 2006). E2 plays a role in regulating viral transcription from the early promoter and viral genome segregation during cell division (Haugen et al., 1987 as cited in Longworth & Laimins, 2004, Munger et al., 2004).

E6 and E7 oncoproteins, encoded by the oncogenic HPV types, are responsible for malignant transformation. These proteins disrupt normal cell growth and proliferation by binding to tumor suppressors proteins such as p53 and retinoblastoma (pRb) (Burd, 2003, Gammoh et al., 2006). High risk HPV E6 protein interacts with many significant cellular protein. To examplify these cellular protein, EF-hand calcium-binding protein E6-BP (reticulocalbin 2), the interferon regulatory factor IRF-3, and the focal adhesion protein paxillin (Munger et al.,

HPV proteins	Molecular weights	Functions
L1	55 kDa	Major viral capsid protein. Self-assembly in capsomers and capsids, and interacting with L2. Interacting with cell reseptor.
L2	70 kDa	Minor viral capsid protein. Interacting with DNA. Facilitating virion assembly. Interacting with cell receptor.
E1		Viral genome replication. DNA helicase and ATPase activity. Binding to specific DNA elements in the viral origin of replication and assembling into hexameric helicases with the assist of a second viral protein, E2.
E2	42 kDa	Site-specific DNA binding protein. Viral genome replication . Viral genome expression regulation. Viral genome segregation during cell division. Interacting with and recruits E1 to the origin. Playing a role in regulating viral transcription from the early promoter.
E4		Facilitating virus assembly and release. Interacting with the keratin cytoskeleton and intermediate filaments. Inducing G2 arrest.
E1^E4	10 kDa	Binding and collapsing the cytokeratin network. preventing the progression of cells into mitosis by arresting them in the G2 phase of the cell cycle. Binding to mitochondria. Inducing the detachment of mitochondria from microtubules. Induction of apoptosis.
E5	83 residues	Cellular transformation, and initiation of neoplasia. Being able to activate epidermal growth factor receptor (EGFR) and other protein kinases. Inhibiting apoptosis. Interacting with gap junction proteins.
E6	150 aa	Immortalization and transformation of infected epithelial cells . Disrupting normal cell growth and proliferation by binding to protein p53. Associating with EF-hand calcium-binding protein, E6-BP (reticulocalbin 2), the interferon regulatory factor IRF-3, and the focal adhesion protein paxillin, calcium- binding protein ERC 55 hDLG (the mammalian homologue of the Dropsophila discs large tomour suppressor protein), hScrib and MUPP control cell polarity. Leading to the disruption of the actin cytoskeleton and cell matrix interactions. Inducing telomerase. Preventing cell differentiation.
E7	100 aa	Immortalization and transformation of infected epithelial cells. Disrupting normal cell growth and proliferation by binding to protein pRb. Leading to the delocalization of dynein from mitotic spindles via an association with Nuclear Mitotic Apparatus Protein 1 (NuMA). Destabilising centrosomes and causes mitotic defects. Activating cell cycle positive regulators.

Table 1. HPV proteins and their functions.

2004). E6 also binds the p53 as part of a trimeric complex with the cellular ubiquitin ligase, E6AP, leading to the rapid turnover of p53 (Scheffner et al., 1990; Werness et al., 1990 as cited in Longworth & Laimins, 2004).

HPV E7 proteins are low-molecular-weight proteins of approximately 100 amino acids. This oncoprotein encoded by small DNA tumor viruses, they associate with and adjust the functions of cellular protein complexes. The HPV E7 proteins interact with the retinoblastoma (Rb) family of tumor suppressors protein and the related "pocket proteins" p107 and p130. The proteins control the activities of the E2F family of transcription factors that regulate multiple cell cycle transitions as well as other cellular activities (Munger et al., 2004). E7 also binds to other proteins such as p130, p21, p27, cyclin A, cyclin E, the cyclin dependent kinase inhibitor (CKI), TBP,P300/CBP, MPP2,IGFBP-3, Mi2, NuMA (nuclear mitotic apparatus protein 1), p600. and a cellular protein kinase activity (Dyson et al., 1989 as cited in Longworth & Laimins, 2004; Jones and Munger, 1996; Pim and Banks, 2010).

HPV-16 may not only inactivate the tumor suppressor proteins p53 and pRB with its E6 and E7 oncoproteins, respectively, but could also alter other cellular functions through E7 interaction with the cytoskeleton or associated proteins (Rey et al.,2000). Causing both benign and malignant lesions, HPV must first infect the divisible basal cell to induce papilloma formation (Burd, 2003; Flores et al., 2000; Howley 1996; Stanley, 2001). Viral replication occurs concomitantly with epithelial cell differentiation. Entering the basal cell, HPV replicates simultaneously with epithelial cell differentiation and reaches the keratinized cell (Andersson et al., 2005; Burd, 2003; Flores et al., 2000; Hoory et al., 2008; Howley 1996; Stanley, 2001).

The E4 protein is the most abundantly expressed HPV protein. HPV E1^E4 accumulates in differentiating cells of the upper epithelial layers. It is synthesized from a spliced mRNA, E1^E4, which encodes five amino acids from the E1 ORF spliced to the protein encoded by the E4 ORF (Chow et al.,1987, Doorbar et al., 1990, Nasseri et al., 1987 as cited in Raj et al., 2004). The first activity described for the 10-kDa HPV type 16 (HPV16) E1^E4 protein was its ability to bind and collapse the cytokeratin network (Doorbar et al., 1991 as cited in Raj et al., 2004). Although all of the role of HPV16 E1^E4 is unclear, previous work has revealed that HPV16 E1^E4 can interact with keratins and cause the reorganization of the keratin intermediate-filament network (Doorbar et al., 1991 as cited in Wang et al., 2004). The HPV 16 E1^E4 protein binds to keratins directly and interacts strongly with keratin 18, a member of the type I intermediate-filament family. By contrast, HPV16 E1^E4 bound only weakly to keratin 8, a type II intermediate-filament protein, and showed no detectable affinity for the type III protein, vimentin (Wang et al., 2004).

The product of the E5 oncogene in HPVs contributes to cellular transformation. HPV16 E5 is a highly hydrophobic protein. It found mainly at the Golgi apparatus and internal membranes (Conrad et al., 1993 as cited in Alonso and Reed, 2002). Little is known about the biological activities of the HPV16 E5 protein or the source of its oncogenicity. It has been shown that E5 is able to regulate epidermal growth factor receptor (EGFR) activation in the presence or absence of ligand, and that expression of the protein in human keratinocytes results in altered gap junction-mediated cell–cell communication (Alonso and Reed, 2002). HPV E5 is also known to interact with growth factor receptors and gap junction proteins and is believed to play a role during the initiation of neoplasia (Yang et al., 2003).

Most benign and low-grade cervical lesions contain HPV DNA in an extrachromosomal state (Durst et al., 1985 as cited in Martineza 2007). However, in most cases of cervical carcinomas the HPV DNA is usually found integrated into the host chromosomes, frequently disrupting the E1 and E2 genes (zur hausen, 2000, 2002; Durst et al., 1985; Meissner et al., 1989 as cited in Martinez 2007). This process result in increased expression of the viral E6 and E7 oncogenes (Yee et al., 1985 as cited in Martinez 2007).

A common feature of Human papillomavirus infection is the appearance of koilocytosis in the differentiated layers of squamous epithelium. Koilocytosis is the most common cytopathic effect and is considered by pathologists to be the major histopathological aspect for determination of HPV infection. Koilocytosis is composed of the presence of abnormal koilocytes. The greatest change caused by HPV in the epithelial cell cytoplasm is called koilos. Koilos means "hollow" in Greek. These koilocytes are squamous epithelial cells that may contain an acentric hyperchromatic nucleus and large clear perinuclear halos that usually occupy a greater volume than that of the cytoplasm (Fornatora et al., 1996; Krawczyk et al., 2008; Miyahara et al., 2011, Safi Oz et al., 2009, Safi Oz, 2010). The multiple nuclei of koilocytes are in fact multilobation of a single nucleus, and this phenomenon is associated with upregulation of gene products related to the G2 chectpoint. On restoration of 3D confocal images, the multinucleated feature of koilocytes was revealed to be multilobation of a single nucleus, as opposed to true multinucleation (Cho, 2005, 2006).

HPV causes various changes through its structural proteins in the cytoplasms and nuclei of the cells and tissues it infects (Krawczyk et al., 2008, Safi Oz et al., 2009, Safi Oz, 2010, Fornatora et al. 1996 as cited in Miyahara et al., 2011). The formation of koilos is influenced by the structural proteins of the virus, cell skeletal filaments, and tumour suppressor genes. Modifications of the cytoskeleton as a result of viral protein expression have been associated with oncogenic transformation by papillomaviruses. HPV proteins are interacted with cell skeletal filaments. Some of these proteins are E6 (HPV16,18), E7 (HPV16,18,38), E5 (high and low risk HPV types), E1^E4 (HPV16), E4 proteins (Lee & Dominguez, 2010; McIntosh et al., 2010; Nguyen 2008; Rey et al., 2000, Safi Oz, 2010; Stanley, 2001; Uribe & Jay., 2009; Yue et al., 2011).

3. HPV proteins in relation with cytoskeletal filaments and interaction mechanisms

Malignant transformation occurs with the alteration of cytoskeleton (Ben-Ze'ev 1997 as cited in Akgul et al., 2009). All these chances occur in different stages of cell cycle. Disruption of cytoskeleton not only means disruption of cytoskeletal organization but also disruption of many cellular functions. In this section, first of all cytoskeleton, its members and functions will be mentioned briefly. Then HPV proteins which are known and thought to have relation with cytoskeleton due to studies carried out until today will be explained. HPV proteins and cellular molecules interacted with cytoskeletal filament disruption were documented in Table 2)

The cytoskeleton is a network of fibers throughout the cell's cytoplasm that helps the cell maintain its shape and gives support to the cell. In addition to providing support for the cell, the cytoskeleton is also involved in cellular motility and in moving vesicles within a cell, as well as assisting in the formation of food vacuoles in the cell. A variety of cellular organelles are held in place by the cytoskeleton. The cytoskeleton is made up of three different types of protein filaments: microtubules, actin filaments (microfilament) and intermediate filaments. Each type of filament has different mechanical possestions and dynamics, but certain fundamental principles are common to them all (Alberts et al.,2002; http://biology.about.com/od/cellanatomy/a/aa013108a.htm).

Actin filaments determine the shape of the cell's surface and are necessary for whole cell locomadation. The actin cytoskeleton is a critical part of the cellular activities such as cell shape, cell division, motility, contraction, focal adhesion, phagocytosis, protein sorting and signal transduction (Lee & Dominguez 2010; Uribe & Jay 2009). Actin filament's usefullness to the cell depends on a large number of accessory proteins that link the filaments to other cell component. These proteins are essential for the control assembly of the cytoskeletal filaments in particular locations (Alberts et al., 2002). Cell movement is an important phenomenon in embryonic morphogenesis, immune surveillance, angiogenesis and tissue repair and regeneration (Hussey et al., 2006; Itoh and Yumura, 2007; McMahon and Gallop, 2005; Puppo et al., 2008; Yamaguchi and Condeelis, 2007 as cited in Lee & Dominguez, 2010). Two transition types (monomeric or G actin and filamentous or F actin) of actin filaments are in cells (Uribe & Jay 2009). Schematic representation of monomeric and filamentous actin were seen in Figure. 1.

The actin filament is asymmetric; actin monomers join the barbed (or +) fast growing end of the filament in the ATP-bound state and depart the filament preferentially from the pointed (or -) end primarily in the ADP state, giving rise to a process known as actin filament threadmilling. The transition between two types of actin is tighty regulated in cells by a large number of Actin-Binding Proteins (ABPs) (Lee & Dominguez, 2010; Uribe & Jay 2009). ABPs carry out a wide range of functions, including actin filament nucleation, elongation, severing, capping, and crosslinking and actin monomer sequestration (Lee & Dominguez 2010). The reorganization of the actin cytoskeleton is regulated in time and space by multiple factor, most notably Rho family GTPases that act as GTP-dependent molecular switches (Raftopoulou and Hall, 2004 as cited in Lee & Dominguez 2010). Among the small GTPases of the Rho family, Cdc42, Rac, and Rho are recognized as the most important regulators of actin assembly, controlling respectively the formation of filopodia, lamellipodia, and stress fibers (Etienne- Manneville and Hall, 2002 as cited in Lee & Dominguez 2010). Signals transmitted through these GTPases lead to localized actin cytoskeleton assembly/disassembly at the plasma membrane, with the actin filaments acting to push the cellular membrane (Hall, 1994 as cited in Lee & Dominguez 2010).

By interacting with paxillin, E6 protein facilites transformation by disrupting the normal links between paxillin and the actin cytoskeleton by displacing paxillin-LD motif-binding proteins, disrupts the actin filament formation and the regulation of cytoskeleton (Cooper et al., 2007; Safi Oz et al., 2009, Rapp & Chen, 1998, Turner, CE., 2000). In the light of this information, the disruption of actin filament formation and thus, cytoskeleton disruption are believed to affect the formation of koilos around the nucleus (Safi Oz et al., 2009, Rapp & Chen, 1998, Cooper et al., 2007). With HPV disrupting actin filament formation, it is thought that cell shape and division, motility, contraction, focal adhesion and phagocytosis may be influenced.

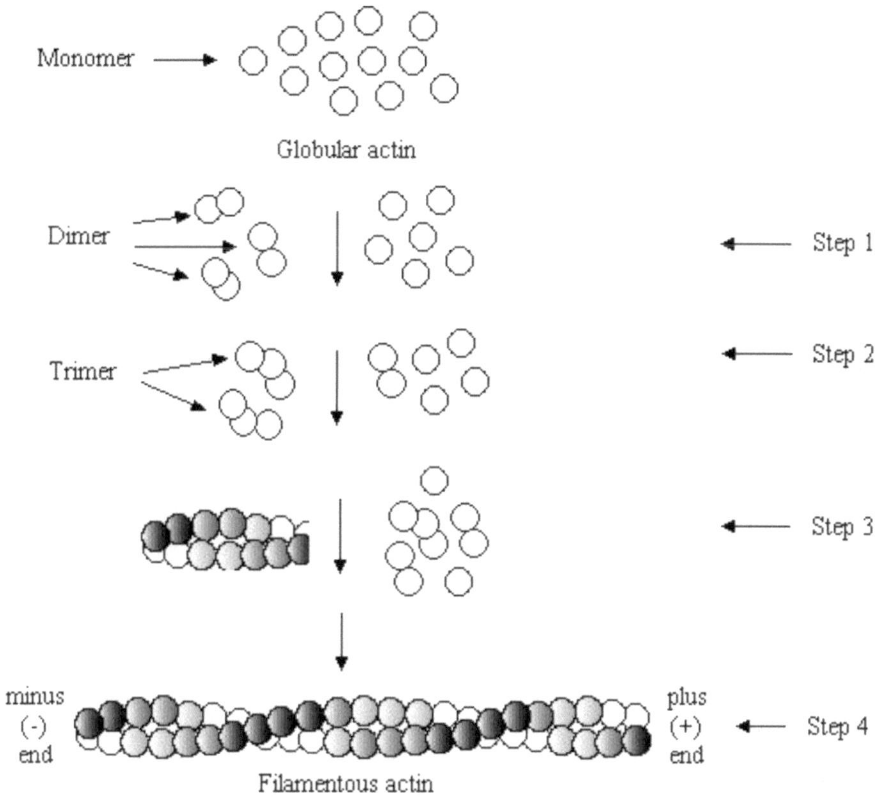

Fig. 1. Schematic representation of monomeric and filamentous actin

The bovine papillomavirus (BPV) E6 oncoprotein also interacts with paxillin and disrupt the actin cytoskeleton. HPV16 E6 binding to paxillin may contribute to the carcinogenic potential of the human papillomavirus (HPV). The association of HPV16 E6 with paxillin was affected by depolymerization of the actin fiber network. Disruption of the actin cytoskeleton is a characteristic of many transformed cells. (Tong & Howley, 1997).

HPVE6 interacted with numerous proteins involved in adhesion, cell architecture and polarity. hDLG (the mammalian homologue of the Dropsophila discs large tomour suppressor protein), hScrib and MUPP control cell polarity and cellular scaffolds, and their interaction with E6 would lead to deregulation of cytoskeletal organization and cell-cell interactions (Campo, 2005). E6 also interact with the calcium binding protein ERC 55 and the paxillin, interactions that could lead to the disruption of the actin cytoskeleton and cell matrix interactions. Paxillin is a protein associated with focal adhesion kinase (FAK), a kinase that plays a regulatory role in cell migration, and vinculin and involved in the regulation of the cytoskeleton. Paxillin takes role in the regulation of actin cytoskeleton by interacting with other adhesion proteins in the cell such as actopaxin and vinculin. When Human Papillomavirus E6 protein is associated with paxillin, interaction of paxillin with other adhesion proteins therefore formation of actin cytoskeleton is disrupted. (Table 2)

<table>
<tr><th>HPV proteins</th><th>Cellular molecules</th><th>Types of cytoskeletal filamets</th><th>Effects</th></tr>
<tr><td>HPV 16 E5</td><td>Golgi apparatus
Endoplasmic reticulum
Cellular membrane</td><td rowspan="7">Actin filament</td><td>Inhibits endocytotic activity</td></tr>
<tr><td rowspan="4">HPV 16 E6</td><td>Paxillin
(disrupt paxillin and vinculin, actopaxin interaction)</td><td rowspan="4">Disruption of actin filament</td></tr>
<tr><td>ERC55 (calcium binding protein)</td></tr>
<tr><td>hDLG (the mammalian homologue of the Dropsophila discs large tomour suppressor protein)
hScrib
MUPP</td></tr>
<tr><td>Tight junction complex</td></tr>
<tr><td>HPV 16 E7</td><td rowspan="2">Unknown</td><td rowspan="2">Disruption of actin filament</td></tr>
<tr><td>HPV 38 E7</td></tr>
<tr><td>HPV 16 E7</td><td>Microtubule network (attaches to microtubule network via the motor protein complex dynein)
NuMA (Nuclear Mitotic Apparatus Protein 1) / dynein network</td><td rowspan="2">Microtubule</td><td>Disruption of microtubule motors and HPV associated tumorigenesis.
Mitotic errors</td></tr>
<tr><td>HPV 16 L2</td><td>Microtubule network (attaches to microtubule network via the motor protein complex dynein)</td><td>Disruption of microtubule motors</td></tr>
<tr><td>HPV E4</td><td>Cytokeratin</td><td rowspan="2">Intermediate filament</td><td rowspan="2">Total collapse of the cytokeratin matrix</td></tr>
<tr><td>HPV E1^E4</td><td>Cytokeratin
DEAD-BAX protein</td></tr>
</table>

Table 2. HPV proteins and cellular molecules interacted with cytoskeletal filament disruption

HPVE6, specifically targets p53 for inactivation in order to promote cell growth and transformation and tumor supressors such as MAGI-1 and SAP97/hDlg for degradation. HPVE6 also targets numerous cellular proteins involved in a variety of cellular processes such as calcium signaling, cell adhesion, transcriptional control, DNA synthesis, apoptosis, cell cycle control, DNA repair, and small G-protein signaling. (Das et al., 2000, Degenhardt & Silverstein, 2001, Filippova et al, 2002, Gao et al., 1999, Gao et al., 2000, Iftner et al., 2002, Kuhne & Banks, 1998 Tong and Howley, 1997 as cited in Zhang et al., 2007). Cellular targets for the E6 proteins from high-low risk HPV types are Bak, myc, E6AP, E6BP/ERC55, P300 /CBP, PDZ proteins, hTERT, Tyk2, hAda3 (Pim and Banks, 2010). HPV E6 interacts with tight junction complex (Zhang et al., 2007). Tight junction acts as an impermeable barrier that divides epithelial cells into functionally distinct apical and basolateral membrane domains (Yeaman et al., 1999 as cited in Zhang., 2007). Tight junctions consist of several transmembrane proteins (occludin, claudins, and junctional adhesion molecule). All these proteins are associated with at least one of the Zonula occludens proteins (ZOPs). ZOPs bind to the junctional transmembrane proteins linking them to the actin cytoskeleton. So, ZOPs establish a link between the junction site and the cytoskeleton by interacting directly with actin filaments (Fanning et al., 1998, Itoh et al., 1997, Wittchen et al., 1999 as cited in Traweger et al., 2003). ZOPs currently comprising ZO-1, ZO-2, and ZO-3, belong to the family of membrane-associated guanylate kinase homologue (MAGUK) proteins. MAGUK proteins are involved in the organization of epithelial and endothelial intercellular junctions (Traweger et al., 2003 as cited in Bauer et al., 2010). HPV E6 polypeptide binds to MAGUK Proteins (Zhang et al., 2007). The ZO-2 protein is targeted by HPVE6. ZO-2, a 160-kDa phosphoprotein and was found to co-precipitate with ZO-1 in epithelial cells (Gumbiner et al., 1991, Jesaitis and Goodenough, 1994 as cited in Traweger et al., 2003).

ZOPs not only associate with each other but also with components of adherens junctions and gap junctions in cells lacking (Gumbiner et al., 1991, Howarth and Stevenson, 1995 as cited in Traweger et al., 2003). Adherens junction is responsible for cell-cell adhesion (Gumbiner, 1996 as cited in Zhang., 2007). The disruption of adherens junction decreases the phosphorylation of E-cadherin by protein kinase CK2, and this process of downregulation is treated as a common event in carcinogenesis (Serres et al., 2000 as cited in Zhang., 2007). Tight junction disruption and apobasical activity directly contribute to carcinogenesis by deregulating normal proliferation and differentiation programs in epithelial cells (Matter & Balda et al., 2003 as cited in Zhang., 2007). It is also thought that the damage caused by HPV on E6 proteins and tight junctions on carcinogenesis process is important.

HPV-16 may not only inactivate the tumor suppressor proteins p53 and pRB with its E6 and E7 oncoproteins, respectively, but could also alter other cellular functions through E7 interaction with the cytoskeleton or associated proteins. The E7 oncoprotein of Human Papillomavirus type 16 interacts with F-Actin in vitro and in vivo. F-actin is part of cellular structures such as microfilaments and the cell cortex and interacts with several structural and regulatory components. F-actin modifications resulting from viral protein expression will not only affect cytoskeletal organization but can also disrupt several cellular functions (Rey et al, 2000).

Yue et al. showed that HPV38 E7 induces actin stress fiber disruption, and this phenomenon correlates with its ability to down-regulate Rho activity. In addition, HPV38 E7 is able to induce actin fiber disruption by directly binding to the eukaryotic elongation factor 1A (eEF1A) and abolishing its effects on actin fiber formation. Their data support the conclusion that HPV38 E7 promotes keratinocyte proliferation in part by negatively regulating actin cytoskeleton fiber formation and by binding to eEF1A and inhibiting its effects on actin cytoskeleton remodeling (Yue et al., 2011).

The second type of cytoskeletal filament is the microtubule. Microtubules determine the positions of membrane-enclosed organelles and direct intracellular transport. Microtubules are formed from protein subunits of tubulin (alpha-tubulin and beta-tubulin) (Alberts et al., 2002). Construction of microtubules was seen in Figure 2.

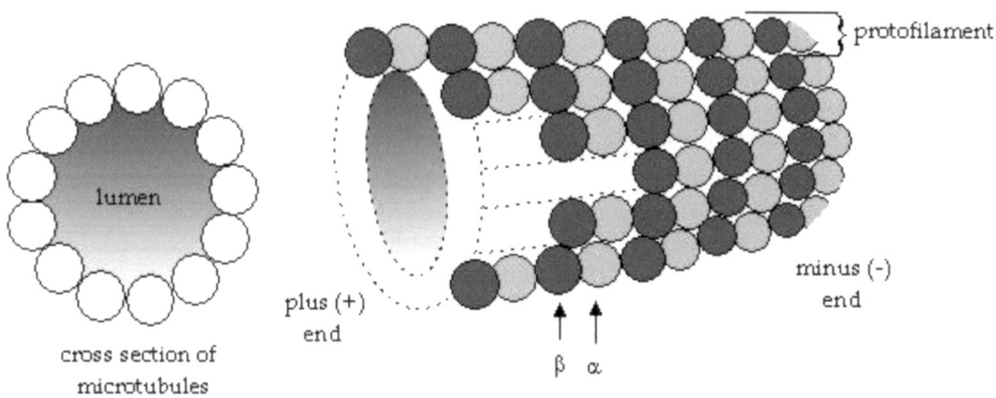

Fig. 2. Construction of microtubules from α and β tubulins

Romani et al. showed that the effect of HPV transformation on cellular cytoarchitecture. Cells from laryngeal papillomas and normal epithelium were cultured *in vitro*. Cytoskeletal components of both types of cells were visualized by immunofluorescence, to determine whether there were any differences in the structure or distribution of the cytoskeleton. The intermediate filaments and actin filaments are altered in the papilloma cells but there isn't significant change in microtubules (Romani et al., 1987). (Table 2) Most of the studies carried out up-to-now are about HPV proteins and motor proteins. HPV16 E7 expresion leads to an increased population of mitotic cells with dynein, a minus end–directed microtubule motor protein, delocalized from the mitotic spindle. Dynein is composed of several subunits. The dynein motor complex aids in the positioning of the Golgi complex and mitochondria, along with other organelles, and transports cargo from the endoplasmic reticulum, endosomes, and lysosomes. It is possible that the disruption of microtubule motors by high-risk HPV may contribute to HPV associated tumorigenesis (Nguyen et al., 2008). The other type of motor protein is kinesin. Kinesin uses the energy of ATP hydrolysis to move along a microtubule. These proteins have legs and feet that change conformations by binding and hydrolyzing ATP to walk along the microtubules.

Also HPV16 L2 protein attaches to microtubule network via the motor protein complex dynein (Florin et al., 2006; Schneider et al., 2011). The viral capsid play a critical role in the establishment of the viral infection. The L2 protein is an internally located multifunctinal protein with roles in genome encapsidation (Schelhaas et al., 2008, Holmgren et al., 2005 as cited in Horvath et al., 2010). Papillomaviruses enter cells via endocytosis. After endocytic cell entry and egress from endosomes, HPV16L2 goes along with the viral DNA to the nucleus. HPV16 L2 protein may be involved in the intracytoplasmic transport of the viral genome (Florin et al., 2006; Schneider et al., 2011).

The high-risk HPV16 E7 expression leads to the delocalization of dynein from mitotic spindles via an association with Nuclear Mitotic Apparatus Protein 1 (NuMA). The disruption of the NuMA/dynein network may result in mitotic errors (Nguyen, 2008, 2009). It is hypothesized that these event may important role in chromosome alignment and viral persistance (Nguyen & Munger., 2009).

The third type of cytoskeletal filament is the intermediate filament. Intermediate filaments (IFs) provide mechanical strenght and resistance to share stres (Alberts et al., 2002). Intermediate filament-associated diseases clearly represent a significant group of human pathologies, and these pathologies that have given us the best clues to the function of this type of cytoskeleton component (Penky & Lane, 2007). Intermediate filaments are composed of smaller subunits that are themselves elongated and fibrous, but actin filaments and microtubules are made of compact and globular subunits (Alberts et al., 2002).

IFs is a highly elongated, rod-like dimer based on an α-helical coiled-coil structure. Assembly of cytoplasmic IF proteins, such as vimentin, begins with a lateral association of dimers into tetramers and gradually into the so-called unit-length filaments (ULFs) (Strelkov et al., 2003). The molecular organisation of the intermediate filaments is specific for the cell type, the developmental stage and the type of differentiation (McIntosh et al., 2010). Major types of intermediate filament proteins in vertebrate cell are nuclear, vimentin-like, epithelial and axonal IF. Nuclear IF are composed of lamin A, B and C. The nuclear lamins are filamentous proteins, providing the nucleus with a putative skeleton for chromatin attachment (Alberts et al., 2002, Carmo-Fonseca &David-Ferreira , 1990).

Different families of intermediate filaments are keratins, neurofilaments, vimentin-like filaments. Neurofilaments are found in concentrations along the axons of vertebrate neurons. Neurofilament proteins are NF-L, NF-M, NF-H. The vimentin-like filaments are found in muscle, glial cells, many cells of mesenchymal origin and some neurons (Alberts et al., 2002). The most diverse intermediate filament family is that of the keratins. Keratins are major structural proteins in epithelial cells and form the cytoplasmic network of intermediate filaments (Fuchs et al., 1998 as cited in Wang et al., 2004). Every keratin filament is made up of type I (acidic) and type II (neutral/basic) keratin chains (Alberts et al., 2002). The keratin IF network of epidermal keratinocytes provides a protective barrier against mechanical insult, it is also a major player in absorbing stress in these cells (McIntosh et al., 2010). They contain at least 20 members, called keratin 1 (K1) to K20, which are divided into two types according to the sequence and isoelectric point (pI). K9 to K20 are type I (acidic) keratins. The type II keratins, K1 to K8, are neutral or basic. Type I and type II keratins form noncovalent heteropolymers at a 1:1 ratio (Moll et al., 1998 as cited in Wang et al., 2004). Recently, several new functions of keratins have emerged. K8 and K18 prevent Fas- and possibly tumor necrosis factor-induced apoptosis (Caulin et al., 1998, Gilbert et al., 2001, Inada et al., 2001, Ku et al., 2003 as cited in Wang et al., 2004). Keratin intermediate filaments are highly dynamic structures and are reorganized during cellular events such as mitosis and apoptosis (Wang et al., 2004). Diversity of keratins is clinically useful in the diagnosis of epithelial carcinomas, as the particular set of keratins expressed gives an indication of the epithelial tissue in which the cancer originated and thus can help to guide to choise of treatment (Alberts et al., 2002). HPVE4 interacts with the keratin cytoskeleton and intermediate filaments (Campo, 2005). Recent studies have introduced a new protein named E1^E4 of HPV16 that could disrupt the epithelial cytoskeleton. This protein is encoded by spliced mRNAs that fuse the two early genes, E1 and E4, which encodes five amino acids from the E1 ORF spliced to the protein encoded by the E4 ORF , and is the most abundantly expressed viral protein in HPV-infected epithelia (Doorbar et al., 1991 as cited in Ohta & Nishiyama, 2011). It has been reported that this protein degrades the cytoskeleton by interacting with epithelial cell proteins (Davy et al., 2002, Nakahara et al.,2002). (Table 2) Doorbar et al showed that expression of the HPV-16 E1^E4 protein in human keratinocytes (the natural host cell for HPV infection) results in the total collapse of the cytokeratin matrix. Tubulin and actin networks are unaffected by E1-E4, as are the nuclear lamins (Doorbar et al., 1991). The human HPV16 E1^E4 protein is associate with and reorganise the keratin IF network in cells in culture. HPV16 E1^E4 was found to effect a dramatic cessation of keratin IF network dynamics by associating with both soluble and insoluble keratin. These observations shed new light on the mechanism of keratin IF network reorganisation mediated by HPV16 E1^E4 (McIntosh et al., 2010). E1^E4 also translocates to mitokondria via an N-terminal leucine-rich region and induces the detachment of mitocondria from microtubules. The detached mitochondria then aggregate adjacent to the nucleus (Ohta & Nishiyama, 2011).

HPV16 E1^E4 protein is the most abundantly expressed viral protein in HPV infected epithelia. HPV E1^E4 possesses the ability to bind to the cytokeratin network by interacting directly with cytokeratins and to DEAD-box proteins. Keratin association leads to the eventual reorganization of the cytokeratin network *in vivo* as well as *in vitro* (Wang et al., 2004 as cited in Raj et al., 2004). Interestingly, the collapse of the network appears to initiate from the plasma membrane. Once collapsed, the cytokeratin appears as a cluster beside the nucleus.

HPV16 E1^E4 is also able to prevent the progression of cells into mitosis by arresting them in the G2 phase of the cell cycle.

HPV16 E1^E4 protein binds to mitochondria after binding to and collapsing the cytokeratin network and induces the detachment of mitochondria from microtubules, causing the organelles to form a single large cluster adjacent to the nucleus. This is followed by a severe reduction in the mitochondrial membrane potential and an induction of apoptosis (Raj et al., 2004).

In addition to the proteins mentioned above, it is expressed that HPV E5 protein contributes to the formation of koilocytes together with E6. The HPV E5 proteins are small (83 amino acids) hydrophobic proteins whose biological functions remain unresolved. These proteins are localized to endosomal membranes and the Golgi but on occasion are found in the cellular membranes (Longworth & Laimins, 2004). This protein associates with Golgi apparatus, endoplasmic reticulum and cellular membrane and inhibits endocytic activity by linking actin cytoskeleton. Although the role of HPV E5 in the cell-cycle is not known completely, it was shown with studies carried out on rodents that it shows low oncogenic activity in addition to major oncoproteins E6 and E7 (Kabsch & Alonso, 2002; Suprynowicz et al., 2008; Yang et al., 2003 as cited in Safi Oz., 2010). E6 protein in low and high risk HPV types aims at p53 and PDZ protein which organizes membrane transport in polarized epithelial cell membrane and may be damaging cell cytoskeleton (Safi Oz 2009, Krawczyk et al., 2008). HPV E5 - cell cytoskeleton association is an issue which requires more detailed biochemical and cellular studies.

4. Conclusion

Here, I summarize recent progress in my understanding of the interaction between Human papillomavirus proteins and their ability to disrupt cytoskeletal filaments. Disruption of cell cytoskeleton causes the occurrence of some important diseases such as cancer. Disruption of cell cytoskeleton both causes the disruption of cellular motility and cellular integrity and failure of important biological events such as cell division, contraction and phagocytosis. Association of various viruses with cell cytoskeleton is a study issue which has been gaining importance in recent years. HPV is included in this group of virus. In the studies of cell cytoskeleton - HPV, HPV16 and 18 which are among the risky group in the sense of cancer formation, become prominent. E6 protein of HPV16 and 18, E5 protein of HPV 16 and E7 protein of HPV38 associate with the members of actin cell cytoskeleton and damages cell cytoskeleton. Moreover, HPV E6 associates through MAGUK (membrane-associated guanylate kinase homologue) proteins with tight junctions which form impermeable barrier between apical and basal membrane domains. Although studies show that actin and intermediate filaments in papilloma cells alter but there are no significant alterations in microtubules; more detailed studies are required on this subject. In association of HPV - microtubule, some studies have been shown in which HPV16 minor capsid protein L2 and E7 link with microtubule network via motor protein dynein. Moreover it was stated that HPV16 E7 causes dynein delocalization via Nuclear mitotic apparatus (NuMa). I am of the opinion that there are few studies upon HPV and kinesine from motor proteins; enlightenment of this subject will direct the association of HPV–microtubule. Comprehensive understanding of HPV-cytoskeleton interaction will offer new insights into the HPV life cycle as well as karcinogenesis. This virus- cytoskeleton interaction will also provide a paradigm for investigating other DNA tumor viruses that share a similar mechanism for interacting with cytokeratin filaments.

5. Acknowledgement

I am very grateful to my husband, Burak Oz, for his drawings and encouragement.

6. References

Akgul B., Zigrino, P., Frith, D., Hanrahan & S., Storey A. (2009). Proteomic analysis reveals the actin cytoskeleton as cellular target for the human papillomavirus type 8. Virology Vol .386 pp. 1–5 ISSN: 0042-6822

Alberts B , Johnson A, Lewis J , Raff M , Roberts K , Walter P. (2002). The cytoskeleton, In: Molecular Biology of the Cell (4th Edition), p: 907-982 Garland Science Taylor&Francis group, ISBN 0-8153-3218-1, United States of America

Alonso A & Reed J. (2002). Modelling of the human papillomavirus type 16 E5 protein. *Bichimica et Biophysica Acta* Vol. 1601 pp. 9-18 ISSN ·0006-3002

Andersson, S., Safari, H., Mints, M., Lewensohn- Fuchs, I., Gyllensten, U & Johansson, B. (2005). Type distribution, viral load and integration status of high-risk human papillomaviruses in pre-stages of cervical cancer (CIN) *British Journal of Cancer* Vol. 92, pp.2195 - 2200 ISSN (printed): 0007-0920. ISSN (electronic): 1532-1827

Bailey, R. The cytoskeleton, In: About.com Biology, 2011, http: //biology.about.com/od/cellanatomy/a/aa013108a.htm

Bauer, H., Zweimueller-Mayer, J, Steinbacher, P., Lametschwandtner, A & Bauer, HC. (2010). The Dual Role of Zonula Occludens (ZO) Proteins. *Journal of Biomedicine and Biotechnology* Volume 2010, Article ID 402593, 11 pages ISSN (printed): 1110-7243, ISSN (electronic): 1110-7251

Ben-Ze'ev, A. (1997). Cytoskeletal and adhesion proteins as tumor suppressors. Curr. Opin. Cell Biol. Vol.9 No.1, pp. 99–108, (Online); ISSN:0955-0674

Blachon, S & Demeret, C. (2003). The regulatory E2 proteins of human genital papillomaviruses are pro-apoptotic. *Biochimie* Vol. 85, pp. 813-819 ISSN: 0300-9084

Bosch, FX., Lorincz, A., Munoz, N., Meijer, CJ & Shah KV. (2002). The causal relation between human papillomavirus and cervical cancer. *J Clin Pathol* Vol.55 pp. 244–65. ISSN (printed): 0021-9746. ISSN (electronic): 1472-4146.

Brentjens, MH., Yeung-Yue, KA., Lee, PC &Tyring, SK. (2002). Human papillomavirus: a review. *Dermatol Clin* Vol.20 pp. 315–31. ISSN: 0738-081X (Print) 1879-1131 (Electronic

Burd E. (2003). Human Papillomavirus and Cervical Cancer. *Clin Microbiol Rev* Jan pp. 1-17 ISSN: 0983-8512

Campo, S. (2005). The essential transforming proteins of HPV: E5, E6 and E7. News letter on Human Papillomavirus. HPV Today 2005: 8-10 website: www.hpvtoday.com

Carmo-Fonseca M & David-Ferreira JF. (1990). Interactions of intermediate filaments with cell structures. *Electron Microscopy Reviews* Vol. 3, Issue 1, pp. 115-141, ISSN: 0892-0354

Caulin, C., C. F. Ware, T. M. Magin, & R. G. Oshima. (2000). Keratindependent, epithelial resistance to tumor necrosis factor-induced apoptosis. *J. Cell Biol.* Vol. 149 pp.17–22, ISSN (printed): 0021-9525. ISSN (electronic): 1540-8140

Cho, NH., Kang, S., Hong, S., Jeong, GB., Choi, IW., Choi, HJ & Choi HK. (2005). Multinucleation of koilocytes is in fact multilobation and is related to aberration of the G2 checkpoint. *J Clin Pathol* Vol. 58 pp. 576-582 ISSN (printed): 0021-9746. ISSN (electronic)

Cho, NH., Kang, S., Hong, S., Jeong, GB., Choi, IW., Choi, HJ & Choi HK. (2006). Multinucleation of koilocytes is actually multilobation. *Int J Gynecol Cancer.* (Mar-Apr) Vol. 16 No. 2 pp.686-9 ISSN (printed): 1048-891X

Chow, LT., Reilly SS, T. R. Broker TR, & L. B. Taichman LB. (1987). Identification and mapping of human papillomavirus type 1 RNA transcripts recovered from plantar warts and infected epithelial cell cultures. *J. Virol.* Vol. 61 pp. 1913–1918. Online ISSN: 1098-5514; Print ISSN: 0022-538X .

Conrad M, Bubb VJ, Schlegel R. (1993). The human papillomavirus type 6 and 16 E5 proteins are membrane- associated proteins which associate with the 16 kilodalton pore-forming protein, *J. Virol.* Vol.67 pp. 6170– 6178. Online ISSN: 1098-5514; Print ISSN: 0022-538X ...

Cooper, B., Brimer, N & Vande Pol SB. (2007). Human Papillomavirus E6 Regulates the Cytoskeleton Dynamics of Keratinocytes through Targeted Degradation of p53. *Journal of Virology* (Nov) Vol. 81, No. 22 pp. 12675–12679, Online ISSN: 1098-5514; Print ISSN: 0022-538X

Dao, LD., Duffy, A., Van Tine, BA., Wu, SY., Chiang, CM., Broker, TR & Chow LT. (2006). Dynamic Localization of the Human Papillomavirus Type 11 Origin Binding Protein E2 through Mitosis While in Association with the Spindle Apparatus. *Journal of Virology* Vol.80, No.10 (May) pp. 4792-4800 Online ISSN: 1098-5514; Print ISSN: 0022-538X

Das, K., Bohl, J & Vande Pol, SB. (2000). Identification of a second transforming function in bovine papillomavirus type 1 E6 and the role of E6 interactions with paxillin, E6BP, and E6AP. *J. Virol.* Vol. 74 pp. 812–816, ISSN: 0022-538X

Davy CE, Jackson JD, Wang Q et al. Identification of a G2 arrest domain in the E1^E4 of Human Papillomavirus type 16. 2002. *J Virol* Vol.76, pp.9806-9818, Online ISSN: 1098-5514; Print ISSN: 0022-538X

de Villiers, EM., Fauquet, C., Broker, TR., Bernard, HU & zur Hausen, H. (2004). Classification of papillomaviruses. *Virology* Vol. 324:17–27. ISSN: 0042-6822

Degenhardt, YY & Silverstein, SJ. (2001). Gps2, a protein partner for human papillomavirus E6 proteins. *J. Virol.* Vol. 5 pp.151–160, ISSN: 0022-538X

Doorbar J. (2005). The papillomavirus life cycle. *Journal of Clinical Virology* vol. 32S pp. S7–S15 ISSN: 1386-6532

Doorbar, J., Ely, S., Sterling, J., McLean, C & Crawford L. (1991). Specific interaction between HPV-16 E1-E4 and cytokeratins results in collapse of the epithelial cell intermediate filament network. *Nature*. (Aug) Vol. 29 No. 352 (6338) pp. 824-7. ISSN : 0028-0836

Doorbar, JA. Parton, K., Hartley, K., Banks, L., Crook, ., Stanley, & Crawford.L. (1990). Detection of novel splicing patterns in an HPV16-containing keratinocyte cell line.*Virology* Vol. 178 pp. 254–262. ISSN: 0042-6822

Durst, M., Kleinheinz, A., Hotz, M. & Gissmann, L. (1985. The physical state of human papillomavirus type 16 DNA in benign and malignant genital tumors. *J Gen Virol* Vol. 66 pp.1515–22 Print ISSN: 0022-1317; Online ISSN: 1465-2099

Dyson, N., Howley, PM., Munger, K & Harlow E. (1989). The human papilloma virus-16 E7 oncoprotein is able to bind to the retinoblastoma gene product. *Science* Vol. 243, pp.: 934–937. ISSN 0036-8075 (print), 1095-9203 (online)

Etienne-Manneville, S & Hall, A. (2002). Rho GTPases in cell biology. *Nature* Vol. 420 pp. 629-635, ISSN : 0028-0836

Fanning, A. S., Jameson, BJ., Jesaitis, LA., & Anderson, JM. (1998). The tight junction protein ZO-1 establishes a link between the transmembrane protein occludin and the actin cytoskeleton. *J. Biol. Chem.* Vol. 273, pp.29745–29753, Print ISSN 0021-9258; Online ISSN 1083-351X

Filippova, M., Song, H., Connolly, JL., Dermody, TS & Duerksen- Hughes, PJ. (2002). The human papillomavirus 16 E6 protein binds to tumor necrosis factor (TNF) R1 and protects cells from TNF-induced apoptosis. *J. Biol. Chem.* Vol. 277 pp.21730–21739, Print ISSN 0021-9258; Online ISSN 1083-351X

Flores, E., Allen-Hoffmann, L., Lee, D & Lambert P. (2000). The Human Papillomavirus type 16 E7 oncogene is required for the productive stage of the viral life cycle. *J Virol* Vol. 74 pp. 6622-6631 Online ISSN: 1098-5514; Print ISSN: 0022-538X

Florin, L., Becker, KA., Lambert, C., Nowak, T., Sapp, C., Strand, D., Streeck, RE & Sapp, M. (2006). Identification of a Dynein interacting domain in the papillomavirus minor capsid protein *J Virol. (Jul) Vol.80, No.13, pp.6691-6* 16775357, Online ISSN: 1098-5514; Print ISSN: 0022-538X

Fornatora, M., Jones, AC., Kerpel, S & Freedman P. (1996). Human papillomavirus-associated oral epithelial dysplasia (koilocytic dysplasia): an entity of unknown biologic potential. *Oral Surg Oral Med Oral Pathol Oral Radiol Endod* Vol. 82 pp. 47-56 ISSN (printed): 1079-2104. ISSN (electronic): 1528-395X

Fuchs, E., & K. Weber. (1994). Intermediate filaments: structure, dynamics, function, and disease. *Annu. Rev. Biochem.* Vol. 63 pp. 345–382, ISSN: 0066-4154

Gammoh, N., Grm, HS., Massimi, P & Banks, L. (2006). Regulation of Human papillomavirus type 16 E7 activity through direct protein interaction with the E2 transcriptional activator. *J Virol* pp. 1787-1797 Online ISSN: 1098-5514; Print ISSN: 0022-538X

Gao, Q., Kumar, A., Srinivasan, S., Singh, L., Mukai, H., Ono, Y., Wazer, DE, & Band V. (2000). PKN binds and phosphorylates human papillomavirus E6 oncoprotein. *J. Biol. Chem.* Vol. 275 pp. 14824–14830, Print ISSN 0021-9258; Online ISSN 1083-351X

Gao, Q., Srinivasan, S., Boyer, SN., Wazer, DE & Band, V. (1999). The E6 oncoproteins of high-risk papillomaviruses bind to a novel putative GAP protein, E6TP1, and target it for degradation. *Mol. Cell. Biol.* Vol.19 pp.733–744, Online ISSN: 1098-5549; Print ISSN: 0270-7306

Gilbert, S., A. Loranger, N. Daigle, & N. Marceau. (2001). Simple epithelium keratins 8 and 18 provide resistance to Fas-mediated apoptosis. The protection occurs through a receptor-targeting modulation. *J. Cell Biol.* Vol. 154 pp.763– 773, ISSN (printed): 0021-9525. ISSN (electronic): 1540-8140

Gumbiner, B., Lowenkopf T & Apatira D. (1991). Identification of a 160- kDa polypeptide that binds to the tight junction protein ZO-1. *Proc. Natl. Acad. Sci. USA* Vol. 88 pp.3460–3464, ISSN:0027-8424 (Print) ; 1091-6490 (Electronic) ; 0027-8424 (Linking).

Gumbiner, BM. (1996). Cell adhesion: the molecular basis of tissue architecture and morphogenesis. *Cell* Vol.84 pp.345–357, ISSN: 0092-8674

Hall, A. (1994). Small GTP-binding proteins and the regulation of the actin cytoskeleton. *Annu. Rev. Cell Biol.* Vol.10 pp. 31-54, ISSN: 0743-4634

Haugen, CTPTH., Turk, JP., Tabatabai, F., Schmid III, PG., Durst, M., Gissmann, L., Roman A & Turek LP. (1987). Transcriptional regulation of the human papillomavirus-16 E6–E7 promoter by a keratinocyte- dependent enhancer, and by viral E2 trans-activator and repressor gene products: implications for cervical carcinogenesis. *EMBO* J. Vol.6 pp.3745–3753 ISSN 0261-4189

Holmgren, SC., Patterson, NA., Ozbun, MA & Lambert PF. (2005). The minor capsid protein L2 contributes to two steps in the human papillomavirus type 31 life cycle. *J Virol*, Vol.79 pp.3938-3948, Online ISSN: 1098-5514; Print ISSN: 0022-538X

Hoory, T., Monie, A., Grawitt, P & Wu TC. (2008). Molecular epidemiology of human papillomavirus. *J Formos Med Assoc* Vol. 107 pp. 198-217 ISSN: 0929-6646

Horvath, CAJ., Gaëlle, AV., Boulet, GAV., Renoux, VM., Philippe, O., Delvenne, PO., John-Paul, J & Bogers, JPJ. (2010). Mechanisms of cell entry by human papillomaviruses: an overview. *Virology Journal* Vol.7:No.11, pp.1-7 ISSN: 1743-422X

Howarth AG & Stevenson BR. (1995). Molecular environment of ZO-1 in epithelial and non-epithelial cells. *Cell Motil. Cytoskeleton.* Vol.31, No.4, pp.323-332, ISSN (printed): 0886-1544. ISSN (electronic): 1097-0169

Howley PM: Papillomavirinae: The viruses and Their Replication. In: Fields BN, Knipe DM, Howley PM (Eds): Fundamental Virology. 3th ed. Philadelphia, JB Lippincott Company, 1996;947-978

Hughes, FJ & Romanos, MA. (1993). E1 protein of human papillomavirus is a DNA helicase/ATPase. *Nucleic Acids Research* Vol.21, No.25 pp. 5817-5823 Online ISSN 1362-4962 Print ISSN 0305-1048

Iftner, T., Elbel, M., Schopp, B., Hiller, T., Loizou, JI., Caldecott, KW & Stubenrauch, F. (2002). Interference of papillomavirus E6 protein with singlestrand break repair by interaction with XRCC1. *EMBO J.* Vol. 21 pp.4741–4748, ISSN 0261-4189

Inada, H., I. Izawa, M. Nishizawa, E. Fujita, T. Kiyono, T. Takahashi, T. Momoi, & M. Inagaki. (2001). Keratin attenuates tumor necrosis factorinduced cytotoxicity through association with TRADD. J. Cell Biol. 155:415- 426, ISSN (printed): 0021-9525. ISSN (electronic): 1540-8140

Itoh, M., Nagafuchi, A., Moroi, S., & Tsukita, S. (1997). Involvement of ZO-1 in cadherin-based adhesion through its binding to-catenin and actin filaments. *J. Cell Biol.* Vol.138 pp. 181–192, ISSN (printed): 0021-9525. ISSN (electronic): 1540-8140

Jesaitis, LA & Goodenough DA. (1994). Molecular characterization and tissue distribution of ZO-2, a tight junction protein homologous to ZO-1 and the Drosophila discs-large tumor suppressor protein *J. Cell Biol* Vol.124 pp.949-961, ISSN (printed): 0021-9525. ISSN (electronic): 1540-8140

Jones, DL & Munger, K. (1996). Interactions of the human papillomavirus E7 protein with cell cycle regulators. *Seminars in Cancer Biology* Vol.7: 327-337 ISSN: 1044-579X

Kabsch K, Alonso A. (2002). The Human Papillomavirus Type 16 E5 Protein Impairs TRAIL and FasLMediated Apoptosis in HaCaT cells by different mechanisms. J Virol Vol.76 pp.12162-12172, Online ISSN: 1098-5514; Print ISSN: 0022-538X ...

Koning MNC, Khoe LV, Eekhof JAH, Kampa M, Gussekloo J, Ter Schegget J, Bouwes Bavinck JNB & Quint WGV. (2011). Lesional HPV types of cutaneous warts can be reliably identified by surface swabs. *J Clin Virol.* ISSN: 1386-6532

Krawczyk, E., Suprynowicz, FA & Liu, X et al. (2008). Koilocytosis, A cooperative interaction between the Human Papillomavirus E5 and E6 oncoproteins. *Am J Pathol* Vol. 173 pp. 682-688 ISSN: 0002-9440 (Print) 1525-2191 (Electronic)

Ku, N. O., R. M. Soetikno, & M. B. Omary. (2003). Keratin mutation in transgenic mice predisposes to Fas but not TNF-induced apoptosis and massive liver injury. *Hepatology* Vol. 37 pp.1006–1014, Online ISSN: 1527-3350

Ku¨hne, C & L. Banks L. (1998). E3-ubiquitin ligase/E6-AP links multicopy maintenance protein 7 to the ubiquitination pathway by a novel motif, the L2G box. *J. Biol. Chem.* Vol. 273 pp.34302–34309, Print ISSN 0021-9258; Online ISSN 1083-351X

Lee, SH & Dominguez, R. (2010). Regulation of actin cytoskeleton dynamics in cells. *Mol Cells.* (Apr) Vol.29 No. 4 pp. 311-25 ISSN 1097-2765 (printable version).

Longworth, MS. & Laimins, LA. (2004). Pathogenesis of Human Papillomaviruses in Differentiating Epithelia. *Microbiology and Molecular Biology Reviews.* Vol. 68, No. 2, (June) pp. 362–372 Online ISSN: 1098-5557; Print ISSN: 1092-2172

Martineza, I., Wangb, J., Hobsona, KF., Robert, L., Ferrisb, RL., Saleem, A & Khana SA. (2007). Identification of differentially expressed genes in HPV-positive and HPV-negative oropharyngeal squamous cell carcinomas. *European Journal of Cancer* Vol. 43 pp. 415 -432 ISSN: 0959-8049

Matter, K & Balda MS. (2003). Signalling to and from tight junctions. *Nat. Rev. Mol. Cell Biol.* Vol. 4 pp.225–236, ISSN (printed): 1471-0072. ISSN (electronic): 1471-0080.

McIntosh, PB, Laskey P, Sullivan K, Davy C, Wang Q, Jackson DJ, Griffin HM, & John Doorbar. J. (2010). E1^E4-mediated keratin phosphorylation and ubiquitylation: a mechanism for keratin depletion in HPV16-infected epithelium. *J Cell Sci.* (August) Vol. 15; No. 123(16) pp. 2810–2822 Online ISSN: 1477-9137; Print ISSN: 0021-9533

Meissner, JD. (1999). Nucleotide sequences and further characterization of human papillomavirus DNA present in the CaSki, SiHa and HeLa cervical carcinoma cell lines. *J Gen Virol* Vol. 80 pp.1725–33 Print ISSN: 0022-1317; Online ISSN: 1465-2099

Miyahara, GI., Simonato, LE., Mattar, NJ., Camilo, Jr DJ & Biasoli ER. (2011). Correlation between koilocytes and human papillomavirus detection by PCR in oral and oropharynx squamous cell carcinoma biopsies. *Mem Inst Oswaldo Cruz, Rio de Janeiro,* (March) Vol. 106 No. 2 pp. 166-169 Print version ISSN 0074-0276

Moll, R., W. W. Franke, D. L. Schiller, B. Geiger, & R. Krepler. (1982). The catalog of human cytokeratins: patterns of expression in normal epithelia, tumors and cultured cells. *Cell* Vol. 31 pp.11–24, ISSN: 0092-8674

Mu¨nger, K., Baldwin, A., Edwards, KM., Hayakawa, H., Nguyen, CL., Owens, M., Grace, & M, Won Huh, K. (2004). Mechanisms of Human Papillomavirus-Induced Oncogenesis. *Journal of Virology* (Nov) pp. 11451–11460 Online ISSN: 1098-5514; Print ISSN: 0022-538X

Myers, G., Bernard, H-U., Delius, H., Favre, M., Icenogel, J., Van Ranst, M., Wheeler C, editors. Human papillomaviruses a compilation and analysis of nucleic acid and amino acid sequences. 1st ed. Los Alamos, USA: Theoretical Biology and biophysics group T-10, Los Alamos National Laboratory; 1994.

Nakahara T, Nishimura A, Tanaka M, Ueno T, Ishimoto A, Sakai H. Modulation of the cell division cycle by Human Papillomavirus type 18 E4. *(2002). J Virol* . Vol. 76, pp.10914-10920, Online ISSN: 1098-5514; Print ISSN: 0022-538X

Nasseri, M., Hirochika, R., Broker TR, & Chow LT. (1987). A human papillomavirus type 11 transcript encoding an E1∧E4 protein. *Virology* Vol. 159 pp.433–439. ISSN: 0042-6822

Nguyen CL & Mu¨nger K. (2009). Human Papillomavirus E7 Protein Deregulates Association with Nuclear Mitotic Apparatus. *Journal Of Virology* (Feb) pp. 1700–1707, Online ISSN: 1098-5514; Print ISSN: 0022-538X

Nguyen, CL., McLaughlin-Drubin, ME & Munger K. (2008). Delocalization of the microtubule motor dynein from mitotic by the Human Papillomavirus E7 oncoprotein is not induction of multipolar mitoses. *Cancer Res* Vol. 68 No.21 pp. 8715-8722 Online ISSN: 1538-7445; Print ISSN: 0008-5472

Ohta A & Nishiyama Y. (2011). Mitochondria and viruses. *Mitochondrion* Vol.11 pp.1-12, ISSN: 1567-7249

Ozbun, MA &Meyers, C. (1998). Temporal usage of multiple promoters during the life cycle of human papillomavirus type 31b. *J Virol* Vol. 72 pp.2715–22 Online ISSN: 1098-5514; Print ISSN: 0022-538X

Penky, M & Lane EB. (2007). Intermediate filaments and stress. *Experimental Cell Research* Vol. 313;2244-2254, ISSN: 0014-4827

Pim, D & Banks, L. (2010). Interaction of viral oncoproteins with cellular target molecules: infection with high-risk vs low-risk human papillomaviruses *APMIS* Vol. 118 pp. 471–493 Online ISSN: 1600-0463

Prétet, JL., Charlot, JF & Mougin, C. (2007). Virological and carcinogenic aspects of HPV. *Bull Acad Natl Med.* Vol.191, No.3 (Mar) pp. 611-23 ISSN: 0001-4079 (Print)

Raftopoulou, M & Hall, A. (2004). Cell migration: Rho GTPases lead the way. *Dev. Biol.* Vol. 265, pp. 23-32, ISSN: 1054-5476

Raj, K., Berguerand, S., Southern, S., Doorbar, J., & Beard P. (2004). E1^E4 Protein of Human Papillomavirus Type 16 Associates with Mitochondria. *Journal of Virology,* (July) Vol. 78, pp. 7199–7207 Online ISSN: 1098-5514; Print ISSN: 0022-538X

Ramoz, N., Rueda, LA., Bouadjar, B., Montoya, LS., Orth, G &Favre M. (2002). Mutations in two adjacent novel genes are associated with epidermodysplasia verruciformis. *Nat Genet* Vol.32 pp.579–81. ISSN : 1061-4036

Rapp L & Chen J. (1998). The papillomavirus E6 proteins. *Biochim Biophys Acta* (Aug) Vol. 19 pp. F1-19, ISSN 0006-3002

Rey, O., Lee, S., Marcel, A., Baluda, MA., Swee, J., Ackerson, B., Chiu, R & Park NH. (2000). The E7 Oncoprotein of Human Papillomavirus Type 16 Interacts with F-Actin in Vitro and in Vivo. *Virology* Vol. 268 pp. 372- 381 ISSN: 0042-6822

Romani VG, Abramson AL & Steinberg BM. (1987). Laryngeal papilloma cells in culture have an altered cytoskeleton. *Acta Otolaryngol.* (Mar-Apr) Vol. 103 No. (3-4) pp. 345-52, ISSN (printed): 0001-6489. ISSN (electronic): 1651-2251

Safi Oz Z. (2010). Approach to koilocytosis mechanism by HPV proteins. *Marmara Medical Journal* Vol. 23 No. 1 pp;60-66 Online ISSN: 1309 - 9469. Print ISSN: 1019 - 1941

Safi, Z., Demirezen, S., Mocan Kuzey, G., Beksac, MS & Ustacelebi S. (2009). Cytologic and Clinical Evaluation of Human Papillomavirus in Women Underwent Routine Gynecologic Examination. *Gynecol Obstet Reprod Med.* Vol.15 No.2 pp.94-99 (ISSN 1300-4751),

Scheffner, M., Werness, BA., Huibregtse, JM., Levine, AJ & Howley PM. (1990). The E6 oncoprotein encoded by human papillomavirus types 16 and 18 promotes the degradation of p53. *Cell* Vol. 63 pp.1129–1136. ISSN: 0092-8674

Schelhaas, M., Ewers, H., Rajamäki, ML., Day, PM., Schiller, JT & Helenius A. (2008). Human papillomavirus type 16 entry: retrograde cell surface transport along actin-rich protrusions. *PLoS Pathog* (Sep) Vol.5 No.4,e1000148, ISSN 1553-7366

Schneider, MA., Spoden, GA., Florin, L & Lambert, C. (2011). Identification of the Dynein Light Chains required for Human Papillomavirus Infection. *Cell Microbiol.* (Aug) Vol.13 No.1,pp.32-46, ISSN (printed): 1462-5814. ISSN (electronic): 1462-5822.

Serres, M., Filhol O, Lickert H, Grangeasse C, Chambaz EM, Stappert J, Vincent, C & Schmitt D. (2000) The disruption of adherens junctions is associated with a decrease of E-cadherin phosphorylation by protein kinase CK2. Exp. *Cell Res.* Vol.257 pp.255–264, ISSN: 1001-0602

Stanley M. (2001). Human Papillomavirus and cervical carcinogenesis. *Best Pract Res Clin Obstet Gynecol* Vol. 15 pp. 663-676 ISSN: 1521-6934

Strelkov SV, Herrmann H & Aebi U. (2003). Molecular architecture of intermediate filaments. *BioEssay* Vol.3 pp. 243-251, ISSN: 1809-8460

Suprynowicz FA, Disbrow GL, Krawczyk E, Simic V, Lantzky K & Schlegel R. (2008). HPV 16 E5 oncoprotein upregulates lipid raft components caveolin-1 and ganglioside GM1 at the plasma membrane of cervical cells. Oncogene Vol. 27 pp. 1071-1078, ISSN: 0950-9232

Tong, X & Howley, PM. (1997). The bovine papillomavirus E6 oncoprotein interacts with paxillin and disrupts the actin cytoskeleton. *Proc Natl Acad Sci U S A.* (Apr) Vol. 29 No.94 (9) pp. 4412-7, ISSN:0027-8424 (Print); 1091-6490 (Electronic); 0027-8424 (Linking)

Tong, X & Howley, PM. (1997). The bovine papillomavirus E6 oncoprotein interacts with paxillin and disrupts the actin cytoskeleton. *Proc. Natl. Acad. Sci. USA* Vol. 94 pp. 4412–4417, ISSN:0027-8424 (Print) ; 1091-6490 (Electronic) ; 0027-8424 (Linking)

Traweger, A., Fuchs, R., Krizbai, IA., Weiger, TM., Bauer, HC & Bauer, H. (2003). The Tight Junction Protein ZO-2 Localizes to the Nucleus and Interacts with the Heterogeneous Nuclear Ribonucleoprotein Scaffold Attachment Factor-B. *The Journal of Biological Chemistry* Vol. 278, No. 4, (Issue of January 24), pp. 2692–2700, Print ISSN 0021-9258; Online ISSN 1083-351X

Turner CE. Paxillin interactions. (2000). Cell Science at a glance. J Cell Sci Vol.113, pp.4139-4140 www.biologists.com/jcs, Online ISSN: 1477-9137; Print ISSN: 0021-9533.

Uribe R & Jay D. (2009). A review of actin binding proteins: new perspectives. *Mol Biol Rep.* Vol. 36 pp.121-125 ISSN (printed): 0301-4851. ISSN (electronic): 1573-4978

Walboomers, J., Jacobs, M., Manos, MM., Bosch, F., Kummer, J & Shah K, et al. (1999). Human papillomavirus is a necessary cause of invasive cervical cancer worldwide. *J Pathol* Vol. 189 pp.12–9. ISSN: 0022-3417 Online ISSN: 1096-9896

Wang, Q., Griffin, H., Southern, S., Jackson, D., Martin, A., McIntosh, P., Clare Davy, C., Phillip J. Masterson PJ., Philip A. Walker PA., Laskey, P., Omary MB., & Doorbar1 J. (2004). Functional Analysis of the Human Papillomavirus Type 16 E1^E4 Protein Provides a Mechanism for In Vivo and In Vitro Keratin Filament Reorganization. *Journal of Virology* (Jan) Vol.78 No.2 pp.821–833 Online ISSN: 1098-5514; Print ISSN: 0022-538X

Wang, Q., Griffin, S., Southern, S., Jackson, D., Martin, A., McIntosh, P., Davy, C., Masterson, P., Walker, P., Laskey, P., Omary, M., & Doorbar J. (2004). Functional analysis of the human papillomavirus type 16 E1^E4 protein provides a mechanism for in vivo and in vitro keratin filament reorganization. *J. Virol.* Vol.78 pp. 821–833. Online ISSN: 1098-5514; Print ISSN: 0022-538X ...

Werness, BA., Levine, AJ & Howley PM. (1990). Association of human papillomavirus types 16 and 18 E6 proteins with p53. *Science* Vol. 248 pp.76-79

Wilson, VG., West, M., Woytek, K & Rangasamy D. (2002). Papillomavirus E1 proteins: Form, Function, and Features. *Virus Genes* Vol.24, No. 3, pp. 275-290 ISSN: 0920-8569

Wittchen, ES., Haskins, J & Stevenson, BR. (1999). Protein interactions at the tight junction. Actin has multiple binding partners, and ZO-1 forms independent complexes with ZO-2 and ZO-3. *J. Biol. Chem.* (Dec 3) Vol. 274 No. 49 pp. 35179–35185, Print ISSN 0021-9258; Online ISSN 1083-351X

Yang, DH., Wildeman, AG & Sharom FJ. (2003). Overexpression, purification, and structural analysis of the hydrophobic E5 protein from human papillomavirus type 16. *Protein Expression and Purification* Vol. 30 pp. 1–10 ISSN (printed): 1046-5928. ISSN (electronic): 1096-0279

Yeaman, C., Grindstaff, KK & Nelson, WJ. (1999). New perspectives on mechanisms involved in generating epithelial cell polarity. *Physiol. Rev.* Vol. 79 pp.73–98, ISSN: 0031-9333

Yee, C., Krishnan, HI., Baker, CC., Schlegel, R & Howley PM. (1985). Presence and expression of human papillomavirus sequences in human cervical carcinoma cell lines. *Am J Pathol* Vol.119 pp.361–6 ISSN: 0002-9440 (Print) 1525-2191 (Electronic)

Yue, J., Shukla, R., Accardi, R., Zanella-Cleon, I., Siouda, M., Cros, MP., Krutovskikh, V., Hussain, I., Niu, Y., Hu, S., Becchi, M., Jurdic, P., Tommasino, M & Sylla, BS. (2011). Cutaneous HPV 38 E7 Regulates Actin Cytoskeleton Structure for Increasing Cell Proliferation through CK2 and the Eukaryotic Elongation Factor 1A. *J Virol.* (Jun 22) [Epub ahead of print) ISSN: 0022-538X

Zhang, Y, Dasgupta, J., Ma, RZ., Banks, L., Thomas, M & Chen, XS. (2007). Structures of a Human Papillomavirus (HPV) E6 Polypeptide Bound to MAGUK Proteins: Mechanisms of Targeting Tumor Suppressors by a High-Risk HPV Oncoprotein. *Journal of Virology* (Apr) Vol. 81, No. 7 pp. 3618–3626, Online ISSN: 1098-5514; Print ISSN: 0022-538X

zur Hausen H. (2000). Papillomaviruses causing cancer: Evasion from host-cell control in early events in carcinogenesis. *J Natl Cancer* Inst Vol. 92 pp.690–8 ISSN: 0027-8874, online ISSN : 1460-2105

zur Hausen H. (2002). Papillomaviruses and cancer: from basic studies to clinical application. *Nature Rev Cancer* Vol.2 pp. 342–50 (ISSN: 1474-175X, 1474-1768).

12

A Functional RNAi-Based Knockdown System: A Tool to Investigate HPV Entry?

Caroline Horvath[1], Gaelle Boulet[1], Shaira Sahebali[1], John-Paul Bogers[1,2] and Davy Vanden Broeck[1,2*]

[1]*Applied Molecular Biology Research Group (AMBIOR), University of Antwerp, Antwerp*
[2]*International Centre for Reproductive Health (ICRH), Ghent University, Ghent*
Belgium

1. Introduction

Worldwide, cervical cancer is an important health issue leading to high morbidity and mortality rates. The HPV virus plays an essential in the development of this disease. Of the more than 100 different HPV types identified, 40 are known to infect the genital tract (Woodman et al., 2007). These mucosal HPV types are classified as "low-risk" and "high-risk" types based on the prevalence ratio in cervical cancer and its precursors. Low-risk HPV types, such as 6 and 11, induce benign lesions with minimum risk of progression to malignancy. In contrast, high-risk HPVs have higher oncogenic potential (Fehrmann & Laimins, 2003). Approximately 99% of cervical cancers contain HPV DNA of high-risk types, with type HPV16 being the most prevalent, followed by types 18, 31, 33, and 45. Cervical HPV infection is one of the most common sexually transmitted infections (Walboomers et al. 1999; Woodman et al., 2007).

HPVs are obligatory intracellular parasites that must deliver their genome and accessory proteins into host cells and subsequently make use of the biosynthetic cellular machinery for viral replication. The journey of a HPV particle from the cell surface to the cytosol and nucleus consists of a series of consecutive steps that move it closer to its site of replication (Day & Schiller, 2006; Marsh & Helenius, 2006). Host cell entry of HPV is initiated by binding of the virus particle to cell surface receptors followed by internalization. Since HPV replication and assembly requires infected basal keratinocytes to undergo the stepwise differentiation program of the epithelium, HPV propagation in cell culture is a major challenge. This has prompted many researchers to study the HPV-host cell interactions by generating VLPs, PsVs and QVs. Because of many difficulties, including viral particle heterogeneity due to the maturity state of the "artificial" viral particles used in many studies, data concerning the HPV entry mechanisms are contradictory and still a subject of scientific debate (Horvath et al., 2010).

To prevent and cure HPV infections and its complications, it is important to identify the viral infection mechanisms by means of investigating the viral biology. Viral attachment and

---

* Corresponding author

internalization are first fundamental steps in the infection process and therefore, the ideal points to interfere with the progression of the viral life cycle. Identifying HPV uptake mechanisms may lead to a more specific pharmacological control of viral processing hereby improving therapeutic and prevention strategies.

The design of a tool to study HPV internalization is the important goal in this research project. HPVs are small, non-enveloped DNA viruses that generally enter through clathrin-coated endocytic vesicles or via the clathrin-independent caveolae system (Day et al., 2003). To date, most of the studies proved that different types of HPVs entered cells in distinct pathways, including clathrin-mediated endocytosis, caveolar endocytosis and clathrin- and caveolae-independent uptake mechanisms, although it was found that clathrin-mediated endocytosis was the major cellular entry route (Horvath et al., 2010). Therefore, it is important to design an experimental model to study the exact role of clathrin-mediated endocytosis in the uptake of HPV.

The use of molecular tools with such precise specificity to individual cellular functions allows the defined examination of endocytic pathways (Day et al., 2006). In an experimental setting, it is challenging to identify a particular endocytotic pathway that is unique for the uptake of a specific ligand. It is important that the internalization route of interest is exclusively suppressed without affecting other endocytotic pathways. Chemical inhibitors like cholesterol extracting or sequestrating drugs such as cyclodextrins, filipin and nystatin not only disrupt caveolae/lipid rafts, but also lead to the destabilization of CCPs (Rodal et al., 1999; Subtil et al., 1999). The development of molecular inhibitors in the form of dominant negative molecules has surpassed the use of these pharmacological inhibitors in terms of decreasing non-specific effects (Day et al., 2003). Different accessory proteins such as dynamin, amphiphysin and Eps15 have been subjected to dominant negative overexpression (Benmerah et al., 1998; Benmerah et al., 1999; Yao et al., 2005).

Targeting viral mRNA is one of the most active areas of research and development. Several strategies have emerged over the years such as antisense-oligonucleotides, ribozymes and RNA interference (RNAi). All these strategies share the features of conceptual simplicity, straightforward drug design and quick route to identify drug leads (Le Calvez et al., 2004). RNA interference is the inhibition of expression of specific genes by double-stranded RNAs (dsRNAs). It is becoming the method of choice to knockdown gene expression rapidly and robustly in mammalian cells. Comparing to the traditional antisense method, RNAi technology has the advantage of significantly enhanced potency, therefore, only lower concentrations may be needed to achieve the same level of gene knockdown. RNAi gained rapid acceptance by researchers after Tuschl *et al.* discovered that *in vitro* synthesized small interfering RNAs (siRNAs) of 21 to 23 nucleotides in length can effectively silence targeted genes in mammalian cells without triggering interferon production (Le Calvez et al., 2004; Tuschl et al., 1999).

The transient nature of siRNA, due to the short lifespan of synthetic RNA molecules and the absence of a RNA-dependent RNA polymerase in mammalian cells, limits its applications (Dykxhoorn et al., 2008; Kim & Rossi, 2007; Rao et al., 2009). To overcome these limitations, a vector-based production of short hairpin RNA (shRNA) is used, hereby mediating a long-term and stable knockdown of the target transcripts for as long as transcription of the shRNAs takes place (Brummelkamp et al., 2002, Kim & Rossi, 2007; Paddison et al., 2002).

As described above, epsin is an essential accessory protein involved in clathrin-mediated endocytosis. Therefore, epsin is the target protein to generate a shRNA-based knockdown construct to investigate the role of clathrin-mediated endocytosis in the uptake of HPV.

Another approach to investigate the role of clathrin-mediated endocytosis in the uptake of HPV, is the use of dominant-negative inhibitors of Eps15. Eps15 (epidermal growth factor pathway substrate 15) is a protein that is associated with clathrin-mediated endocytosis and consists of three different domains. The N-terminal region contains three copies of the conserved Eps15 homology domain (EH-domain). The central region of the protein is important in the homodimerization/oligodimerization of Eps15 and the C-terminal region contains binding sites for AP2. Overexpression of the C-terminal region (GFP-Eps15 DIII mutant) has a strong inhibitory effect on the uptake of the clathrin markers transferrin and epidermal growth factor receptor (EGFR) (figure 1) (Benmerah et al., 1998). Another Eps15 mutant (GFP-Eps15 EΔ95/295), missing the second and third EH-domain in its N-terminal region has a negative influence on clathrin-mediated internalization (figure 1) (Benmerah et al., 1999). Both vectors, in combination with a control plasmid (GFP-Eps15 D3Δ2), can be used in order to study the involvement of clathrin-mediated endocytosis in the uptake of HPV.

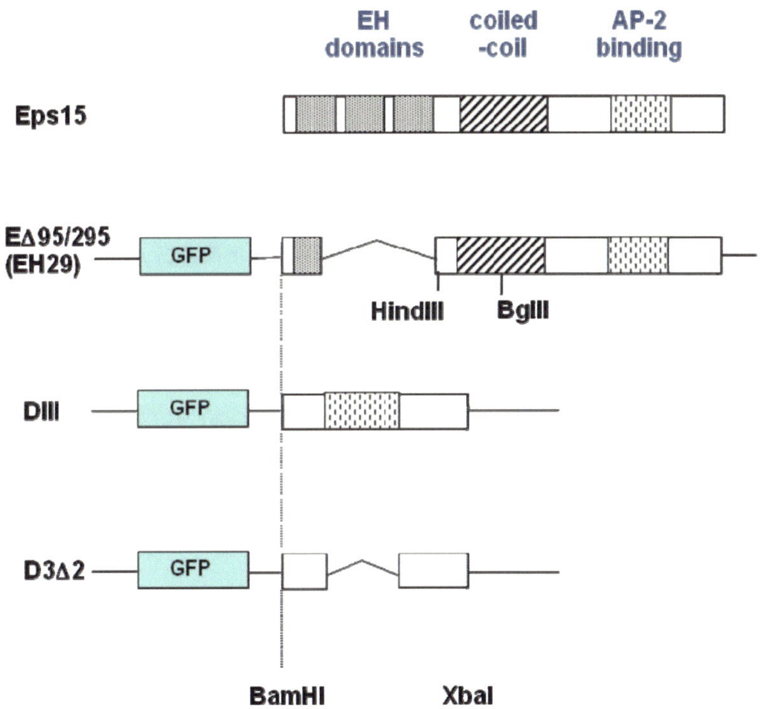

Fig. 1. Eps15 mutants
The EH29 mutant was generated by deleting 537 nucleotides (+288/+825) resulting in a construct length of 2163 nucleotides versus 2700 for wild type Eps15. This construct has been cloned between the BamHII/XbaI sites of the EGFP-C2 vector.
The DIII construct corresponds to the C-terminal domain of Eps15 (+1587/+2700) resulting in a construct length of 1200 bp. The D3D2 construct corresponds to DIII from which AP-2 binding sites has been removed (+1863/+2217) resulting in a 760 nucleotides long insert (Benmerah et al,, 1998; Benmerah et al., 1999).

2. Materials & methods

2.1 Cell culture

The human cervical cell line HeLa (ATCC CCL-2), which contains 10-50 copies of integrated HPV-18 and the human keratinocyte cell line HaCaT (Prof. Boukamp, Deutsches Krebsforschungszentrum (DKFZ), German Cancer Research Centre, Heidelberg, Germany), were grown under a humidified carbon dioxide atmosphere in Dulbecco's Modified Eagle's Medium (DMEM) supplemented with 10% fetal bovine serum, 200mM L-glutamin, 50mg/L penicillin/streptomycin, 50mg/L gentamicin, non-essential amino acids (Gibco, Carlsbad, CA, USA) and 50mg/L amphotericin (Sigma-Aldrich, Milan, Italy).

Human intestinal colon carcinoma cells, Caco-2 cells (ATCC HTB-37) were cultured in Modified Eagle's Medium (MEM) supplemented with 10% fetal bovine serum, non essential amino acids, 50mg/L penicillin/streptomycin, 50mg/L gentamicin, 55mg/L sodium pyruvate (Gibco, Carlsbad, CA, USA) and 1mg/L amphotericin (Sigma-Aldrich, Milan, Italy).

2.2 RNAi selection and plasmid preparation

Based on the primary sequences of the different epsin isoforms a multiple alignment and homology search was performed using ClustalW (searchlauncher.bcm.tmc.edu/multi-align/.html). A stretch of 21 nucleotides was selected from the conserved ENTH region located <0.2 kb after the start codon, according to the guidelines and parameters (Tuschl et al., 1999). (table 1).

pRNATin-H1.2/Neo is a siRNA inducible expression vector (GenScript). The H1.2 promotor is an engineered inducible H1 promotor (RNA polIII) containing a tetracycline operator (TetO1). The tetracycline operator itself has no effect on expression. When the tetracycline repressor (TetR) is present, it effectively binds the TetO1 and blocks the transcription. In the presence of tetracycline or doxycycline, the inducer binds TetR and causes the TetR protein to release the TetO1 site, and derepressing the transcription from the H1 promotor. The pRNATin-H1.2/Neo vector is designed for mammalian transfection and carries a neomycin resistance gene which can be used for establishing stable cell lines and a cGFP (coral GFP) marker under CMV promotor control to track the transfection efficiency. The insert is cloned after the H1 promotor and transcribed into short double stranded RNA (dsRNA) with a hairpin structure.

The parental plasmid was digested with *Bam*H1 and *Hin*dIII, separated on a 1% agarose gel and purified using the Qiagen Extraction kit. The shRNA insert was designed by using siRNA construct builder (GenScript; http://www.genscript.com/rnai.html). The shRNA sequences (table 1) were allowed to anneal and ligated into the digested vector using Ready-to-Go T4 ligase. In parallel, a functional non-targeting shRNA, a sequence with no matching mRNA (scrambled sequence) (table 1), was ligated into the same vector.

Correct insertion of the construct was confirmed by sequencing (data not shown). After transformation of *E.coli*, ampicillin recombinant strains were selected by using Fast-Media® Amp XGal Agar. Bacterial cells were grown in medium supplemented with 5µl/ml ampicillin and plasmids were purified using the PureYield Plasmid Midiprep System (Promega, Madison, WI, USA). Transformation and purification for the Eps15 mutant vectors was performed in a similar way, hereby selecting recombinant strains by using kanamycin selection.

Name	Sequence (5′→3′)
siRNA epsin	Forward: GAAGAACATCGTCCACAACTA Reverse: CTTCTTGTAGCAGGTGTTGAT
siRNA scrambled	Forward: GCATATGTGCGTACCTAGCAT Reverse: CGTATACACGCATGGATCGTA
shRNA epsin	GGATCCCGAAGAACATCGTGCACAACTATTCAAGAGATAGTTGTGC ACGATGTTCTTCTTTTTCCAAAAGCTT
shRNA scrambled	GGATCCCGCATATGTGCGTACCTAGCATTTCAAGAGAATGCTAGGTA CGCACATATGCTTTTTTCCAAAAGCTT

Table 1. siRNA and shRNA sequences

2.3 Transfection and selection

Liposomal transfection using Lipofectamine2000 (Invitrogen, San Diego, CA, USA) was performed according to the manufacture's protocol. In brief, 4 µg plasmid DNA was added to 250µl OptiMEM and gently mixed, 5µl Lipofectamine2000 was suspended in 250µl OptiMEM, both mixtures were combined after a 5 minute incubation at room temperature and added to HeLa and HaCaT cells, with a 90-95% cell density, in a 6-well plate.

HeLa and HaCaT cells were trypsinized 24h after transfection and seeded into a selection medium containing 100 µg/ml G418 as a starting point. A kill curve was created by doubling the G418 concentration with each medium change eventually culturing the HeLa and HaCaT cells in selection medium containing 1500 µg/ml G418.

To estimate the transfection efficiency through GFP expression, cells were grown in MatTek glass bottom dishes (MatTek Corp., Ashland, MA, USA), fixed with 4% paraformaldehyde for 30 min at RT and mounted in Citifluor. Confocal fluorescence microscopy (Zeiss CLSM 510) was used to discriminate between transfected and non-transfected cells. GFP-positive cells were counted by fluorescence microscopy and expressed as the percentage of the total amount of cells visualized by light microscopy.

2.4 Real-time RT-PCR

The effect of shRNA against epsin was evaluated by monitoring the epsin mRNA expression level.

Total RNA was isolated using the reagent-based method TRIzol® (Invitrogen, Carlsbad, CA, USA) and RNA concentration and purity were monitored by UV-spectrophotometry. Prior to cDNA synthesis, DNA was removed from the total RNA extracts. An amount of 12µl DNase-treated total RNA was reversed transcribed in a 20µl reaction volume using the

Transcriptor First Strand cDNA synthesis kit (Roche Applied Science, Indianapolis, IN, USA) according to the manufacturer's instructions.

Real-time RT-PCR analyses were performed using the LightCycler system based on the TaqMan methodology (Roche Applied Science, Indianapolis, IN, USA). PCR-efficiencies (E) were tested for hypoxanthine phosphoribosyltransferase (HPRT) and epsin (EPN), ranging from 92%-132%. Specific primers and probes for these genes were designed using Primer Express 2.0 software (Applied Biosystems, Foster City, CA, USA) (table 2).

For the LightCycler reaction a Mastermix of the following reaction components was prepared to the indicated end-volume (20µl): 7µl PCR-H_2O, 1µl forward primer (0.5µM), 1µl reverse primer (0.5µM), 2µl probe (0.2µM), 4µl LightCycler Mastermix (LightCycler TaqMan Master kit; Roche Applied Science, IN, USA) was filled in the LightCycler glass capillaries and 5µl cDNA was added as PCR template. The following protocol was used: denaturation program (95°C for 10min), amplification and quantification program repeated 50 cycles (95°C for 10s, 58°C for 10s, 72°C for 10s with a single fluorescence measurement), melting curve program (55-95°C, with a heating step of 0.1°C per second and a continuous fluorescence measurement) and finally a cooling step to 40°C.

Name	Sequence 5'→3'
	Forward: ACTTCCAGTACGTGGACCGC
EPN	Reverse: GCTGCTTAGCTTTCTCACGCA
	TaqMan probe: FAM-ACGGCAAGGACCAGGGCGTGA-Dabcyl
	Forward: GGCAGTATAATCCAAAGATGGTCA A
HPRT	Reverse: GTCTGGCTTATATCCAACACTTCGT
	TaqMan probe: FAM-CAAGCTTGCTGGTGAAAAGGACCCC-Dabcyl

Table 2: Epsin and HPRT primer and probe sequences

2.5 Western blotting

Cells were lysed 60 min on ice in standard lysis buffer (50 mM NaCl, 10 mM HEPES, 3 mM $MgCl_2$, 300 mM sucrose and 0.5% Triton X-100) supplemented with Complete Mini EDTA-free protease inhibitor (Roche). Lysates were centrifuged at 15,000xg for 20 min at 4°C and supernatans was collected.

Protein A/G agarose beads were coated with goat-anti-epsin polyclonal antibodies (Santa Cruz Biotechnology, 1:1000) and incubated overnight with the cell lysate on ice. After centrifugation at 15,000xg for 5 min at 4°C, the sediment was suspended in NuPAGE LDS Sample Buffer (Invitrogen), heat denaturated for 10 min at 95°C and loaded on a NuPAGE 12% bis-tris polyacrylamide gel (Invitrogen). After electrophoresis in NuPAGE MOPS SDS running buffer using the NOVEX XCell II unit (40 min, 200V, 120mA), proteins were transferred to Immun-Blot® I PVDF membranes (Bio-Rad) (1h, 30V, 170mA). Membranes were blocked in Tris buffered saline containing 0.05% Tween-20 (TBST) and 5% non-fat dry milk for 1h. After blocking, membranes were probed overnight at 4°C with polyclonal goat-anti-epsin in TBST containing 5% dry non-fat milk. Membranes were washed five times with TBST during 5 minutes and incubated with TBST containing 5% dry non-fat milk and mouse anti-goat peroxidase conjugated antibody (Calbiochem, 1:2500) for 2h at room temperature.

After several washing steps, 5 times for 5 minutes, immunoblots were detected using the ECL® Plus Western blot detection system by the ChemiGenius2.

3. Results

3.1 Transfection efficiency

Efficiency of transfection with pRNATin-H1.2/Neo was measured by confocal fluorescence microscopy and the amount of GFP-positive cells were counted by fluorescence microscopy and expressed as the percentage of the total amount of cells visualized by light microscopy. Figure 2 shows the efficiency of transfection with pRNATin-H1.2/Neo in HeLa cells which amounted to 81%.

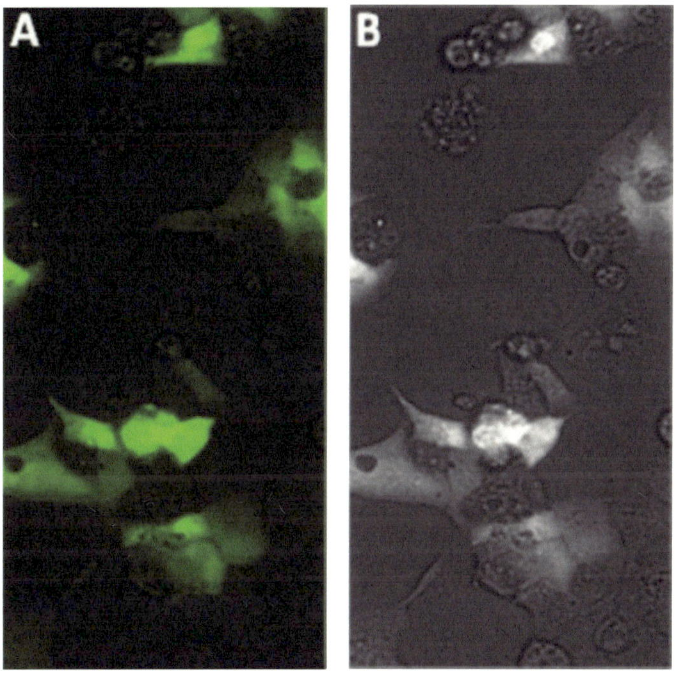

Fig. 2. Efficiency of transfection with pRNATin-H1.2/Neo in HeLa cells. The amount of transfected cells was determined by counting GFP-positive cells versus the total amount of cells, determined by fluorescence **(A)** and light microscopy **(B)** respectively

3.2 Real-time RT-PCR and western blotting

3.2.1 Synthetic siRNA

The synthetic siRNA (table 3) reduced the epsin expression with a factor >10^3 (figure 3 A) without affecting expression profiles of the housekeeping gene. In negative controls (HeLa scrambled) the expression of epsin was barely affected, an indication that the transfection procedure did not elicit non-specific effects (figure 3 A).

Western blot analysis shows a reduction of the epsin protein in HeLa epsin deficient cells (HeLa eps-; figure 3 B) compared to HeLa control and HeLa scrambled.

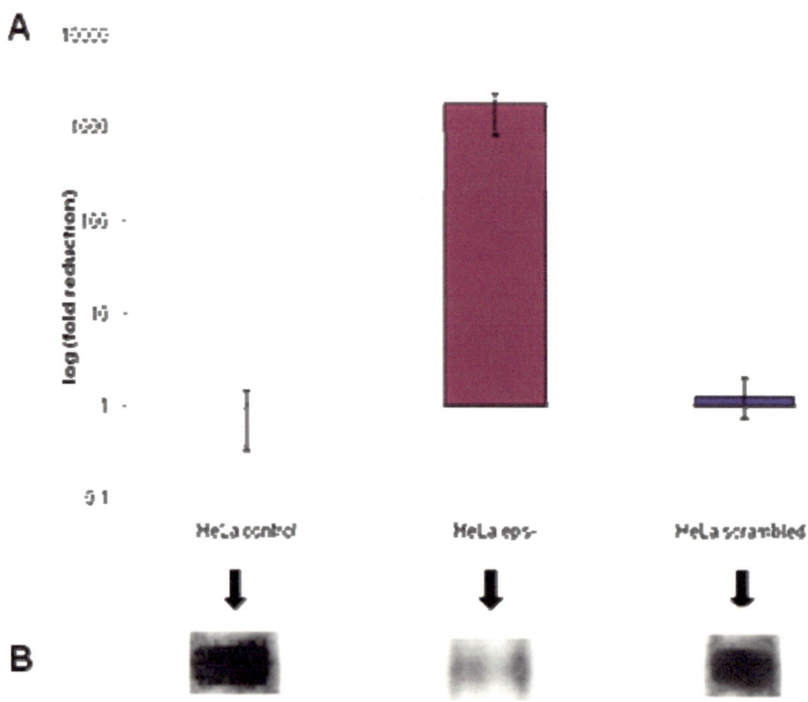

Fig. 3. **A.** The synthetic siRNA reduced the epsin expression with a factor >10^3. **B.** Western blot analysis shows a reduction of the epsin protein in HeLa epsin deficient cells (HeLa eps-).

3.2.2 Plasmid transfection shRNA

The extent of siRNA-mediated silencing of epsin expression in HeLa cells (both control and transfected cells) by using a shRNA-based knockdown construct, was controlled by means of real-time RT-PCR and Western blotting (figure 4-5).

Real-time RT-PCR for epsin and HPRT expression was performed on HeLa control cells and on HeLa cells transfected with a vector expressing siRNA against epsin (HeLa eps-) and a scrambled sequence (HeLa scrambled). In order to exclude secondary transfection effects, the expression profile of a housekeeping gene HPRT was compared in both transfected cells and control cells. The real time RT-PCR curves of HeLa control, HeLa scrambled and HeLa eps- nearly coincided, resulting in almost identical C_P values. These data reveal that neither the carbohydrate nor nucleic acid metabolism were compromised by the transfection procedure, an essential requisite for application of siRNA-induced silencing of specific target genes (figure 4 A). However, the same results were obtained for epsin, indicating that there is no suppression of epsin in cells transfected with the vector expressing siRNA against epsin (figure 4 B).

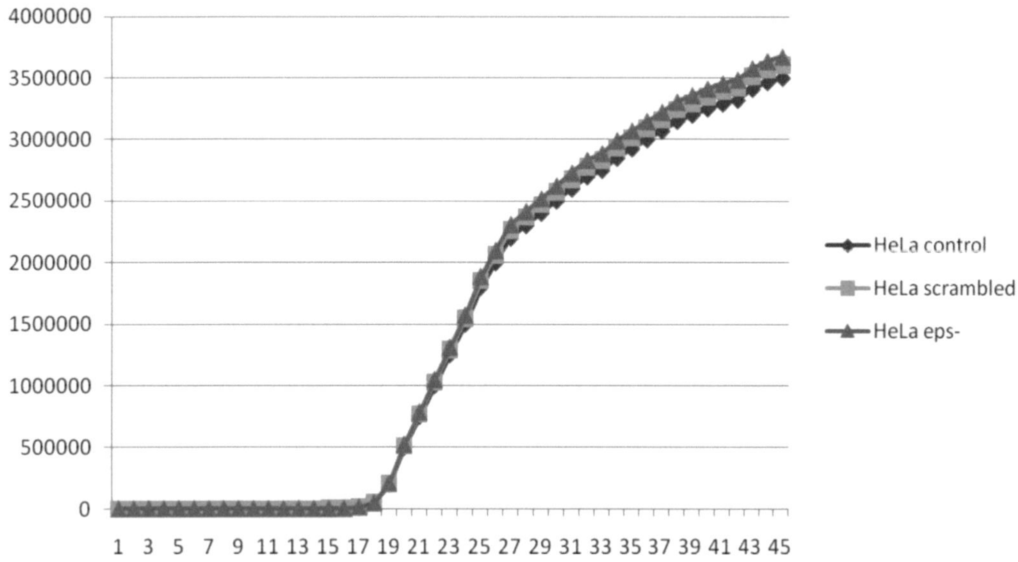

A

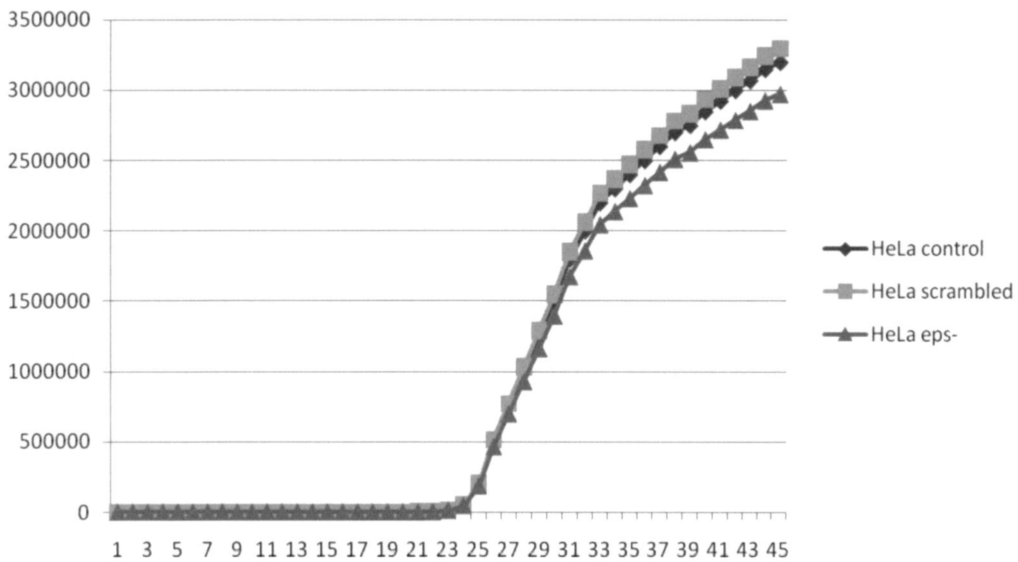

B

Fig. 4. The extent of siRNA-mediated silencing of epsin expression in HeLa control and transfected cells (HeLa scrambled/HeLa eps-) by using a shRNA-based knockdown construct, control by means of real-time RT-PCR. Real-time RT-PCR was performed on HeLa control cells and cells transfected with a vector expressing siRNA against epsin and a scrambled sequence. Total RNA was isolated and used for real-time RT-PCR with primers against the housekeeping gene HPRT (**A**) and against epsin (**B**).

In order to evaluate expression of epsin at the protein level, Western blotting was performed. These results revealed that there was no reduction of cellular epsin in transfected HeLa cells versus controls (figure 5).

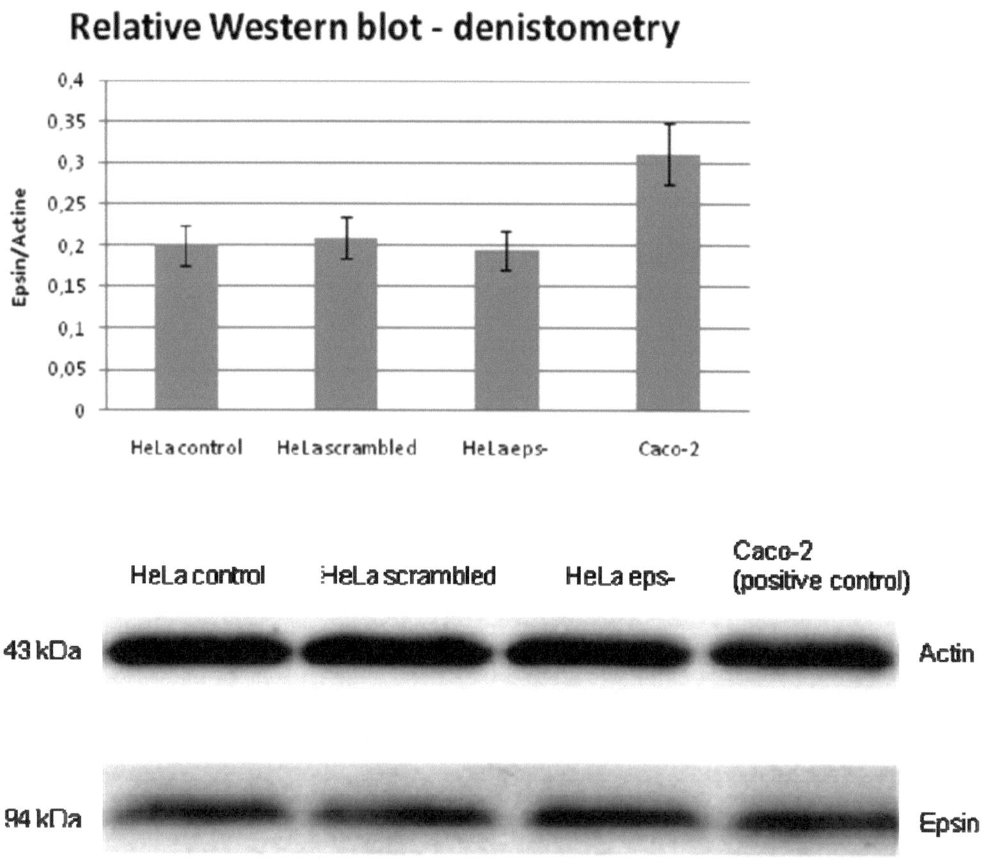

Fig. 5. Western blotting was performed on HeLa control and transfected cells. Caco-2 cells were used as a positive control. Densitometric scans of the protein bands were performed and normalized. There was no reduction of epsin at the protein level measured.

4. Discussion

Despite the significant advances and the emergence of a general picture of the infectious HPV entry pathway, many details remain to be clarified. This study intended to design an experimental model to study the exact role of clathrin-mediated endocytosis in the uptake of HPV, hereby exploiting the technique of RNAi. Because proteins as clathrin heavy chain (CHC) and AP2 suffer from cross reaction phenomena with other endocytotic pathways (Hinrichsen et al., 2003), the essential accessory protein of clathrin-mediated endocytosis, epsin was used as the target protein to generate a shRNA-based knockdown construct.

CHC is inherently specific for clathrin-mediated endocytosis, although it is not unique for internalization at the plasma membrane, because of its involvement in vesicular transport at the trans-Golgi network (TGN) (Alberts et al., 2002). AP2 has an important function in the recognition of certain cargo motifs, although it is not recognized by all cargo molecules that are internalized via coated pits. Moreover, coated pits can be formed independently of AP2 interaction with cargo (Nesterov et al., 1999; Rappoport et al., 2004). To date, for epsin there are no specific restrictions in specificity for clathrin-mediated endocytosis at the plasma membrane reported.

It is important to know that complete inhibition of clathrin-mediated uptake would undoubtedly lead to induction of apoptosis, hence partial blocking of clathrin-mediated endocytosis has the advantage that cell viability is not significantly reduced. Hinrichsen *et al.*, have shown that a reduction of clathrin to 20% is the absolute limit to ensure cell viability (Hinrichsen et al., 2003). In addition, it has been reported that the uptake of the transferrin receptor, which is an important marker for clathrin-mediated endocytosis, can never be abolished completely in living cells (Iversen et al., 2003).

In this study, a inducible shRNA-based epsin knockdown construct was used. Transient or constitutive expression of either siRNA or shRNA results in temporal or persistent inhibition of gene expression, respectively. A tightly regulated and reversibly inducible RNAi-mediated gene silencing approach could conditionally control gene expression in a temporal or spatial manner that provides an extremely useful tool for studying gene function. It provides an ideal genetic switcher allowing the inducible and reversible control of specific gene activity in mammalian cells (Wu et al., 2007). Moreover, it is less likely that the use of such a system would compromise cell viability.

In our experiments, there was no reduction of the epsin expression in HeLa cells on both mRNA and protein level. However, Vanden Broeck *et al.*, showed a highly specific reduction of epsin in Caco-2 cells using a constitutive shRNA-based knockdown construct. Epsin expression at the protein level was reduced by ~75%, resulting in an equal inhibition of clathrin-mediated endocytosis (Vanden Broeck & De Wolf, 2006).

There are different reasons to explain to obtained results in this study. First of all there might be some cell type specific differences that could clarify these data. Different cells express different genes and feature different cellular pathways. It is likely that different cell types will reveal different results. Moreover, certain cell types could have more profound off-target effect compared to other cell types. Although HeLa cells are probably the most frequently used cell type in published RNA studies, Koller *et al.*, showed that in general, higher concentration of siRNA were needed to see effects in HeLa cells compared to other cell types (Koller et al., 2006).

Furthermore, the copy number of the plasmid could be too low in transfected HeLa cells or the reduction of epsin is detrimental to the cells, leading to the selection against those with reduced levels of expression (counter-selection of knockdown cells). Although we have used high concentration of antibiotics in our experiments, even much higher concentrations of antibiotics may lead to survival of those cells with higher integration numbers and therefore probably more knockdown efficiency.

5. Future perspectives

To prevent and cure HPV infections and its complications, it is important to identify the viral infection mechanisms by means of investigating the viral biology. Viral attachment and internalization are first fundamental steps in the infection process and therefore, the ideal points to interfere with the progression of the viral life cycle.

The use of molecular tools with such precise specificity to individual cellular functions allows the defined examination of endocytic pathways. The use of an inducible vector system, expressing shRNA against pathway-specific markers is an important step in achieving this goal. This study used such an inducible system in order to knockdown epsin in HeLa, herby interfering with clathrin-mediated endocytosis. Although no reduction of epsin has been achieved, it is important to adjust and optimize the experimental setting, hereby using different vector systems and multiple cell types.

The use of live cell imaging and single virus tracking are important means to dissect multiple infection pathways and multiple infection steps.

Finally, it is important to note that cultured cells are simplified model system. A complete understanding of viral infection would greatly benefit from *in vivo* experiments. It is therefore particularly exciting to track virus particles in live tissues and animals to see how viruses break host defence barriers to reach target cells for infection.

6. References

Alberts, B., Johnson, A., Lewis, J., Raff, M., Roberts, K. & Walter, P. (2002). Intracellular vesicular traffic, In *Molecular Biology of the Cell*, Alberts, B., pp.711-766. Garland Science, ISBN 9780815332183, New York.

Benmerah, A., Bayrou M., Cerf-Bensussan N. & Dautry-Varsat A. (1999). Inhibition of clatrhin-coated pit assembly by an Eps15 mutant. *Jounral of Cell Science*, Vol.112 No.9, (May 1999), pp.1303-1311, ISSN 0021-9533.

Benmerah, A., Lamaze, C., Bègue, B., Scmid, S.L., Dautry-Varsat, A. & Cerf-Bensussan, N. (1998). AP-2/Eps15 interaction is required for receptor-mediated endocytosis. *The Journal of Cell Biology*, Vol.140 No.5, (March 1998), pp.1055-1062, ISSN 0021-9525.

Brummelkamp, T.R., Bernards, R. & Agami, R. (2002). A system for stable expression of short interfering RNAs in mammalian cells. *Science*, Vol.296 No.5567, (April 2002), pp.550-553, ISSN 0036-8075.

Day, P.M. & Schiller, J.T. (2006). Early events in the papillomavirus life cycle, In: *Papillomavirus research: from natural history to vaccines and beyond*, Campo, S.M., pp.175-192, Caister Academic Press, ISBN 9781904455042, Norfolk.

Day, P.M., Lowy, D.R. & Schiller, J.T. (2003). Papillomaviruses infect cells via a clathrin-dependent pathway. *Virology*, Vol.307 No.1, (March 2003), pp.1-11, ISSN 0042-6822.

Dykxhoorn, D.M., Chowdhury, D. & Lieberman, J. (2008). RNA interference and cancer: endogenous pathways and therapeutic approaches. *Advances in Experimental Medicine and Biology*, Vol.615, pp.299-329, ISSN 0065-2598.

Fehrmann, F. & Laimins, L.A. (2003). Human papillomaviruses: targeting differentiating epithelial cells for malignant transformation. *Oncogene*, Vol.22 No.33, (August 2003), pp.5201-5207, ISSN 0950-9232.

Hinrichsen, L., Harborth, J., Andrees, L., Weber, K. & Ungewickell, E.J. (2003). Effect of clatrhin heavy chain- and α-adaptin-specific small inhibitory RNAs on endocytic accessory proteins and receptor trafficking in HeLa cells. *The Journal of Biological Chemistry*, Vol.278 No.46, (November 2003), pp.45160-45170, ISSN 0021-9258.

Horvath, C.A., Boulet, G.A., Renoux, V.M., Delvenne, P.O. & Bogers, J.J. Mechanisms of cell entry by human papillomaviruses: an overview. *Virology Journal*, Vol.7, (January 2010), 11, ISSN 0022-538X.

Iversen, T.G., Skretting, G., Van Deurs, B. & Sandvig, K. (2003). Clathrin-coated pits with long, dynamin-wrapped necks upon expression of a clathrin antisense RNA. *Proceedings of the National Academy of Sciences of the United States of America*, Vol.100 No.9, (April 2003), pp.5175-5180, ISSN 0027-8424.

Kim, D.H. & Rossi, J.J. (2007). Strategies for silencing human diseases using RNA interference. *Nature Reviews. Genetics*, Vol.8 No.3, (March 2007), pp.173-184, ISSN 1471-0056.

Koller, E., Propp, S., Murray, H., Lima, W., Bhat, B., Thaza, P.P., Allerson, C.R., Swayze, E.E., Marcusson, E.G. & Dean, N.M. (2006). Competiotion for RISC binding predicts in vitro potency of siRNA. *Nucleic Acids Research*, Vol.34 No.16, (August 2006), pp.4467-4476, ISSN 0305-1048.

Le Calvez, H., Yu, M. & Fang, F. (2004). Biochemical prevention and treatment of viral infections - a new paradigm in medicine for infectious treatment. *Virology Journal*, Vol.1, (November 2004), 12, ISSN 0022-538X.

Marsh, M. & Helenius, A. (2006). Virus entry: open sesame. *Cell*, Vol.124 No.4, (February 2006), pp.729-740, ISSN 0092-8674.

Nesterov, A., Carter, R.E., Sorina, T., Gill, G.N. & Sorkin, A. (1999). Inhibition of the receptor-binding function of clathrin adaptor protein AP-2 by dominant-negative mutant mu2 subunit and its effects on endocytosis. *The EMBO Journal*, Vol.18 No.9, (May 1999), pp.2489-2499, ISSN 0261-4189.

Paddison, P.J., Caudy, A.A., Berstein, E., Hannon, G.J. & Conklin, D.S. Short hairpin RNAs (shRNAs) induce sequence-specific silencing in mammalian cells. (2002). *Genes & Development*, Vol.16 No.8, (April 2002), pp.948-958, ISSN 0890-9369.

Rao, D.D., Vorhies, J.S., Senzer, N. & Nemunaitis, J. (2009). SiRNA vs. shRNA: similarities and differences. *Advanced Drug Delivery Reviews*, Vol.61 No.9, (July2009), pp.746-759, ISSN 0169-409X.

Rappoport, J.Z., Simon, S.M. & Benmerah, A. (2004). Understanding living clathrin-coated pits. *Traffic*, Vol.5 No.5, (May 2004), pp.327-337, ISSN 1398-9219.

Rodal, S.K., Skretting, G., Garred, O., Vilhardt, F., van Deurs, B. & Sandvig, K. (1999). Extraction of cholesterol with metyl-beta-cyclodextrin perturbs formation of clathrin-coated endocytic vesicles. *Molecular Biology of the Cell*,Vol.10 No.4, (April 1999), pp.961-974, ISSN 1059-1524.

Subtil, A., Gaidarov, I., Kobylarz, K., Lampson, M.A., Keen, J.H. & McGraw, T.E. (1999). Acute cholesterol depletion inhibits clathrin-coated pit budding. *Proceedings of the National Academy of Sciences of the United States of America*, Vol.96 No.12, (June 1999), pp.6775-6780, ISSN 0027-8424.

Tuschl, T., Zamore, P.D., Lehmann, R., Bartel, D.P. & Sharp, P.A.. (1999). Targeted mRNA degradation by double-stranded RNA in vitro. *Genes & Development*, Vol.12 No.24, (December 1999)pp.3191-3197, ISSN 0890-9369.

Vanden Broeck, D. & De Wolf, M. (2006). Selective blocking of clathrin-mediated endocytosis by RNA interference: epsin as target protein. *Biotechniques*, Vol.41 No.4, (October 2006), pp.475-484, ISSN 0736-6205.

Walboomers, J.M.M., Jacobs, M.V., Manos, M.M., Bosch, F.X., Kummer, J.A., Shah, K.V., Snijders, P.J.F., Peto, J., Meijer, C.J.L.M. & Muñoz, N. (1999). Human papillomavirus is a necessary cause of invasive cervical cancer worldwide. *Journal of Pathology*, Vol.189 No.1, (September 1999), pp.12-19, ISSN 1096-9896.

Woodman, C.B.J., Collins, S.I. & Young, L.S. (2007). The natural history of cervical HPV infection: unresolved issues. *Nature Reviews. Cancer*, Vol.7 No.1, (January 2007), pp.11-22, ISSN 1474-175X.

Wu, R.H., Cheng, T.L., Lo, S.R., Hsu, H.C. , Hung, C.F., Teng, C.F., Wu, M.P., Tsai, W.H. & Chang, W.T. (2007). A tightly regulated and reversibly inducible siRNA expression system for conditional RNAi-mediated gene silencing in mammalian cells. *Journal of Gene Medicine*, Vol.9 No.7, (July 2007), pp.620-634, ISSN 1099-498X.

Yao Q, Chen J, Cao H, Orth JD, McCaffery JM, Stan RV & McGiven MA. (2005). Caveolin-1 interacts directly with dynamin-2. *Journal of Molecular Biology*, Vol.348 No.2, (April 2005), pp.491-501, ISSN 0022-2836.

13

Molecular Events Towards Wnt Pathway Activation in Cervical Cancer: Changing the Balance on NKD/DVL Signals

Carlos Pérez-Plasencia[1,2,3], Patricia Piña-Sánchez[4], Felipe Vaca-Paniagua[1,2], Verónica Fragoso-Ontiveros[1,2], Nadia Jacobo-Herrera[5], César López-Camarillo[6] and Omar Vargas-Hernández[1,2]

[1]*Universidad Nacional Autónoma de México UNAM, FES-Iztacala, UBIMED Tlalnepantla, Estado de México*
[2]*Instituto Nacional de Cancerología, Laboratorio de Genómica*
[3]*Instituto Nacional de Cancerología, Unidad de Genómica y Secuenciación Masiva (UGESEM-INCan). Tlalpan, D. F.*
[4]*Instituto Mexicano del Seguro Social, CMNSXXI, UIMEO. Cuauhtemoc, D. F.*
[5]*INCMNSZ, Unidad de Bioquímica. Tlalpan, D. F.*
[6]*UACM, Posgrado en Ciencias Genómicas. Benito Juárez, D. F.*
México

1. Introduction

The Wnt signaling pathway is a key regulator of developmental and homeostatic processes, including embryogenesis, stem cell maintenance, cell fate specification, cell polarity, migration, and, when is aberrantly activated, cancer progression. The Wnt pathway is a highly conserved mechanism during evolution, hence homologues of this via can be found in metazoan organisms, showing a crucial role in the developmental processes of metazoan body (Pang et al., 2010).

The aim of the current chapter is to review and analyze recent data pointing to specific alterations in Wnt pathway components occurring during Cervical Cancer (CC) progression. We address an overall discussion about the feasible role of E6/E7 proteins as chromatin remodelers, hence turning off by promoter silencing or turning on, by recruiting co-activators and transcription factors to genes that promote malignant progression. We also present our results, highlighting Wnt aberrant activation in cervical biopsies. Therefore, we propose that cervical neoplasms caused by high-risk human papillomavirus (HPV) activate the Wnt/beta-catenin pathway in order to establish and progress.

2. HPV viral cycle and cervical cancer development

Epidemiological and molecular studies have shown a causal relationship between high-risk HPV infection and CC development (Walboomers et al., 1999). However, HPV is a necessary agent, but not sufficient cause of cervical intraepithelial neoplasia and CC. The above mentioned arises from epidemiological studies that demonstrated that HPV is one of the most common sexually transmitted agents with prevalence between 10-40 percent in women who have no cytological abnormalities (Jacobs et al., 2000; Molano et al., 2002). There is enough evidence suggesting that is very likely that most of people could have an HPV sub-clinical infection, especially increasing the risk at juvenile ages (younger than 25 years old). This is due to many factors, for instance, in the case of older women could be the acquired immunity to HPV from previous exposures, likewise the alcohol consumption and the number of sexual partners can increase specific risk (Burk et al., 1996; Kjaer et al., 1997; Ho et al., 1998; Lazcano-Ponce et al., 2001.).

Moreover, other cohort and multi-center studies have shown that the presence of the viral sequence can reach up to 85% in women who have no cytological abnormalities detected by pap-smear (Roteli-Martins et al., 2011). Apparently the median duration of HPV infection is around eight months with a high consistence between different populations (Ho et al., 1998; Franco et al., 1999.; Molano et al., 2002.). Thus, we can conclude that in the CC multistep carcinogenesis process HPV persistent infection is the initial step, however, other factors are involved towards the development of malignant phenotype.

Regarding HPV molecular events towards carcinogenesis, there are three key events during HPV course of infection associated with cancer: 1) viral DNA integration to host genome; 2) expression of viral proteins (namely E1, E2, E4, E5, E6 and E7), and 3) the complex interactions between E2, E6/E7 and cellular proteins (Figure 1). Cervical cancer is a complex disease elicited by the interaction of viral, host, and environmental factors, exerting an influence on the risk of disease progression from early cervical abnormalities to invasive cancer; thus the proper identification of involved factors will lead us to a better knowledge of the natural history of HPV infection.

Once HPV has infected basal cells, the viral genome is actively replicated as episome and early genes (E1–E7) are expressed. E1 and E2 are essential proteins for viral genome replication and viral cycle completion (Matsukura et al., 1989). E1 is an ATP-dependent DNA helicase which unwinds the double-stranded viral DNA and interacts with the -primase subunit of the DNA polymerase, to recruit the replication complex to the viral replication origin (Masterson et al., 1998; Conger et al., 1999). E1 also interacts with multiple cyclins and is phosphorylated by cyclin/CDK complexes (Dalton et al., 1995; Cueille et al., 1998.). These interactions require the consensus RxL cyclin binding motif, present in the amino-terminal domain of the E1 protein. Moreover, mutation of RxL motif severely compromises replication of viral genome (Ma et al., 1999), suggesting that E1 is regulating HPV genome replication through interaction with cyclins and CDKs complexes (Deng et al., 2004).

The full-lenght E2 protein is a sequence-specific transcription factor that functions as an activator or repressor to tightly regulate the transcriptional activity of all HPV genes. This is achieved through four consensus E2-binding sites (E2-BSs), ACCGN4CGGT, whose locations within the upstream regulatory region (URR) are highly conserved among genital HPVs (Fig. 1; Hedge, 2002; Hou et al., 2002). It has also been seen that E2 participates in viral DNA replication via interaction with the protein E1 (Chiang et al., 1992). Hence, the versatile role of E2 protein functioning as a transcriptional repressor/activator and promoting genome DNA replication could be explained by E2-BSs occupancy in a context-dependent fashion. In this respect, E2 binding to E2-BS4 can especifically up-regulate viral early gene expression, including the expression of oncogenes E6 and E7. In contrast, E2 binding at the promoter-proximal sites E2-BS1 and E2-BS2 leads to transcriptional repression of the early genes, including E6 and E7, whereas the E2-BS3 site is important for viral DNA replication (Steger & Corbach, 1997; Stubenrauch & Pfister, 1994; Stubenrauch et al., 1998). In this way, E2 contributes to the cell cycle control by regulating the expression of E6 and E7. Repression of HPV-early genes mediated by E2 appears to involve the displacement of cellular transcription factors from the viral promoter (Tan et al., 1994). Therefore, viral DNA replication and viral gene expression reflect the relative occupancy of different E2 binding sites, finely modulated by the concentration of the E2 protein (Figure 2A).

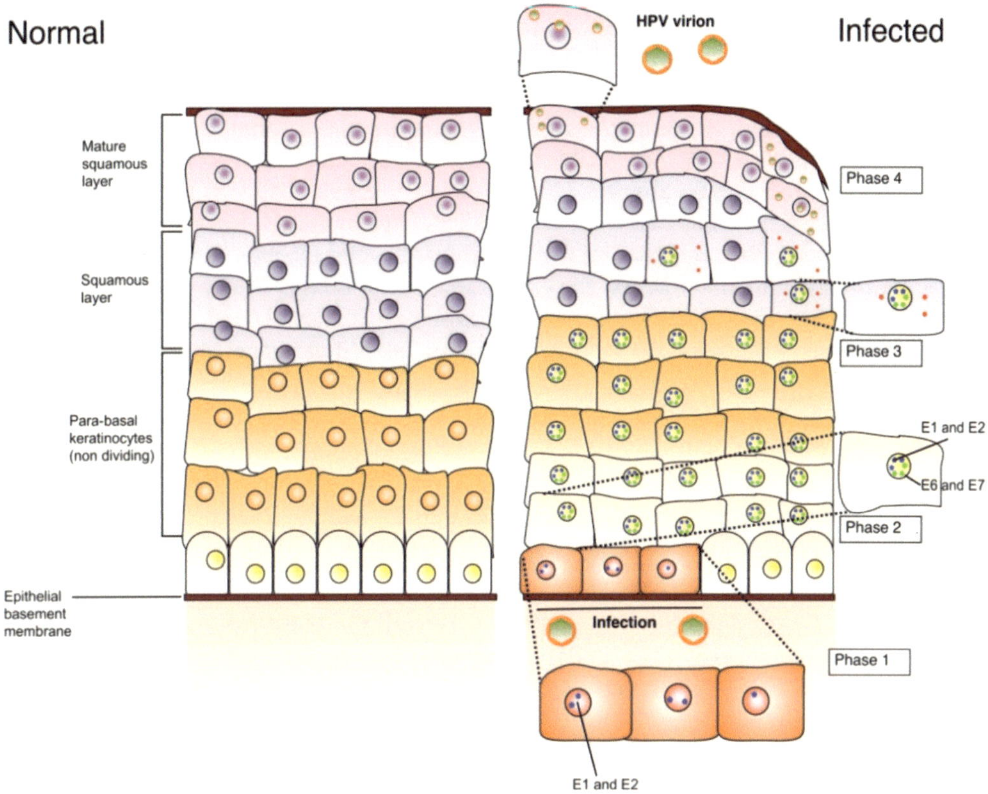

Fig. 1. HPV viral cycle and cervical cancer development.
Human papillomavirus infect epithelial basal cells through mechanical microabrassions or by infecting the transformation zone, an abrupt transition from a columnar to a squamous epithelium (Phase 1). Infected cells actively express the early genes E1, E2, E4 and E5 (Phase 2). E6 and E7 are expressed in limited amounts due to transcriptional modulation exert by E2, which permits to cells have a higher cell cycle rate. Infected basal cells migrate to the lumen as they differentiate expressing the late capside genes L1 and L2 (Phase 3). Viral genome is replicated as an episome in sub-clinical infections or low grade intra-epithelial-lesions (LGSIL), and is encapsidated in the nucleus of the upper layer epithelium (Phase 4). Shed viral particles then can infect new zones of epithelium or be sexually transmitted. Only a limited number of infections progress to high grade intra-epithelial-lesions (HGSIL) and cervical carcinoma (CC). The progression of LGSIL to CC is associated with the integration of the HPV genome into the host genome and the loss of transcriptional repression exerted by E2.

However, E2 is not only a transcription factor, but can also induce apoptosis in absence of any other HPV open reading frame by its association to the DED motif of caspase-8. HPV-18 E2 protein induces caspase oligomerization through its amino-terminus motif containing a 27 amino-acid -helix (Demeret et al., 2003; Thierry & Demeret C., 2008). In this context, HPV-16 E2 protein induces apoptosis by means of the binding to p53; this interaction has important implications in the viral cycle. Fo example, it has been reported elsewhere that p53-E2 heterodimer can down-regulate HPV-16 DNA replication (Webster et al., 2000; Brown et al., 2008). It is known that E2 regulates the cell cycle progression through two main mechanisms: a) by means of apoptosis either p53-dependent or caspase induction pathway; and by b) balancing the expression/repression of oncoviral proteins E6 an E7. That balance executed by E2 is broken upon HPV integration onto the host genome.

HPV genome replicates as episome or extrachromosomic molecule in benign cervical precursor lesions. However, cancer tissues can contain both episomal and integrated HPV DNA that has been covalently incorporated into the host cell chromosomal DNA (Cullen et al., 1991; Hudelist et al., 2008). Because the HPV genome is a ring molecule, it requires to be open in order to be integrated; this process involves a breakage in the E1–E2 open reading frames region and deletion of E2 and adjacent regions E2–E4, E5, and L2, after integration. Hence, as we discussed above the fine tune on the expression levels of E6 and E7 exerted by E2 is lost and viral oncogenes E6 and E7 are actively expressed in CC tissue (Ueda et al., 2003). It has been suggested that common sites of viral integration are cellular genes that could contribute essentially to the enhanced progression risk of HPV-induced premalignant lesions to neoplastic lesions. Thus, it has been reported that frequent integration sites are near to *MYC, NR4A2, hTERT, APM-1, FANCC,* and *TNFAIP2* (reviewed by Wentzensen et al., 2004).

2.1 Effect of protein-protein interactions of E6 and E7 with nuclear proteins in the regulation of transcription

The active expression of E6 and E7 is required to increase the proliferation capacity of malignant cells and uncoupling differentiation through targeting prominent regulators of cell cycle control progression. E6 and E7 epithelial expression and its interactions with cellular proteins have been at the center of the HPV biomedical research scenario probably for the past 20 years. The central core of the classic E6/E7 model is the binding and inactivation of tumour suppressor proteins p53 and pRb, respectively; which was established between the late 1980's and the early 1990's (Dyson et al., 1989; Scheffner et al., 1990). Currently, it is well-known that E6 and E7 interact with a plethora of cellular proteins, in the nucleus and in the cytoplasm, that participate in molecular pathways involved in the activation and establishment of the malignant phenotype. We will not discuss about the cytoplasmic interactions between E6/E7 with cellular proteins but there are some available reviews previously published that are highly recommended, with extensive and comprehensive content (Moody & Laimins, 2010; Lavia et al., 2003).

It has been well described that E6 and E7 do not posses DNA-binding domains (Mallon et al., 1987; Grossman et al., 1988). However, in the nucleus these viral products interact with chromatin remodeling proteins, such as the histone acetyl transferase CREB-binding protein CBP/P300; with transcriptional coactivators, such as hADA3; with transcription factors, such as AP1, IRF3, E2F1, TBP, MPP2, SRC-1 and pCAF; DNA-methyl transferases, and the telomerase (Antinore et al., 1996; Phillips & Vousden, 1997; Ronco et al., 1998; Lüscher-Firzlaff et al., 1999; Huang & McCance, 2002; Hwang et al., 2002; Maldonado et al., 2002;

Baldwin et al., 2006; ; Burgers et al., 2007; Liu et al., 2009.). These protein-protein interactions may conduct important changes in transcriptional regulation by the direct action of these viral oncoproteins upon specific genes. For instance, E6 and E7 recruit c-Jun, c-Fos and CBP/p300, and also inhibit the binding of the repressive histone deacetylase NCoR to the promoter of COX-2. This corepressor/coactivator exchange caused by E6 and E7 induce the expression of this target gene (Subbaramaiah and Dannenberg, 2007; Haertel-Wiesmann et al., 2000; Howe et al., 1999). In addition, the over-expression of COX-2 could accentuate the malignant phenotype induced by Wnt hyper-activation and correlates with the progression of cervical epithelial lesions and lymph node metastasis in cervical cancer patients (Liu et al., 2011; Balan et al., 2011). Likewise, the interaction between E6 and E7 with CBP/p300 has been described in the context of the promoters of *TP53* and the proinflammatory IL-8. This event inhibits the histone acetylation of *TP53* promoter region and prevents the interaction between CBP/p300 with NFkappa-B and SRC-1 in the promoter of IL-8, which results in the inhibition of the expression of p53 and IL-8 (Bernat et al., 2003). Altogether, this aberrant repression contributes to hinder apoptosis, induce malignant transformation and could compromise the immune response against HPV. Aditionally, the E6-hADA3 interaction prevents the transactivation of *TP53* and the transcriptional induction mediated by the retinoic X receptor (Hu et al,. 2009; Zeng et al., 2002, Kumar et al., 2002). Moreover, the binding between E7 and DNMT1 stimulate the methyltransferase activity of this enzyme, producing an aberrant hypermethylation state, which could lead to the silencing of tumour suppressor genes and cellular transformation (Burgers et al., 2007). Similarly, the promoter of the catalytic subunit of hTERT has E6 and cellular transcription factor Myc consensus sequences both actively participating in the induction of this gene (Sekaric et al., 2008). This effect is consistent with the increased hTERT activity observed in primary epithelial cells transfected with E6 and provides a molecular basis for the immortalization of these cells (Klingelhutz et al., 1996). Furthermore, E6 can interact directly with hTERT, this interaction upregulates the activity of hTERT which could be determinant for cellular immortalization and progression to cancer (Liu et al., 2009).

As we have described above, E2 has a functional DNA-binding domain and regulates viral gene expression. In addition, E2 can also regulate the expression of relevant cellular genes. In this regard, E2 binds to and transactivates the promoter of the splicing factor SF2/ASF. SF2/ASF participates in the regulation of the alternative splicing, and its overexpression mediated by E2 could be related to the production of the viral alternative transcripts of L1 and L2 in the replicative cycle (Mole et al., 2009). E2 also interacts with the transcription factor Sp1 in the promoter of hTERT to repress its expression (Lee et al., 2002). This fact is consistent with the increased hTERT transcription observed in cells that have lost E2 as a result of viral genome integration, and is independent of E6 co-activation of the hTERT promoter (Lee et al., 2002; Sekaric et al., 2008). Additionaly, E2 can interact with C/EBP to promote keratinocyte differentiation (Hadaschick et al., 2003). Altogether, these findings illustrate mechanisms that participate in differentiation, growth inhibition and senescence induction, which are associated to E2 function (Dowhanick et al., 1995).

These findings reveal that the interaction of E6, E7 and E2 with nuclear proteins could constitute a hallmark of transcriptional regulation. This direct trans regulation exerted by the presence *in situ* of these viral proteins in human promoters, in the form of co-regulatory complexes (E6 and E7) or by direct binding to DNA (E2), could occur at a global, genomic level. These events provide new molecular mechanisms of aberrant phenotype development, where E2 and E6/E7 have counteracting forces. Therefore, the new horizon in the comprehension of the molecular pathology of HPV must address this complex nuclear scenario, in which cellular and viral proteins are partners in the promotion of the malignant phenotype (Figure 2B).

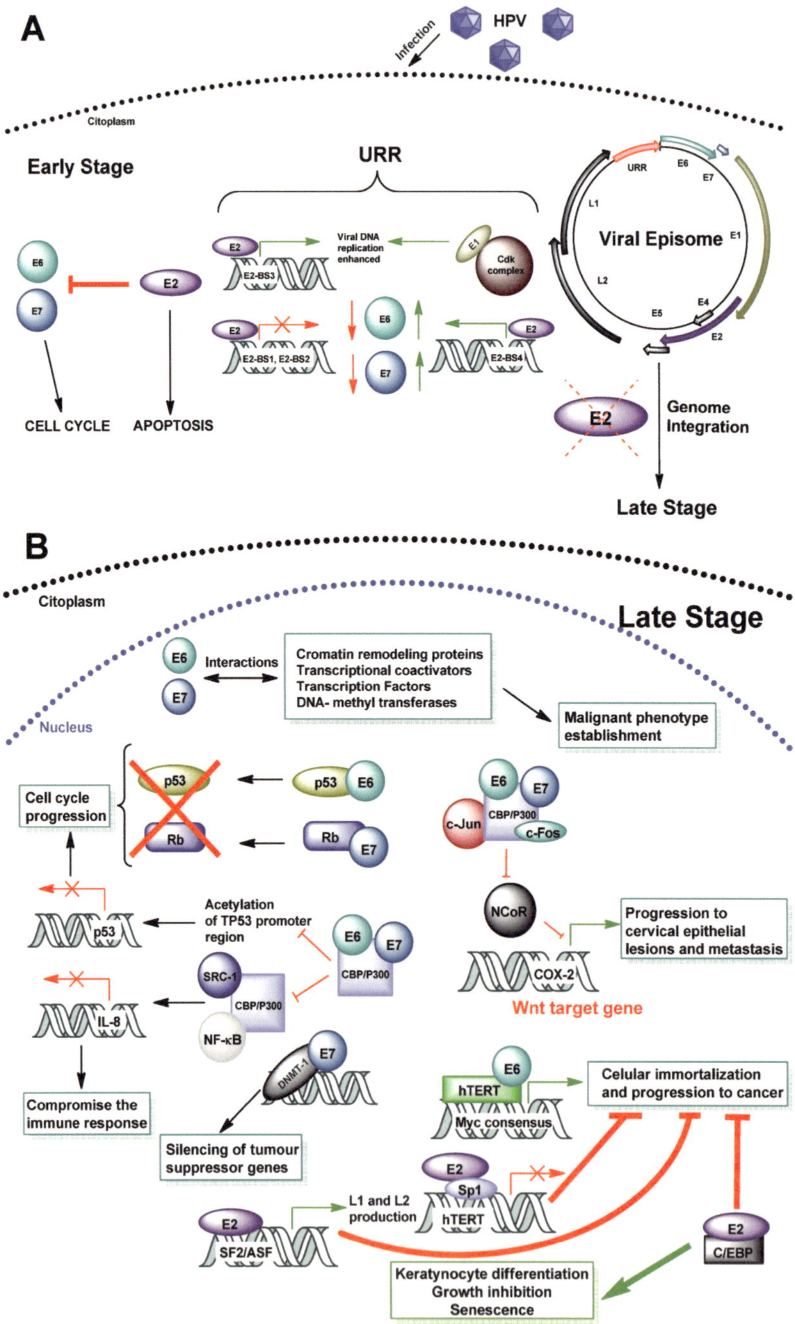

Fig 2. Molecular mechanisms induced by HPV early-expressed proteins.
A. Meanwhile HPV is maintained as episome, E1 and E2 are actively expressed, which are

essential proteins for viral genome replication and viral cycle completion. E2 is a sequence-specific transcription factor which regulates the E6 and E7 rate of expression; depending on E2-BSs occupancy sites.
B. Human papilloma virus E6 and E7 interact with nuclear proteins such as transcription factors, chromatin remodelers, co-activators and DNA methyl-transferases to influence gene expression and cellular processes towards malignant phenotype and tumoral progression. In the late stage of the infection E2 expression is reduced with a concomitant increase in hTERT expression and reduction of differentiation, therefore the oncogenic activity of E6 and E7 are up-regulated (for details see text).

3. Wnt cell signalling pathway

One of the most relevant signaling pathways in tumourigenesis that has been proposed as a hallmark of CC initiation and progression is the Wnt/beta catenin pathway (Uren et al., 2005; Kloth, 2005; Pérez-Plasencia et al., 2007; Pérez-Plasencia et al., 2008). The proto-oncogenic effects of Wnt were discovered almost 30 years ago in C3H mice bearing mammary tumours induced by a viral agent, the mouse mammary tumour virus (MMTV), which genomic sequences were integrated in the host genome. After this seminal work it was clear that common sites of MMTV integration were *int-* called sequences, which were transcriptionally activated in C3H mice breast tumours and inactivated in their normal counterparts (Nusse et al., 1984). Since then, a wealth of evidence has put in the scene the significance of Wnt activation during neoplasm progression in a vast majority of tumour types. The activity of Wnt proteins encompass the regulation of three pathways: 1) the planar cell polarity (PCP) pathway, which controls the polarization and differentiation of cells within a plane of an epithelium and is essential in the neural tube closure and alignment of the neurosensory hair cells of the cochlea (Curtin et al., 2003; Quian et al., 2007.); 2) the Wnt/Ca+2 pathway that regulates cell movement and adhesion (Kuhl et al., 2000); and 3) the Wnt/beta-catenin or "canonical" pathway, which we will further discuss in this chapter, and that is involved in the regulation of proliferation and that is considered as a hallmark of cancer as well (Ying & Tao, 2009; Hu & Li, 2010; Morris et al., 2010.).

Wnt glycoproteins are extracellular ligands found in many species, ranging from the ctenophore *Mnemiopsis leidyi* to humans (Pang et al., 2010). In mammals, Wnt signalling regulates the establishment of the anterior-posterior (A-P) axis, which was demonstrated by gene depletion in mouse (Zeng et al., 1997). In the adult body, Wnts are involved in the regulation of several biological processes, for instance, cell fate specification, proliferation, migration, cell adhesion, cell polarity, tissue architecture, organogenesis, and angiogenesis, among other. (Wodarz et al., 1988; Peifer et al., 2000; Ross et al., 2000; Gong et al., 2001; Goodwin et al., 2002.).

In tumours, the Wnt/beta-catenin pathway is activated and regulates the expression of genes involved in cell cycle progression, such as cyclin D1 (Tetsu & McCormick, 1999); transcription factors, such as cMyc, that enhance the shift to aberrant tumoural metabolism towards aerobic glycolisis (He et al., 1998); antiapoptotic proteins, such as survivin (Zhang et al., 2001a); proangiogenic factors including VEGF (Zhang et al., 2001b); and metalloproteinases related to tumour progression, invasion and metastasis (Brabletz et al., 1999; Crawford et al., 1999). The alterations in Wnt canonical pathway have been well characterized in colorectal cancer, in which the via is activated in 80% of cases due to a high rate of mutations in the negative regulators, including axin, APC and GSKb1 and activating mutations on -catenin (Miyoshi et al., 1992; Bienz & Clevers, 2000; Segditsas & Tomlinson, 2009)(Figure 3).

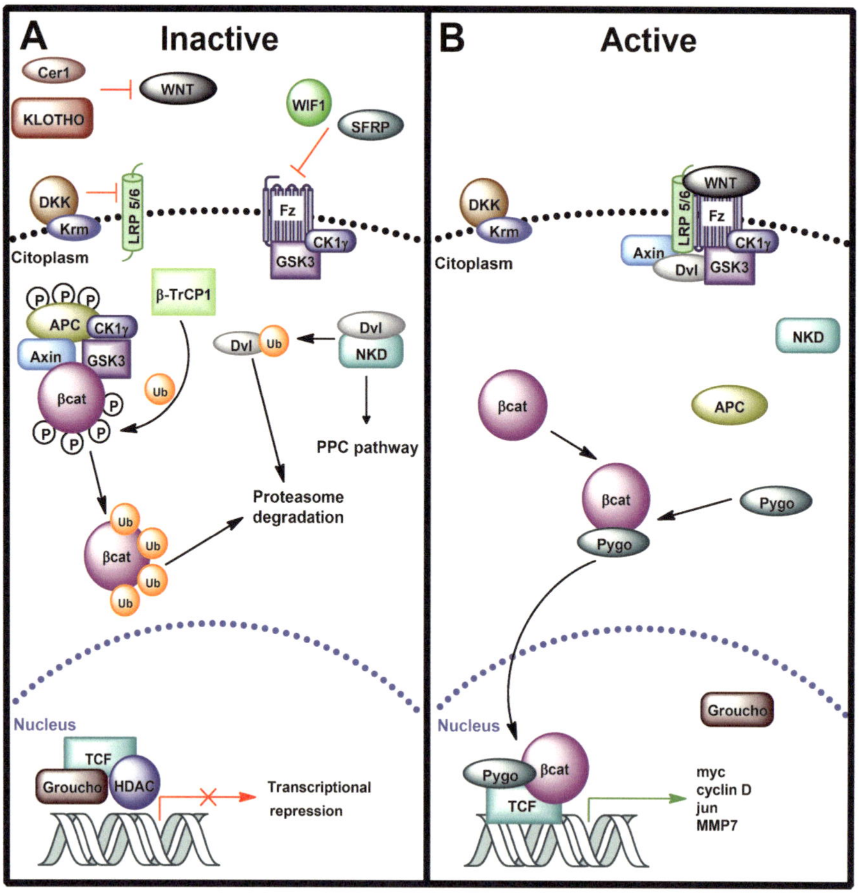

Fig. 3. Wnt canonical signaling pathway.

A. WNT Pathway not active.

When the wnt signaling pathway is not active, β-catenin binds to the degradation complex composed by APC, axin, and the serine/theronine kinases CK1 and GSK3. The main role of the degradation complex is to phosphorylate β-catenin leading to its degradation by means of the proteasome-ubiquitin pathway. βTrCp1 functions as an ubiquiting-ligase protein. The pathway can be regulated by several proteins that operate at the receptor-ligand level; such as, Cer1, DKK, WIF1 and sFRP, whose function is to modulate positive signals induced by Wnts. Planar Cell Polarity pathway (PCP) is regulated by NKD genes which interacts to DVL and degrade it by ubiquitination.

B. WNT Pathway activated.

The contact of wnt with its receptors leads to the stabilization of β-catenin and its accumulation in cytoplasm and nucleus. β-catenin displaces the transcriptional repressor groucho from the LEF/TCF complex, leading to the activation of target genes, such as c-myc and cyclinD1, which are involved in cell proliferation and cell cycle progression.

Wnt binds to and activate the seven-transmembrane domain specific receptors denominated Frizzled (FZD). The secretion and post-translational modification of Wnt proteins are attained by accompaning molecules, such as porcupine and Wntless (WIs), a process needed to the optimal release and Wnt binding to their receptors and co-receptors (reviewed at Coudreuse & Korswagen, 2007). The broad range of cellular processes regulated by the Wnt pathway can be explained -at least in part- by the high diversity between Wnt proteins and FZD receptors: nineteen members of Wnt family and ten FZD genes have been identified in higher vertebrates (Wordaz & Nusse R, 1988). Besides, interactions between Wnt proteins and their receptors show an important rate of promiscuity (Bahnot et al., 1996). The interaction between Wnt and Fzd requires the cooperation of LRP-5/6 co-receptors, which are long single-pass transmembrane proteins (Wehrli et al., 2000). In this light, mutational studies have shown that both genes are involved in developmental processes; for instance, dorsal thalamic development, skeletal and neural tube abnormalities, decrease in osteoblast proliferation, osteopenia, and persistent embryonic eye vascularization (Kokubu et al., 2004; Zhou et al., 2004; Lindvall, 2006.).

Another level of regulation operating on the interaction between LRP5/6, FZDs, and Wnts is achieved by secreted proteins acting as antagonists such as the secreted frizzled-related protein (sFRP), Dickkopf (Dkk), Cerberus1 (Cer1), and KLOTHO, which can inhibit Wnt signaling through direct binding to Wnt or co-receptor molecules. Dkk binds to LDL receptor-related protein (LRP) with other transmembrane proteins, the Kremens (Krm); thus promoting LRP internalization and inactivation (Mao et al., 2002; Pinson et al., 2000). It has been observed that the lack of expression of the sFRP1 is common in cervical, breast, ovary and kidney neoplasms, by mechanisms that include the loss of the *sFRP1* locus in chromosome 8p21 and promoter hipermethylation; moreover, sFRP1 downregulation is associtated with tumour progression and invasion (Klopocki et al., 2004; Ko et al., 2002; Ugolini et al., 2001). Similarly, in primary colorectal carcinomas it has been detected a high frequency of hypermethylation on *sFRP1, sFRP2, sFRP4* and *sFRP5* promoters, which correlates to a reduced expression of these genes (Suzuki et al., 2002). In addition, *in vitro* experiments showed that Dkk-3 has reduced expression in immortalized and tumour cells and it is frequently downregulated in non-smal cell lung cancer (Tsuji et al., 2000).

After Wnt binds to their receptor co-receptor complex, FZD recruits Disheveled (Dvl), which transduces the Wnt signal into the cell through interaction with several pathway components. Indeed, Dvl has a key role in the Wnt signal routing and amplification through pathway-specific effectors, by its interaction with axin, which performs a scaffolding function in the Wnt pathway by its association with key proteins for β-catenin phosphorylation and poly-ubiquitination, including GSK-3β, CK1, APC, and β-catenin itself (Zeng et al., 2005; Davidson et al., 2005; McDonald et al., 2009). The consequence of axin phosphorylation is inactivation of "degradation complex" and the subsequent activation of β-catenin (Xing et al., 2003). Degradation complex is a multi-protein assembly activated in the absence of Wnt signaling, whose main task is to add ubiquitins to β-catenin resulting in its inactivation by means of the ubiquitin-proteasome pathway (Peifer & Polakis, 2000). A key component of the degradation complex is APC. When β-catenin binds to APC, it displaces the bound to axin because the binding affinity of β-catenin increases dramatically upon phosphorylation and because the binding motifs of APC to axin and β-catenin overlap. Most colorectal tumours contain truncating mutations on APC, which leads to an inability to bind Axin or degrade β-catenin (Kinzler & Vogelstein, 1996; Xing et al., 2003).

Finally, stabilized non-phosphorylated β-catenin tends to accumulate in the cytoplasm leading to its nuclear translocation, where it is associated with lymphoid enhancer-binding factor 1/Tcell-specific transcription factor (LEF/TCF) and transcriptional activator Pygopus (Pygo). Pygo contains a PHD domain, which is shared by many nuclear proteins with a role in chromatin remodeling and transcriptional co-activation (Belenkaya et al., 2002). Several genes activated by the Wnt signaling pathway, which are involved in cell proliferation and differentiation processes have been identified (Daniels & Weis, 2005) (Figure 3).

The Naked cuticle (Nkd) protein family (NKD1,2), whose activity is required to restrict Wnt signaling during *Drosophila* embryonic segmentation, thus establishing a negative-feedback loop and ameliorating canonical Wnt signaling by binding and destabilizing Dsh/Dvl proteins (Rousset et al., 2001). NKD was the first Wnt antagonist found to be induced by the Wnt pathway (Zeng et al., 2000). Besides, Naked cuticle is proposed to function as a switch, acting to restrict classical Wnt signaling and to activate a second Wnt signaling pathway that controls planar cell polarity (PCP) during gastrulation movements in vertebrates (Wharton et al., 2001). Recently, it has been shown mutations in NKD1 in a subset of DNA mismatch repair-deficient colorectal tumours that are not known to harbor mutations in other Wnt-pathway genes. The mutant Nkd1 proteins were defective at inhibiting Wnt signaling; in addition, the mutant Nkd1 proteins stabilize β-catenin and promote cell proliferation, in part due to a reduced ability of each mutant Nkd1 protein to bind and destabilize Dvl proteins (Guo et al., 2009). Those results suggest that NKD1 is a negative regulator of Wnt and an important target of mutations during the carcinogenesis process.

3.1 Wnt pathway and Cervical Carcinoma

Wnt/-catenin pathway activation is an established hallmark of cancer; hence, mutations in distinct components of this pathway have been studied and identified in nearly all human cancers. In contrast to what is observed in other tumours, Wnt canonical pathway activation caused by mutations is meaningless in CC. In this regard, cervical high grade lesions have an increased expression and nuclear localization of β-catenin with no mutations of CTNNB1 nor Axin (Shinohara et al., 2001; Pereira-Suárez et al., 2002; Su et al., 2003). Thus, in CC it is possible that activation of β-catenin occurs independently of activating mutations by an upstream level mechanism, which could be accomplished by the inactivation of negative regulators. It is well-known that during carcinogenesis aberrant CpG island methylation inactivates distinct tumour suppressor genes, a mechanism that could be explained by means of an increase in DNA methyltransferase (DNMT) activity (Robertson, 2001). In this context HPV16/E7 has the capacity to bind and increase the DNMT1 activity, (Burgers et al., 2007); thus, it is feasible that negative Wnt/β catenin-pathway regulators are inactivated by methylation. In this respect, sFRPs, axin, DICKKOPF (Dkk), KLOTHO and APC genes have enriched CpG islands in their promoters which can be found as hypermethylated in CC (Mikheev et al., 2004; Chung et al., 2009a; Chung et al., 2009b; Lee et al., 2009; Okino et al., 2003; Lee et al., 2010; Song et al., 2009). Therefore, it is probable that inactivation of these genes by promoter hypermethylation induce activation of Wnt canonical pathway during cervical carcinogenesis.

On the other hand, respecting the upstream activation of Wnt/β-catenin pathway, the over-expression of pathway activators such as Wnt ligands, frizzled receptors, and disheveled has been described. There is evidence showing over-expression of WNT10B, -14, FZD10, and

DVL-1 in cervical cell lines (Kirikoshi & Katoh, 2002; Kirikoshi et al., 2001; Koike et al., 1999; Okino et al., 2003); nonetheless, this has not been explored in pathological specimens.

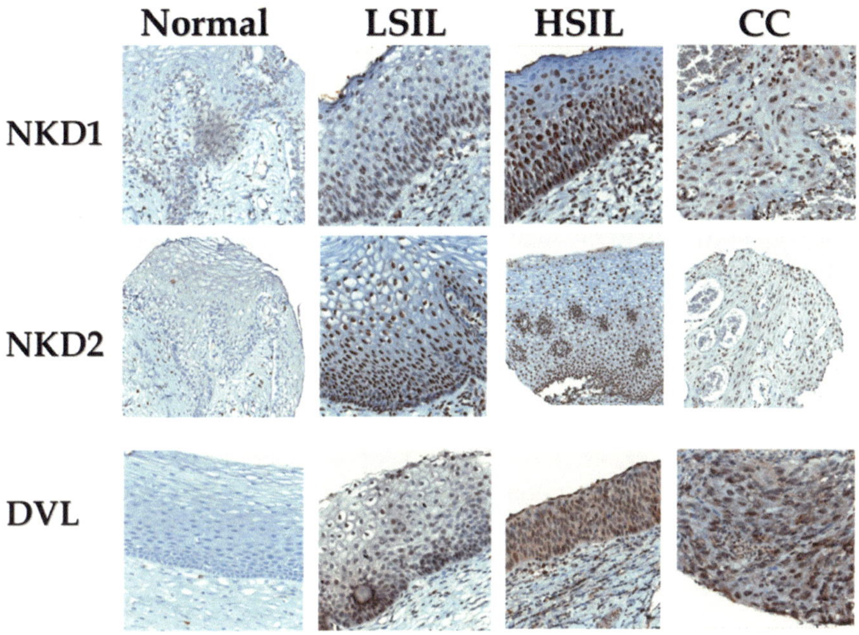

Fig. 4. NKD and DVL are over-expressed from early staged lesions.

Levels of Wnt regulators were assessed in cervical epithelial lesions by means of Immune-histochemistry. Unexpectedly NKD1 and 2 were over-expressed showing an aberrant nuclear staining. As expected, DVL is over-expressed in cervical lesions.

We have reported by genome-wide expression analysis in HPV16 CC tissues that one of the most altered pathways is Wnt/β-catenin. In our study, we observed a significant increment of Wnt4, -8a, Fzd2, GSK3β, and β-catenin in tumours. In addition, genes also belonging to this pathway are actively expressed in normal cervical epithelia, such as sFRP4, PPP2C, and FZD7 (Pérez-Plasencia et al., 2007). This evidence demonstrates two important facts: first, the deregulation in specific genes belonging to Wnt/β-catenin pathway could play an important role in cervical carcinogenesis, and second, the presence of some Wnt/β-catenin-related genes in normal tissues suggests that this pathway is involved in cervical epithelial differentiation. Interestingly, gene components of the planar cell polarity (PCP) pathway were actively expressed in normal cervices, indicating that this branch of Wnt signaling is down regulated in CC. In vertebrates, PCP is considered as any process affecting cell polarity within an epithelial plane and involving one or more core PCP genes. PCP has shown to be an important developmental and adult tissue differentiation process (Wang & Nathans, 2007). To our knowledge, there are no previous reports showing active PCP genes in normal cervical epithelia. This result demonstrates that during the carcinogenesis process, infected cervical cells turn off the PCP pathway, activating the canonical pathway with a concurrent increase of genes participating in it, for instance, Wnt4, -8A, FZD2, CTNNB1, among others. The activation of the canonical pathway leads to the upregulation of target genes such as MYC, JUN, FOS, and RRAS, which are related to growth promotion (Pérez-

Plasencia et al., 2007). Notwithstanding, NKD1 and NKD2 expression in CC specimens show an increased expression and aberrant nuclear localization as an early event, occurring from low grade squamous intraepithelial lesions to carcinoma (Figure 4). Apparently, the aberrant localization is due to a lack of 300 bp in transcripts sequence (Pérez-Plasencia unpublished results), indicating a key role of NKD genes in Wnt pathway regulation on CC tumour progression.

Additionaly, some experiments *in vitro* have shown that high-risk HPV16 E6 oncoprotein was capable of activate Wnt/beta-catenin pathway in an E6AP dependent fashion (Lichtig et al., 2010). Altogether, these data are in concordance with the fact that human genital keratinocytes immortalized with high-risk HPV need the activation of Wnt canonical pathway to be transformed and suggest that this event is essential in the cervical tumourigenesis (Uren et al., 2005).

4. Conclusions

The extensive use of the Papanicolau smear and colposcopy examination have significantly decreased the CC mortality rates; however, this neoplasm still remains as the second cause of death in women worldwide. Concordantly, HPV presence has been found in more than 99% of CC, hence HPV infection is considered as the most important etiologic factor in cervical carcinogenesis. Even though HPV infection is very common among the young sexually active population, only a small fraction of infected individuals develop cervical carcinoma later in life. Thus, HPV is considered only as an initial hit in the multistep carcinogenesis that leads to the development of CC. The molecular pathways involved in the progression of HPV-infected cells to CC have not been accurately identified. Here, we reviewed the role of Wnt/β-catenin pathway over-activation and the inactivation of planar cell polarity pathway in CC cells as a second hit to develop CC; moreover, one key regulator of PCP, NKD, is aberrantly localized in nucleus and overexpressed in CC. In this regard, many reports have described that Wnt/β-catenin pathway is aberrantly active in CC, where common tumour-causing mutations on the genes of this pathway, such as APC, Axin and CTNNB1 have not been found. Thus Wnt/β-catenin pathway over-activation could be caused by disregulation in upstream modulators, by means of negative regulators inactivation or over-expression of activators. On the other hand, an additional branch in Wnt signaling pathway, that could be determinant during CC pathogenesis, is the planar cell polarity (PCP) pathway, which is involved in cellular differentiation. PCP is a key via in differentiation and the morphogenetic process involved in development of epithelia. In normal cervical epithelia, cells are polarized and migrate from basal to the luminal space as they differentiate. Interestingly, PCP component genes are repressed in CC, indicating that this pathway could be abated prior the establishment of the neoplasia. From the diagnostic point of view, this fact could be of great importance because the possibility to reveal PCP downregulation as an early tumourigenic process could provide for potential methods of early molecular markers detection in patients who have HPV and will develop CC.

5. Acknowledgments

This work was supported in part by UNAM (Grant IACOD-TB200111, Grant PAPCA-2010-2011 No.21) and by CONACyT (Grant SALUD-2009-01-113948).

6. References

Antinore M, Birrer MJ, Patel D, Nader L, McCance DJ. (1996). The human papillomavirus type 16 E7 gene product interacts with and trans-activates the AP1 family of transcription factors. *EMBO J*. 15(8):1950-60.

Balan R, Amălinei C, Giuşcă SE, Ditescu D, Gheorghiţă V, Crauciuc E, Căruntu ID. (2011). Immunohistochemical evaluation of COX-2 expression in HPV-positive cervical squamous intraepithelial lesions. *Rom J Morphol Embryol*. 52(1), 39-43.

Baldwin A, Kyung-Won H, Münger K. (2006). Human papillomavirus E7 oncoprotein dysregulates steroid receptor coactivator 1 localization and function. *Journal of virology*. 80(13):6669-77.

Belenkaya TY, Han C, Standley HJ, Lin X, Houston DW, Heasman J, Lin X. (2002). Pygopus encodes a nuclear protein essential for Wingless/Wnt signaling. *Development*.129:4089–4101.

Bernat A, Avvakumov N, Mymryk JS, Banks L. (2003). Interaction between the HPV E7 oncoprotein and the transcriptional coactivator p300. *Oncogene*. 22(39):7871-81.

Bhanot P, Brink M, Samos CH, Hsieh JC, Wang Y, Macke JP, Andrew D, Nathans J, Nusse R. (1996). A new member of the frizzled family from Drosophila functions as a Wingless receptor. *Nature*. 382(6588):225–230.

Bienz M, Clevers H. (2000). Linking colorectal cancer to Wnt signaling. Cell.103:311–320.

Brabletz T, Jung A, Dag S, Hlubek F, Kirchner T. (1999). beta-catenin regulates the expression of the matrix metalloproteinase-7 in human colorectal cancer. *Am J Pathol*. 155(4):1033-8.

Brown C, Kowalczyk AM, Taylor AR, Morgan IM, Gaston K. (2008). P53 represses human papillomavirus type 16 DNA replication via the viral E2 protein. *J. Virol*. 5:5.

Burgers WA, Blanchon L, Pradhan S, de Launoit Y, Kouzarides T, Fuks F. (2007). Viral oncoproteins target the DNA methyltransferases. *Oncogene*. 26(11):1650-5.

Burk RD, Kelly P, Feldman J, Bromberg J, Vermund SH, DeHovitz JA, Landesman SH. (1996). Declining prevalence of cervicovaginal human papillomavirus infection with age is independent of other risk factors. *Sex Transm Dis*. 23:333-341

Chiang CM, Ustav M, Stenlund A, Ho TF, Broker TR, Chow LT. (1992). Viral E1 and E2 proteins support replication of homologous and heterologous papillomaviral origins. *Proc Natl Acad Sci U S A*. 89:5799-803.

Chung MT, Lai HC, Sytwu HK, Yan MD, Shih YL, Chang CC, Yu MH, Liu HS, Chu DW, Lin YW. SFRP1 and SFRP2 suppress the transformation and invasion abilities of cervical cancer cells through Wnt signal pathway. (2009a). *Gynecol Oncol* 112(3):646-53.

Chung MT, Sytwu HK, Yan MD, Shih YL, Chang CC, Yu MH, Chu TY, Lai HC, Lin YW. (2009b). Promoter methylation of SFRPs gene family in cervical cancer. *Gynecol Oncol*. 112(2):301-6.

Conger KL, Liu JS, Kuo SR, Chow LT, Wang TS. (1999). Human papillomavirus DNA replication. Interactions between the viral E1 protein and two subunits of human dna polymerase alpha/primase. *J Biol Chem*. 274:2696-705.

Coudreuse D, Korswagen HC. (2007). The making of Wnt: new insights into Wnt maturation, sorting and secretion. *Development*. 134(1):3-12.

Crawford HC, Fingleton BM, Rudolph-Owen LA, Goss KJ, Rubinfeld B, Polakis P, Matrisian LM. (1999). The metalloproteinase matrilysin is a target of beta-catenin transactivation in intestinal tumors. *Oncogene*.18(18):2883-91.

Cueille, N., R. Nougarede, F. Mechali, M. Philippe, and C. Bonne-Andrea. (1998). Functional interaction between the bovine papillomavirus virus type 1 replicative helicase E1 and cyclin E-Cdk2. *J. Virol.* 72:7255-7262.

Cullen AP, Reid R, Campion M, Lorincz AT. (1991). Analysis of the physical state of different human papillomavirus DNAs in intraepithelial and invasive cervical neoplasm. *J Virol.* 65:606–12.

Curtin JA, Quint E, Tsipouri V, Arkell RM, Cattanach B, Copp AJ, Henderson DJ, Spurr N, Stanier P, Fisher EM, Nolan PM, Steel KP, Brown SD, Gray IC, Murdoch JN. (2003). Mutation of Celsr1 disrupts planar polarity of inner ear hair cells and causes severe neural tube defects in the mouse. *Curr Biol.* 13(13):1129-33.

Dalton, S., and L. Whitbread. (1995). Cell cycle-regulated nuclear import and export of Cdc47, a protein essential for initiation of DNA replication in budding yeast. *Proc. Natl. Acad. Sci. USA.* 92:2514-2518.

Daniels DL, Weis WI. (2005). Neta-catenin directly displaces Groucho/TLE repressors from Tcf/Lef in Wnt-mediated transcription activation. *Nat Struct Mol Biol.* 12:364–371.

Davidson G, Wu W, Shen J, Bilic J, Fenger U, Stannek P, Glinka A, Niehrs C. (2005) Casein kinase 1 gamma couples Wnt receptor activation to cytoplasmic signal transduction. *Nature*.438(7069):867-72.

Demeret C, Garcia-Carranca A, Thierry F. (2003). Transcription-independent triggering of the extrinsic pathway of apoptosis by human papillomavirus 18 E2 protein. *Oncogene.* 22(2):168-75.

Deng W, Lin BY, Jin G, Wheeler CG, Ma T, Harper JW, Broker TR, Chow LT. (2004). Cyclin/CDK regulates the nucleocytoplasmic localization of the human papillomavirus E1 DNA helicase. *J Virol*.78(24):13954-65.

Dowhanick JJ, McBride AA, Howley PM. (1995). Suppression of cellular proliferation by the papillomavirus E2 protein. *J Virol.* 69(12):7791-9.

Dyson N, Howley PM, Munger K, Harlow E. (1989). The human papilloma virus-l6 El oncoprotein is able to bind to the retinoblastoma gene product. *Science.* 243:934-940.

Franco EL, Villa LL, Sobrinho JP, Prado JM, Rousseau MC, Désy M, Rohan TE. (1999). Epidemiology of acquisition and clearance of cervical human papillomavirus infection in women from a high-risk area for cervical cancer. *J Infect Dis*.180:1415–23.

Gong Y, Slee RB, Fukai N, Rawadi G, Roman-Roman S, Reginato AM, Wang H, Cundy T, Glorieux FH, Lev D, Zacharin M, Oexle K, Marcelino J, Suwairi W, Heeger S, Sabatakos G, Apte S, Adkins WN, Allgrove J, rslan-Kirchner M, Batch JA, Beighton P, Black GCM, Boles RG, Boon LM, Borrone C, Brunner HG, Carle GF, Dallapiccola B, De Paepe A, Floege B, Halfhide ML, Hall B, Hennekam RC, Hirose T, Jans A, Juppner H, Kim CA, Keppler-Noreuil K, Kohlschuetter A, LaCombe D, Lambert M, Lemyre E, Letteboer T, Peltonen L, Ramesar RS, Romanengo M, Somer H, Steichen-Gersdorf E, Steinmann B, Sullivan B, Superti-Furga A, Swoboda W, van den Boogaard MJ, Van Hul W, Vikkula M, Votruba M, Zabel B, Garcia T, Baron R,

Olsen BR, Warman ML. (2001). LDL Receptor-Related Protein 5 (LRP5) Affects Bone Accrual and Eye Development. *Cell*. 107:513–523.

Goodwin AM, D'Amore PA. (2002). Wnt signaling in the vasculature. *Angiogenesis*.5:1–9.

Grossman SR, Mora R, Laimins LA. (1989). Intracellular localization and DNA-binding properties of human papillomavirus type 18 E6 protein expressed with a baculovirus vector. *J Virol*. 63(1):366-74.

Guo J, Cagatay T, Zhou G, Chan CC, Blythe S, Suyama K, Zheng L, Pan K, Qian C, Hamelin R, Thibodeau SN, Klein PS, Wharton KA, Liu W. (2009). Mutations in the human naked cuticle homolog NKD1 found in colorectal cancer alter Wnt/Dvl/beta-catenin signaling. *PLoS One*. 4(11):e7982.

Hadaschik D, Hinterkeuser K, Oldak M, Pfister HJ, Smola-Hess S. (2003). The Papillomavirus E2 protein binds to and synergizes with C/EBP factors involved in keratinocyte differentiation. *J Virol*. 77(9):5253-65.

Haertel-Wiesmann M, Liang Y, Fantl WJ, Williams LT. (2000). Regulation of cyclooxygenase-2 and periostin by Wnt-3 in mouse mammary epithelial cells. *J Biol Chem*. 275(41):32046-51.

He TC, Sparks AB, Rago C, Hermeking H, Zawel L, da Costa LT, Morin PJ, Vogelstein B, Kinzler KW. (1998). Identification of c-MYC as a target of the APC pathway. *Science*. 281(5382):1509-12.

Hegde RS. (2002). The papillomavirus E2 proteins: structure, function, and biology. *Annu Rev Biophys Biomol Struct*.31:343-60.

Ho GY, Bierman R, Beardsley L, Chang CJ, Burk RD. (1998). Natural history of cervicovaginal papillomavirus infectionin young women. *N Engl J Med*. 338:423-428.

Hou SY, Wu SY, Chiang CM. (2002). Transcriptional activity among high and low risk human papillomavirus E2 proteins correlates with E2 DNA binding. *J Biol Chem*. 277(47):45619-29.

Howe LR, Subbaramaiah K, Chung WJ, Dannenberg AJ, Brown AM. (1999). Transcriptional activation of cyclooxygenase-2 in Wnt-1-transformed mouse mammary epithelial cells. *Cancer Res*. 59(7):1572-7.

Hu T, Li C. (2010). Convergence between Wnt-β-catenin and EGFR signaling in cancer. *Mol Cancer*. 9:236.

Hu Y, Ye F, Lu W, Hong D, Wan X, Xie X. (2009). HPV16 E6-induced and E6AP-dependent inhibition of the transcriptional coactivator hADA3 in human cervical carcinoma cells. *Cancer Invest*. 27(3):298-306.

Huang SM, McCance DJ. (2002). Down regulation of the interleukin-8 promoter by human papillomavirus type 16 E6 and E7 through effects on CREB binding protein/p300 and P/CAF. *J Virol*. 76(17):8710-21.

Hudelist G, Manavi M, Pischinger KI, Watkins-Riedel T, Singer CF, Kubista E, Czerwenka KF. (2008). Physical state and expression of HPV DNA in benign and dysplastic cervical tissue: different levels of viral integration are correlated with lesion grade. *Gynecol Oncol*. 92:873–880.

Hwang SG, Lee D, Kim J, Seo T, Choe J. (2002). Human papillomavirus type 16 E7 binds to E2F1 and activates E2F1-driven transcription in a retinoblastoma protein-independent manner. *J Biol Chem*. 277:2923-30.

Jacobs MV, Walboomers JM, Snijders PJ, Voorhorst FJ, Verheijen RH, Fransen-Daalmeijer N, Meijer CJ. (2000). Distribution of 37 mucosotropic HPV types in women with cytologically normal cervical smears: the age-related patterns for high-risk and low-risk types. *Int J Cancer*. 87:221–7.

Kinzler KW, Vogelstein B. (1996). Lessons from Hereditary Colorectal Cancer. *Cell*. 87:159–170.

Kirikoshi H, Katoh M. (2002). Expression and regulation of WNT10B in human cancer: up-regulation of WNT10B in MCF-7 cells by beta-estradiol and down-regulation of WNT10B in NT2 cells by retinoic acid. *Int J Mol Med*. 10:507–511.

Kirikoshi H, Sekihara H, Katoh M. (2001). Expression of WNT14 and WNT14B mRNAs in human cancer, up-regulation of WNT14 by IFNgamma and up-regulation of WNT14B by beta-estradiol. *Int J Oncol*. 19:1221–1225.

Kjaer SK, van den Brule AJ, Bock JE, Poll PA, Engholm G, Sherman ME, Walboomers JM, Meijer CJ. (1997). Determinants for genital human papillomavirus (HPV) infection in 1000 randomly chosen young Danish women with normal Pap smear: are there different risk profiles for oncogenic and nononcogenic HPV types? Cancer *Epidemiol Biomarkers Prev*. 6:799–805.

Klingelhutz AJ, Foster SA, McDougall JK. (1996). Telomerase activation by the E6 gene product of human papillomavirus type 16. *Nature*. 380(6569):79-82.

Klopocki E, Kristiansen G, Wild PJ, Klaman I, Castanos-Velez E, Singer G, Stöhr R, Simon R, Sauter G, Leibiger H, Essers L, Weber B, Hermann K, Rosenthal A, Hartmann A, Dahl E. (2004). Loss of SFRP1 is associated with breast cancer progression and poor prognosis in early stage tumors. *Int J Oncol*. 25(3):641-9.

Kloth JN, Fleuren GJ, Oosting J, de Menezes RX, Eilers PH, Kenter GG, Gorter A. (2005). Substantial changes in gene expression of Wnt, MAPK and TNFalpha pathways induced by TGF-beta1 in cervical cancer cell lines. *Carcinogenesis*. 26(9):1493-502.

Ko J, Ryu KS, Lee YH, Na DS, Kim YS, Oh YM, Kim IS, Kim JW. (2002). Human secreted frizzled-related protein is down-regulated and induces apoptosis in human cervical cancer. *Exp Cell Res*. 280(2):280-7.

Koike J, Takagi A, Miwa T, Hirai M, Terada M, Katoh M. (1999). Molecular cloning of Frizzled-10, a novel member of the Frizzled gene family. *Biochem Biophys Res Commun*. 262:39–43.

Kokubu C, Heinzmann U, Kokubu T, Sakai N, Kubota T, Kawai M, Wahl MB, Galceran J, Grosschedl R, Ozono K, Imai K. (2004). Skeletal defects in ringelschwanz mutant mice reveal that Lrp6 is required for proper somitogenesis and osteogenesis. *Development*. 131:5469–5480.

Kuhl M, Sheldahl LC, Park M, Miller JR, Moon RT. (2000) The Wnt/Ca2+ pathway: a new vertebrate Wnt signaling pathway takes shape. *Trends Genet*. 16:279-283.

Kumar A, Zhao Y, Meng G, Zeng M, Srinivasan S, Delmolino LM, Gao Q, Dimri G, Weber F, Wazer DE, Band H, Band V. (2002). Human papillomavirus oncoprotein E6 inactivates the transcriptional coactivator human ADA3. *Mol Cell Biol.* 22(16):5801-12

Lavia P, Mileo AM, Giordano A, Paggi MG. (2003). Emerging roles of DNA tumor viruses in cell proliferation: new insights into genomic instability. *Oncogene.* 22(42):6508-16.

Lazcano-Ponce E, Herrero R, Muñoz N, Cruz A, Shah KV, Alonso P, Hernández P, Salmerón J, Hernández M. (2001). Epidemiology of HPV infection among Mexican women with normal cervical cytology. *Int J Cancer.* 91:412–20.

Lee EJ, Jo M, Rho SB, Park K, Yoo YN, Park J, Chae M, Zhang W, Lee JH. (2009). Dkk3, downregulated in cervical cancer, functions as a negative regulator of beta-catenin. *Int J Cancer.* 124(2):287-97.

Lee D, Kim HZ, Jeong KW, Shim YS, Horikawa I, Barrett JC, Choe J. (2002). Human papillomavirus E2 down-regulates the human telomerase reverse transcriptase promoter. *J Biol Chem.* 277(31):27748-56.

Lee J, Jeong DJ, Kim J, Lee S, Park JH, Chang B, Jung SI, Yi L, Han Y, Yang Y, Kim KI, Lim JS, Yang I, Jeon S, Bae DH, Kim CJ, Lee MS. (2010). The anti-aging gene KLOTHO is a novel target for epigenetic silencing in human cervical carcinoma. *Mol Cancer.* 9:109.

Lichtig H, Gilboa DA, Jackman A, Gonen P, Levav-Cohen Y, Haupt Y, Sherman L. (2010). HPV16 E6 augments Wnt signaling in an E6AP-dependent manner. *Virology.* 396(1):47-58.

Lindvall C, Evans NC, Zylstra CR, Li Y, Alexander CM, Williams BO. (2006). The Wnt signaling receptor Lrp5 is required for mammary ductal stem cell activity and Wnt1-induced tumorigenesis. *J Biol Chem.* 281(46):35081-7.

Liu H, Xiao J, Yang Y, Liu Y, Ma R, Li Y, Deng F, Zhang Y. (2011). COX-2 expression is correlated with VEGF-C, lymphangiogenesis and lymph node metastasis in human cervical cancer. *Microvasc Res.* (In press).

Liu X, Dakic A, Zhang Y, Dai Y, Chen R, Schlegel R. (2009). HPV E6 protein interacts physically and functionally with the cellular telomerase complex. *Proc Natl Acad Sci U S A.* 106(44):18780-5.

Lüscher-Firzlaff JM, Westendorf JM, Zwicker J, Burkhardt H, Henriksson M, Müller R, Pirollet F, Lüscher B. (1999). Interaction of the fork head domain transcription factor MPP2 with the human papilloma virus 16 E7 protein: enhancement of transformation and transactivation. *Oncogene.* 18:5620-30.

Ma T, Zou N, Lin BY, Chow LT, Harper JW. (1999). Interaction between cyclin-dependent kinases and human papillomavirus replication-initiation protein E1 is required for efficient viral replication. *Proc. Natl. Acad. Sci. USA.* 96:382-387.

MacDonald BT, Tamai K, He X. (2009). Wnt/beta-catenin signaling: components, mechanisms, and diseases. *Dev Cell.* 17(1):9-26.

Maldonado E, Cabrejos ME, Banks L, Allende JE. (2002).Human papillomavirus-16 E7 protein inhibits the DNA interaction of the TATA binding transcription factor. *J Cell Biochem.* 85:663-9.

Mallon RG, Wojciechowicz D, Defendi V. (1987). DNA-binding activity of papillomavirus proteins. *J Virol.* 61(5):1655-60.

Mao B, Wu W, Davidson G, Marhold J, Li M, Mechler BM, Delius H, Hoppe D, Stannek P, Walter C. (2002). Kremen proteins are Dickkopf receptors that regulate Wnt/beta-catenin signaling. *Nature*. 417:664-667.

Masterson PJ, Stanley MA, Lewis AP, Romanos MA. (1998). A C-terminal helicase domain of the human papillomavirus E1 protein binds E2 and the DNA polymerase alpha-primase p68 subunit. *J Virol*. 72:7407-19.

Matsukura T, Koi S, Sugase M. (1989). Both episomal and integrated forms of Human Papillomavirus Type 16 are involved in Invasive Cervical cancers. *Virology*. 172:63-72.

Mikheev AM, Mikheeva SA, Liu B, Cohen P, Zarbl H. (2004). A functional genomics approach for the identification of putative tumor suppressor genes: Dickkopf-1 as suppressor of HeLa cell transformation. *Carcinogenesis*. 25(1):47-59

Miyoshi Y, Ando H, Nagase H, Nishisho I, Horii A, Miki Y, Mori T, Utsunomiya J, Baba S, Petersen G, et al. (1992). Germ-line mutations of the APC gene in 53 familial adenomatous polyposis patients. *Proc Natl Acad Sci U S A*. 89: 4452–4456.

Molano M, Posso H, Weiderpass E, van den Brule AJ, Ronderos M, Franceschi S, Meijer CJ, Arslan A, Munoz N; HPV Study Group HPV Study. (2002). Prevalence and determinants of HPV infection among Colombian women with normal cytology. *Br J Cancer*. 87:324–33

Mole S, Milligan SG, Graham SV. (2009). Human papillomavirus type 16 E2 protein transcriptionally activates the promoter of a key cellular splicing factor, SF2/ASF. *J Virol*. 83(1):357-67.

Moody CA, Laimins LA. (2010). Human papillomavirus oncoproteins: pathways to transformation. *Nat Rev Cancer*. 10(8):550-60.

Morris JP 4th, Wang SC, Hebrok M. KRAS, Hedgehog. (2010). Wnt and the twisted developmental biology of pancreatic ductal adenocarcinoma. *Nat Rev Cancer*. 10(10):683-95.

Nusse R, van Ooyen A, Cox D, Fung YK, Varmus H. (1984). Mode of proviral activation of a putative mammary oncogene (int-1) on mouse chromosome 15. *Nature*. 307(5947):131-6.

Okino K, Nagai H, Hatta M, Nagahata T, Yoneyama K, Ohta Y, Jin E, Kawanami O, Araki T, Emi M. (2003). Up-regulation and overproduction of DVL-1, the human counterpart of the Drosophila dishevelled gene, in cervical squamous cell carcinoma. *Oncol Rep*. 10(5):1219-23.

Pang K, Ryan JF. (2010). NISC Comparative Sequencing Program, Mullikin JC, Baxevanis AD, Martindale MQ. Genomic insights into Wnt signaling in an early diverging metazoan, the ctenophore Mnemiopsis leidyi. *Evodevo*. 1(1):10.

Peifer M, Polakis P. (2000). Wnt signaling in oncogenesis and embryogenesis--a look outside the nucleus. *Science*. 287(5458):1606-9.

Pereira-Suárez AL, Meraz MA, Lizano M, Estrada-Chávez C, Hernández F, Olivera P, Pérez E, Padilla P, Yaniv M, Thierry F, García-Carrancá A. (2002). Frequent alterations of the beta-catenin protein in cancer of the uterine cervix. *Tumour Biol*. 23(1):45-53.

Perez-Plasencia C, Duenas-Gonzalez A, Alatorre-Tavera B. (2008). Second hit in cervical carcinogenesis process: involvement of wnt/beta catenin pathway. *Int Arch Med.* 1(1):10.

Pérez-Plasencia C, Vázquez-Ortiz G, López-Romero R, Piña-Sanchez P, Moreno J, Salcedo M. (2007). Genome wide expression analysis in HPV16 cervical cancer: identification of altered metabolic pathways. *Infect Agent Cancer.* 2:16.

Phillips AC, Vousden KH. (1997). Analysis of the interaction between human papillomavirus type 16 E7 and the TATA-binding protein, TBP. *J Gen Virol.* 78:905-9.

Pinson KI, Brennan J, Monkley S, Avery BJ, Skarnes WC. (2000). An LDL-receptor-related protein mediates Wnt signalling in mice. *Nature.* 407:535-538.

Qian D, Jones C, Rzadzinska A, Mark S, Zhang X, Steel KP, Dai X, Chen P. (2007). Wnt5a functions in planar cell polarity regulation in mice. *Dev Biol.* 306:121-133.

Robertson KD. (2001). DNA methylation, methyltransferases, and cancer. *Oncogene.* 20(24):3139–55.

Ronco LV, Karpova AY, Vidal M, Howley PM. (1998). Human papillomavirus 16 E6 oncoprotein binds to interferon regulatory factor-3 and inhibits its transcriptional activity. *Genes Dev.* 12:2061-72.

Roteli-Martins CM, de Carvalho NS, Naud P, Teixeira J, Borba P, Derchain S, Tyring S, Gall S, Diaz A, Blatter M, Shier RM, Romanowski B, Quint WG, Issam J, Galindo C, Schuind A, Dubin G. (2011). Prevalence of human papillomavirus infection and associated risk factors in young women in Brazil, Canada, and the United States: a multicenter cross-sectional study. *Int J Gynecol Pathol.* 30(2):173-84.

Ross SE, Hemati N, Longo KA, Bennett CN, Lucas PC, Erickson RL, MacDougald OA. (2000). Inhibition of Adipogenesis by Wnt Signaling. *Science.* 289:950–953.

Rousset R, Mack JA, Wharton KA Jr, Axelrod JD, Cadigan KM, et al. (2001). Naked cuticle targets dishevelled to antagonize Wnt signal transduction. *Genes Dev.* 15: 658–671.

Scheffner M, Werness BA, Huibregtse JM, Levine AJ, Howley PM. (1990). The E6 oncoprotein encoded by human papillomavirus types 16 and 18 promotes the degradation of p53. *Cell.* 63:1129-1136.

Segditsas S, Tomlinson I. (2006). Colorectal cancer and genetic alterations in the Wnt pathway. *Oncogene.* 25: 7531–7537.

Sekaric P, Cherry JJ, Androphy EJ. (2008). Binding of human papillomavirus type 16 E6 to E6AP is not required for activation of hTERT. *J Virol.* 82(1):71-6.

Shinohara A, Yokoyama Y, Wan X, Takahashi Y, Mori Y, Takami T, Shimokawa K, Tamaya T. (2001). Cytoplasmic/nuclear expression without mutation of exon 3 of the beta-catenin gene is frequent in the development of the neoplasm of the uterine cervix. *Gynecol Oncol.* 82(3):450-5.

Song Y, Zhang C. (2009). Hydralazine inhibits human cervical cancer cell growth in vitro in association with APC demethylation and re-expression. *Cancer Chemother Pharmacol.* 63(4):605-13.

Steger G., Corbach S. (1997). Dose-dependent regulation of the early promoter of human papillomavirus type 18 by the viral E2 protein. *J. Virol.* 71:50–58.

Stubenrauch F, Colbert AM, Laimins LA. (1998). Transactivation by the E2 protein of oncogenic human papillomavirus type 31 is not essential for early and late viral functions. *J. Virol.* 72:8115–23.

Stubenrauch F, Pfister H. (1994). Low-affinity E2-binding site mediates downmodulation of E2 transactivation of the human papillomavirus type 8 late promoter. *J. Virol.* 68:6959–6966.

Su TH, Chang JG, Yeh KT, Lin TH, Lee TP, Chen JC, Lin CC. (2003). Mutation analysis of CTNNB1 (beta-catenin) and AXIN1, the components of Wnt pathway, in cervical carcinomas. *Oncol Rep*. 10(5):1195-200.

Subbaramaiah K, Dannenberg AJ. (2007). Cyclooxygenase-2 transcription is regulated by human papillomavirus 16 E6 and E7 oncoproteins: evidence of a corepressor/coactivator exchange. *Cancer Res*. 67(8):3976-85.

Suzuki H, Gabrielson E, Chen W, Anbazhagan R, van Engeland M, Weijenberg MP, Herman JG, Baylin SB. (2002). A genomic screen for genes upregulated by demethylation and histone deacetylase inhibition in human colorectal cancer. *Nat Genet*. 31(2):141-9.

Tan SH, Leong LE, Walker PA, Bernard HU. (1994). The human papillomavirus type 16 E2 transcription factor binds with low cooperativity to two flanking sites and represses the E6 promoter through displacement of Sp1 and TFIID. *J Virol*. 68(10):6411-20.

Tetsu O, McCormick F. (1999). Beta-catenin regulates expression of cyclin D1 in colon carcinoma cells. *Nature*. 398(6726):422-6.

Thierry F, Demeret C. (2008). Direct activation of caspase 8 by the proapoptotic E2 protein of HPV18 independent of adaptor proteins. *Cell Death Differ*. 15(9):1356-63.

Tsuji T, Miyazaki M, Sakaguchi M, Inoue Y, Namba M. (2000). A REIC gene shows down-regulation in human immortalized cells and human tumor-derived cell lines. *Biochem Biophys Res Commun*. 268(1):20-4.

Ueda Y, Enomoto T, Miyatake T, Ozaki K, Yoshizaki T, Kanao H, Ueno Y, Nakashima R, Shroyer KR, Murata Y. (2003). Monoclonal expansion with integration of high-risk type human papillomavirus is an essential step for cervical carcinogenesis: association of clonal status and human papillomavirus infection with clinical outcome in cervical intraepithelial neoplasia. *Lab Invest*. 83:1517–1527.

Ugolini F, Charafe-Jauffret E, Bardou VJ, Geneix J, Adélaïde J, Labat-Moleur F, Penault-Llorca F, Longy M, Jacquemier J, Birnbaum D, Pébusque MJ. (2001). WNT pathway and mammary carcinogenesis: loss of expression of candidate tumor suppressor gene SFRP1 in most invasive carcinomas except of the medullary type. *Oncogene*. 20(41):5810-7.

Uren A, Fallen S, Yuan H, Usubutun A, Kucukali T, Schlegel R, Toretsky JA. (2005). Activation of the canonical Wnt pathway during genital keratinocyte transformation: a model for cervical cancer progression. *Cancer Res*. 65:6199-6206.

Walboomers JM, Jacobs MV, Manos MM, Bosch FX, Kummer JA, Shah KV, Snijders PJ, Peto J, Meijer CJ, Muñoz N. (1999). Human papillomavirus is a necessary cause of invasive cervical cancer worldwide. *J Pathol*. 189(1):12-9.

Wang Y, Nathans J. (2007). Tissue/planar cell polarity in vertebrates: new insights and new questions. *Development*. 134:647–658.

Webster K, Parish J, Pandya M, Stern PL, Clarke AR, Gaston K. (2000) The human papillomavirus HPV-16 E2 protein induces apoptosis in the absence of other HPV proteins and via a p53-dependent pathway, *J. Biol. Chem*. 275:87–94.

Wehrli M, Dougan ST, Caldwell K, O'Keefe L, Schwartz S, Vaizel-Ohayon D, Schejter E, Tomlinson A, DiNardo S. (2000). Arrow encodes an LDL-receptor-related protein essential for Wingless signaling. *Nature*. 407(6803):527-30.

Wentzensen N, Vinokurova S, von Knebel Doeberitz M. (2004). Systematic Review of Genomic Integration Sites of Human Papillomavirus Genomes in Epithelial Dysplasia and Invasive Cancer of the Female Lower Genital Tract. *Cancer Res*. 64:3878-3884.

Wharton KA Jr, Zimmermann G, Rousset R, Scott MP. (2001) Vertebrate proteins related to Drosophila Naked Cuticle bind Dishevelled and antagonize Wnt signaling. *Dev Biol*. 234: 93–106.

Wodarz, A.; Nusse, R. (1998). Mechanisms of Wnt signaling in development. *Annu Rev Cell Dev Biol*. 14:59-88.

Xing Y, Clements WK, Kimelman D, Xu W. (2003). Crystal structure of a [beta]-catenin//Axin complex suggests a mechanism for the [beta]-catenin Destruction complex. *Genes Dev*. 17:2753–2764.

Ying Y, Tao Q. (2009). Epigenetic disruption of the WNT/beta-catenin signaling pathway in human cancers. *Epigenetics*. 4(5):307-12.

Zeng L, Fagotto F, Zhang T, Hsu W, Vasicek TJ, Perry WL 3rd, Lee JJ, Tilghman SM, Gumbiner BM, Costantini F. (1997). The mouse Fused locus encodes Axin, an inhibitor of the Wnt signaling pathway that regulates embryonic axis formation. *Cell*. 90(1):181-92.

Zeng M, Kumar A, Meng G, Gao Q, Dimri G, Wazer D, Band H, Band V. (2002). Human papilloma virus 16 E6 oncoprotein inhibits retinoic X receptor-mediated transactivation by targeting human ADA3 coactivator. *J Biol Chem*. 277(47):45611-8.

Zeng W, Wharton KA Jr, Mack JA, Wang K, Gadbaw M, Suyama K, Klein PS, Scott MP. naked cuticle encodes an inducible antagonist of Wnt signalling. (2000). *Nature*. 403(6771):789-95.

Zeng X, Tamai K, Doble B, Li S, Huang H, Habas R, Okamura H, Woodgett J, He X. (2005). A dual-kinase mechanism for Wnt co-receptor phosphorylation and activation. *Nature*. 438(7069):873-7.

Zhang T, Otevrel T, Gao Z, Gao Z, Ehrlich SM, Fields JZ, Boman BM. (2001a). Evidence that APC regulates survivin expression: a possible mechanism contributing to the stem cell origin of colon cancer. *Cancer Res*. 61(24):8664-7.

Zhang X, Gaspard JP, Chung DC. (2001b). Regulation of vascular endothelial growth factor by the Wnt and K-ras pathways in colonic neoplasia. *Cancer Res*. 61(16):6050-4.

Zhou CJ, Pinson KI, Pleasure SJ. (2004). Severe defects in dorsal thalamic development in low-density lipoprotein receptor-related protein-6 mutants. *J Neurosci.* 24:7632–7639.

14

Interplay Between HPV Oncoproteins and MicroRNAs in Cervical Cancer

Reshmi G and M.Radhakrishna Pillai*
Rajiv Gandhi Centre for Biotechnology
Thiruvananthapuram, Kerala,
India

1. Introduction

For close to a century, researchers have known that Papillomavirus infections in humans cause a variety of benign proliferations including warts, epithelial cysts, intraepithelial neoplasias, oral laryngeal, pharyngeal papillomas and other types of hyperkeratosis. However the molecular mechanisms involved are far from understood. HPV has been detected in more than 90% of cervical cancers and therefore implicated as the main etiological agents in cervical cancer. The pathogenesis of cervical cancer is well-known to involve a multi-step process that includes the transformation of normal cervical epithelium to pre-neoplastic cervical intraepithelial neoplasia that is subsequently transformed to invasive cervical cancer. Although the causal relationship between high-risk human papillomavirus (HPV) infection and cervical cancer has been well-documented in epidemiologic and functional studies, HPV infection alone is not sufficient to induce the malignant transformation of HPV-infected cells. Hence, other unidentified genetic alterations, such as microRNAs the *master switches,* are required. A class of molecules discovered quite recently, microRNAs (miRNAs), appear to play a significant role in cell proliferation and differentiation, and aberrant miRNAs are associated with several cancers. An new era focusing on micro RNAs, and the studies on HPV and host miRNA interactions will continue shedding more light on understanding of the HPV life cycle and the mechanistic underpinnings of HPV-induced oncogenesis.

These small non-coding RNAs can contribute to the repertoire of host pathogen interactions during viral infection. This interplay has important consequences, both for the virus and the host. There has been reported evidence of host-cellular miRNAs modulating expression of various viral genes, thereby playing a pivotal role in the host–pathogen interaction network. In the hide-and-seek game between the pathogens and the infected host, viruses have evolved highly sophisticated gene-silencing mechanisms to evade host-immune response. Recent reports indicate that virus also encode miRNAs that protect them against cellular antiviral response. Furthermore, they may exploit the cellular miRNA pathway to their own advantage. This chapter aims to summarize our current knowledge about miRNA profiles in cervical cancer cell lines and tissues as well as recapitulate recent updates on miRNA-induced gene-silencing mechanism; modulating host–virus interactions of HPV integrated Cervical Carcinomas.

2. Human papillomaviruses and cervical cancer

Cervical cancer is the second most common life-threatening cancer among women worldwide, with 493,243 new cases and nearly 273,505 deaths per year (Parkin et al., 2005, 2006). In 2010, there were an estimated 12,200 new cases and an associated 4,210 deaths, accounting for approximately 1% of cancer deaths in women (Jemal et al., 2010). In 1995 the World Health Organization (WHO) declared HPV as a known carcinogen for causing factor for cervical cancer, because DNA of mucosal high-risk HPV types could be detected in almost all cervical cancers (Walboomers et al., 1999). Persistent infection with oncogenic high-risk subtypes of human papillomavirus (HPV) leads to cervical cancer (zur Hausen 2002) and over 50% of the cases are HPV-16 (Walboomers et al., 1999). In cancer development, HPV-16 early proteins E6 and E7 are often believed to act as oncoproteins as both are crucial for immortalization and transformation of cervical keratinocytes (Munger et al., 2004). The E6 and E7 oncogenes work synergistically to deregulate cell cycle controls through a variety of mechanisms. The E6 oncogene promotes ubiquitination and proteasomal degradation of the tumor suppressor protein p53 and also deregulates the cell cycle (Thomas et al., 1999). The E7 protein binds to and inactivates the function of retinoblastoma protein Rb and the related tumor suppressor proteins p107 and p130. It disrupts the complex between Rb and the E2F transcription factor family, which controls the expression of genes involved in cell-cycle progression. Thus, destabilization of p53 and hypophosphorylated pRb by the expression of two viral oncoproteins E6 and E7 promotes chromosomal instability, foreign DNA integration, and other mutagenic events in the cell.

2.1 HPV Oncoproteins

HPVs encode two major oncoproteins, E6 and E7, which are consistently expressed in cervical carcinomas. E6 and E7 lack intrinsic enzymatic activities and transform cells by stimulating cell growth and inactivating tumor suppressor pathways. Expression of HPV16 E6/E7 oncoproteins in primary human epithelial cells causes genomic instability.

2.1.1 E6 protein

The E6 protein of HPV is a 18 kDa phosphoprotein, which is localized in the nucleus and in non-nuclear membranes. E6 is a critical factor in tumor formation and acts to destabilize the tumor suppressor p53. The p53 tumor suppressor protein, in turn, regulates the transcription of several genes that keep cell proliferation in check by inducing cell cycle arrest, DNA repair, or apoptosis. The E6 protein forms a complex with p53 and the cellular ubiquitin ligase causing a deregulation of the cell cycle control at the G1/S and G2/M check points, an important step for the replication of HPV, because a productive infection cycle is only possible in cells, which are in the S-phase of the cell cycle. However, this cell cycle manipulation can lead to activation of oncogenes or inactivation of tumor suppressors and consequent DNA damage cannot be repaired. This leads to genetic instability and to malignant transformation of high-risk HPV-infected cells (Fehrmann and Laimins 2003). Another important way how E6 proteins of genital HPV contribute to transformation is the activation of the human telomerase reverse transcriptase promoter, which controls the transcription of the catalytic telomerase subunit. E6 proteins of cutaneous HPV do not interact with p53 or E6-AP and do not degrade p53 (Elbel *et al.* 1997). Furthermore E6 proteins of both cutaneous and anogenital HPV are able to target the proapoptotic protein for ubiquitin-dependent degradation by assembling E6-AP, thereby inhibiting apoptosis.

2.1.2 E7 protein

E7 is a 11 kDa protein with a zinc finger motif. It acts as an oncogene in genital high risk HPV and is able to immortalize primary foreskin keratinocytes. The major part of the transforming potential of E7 is due to binding and induction of ubiquitin-dependent degradation of the tumor suppressor retinoblastoma protein (Rb) (Berezutskaya and Bagchi 1997). The competitive binding of E7 to Rb and its degradation lead to segregation of the transcription factor E2F. In the G1-phase, E2F is inactivated in a complex with Rb. After segregation, E2F can induce the expression of genes, which are important for DNA synthesis and cell cycle control. Additionally E7 can bind the inhibitors of cyclin dependent kinases p21CIP1 and p27KIP1 and inhibit their functions (Münger *et al.*2001). Both events direct the cell into the S-phase and enable the viral replication.

3. MicroRNA biology

One of the most significant recent advances in biomedical research has been the discovery of ~22-nt-long class of noncoding RNAs designated as microRNAs (miRNAs). MicroRNAs are small, non-coding RNAs that regulate gene expression (Ambros et al., 2003) it function by binding to the 3′ UTRs of their target messenger RNA (mRNA), whereby they induce mRNA degradation or repression of translation. The functions of miRNAs are still largely unknown but they appear to be integral to modulation of gene expression and cell behavior. These regulatory RNAs provide a unique level of posttranscriptional gene regulation that modulates a range of fundamental cellular processes.

MiRNAs were first discovered in *C. elegans* (Lee et al., 1993). They have since been found to be conserved across many species, and may regulate thousands of targets via the RNAi pathway (Lewis et al., 2005). Most miRNAs are transcribed by RNA polymerase II, have a Cap, and are polyadenylated (Cai et al., 2004). They are often processed from polycistronic transcripts (Lee et al., 2002). Following transcription, the large primarymiRNA transcripts are processed into precursor-miRNAs by the protein Drosha . Pre-miRNAs are hairpin-like structures with characteristic 2 nt 3′ overhangs (Figure.1). They are exported to the cytoplasm by exportin 5 (Lund et al., 2004), where further processing into miRNA duplexes by the protein Dicer. MicroRNA duplexes associate with the RISC complex but only one strand, the mature miRNA; remains associated with it and are delivered to its target (Schwarz et al., 2003; Khvorova et al., 2003). The fate of target mRNAs depends on the degree of complementarity with the miRNA. Commonly, the 5′ 2-8 nt of the miRNA (called the seed sequence) is complementary to the target, and the remaining miRNA contains many mismatches. A low degree of complementarity results in translational repression, whereas a high degree of complementarity results in cleavage of the mRNA followed by its eventual destruction (Kim, 2005).

To date, more than 10,000 miRNAs have been annotated in 96 species, including over 700 human miRNAs (miRBase v14.0). More than 50% of miRNA genes are located in cancer associated genomic regions or in fragile sites, suggesting that miRNAs should be important in cancer formation (Calin et al., 2004). Some recent studies show that miRNAs control many crucial biological activities, including cellular proliferation, differentiation and apoptosis (Esquela-Kerscher and Slack, 2006; Zhang et al., 2007). The main function of miRNA is to repress the expression of target mRNA by cleavage or translational silencing, which depends on their complementation with the 3'-untranslated region (3'UTR) of target mRNAs (Calin and Croce, 2006; Esquela-Kerscher and Slack, 2006; Garzon et al., 2005). By using highthroughput miRNA microarray analysis, compared with the adjacent normal tissues, deregulation of the expression of miRNAs has been reported in different kinds of human cancer (Zhang et al., 2007; Lee et al., 2008), including cervical cancer (Lui et al., 2007; Lee et al., 2008). The aberrant expression of miRNA in cancer indicates the possible function of miRNAs in cancer development (Calin and Croce, 2006). Current evidence indicates that viruses use these miRNAs to manipulate both cellular and viral gene expression. Furthermore, viral infection can exert a profound impact on the cellular miRNA expression profile.

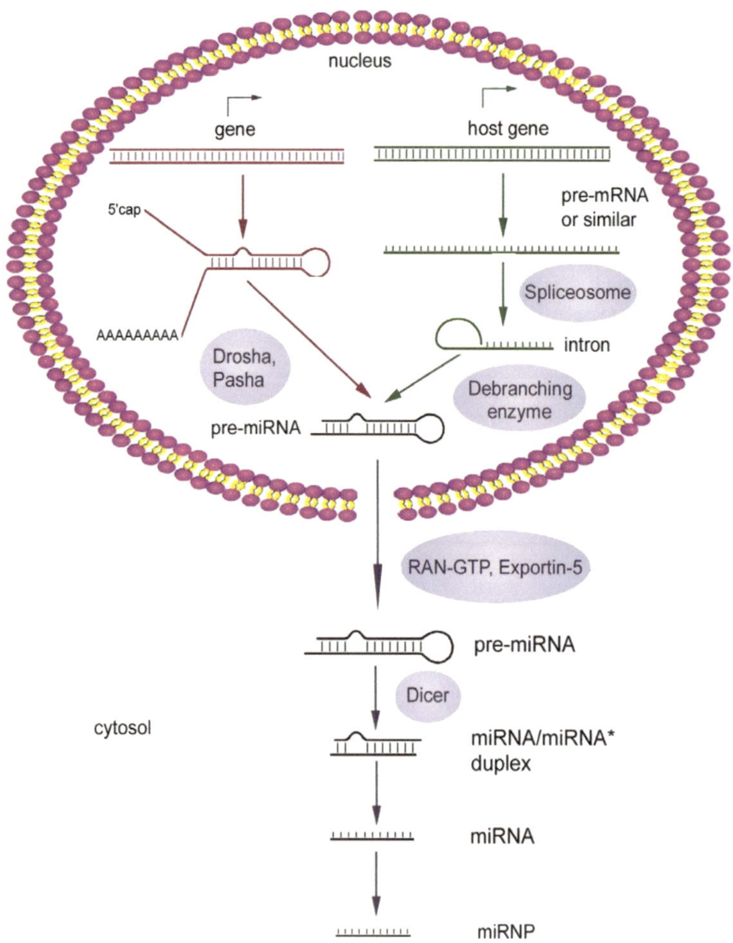

Fig. 1. Biogenesis of MicroRNA

3.1 MicroRNA and cancer

Many studies showed that miRNAs are aberrantly expressed in cancer, suggesting their role as a novel class of oncogenes or tumor suppressor genes. Many studies have been performed to investigate the contribution of miRNAs to carcinogenesis. The findings that miRNAs have a role in cancer are supported by the fact that about 50% of miRNA genes are localized in cancer-associated genomic regions or in fragile sites or integration sites of high-risk HPVs (Calin et al., 2004). Integration may alter miRNA expression via deletion, amplification, or genomic rearrangement. In a recent study, Lu et al., (2005) profiled miRNA expression patterns of human cancers and found differential expression for each cancer type. Depending on the nature of their targets, miRNAs can function as either tumor suppressor genes or oncogenes. For example, overexpression of miRNAs that target oncogenes can lead to increased destruction of these oncogenes and therefore tumor suppression. Conversely, overexpression of miRNAs that target tumor suppressors can result in increased oncogenic activity and tumor formation. Regulation mediated by these genes has possibly a large impact on gene expression because, according to computational predictions, a single miRNA can target dozens of genes. MicroRNAs have been shown to regulate the oncogenes Bcl 2 and Ras, as well as the tumor suppressor pRb. MiR-15 and miR-16 were the first miRNAs shown to be associated with cancer; they are underexpressed in chronic lymphocytic leukemia (CLL) (Calin et al., 2002). They regulate the *Bcl-2* oncogene, which is overexpressed in many cancers (Cimmino et al., 2005). The *let-7* family of miRNAs regulates the Ras oncogenes, which contain activating mutations in about 15-30% of cancers (Johnson SM, et al., 2005) and down regulation of the *let-7* family of miRNAs results in the up regulation of *Ras*, which is most pronounced in lung cancers (Takamizawa J, et al., 2004).

3.2 Altered microRNA signatures in cervical cancer

Many authors have reported that each cancer tissue has a specific microRNA signature and microRNA based cancer classification is a very effective and potential tool (Lu et al., 2005).It is interesting to speculate that miRNA expression signatures have been shown to be promising biomarkers for Cervical Cancer prognosis (Xiaoxia Hu et al.,2010). Thus miRNA expression patterns may serve as potential biomarkers of pre-invasive cervical disease and potential therapeutic targets. Keeping in view the immense impact of microRNAs expressional profile in cancer biology, conducted surveys on expressional patterns of miRNAs in cervical cancer suggested that beyond HPV, microRNAs play a major role in cervical cancer pathogenesis and progression (Reshmi and Pillai 2008). Micro-RNA expression profile in cervical cancer cell lines found that of 174 miRNAs which could be grouped into 46 different miRNA species, miR-21, miR-24, miR-27a, and miR-205 were most abundant in cervical cancer or cervical intraepithelial neoplasia derived cell lines (Wang et al., 2008). MicroRNA array analyses for age-matched normal cervix and cervical cancer tissues, in combination with Northern blot verification identified deregulated miRNAs in cervical cancer tissues. Down regulation of with miR-126, miR-143, and miR-145, miR-218, and miR-424 and up regulation of miR-15b, miR-16, miR-146a, and miR- 155 had shown in Table 1 and 2 respectively. Functional studies showed that both miR-143 and miR-145 are suppressive to cell growth. When introduced into cell lines, miR-146a was found to promote cell proliferation. Another study suggested that overexpression of miR-17-5p, miR-20a, miR-21, miR-92, miR-106a, and miR-155 could be considered a miRNA signature of solid tumors

(Volinia *et al.,* 2006). Eighteen miRNAs were upregulated in solid tumors where 15 were downregulated in cervical cancer tissues. The increased expression of miR-15b, miR-16, miR-146a, miR-155, and miR-223 observed in cervical cancer tissues has also been implicated in the development of other human cancers. Another study suggests that altered miRNA expression patterns seen in early stage invasive squamous cell carcinomas (ISCCs) and normal epithelial tissues of the cervix and findings suggest that miR-127 may be a marker for lymph node metastasis of ISCCs and that miR-199a may be a potential therapeutic target for future cervical cancer therapy (Lee *et al.,* 2008).

miRNA	Chromosome	Putative Function
hsa-miR-210	11	oncogenic
hsa-miR-182	07	og/tsg
hsa-miR-183	08	og/tsg
hsa-miR-200c	12	tumour suppressor
hsa-miR-203	14	og/tsg
hsa-miR-193b	16	oncogenic
hsa-miR-34a	01	og/tsg
hsa-miR-31	11	og/tsg
hsa-miR-210	11	og/tsg
hsa-miR-27a	19	og/tsg
hsa-miR-503	X	og/tsg
hsa-miR-27b	09	og/tsg
hsa-miR-199a	19	og/tsg
hsa-miR-199b	09	og/tsg
hsa-miR-146a	05	og/tsg
hsa-miR-133a	18	og/tsg
hsa-miR-133b	06	og/tsg
hsa-miR-214	01	og/tsg
hsa-miR-127	14	og/tsg

og-oncogene; tsg-tumor suppressor gene

Table 1. MicroRNAs overexpressed in cervical cancer cell lines.

miRNA	Chromosome	Putative function
hsa-miR-126	09	og/tsg
hsa-miR-145	05	og/tsg
hsa-miR-451	17	og/tsg
hsa-miR-195	19	og/tsg
hsa-miR-143	05	og/tsg
hsa-miR-199b	09	og/tsg
hsa-miR-1	01	og/tsg
hsa-miR-495	14	og/tsg
hsa-miR-497	17	og/tsg
hsa-miR-133b	06	og/tsg
hsa-miR-223	X	og/tsg
hsa-miR-126-AS	09	og/tsg
hsa-miR-150	19	og/tsg
hsa-miR-376a	14	og/tsg
hsa-miR-214	01	og/tsg
hsa-miR-487b	14	og/tsg
hsa-miR-10b	02	og/tsg
hsa-miR-218	04	og/tsg
hsa-miR-149	02	og/tsg
hsa-miR-203	14	og/tsg

og-oncogene; tsg-tumor suppressor gene

Table 2. MicroRNAs underexpressed in cervical cancer cell lines.

3.3 Modulation of cellular microRNA regulation by HPV oncoproteins

Deletions or mutations in miRNA genes, as well as aberrant expression of oncogenic or tumor-suppressive miRNAs, are common in human cancers (Calin and Croce 2006; Wang et al. 2008), but the causes for their aberrant expression are poorly understood. Although many human viruses produce their own viral miRNAs in the course of virus infection (Tang S et al., 2008 & Umbach et al. 2008), but recently various studies reported on viral proteins regulation of cellular miRNA expression. Deregulation of oncogenic and tumor suppressive miRNAs in human cervical cancer is associated High-risk human papillomavirus (HPV) integration. Cervical cancer represents a unique tumor model for understanding how viral E6 and E7 oncoproteins deregulate the expression of the microRNA clusters via downstream targets of the transcription factors (Figure.2). It is well recognized that cellular miRNAs play important roles in the regulation of cellular genes. Recent data designate that cellular miRNAs can also target the genetic material of invading viruses. Moreover, Latest host viral interaction studies of HPV integrated cervical cancer samples supports the evidence of interplay between the viral oncoproteins and microRNA expressions in oncogenic HPV-infected cells.

3.3.1 hsa-miR-34a

Recently, miR-34a was identified as a direct transcriptional target of cellular transcription factor p53 (He et al. 2007; Raver-Shapira et al. 2007). This transactivation of miR-34a expression is triggered by the binding of p53 to a consensus p53 binding site identified in the miR-34a promoter region. Since HPV E6 oncoprotein destabilizes p53 during virus infection, one may assume a down-regulation of miR-34a expression in most cervical cancer tissues with oncogenic HPV infection. Interestingly, Wang et al discovery shows that at all stages of pathogenesis induced by the high-risk HPV types, the E6 destabilization of the tumor suppressor p53 down-regulates the tumor-suppressive miR-34a, leading to the elevated expression of cell cycle regulators and cell proliferation (Wang et al., 2009). These intimate interplays among viral E6, p53, miR-34a, and E7 place miR-34a in a central role in a well-known viral oncoprotein–tumor suppressor network.

3.3.2 hsa-miR-23b

Au Yeung et al., suggesting miR-23b is often downregulated in HPV-associated cervical cancer. Interestingly, urokinase-type plasminogen activator (uPA), the miR-23b target, is detected in cervical cancer, but not in normal cervical tissues. Thus, the importance of miR-23b and uPA in HPV-associated cervical cancer development is investigated. HPV-16 E6 oncoprotein was found to decrease the expression of miR-23b, increase the expression of uPA, and thus induce the migration of human cervical carcinoma SiHa and CaSki cells. uPA is the target gene for miR-23b as the miR repressed uPA expression and interacted with the 3'-untranslated region of uPA mRNA. From the above, miR-23b/uPA are confirmed to be involved in HPV-16 E6-associated cervical cancer development (Au Yeung et al., 2011).

3.3.3 hsa-miR-218

MicroRNA-218 (miR- 218) is specifically underexpressed in cell lines, cervical lesions and cancer tissues containing integrated HPV-16 DNA compared to the normal cervix. Martinez et al., studies revealed that exogenous expression of the HPV-16 E6 oncogene reduced miR-218 expression, and conversely, RNA interference of E6/E7 oncogenes in an HPV-16 positive cell line increased miR-218 expression. Exogenous expression of miR-218 in HPV-16 positive cell lines decreased expression of the epithelial-specific gene LAMB3, which is involved in cell migration and tumorigenicity (Martinez et al., 2008)

3.3.4 hsa-mir-29

Yang et al established a putative HPV-associated miRNA–mRNA regulatory network, showing that miR-29 is the most highly enriched. Studies found that YY1 and CDK6 were both positively correlated with E6/E7 RNA expression and targeted by tumour-suppressive miR-29 (Yang et al., 2011). Evidence of miR-29 involvement in HPV infection was further verified in patient samples and by various experimental approaches suggests that HPVs have oncogenic properties at least in part by reshaping the milieu of cellular miRNAs. miR-29 restrains cell cycle progression and induces apoptosis via YY1 and CDK6 promoting malignant transformation induced by HPV, although the abnormality of miR-29 in HPV-infected cells might be regulated in an indirect way.

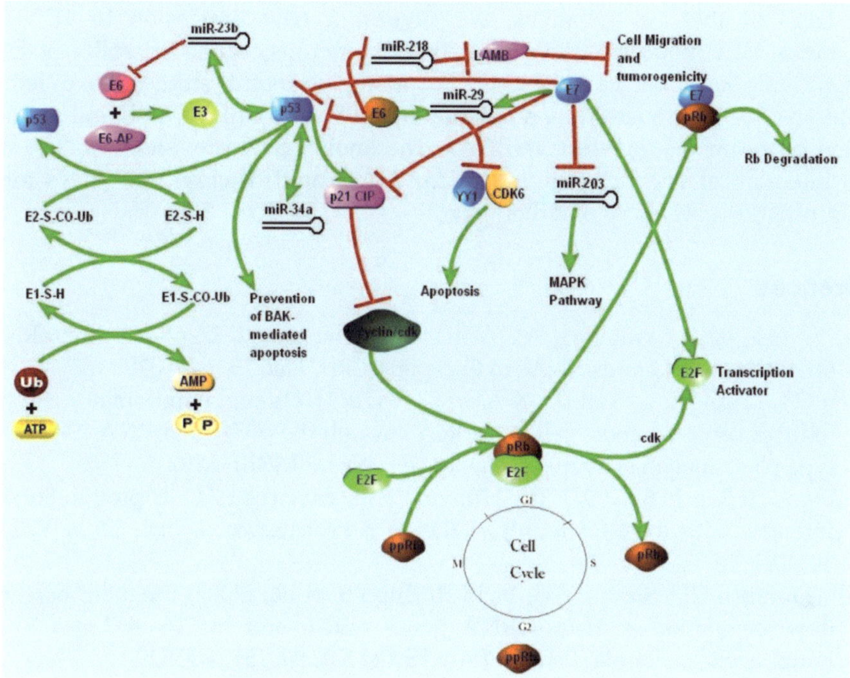

Fig. 2. Interaction of HPV oncoproteins and regulation of MicroRNAs in Cervical Carcinoma

3.3.5 hsa-miR-203

Recent studies indicated that the HPV E7 protein interferes with the normal upregulation of miR-203 expression upon differentiation, which may occur through the mitogen-activated protein (MAP) kinase/protein kinase C (PKC) pathway. Interestingly, the MAPK pathways induce all these transcription factors (Melar et al., 2010). Several downstream targets of p63, CARM-1, p21, and Bax, were also increased in E7-expressing cells, and their levels were inversely correlated with amounts of miR-203.Since the MAPK/protein kinase C (PKC) pathway is also implicated in regulating keratinocyte differentiation, studies suggests that miR-203 levels were affected by the MAPK/PKC pathway signaling and if HPV E7 interfered with the activation of this pathway.

Recent studies indicate that human cellular miRNAs can also target the genetic material of invading HPV viruses. It also gives the virus an opportunity to modulate the host to suite its needs. Thus the range of interactions possible through miRNA-mRNA cross-talk at the host-pathogen interface is large. These interactions can be further fine-tuned in the host by changes in gene expression, mutations and polymorphisms. In the pathogen, the high rate of mutations adds to the complexity of the interaction network. Though evidence regarding microRNA mediated cross-talk in viral infections is just emerging, it offers an immense chance not only to understand the intricacies of host-pathogen interactions but also to develop novel biomarkers and therapeutics.

4. Conclusion

On the basis of these observations, we suggest a new dimension to HPV-initiated carcinogenesis. HPV modulates the expression of numerous cellular microRNAs that are to likely contribute to viral pathogenesis. Surprisingly, recent studies have led to the identification of cellular microRNA regulation by HPV oncoproteins and viral regulation of expression of a tumor suppressor miRNAs. The known data provides evidence that this intimate interplay of oncoproteins and microRNAs could disclose new ways for cancer diagnosis, prognosis evaluator and therapy.

5. References

Ambros, V., Lee, R.C., Lavanway, A., Williams, P.T. & Jewell, D. (2003). MicroRNAs and other tiny endogenous RNAs in *C. elegans*. *Curr. Biol.* 13, 807–818.

Au Yeung C L, Tsang T Y, Yau P L & Kwok T T (2011). Human papillomavirus type 16 E6 induces cervical cancer cell migration through the p53/microRNA-23b/urokinase-type plasminogen activator pathway *Oncogene*. 30, 2401-2410.

Berezutskaya E & Bagchi S. (1997). The Human Papillomavirus E7 Oncoprotein Functionally Interacts with the S4 Subunit of the 26 S Proteasome. *J. Biol. Chem.* 272, 30135–30140.

Calin GA, Dumitru CD, Shimizu M, Bichi R, Zupo S, et al., (2002) Frequent deletions and down-regulation of micro- RNA genes miR15 and miR16 at 13q14 in chronic lymphocytic leukemia. *Proc Natl Acad Sci U S A*. 99, 15524-15529.

Calin, G.A, Calin Dan Dumitru, Terry Hyslop, Evan Noch., et al., (2004). Human microRNA genes are frequently located at fragile sites and genomic regions involved in cancers. *Proc Natl Acad Sci USA*. 101, 2999-3004.

Calin, G. A. & Croce, C. M. (2006). MicroRNA signatures in human cancers. *Nature Rev. Cancer*. 6, 857–866.

Cimmino A, Calin GA, Fabbri M, Iorio MV, Ferracin M, et al., (2005) miR-15 and miR-16 induce apoptosis by targeting BCL2. *Proc Natl Acad Sci U S A*. 102, 13944-13949.

Elbel M, Carl S, Spaderna S & Iftner T (1997). A comparative analysis of the interactions of the E6 proteins from cutaneous and genital papillomaviruses with p53 and E6AP in correlation to their transforming potential. *Virology*. 239, 132–149.

Esquela-Kerscher, A. & Frank, J. Slack. (2006). Oncomirs-microRNAs with a role in cancer. *Nat. Rev. Cancer*. 6, 259–269.

Fehrmann F. & Laimins, L.A. (2003). Human papillomaviruses: Targeting differentiating epithelial cells for malignant transformation. *Oncogene*. 22, 5201-5207.

Garzon, R., Pichiorri, F., Palumbo, T., et al., (2005). MicroRNA fingerprints during human megakaryocytopoiesis. *Proc Natl Acad Sci USA*. 103, 5078–83.

He, L., He X., Lim, L.P. et al., (2007). A microRNA component of the p53 tumour suppressor network. *Nature*. 447, 1130–1134.

Jemal A, Siegel R, Xu J & Ward E. (2010) Cancer statistics, 2010. CA *Cancer J Clin*. 60, 277-300

Johnson SM, Grosshans H, Shingara J, Byrom M, Jarvis R, et al., (2005) RAS is regulated by the let-7 microRNA family. *Cell*. 120, 635-647.

Khvorova, A., Reynolds, A., & Jayasena, S.D. (2003). Functional siRNAs and miRNAs exhibit strand bias. *Cell*. 115(2), 209-216.

Kim, V.N. (2005). MicroRNA biogenesis: coordinated cropping and dicing. *Nat Rev Mol Cell Biol* 6(5), 376-385.

Lee JW, Choi CH,Choi JJ, et al., (2008). Altered microRNA expression in cervical carcinomas. *Clin Cancer Res*.14, 2535–42.

Lee RC, Feinbaum RL, & Ambros V. (1993).The C. elegans heterochronic gene lin-4encodes small RNAs with antisense complementarity to lin-14. *Cell*. 75, 843–54.

Lee,Y. Jeon K, Lee J., Kim S & Kim V.N (2002). MicroRNA maturation: stepwise processing and subcellular localization. *EMBO J*. 21, 4663-4670.

Lewis, B.P., Burge, C.B., & Bartel, D.P. (2005). Conserved seed pairing, often flanked by adenosines, indicates that thousands of human genes are microRNA targets.*Cell*. 120(1), 15-20.

Lui WO, Pourmand N, Patterson BK & Fire A (2007). Patterns of known and novel small RNAs in human cervical cancer. *Cancer Res*. 67, 6031-6043.

Lu, J., Getz, G., Miska, E.A., Alvarez-Saavedra, E., Lamb, J., *et al*., (2005). expression profiles classify human cancers. *Nature*. 435, 834–838.

Lund, E. Guttinger, S., Calado, A., Dahlberg, J.E., & Kutay, U. (2004). Nuclear export of microRNA precursors. *Science*. 303(5654), 95-98.

Martinez I, Gardiner AS, Board KF, FA Monzon FA, Edwards RP & Khan SA (2008). Human papillomavirus type 16 reduces the expression of microRNA-218 in cervical carcinoma cells *Oncogene*. 27(18), 2575–2582.

Melar-New M & Laimins L. (2010). Human papillomaviruses modulate expression of microRNA 203 upon epithelial differentiation to control levels of p63 proteins., *Journal of virology*. 84, 5212-21.

Munger K, Basile JR, Duensing S, et al(2001). Biological activities and molecular targets of the human papillomavirus E7 oncoprotein.*Oncogene* . 20, 7888–98.

Munger K, Baldwin A, Edwards KM, Hayakawa H, Nguyen CL, Owens M, et al., (2004) Mechanisms of human papillomavirus-induced oncogenesis. *J Virol*.78, 11451–6.

Parkin DM, Bray F, Ferlay J & Pisani P (2005) Global cancer statistics, 2002. CA *Cancer J Clin*. 55, 74-108.

Raver-Shapira N, Marciano E, Meiri E., et al., (2007). Transcriptional activation of miR-34a contributes to p53-mediated apoptosis. *Mol Cell*. 26, 731–743.

Reshmi, G. & Radhakrishna P.M. (2008). Beyond HPV: Oncomirs as new players in cervical cancer. *FEBS Letters*. 582, 4113–4116.

Schwarz, D.S., Hutvagner, G., Du, T., Xu, Z., Aronin, N., & Zamore,P.D. (2003).Asymmetry in the assembly of the RNAi enzyme complex. *Cell* 115, 199–208.

Takamizawa J, Konishi H, Yanagisawa K, Tomida S, Osada H, et al., (2004) Reduced expression of the let-7 microRNAs in human lung cancers in association with shortened postoperative survival. *Cancer Res*. 64, 3753-3756.

Tang S, Bertke AS, Patel A, Wang K, Cohen JI & Krause PR(2008). An acutely and latently expressed herpes simplex virus 2 viral microRNA inhibits expression of ICP34.5, a viral neurovirulence factor. *Proc Natl Acad Sci*. 105:10931–10936.

Thomas M, Pim D & Banks L.(1999). The role of the E6-p53 interaction in the molecular pathogenesis of HPV. *Oncogene* .18, 7690–700.

Umbach JL, Kramer MF, Jurak I, Karnowski HW, Coen DM & Cullen BR(2008) MicroRNAs expressed by herpes simplex virus 1 during latent infection regulate viral mRNAs. *Nature* 454:780–783.

Volinia S, Calin GA, Liu CG, Ambs S, Cimmino A, et al., (2006). A microRNA expression signature of human solid tumors defines cancer gene targets. *Proc Natl Acad Sci U S A*. 103, 2257-2261.

Walboomers JM, Jacobs MV, Manos MM, Bosch FX, Kummer JA, et al., (1999) Human papillomavirus is a necessary cause of invasive cervical cancer worldwide. *J Pathol*.189, 12-19.

Wang X, Tang S, Le S.Y., et al., (2008). Aberrant expression of oncogenic and tumorsuppressive microRNAs in cervical cancer is required for cancer cell growth.*PLoS ONE*. 3, e2557.

Wang X, Wang HK, McCoy JP, Banerjee NS, Rader JS, et al., (2009) Oncogenic HPV infection interrupts the expression of tumor-suppressive miR-34a through viral oncoprotein E6. *RNA*. 15, 637-647.

Xiaoxia Hu, Julie K. Schwarz, James S. Lewis, Jr, et al., (2010). A microRNA expression signature for cervical cancer progression. *Cancer Res.* 70, 1441–1448

Yang Li, Fenfen Wang, Junfen Xu, Feng Ye, Yuanming Shen, Jiansong Zhou, Weiguo Lu, Xiaoyun Wan, Ding Ma & Xing Xie. (2011). Progressive miRNA expression profiles in cervical carcinogenesis and identification of HPV-related target genes for miR-29. *The Journal of Pathology*. 224, 484–495.

Zhang B, Pan X, Cobb GP & Anderson TA (2007), microRNAs as oncogenes and tumor suppressors. *Dev Biol*, 302, 1-12.

zur Hausen H (2002). Papillomaviruses and cancer: from basic studies to clinical application. *Nat Rev Cancer*. 2, 342-350.

15

Role of Chronic Inflammation and Resulting DNA Damage in Cervical Carcinogenesis Induced by Human Papillomavirus

Yusuke Hiraku
Department of Environmental and Molecular Medicine, Mie University Graduate School of Medicine Japan

1. Introduction

Cervical cancer is the second most common cancer among women in the worldwide. Especially, in many regions of developing countries, cervical cancer is the most common among women. Infection with human papillomavirus (HPV) is a necessary event preceding the development of premalignant lesions in the cervical epithelium, which can partially progress to cancer. HPV DNA can be identified in almost all specimens of patients with invasive cervical cancer (Chen & Hunter, 2005; Munoz et al., 2003; Tindle, 2002). Molecular epidemiological studies have demonstrated that specific subtypes of HPV are closely associated with cervical cancer, although the risk of cervical cancer varies with HPV types (Bosch et al., 2002; Chen & Hunter, 2005; International Agency for Research on Cancer [IARC] Working Group, 2007; 2011; Munoz et al., 2003; Sisk & Robertson, 2002; Tindle, 2002). IARC has classified several types of high-risk HPV, including HPV-16 and HPV-18, to be carcinogenic to humans (group 1) (IARC Working Group, 2007; 2011).

The molecular mechanisms of HPV-induced carcinogenesis have been extensively investigated by focusing on HPV oncoproteins, E6 and E7 (Yugawa & Kiyono, 2009). E6 and E7 genes are invariably expressed in HPV-positive cervical cancer cells. E6 protein forms a ubiquitin ligase complex with E6-associated protein (E6AP) and promotes the degradation of p53 protein, a tumor suppressor gene product involved in apoptosis, cell cycle arrest and DNA repair. The E6/E6AP complex also induces the transcription of the catalytic subunit of human telomerase reverse transcriptase (hTERT) via degradation of the repressor NFX1-91, leading to cell immortalization (Xu et al., 2008). E7 oncoprotein binds and degrades retinoblastoma protein (RB), a major negative regulator of the cell cycle, and the related family members (Duensing & Munger, 2004). Recent studies demonstrated that E7-mediated degradation of RB requires the calcium-activated calpain, a cysteine protease (Darnell et al., 2007) and involves the interaction with p600, an RB-associated factor (Huh et al., 2005). E7 also inactivates the cyclin-dependent kinase (CDK) inhibitors, p21 and p27 (Duensing & Munger, 2004). E7-induced RB degradation leads to the release of the transcription factor E2F from the RB/E2F transcriptional repressor complex (von Knebel Doeberitz, 2002). Activation of E2F mediates gene transcription with increased expression of cyclin E and cyclin A and aberrant CDK2 activity (Duensing & Munger, 2004). In addition, these oncoproteins cause genomic instability (Duensing & Munger, 2004). E6 and E7 cooperatively induce numerical centrosome aberrations and eventual aneuploidy in cells overexpressing these oncoproteins (Duensing et al., 2000). E7 protein of high-risk type HPV induced chromosome overduplication associated with aberrant multipolar spindle pole formation, while E6 had no immediate effects on centrosome numbers but potentiated mitotic disturbance (Duensing et al., 2000). On the basis of these numerous studies, E6 and E7 oncoproteins are considered to participate in cervical carcinogenesis by inducing cell immortalization, dysregulation of cell proliferation and chromosomal instability.

However, it has been reported that these oncoproteins are insufficient to transform human cells, and additional cellular events are required for cervical carcinogenesis (Duensing & Munger, 2004). The activation of Ha-*ras* in HPV16-immortalized human cervical cells resulted in malignancy, while transfection of HPV-16 DNA alone into cervical cells did not (DiPaolo et al., 1989). Human protooncogenes, including the c-Ha-*ras* gene, can be activated via oxygen radical-induced DNA damage (Du et al., 1994). HPV oncoprotein-expressing cells have an impaired ability to respond to DNA damage (Kessis et al., 1993; Song et al., 1998). These findings raise the possibility that additional factors other than HPV infection mediate DNA damage and participate in carcinogenesis. Recent epidemiological and experimental studies have demonstrated that chronic inflammation contributes to cervical carcinogenesis as described in the following section. In this review, the role of inflammation and resulting DNA damage in cervical carcinogenesis and the molecular mechanisms will be discussed.

2. Involvement of chronic inflammation in cervical carcinogenesis

In 19th century, Rudolf Virchow noted leucocytes in neoplastic tissues and suggested that the "lymphoreticular infiltrate" reflected the origin of cancer at sites of chronic inflammation (Balkwill & Mantovani, 2001). Since then, there has been a growing research interest in the link between chronic inflammation and carcinogenesis. Actually, many malignancies arise from areas of infection and inflammation (Balkwill & Mantovani, 2001; Coussens & Werb, 2002). Epidemiological and experimental studies have provided evidence indicating that chronic infection and inflammatory conditions contribute to a substantial part of environmental carcinogenesis (Coussens & Werb, 2002; IARC, 2003). A recent review has estimated that chronic inflammation accounts for approximately 25 % of human cancers (S. P. Hussain & Harris, 2007). Infection with bacteria, viruses and parasites contributes to a substantial part of chronic inflammation. IARC has estimated that infectious diseases account for approximately 18 % of cancer cases worldwide, which are largely attributed to infection with oncogenic viruses, including HPV (IARC, 2003) (Table 1). Cervical cancer mediated by HPV accounts for approximately 6 % of cancer cases, and the largest part of infection-related carcinogenesis.

Infectious agents*	Cancer site	Number of cancer cases	% of cancer cases worldwide
Bacterial infection			
Helicobacter pylori	Stomach	490,000	5.4
Viral infection			
Human papillomavirus (HPV) (especially high-risk types)	Cervix and other sites	550,000	6.1
Hepatitis B virus Hepatitis C virus	Liver	390,000	4.3
Epstein-Barr virus (EBV)	Lymphoma and nasopharynx	99,000	1.1
Human T-cell lymphotropic virus (HTLV-1)	Leukemia	9,000	0.1
Parasitic infection			
Schistosoma haematobium	Bladder	2,700	0.1
Opisthorchis viverrini (Liver fluke)	Intra- and extrahepatic bile duct	800	
	Total infection-related cancers Total cancers in 1995	1,600,000 9,000,000	17.7 100

*The pathogens listed here have been evaluated as group 1 carcinogens (carcinogenic to humans) by IARC.

Table 1. Burden of infection-related cancer worldwide [Adapted and modified from (IARC, 2003)]

2.1 Epidemiological studies on chronic inflammation and cervical carcinogenesis

Recent epidemiological and experimental studies have revealed that chronic inflammation is associated with HPV-induced cervical carcinogenesis, although it is still unclear whether HPV infection alone or co-infection with HPV and other pathogens induces inflammatory conditions. An epidemiological study in Costa Rica revealed that there was a positive trend of increasing cervical inflammation associated with high-grade lesions in oncogenic HPV-infected women, and proposed a possibility that cervical inflammation is a cofactor for HPV-induced carcinogenesis (Castle & Giuliano, 2003; Castle et al., 2001). Several epidemiological studies have suggested that other pathogens act in conjunction with HPV infection to increase the risk of cervical cancer. *Chlamydia trachomatis* infection increased the risk of squamous cervical cancer among HPV-positive women in Brazil and the Philippines (Smith et al., 2002b). Among the HPV DNA-positive women, seropositivity of herpes simplex virus-2 was associated with increased risks of squamous-cell carcinoma and adeno- or adenosquamous-cell carcinoma (Smith et al., 2002a). In a study using cervical smears, the relative risk of high grade squamous intraepithelial lesions was significantly higher in patients infected with *Gardinerella vaginalis* and *Chramydia* and with dysbacteriosis and non-specific inflammatory changes (leucocytosis) compared with normal subjects (Roeters et al., 2010). In addition, there is a study showing that biopsy specimens of women infected with carcinogenic HPV type had greater inflammation in the epithelium compared with those of women positive for noncarcinogenic HPV type and negative for HPV, although cervical inflammation varies with HPV cofactors, type of HPV infection, and risk of persistence and progression (Kovacic et al., 2008). Recently, meta-analysis showed that bacterial vaginosis is significantly and positively associated with cervical HPV infection (Gillet, et al., 2011), supporting the hypothesis that cervical inflammation is involved in the pathogenesis of HPV-induced cancer.

2.2 Molecular epidemiological studies on cervical carcinogenesis

The expression of inflammation-related molecules in cervical tissues and the association with HPV-induced carcinogenesis have been extensively investigated. Activation of the transcription factor nuclear factor (NF)-κB has been observed in cervical tissues of patients with squamous intraepithelial lesions. In normal cervical tissue and low-grade squamous intraepithelial lesions, NF-κB subunits, p50 and p65, and inhibitor IκBα (IκBα) were mainly localized in the cytosol, whereas in high-grade lesions and squamous cell carcinomas, the p50-p65 heterodimer was translocated into the nucleus and the expression of IκBα protein was concurrently decreased (A. Nair et al., 2003). NF-κB is a key player in inflammation and regulates the expression of various genes involved in controlling the inflammatory response, including inducible nitric oxide synthase (iNOS), cyclooxygenase-2 (COX-2), interleukin (IL)-1β and tumor necrosis factor (TNF)-α (Karin, 2006; Kundu & Surh, 2008). NF-κB also participates in the promotion and progression of inflammation-related cancer (Karin, 2006; Pikarsky et al., 2004). NF-κB mediates the expression of matrix metalloprotease (MMP) 9 and the angiogenic factor, vascular endothelial growth factor (VEGF) (Karin, 2006), which are considered to participate in tumor progression and metastasis.

COX-2 mediates cancer development via various pathogenic events, including inflammatory responses, apoptosis inhibition and angiogenesis (Chun & Surh, 2004; Warner & Mitchell, 2004; Williams et al., 2000). Molecular epidemiological studies have shown the overexpression of COX-2 in cervical cancer (Kim et al., 2004; Kulkarni et al., 2001). Patients positive for both COX-2 and epidermal growth factor receptor (EGFR) had a higher likelihood of locoregional recurrence and worse prognosis than those negative for one or both proteins (Kim et al., 2004).

In biopsy specimens of cervical intraepithelial neoplasia (CIN) 3 patients, activation of signal transducer and activator of transcription (STAT) 3 and coexpression of MMP9 have been detected in perivascular inflammatory cells. STAT3 induced the expression of the chemokine CCL2, followed by MMP9 expression in tumor-instructed monocytes (Schroer et al., 2011). Recently, it has been reported that the plasma levels of cytokines, especially IL-6, IL-8, TNF-α and macrophage inflammatory protein-1α (MIP-1α), were significantly increased in HPV-positive women relative to HPV-negative controls (Kemp et al., 2010). Therefore, the evidence for the participation of inflammatory responses in cervical carcinogenesis has been accumulating, although further studies are required to clarify the precise molecular mechanism.

3. DNA damage mediated by reactive species under inflammatory conditions

DNA damage is a key molecular event causing genetic instability involved in induction of human carcinogenesis. Under inflammatory conditions, reactive oxygen species (ROS) and reactive nitrogen species (RNS), including nitric oxide (NO), are generated from inflammatory and epithelial cells. These species are highly reactive and capable of causing oxidative and nitrative DNA damage, which may contribute to carcinogenesis (S. P. Hussain et al., 2003; J. Nair et al., 2006; Ohshima et al., 2003). ROS can induce the formation of various oxidative DNA lesions, including mutagenic 8-oxo-7,8-dihydro-2'-deoxyguanosine (8-oxodG) (Kawanishi et al., 2001; Tazawa et al., 2003; Wiseman & Halliwell, 1996). If 8-oxodG is not correctly repaired, adenine is preferentially incorporated opposite 8-oxodG during DNA synthesis, leading to G → T transversion (David et al., 2007; Shibutani et al., 1991). Accumulation of 8-oxodG in human body has been demonstrated in patients with cancer and cancer-prone diseases. A significant increase in urinary 8-oxodG levels has been observed in patients with various types of cancer compared with those in control subjects (Erhola et al., 1997; Tagesson et al., 1995; Thanan et al., 2008). The content of 8-oxodG in cervical cells significantly increased with the grade of squamous intraepithelial lesion (Romano et al., 2000), raising the possibility that oxidative DNA damage participates in cervical carcinogenesis.

Whereas ROS are generated from multiple sources, including not only inflammatory cells but also carcinogenic chemicals and electron transport chain in mitochondria, RNS are primarily generated under inflammatory conditions (Kawanishi & Hiraku, 2006). Therefore, RNS-mediated DNA lesions may play an important role in inflammation-related carcinogenesis, and are expected as potential biomarkers to evaluate the cancer risk. 8-Nitroguanine is a nitrative DNA lesion, formed under inflammatory conditions. NO and superoxide ($O_2^{\bullet-}$) are generated from inflammatory and epithelial cells, and react with each other to form peroxynitrite ($ONOO^-$), a highly reactive species causing nitrative and oxidative DNA damage. *In vitro* experiments revealed that the interaction of guanine with $ONOO^-$ led to the formation of 8-nitroguanine (Yermilov et al., 1995a), in addition to 8-oxodG (Inoue & Kawanishi, 1995) (Figure 1). In an *in vivo* experiment, 8-nitroguanine was formed via inflammation in the lung tissues of mice with viral pneumonia (Akaike et al., 2003).

8-Nitroguanine formed in DNA is chemically unstable, and can be spontaneously released, resulting in the formation of an apurinic site (Yermilov et al., 1995b). Adenine is preferentially incorporated opposite an apurinic site during DNA synthesis, leading to G → T transversion (Loeb & Preston, 1986). Translesion DNA synthesis is the process in which error-prone DNA polymerases bypass unrepaired DNA lesions or insert nucleotides opposite the lesions. Cells deficient in subunits of DNA polymerase ζ, were hypersensitive to NO, and translesion DNA synthesis past apurinic site mediated by this polymerase might contribute to extensive point mutations (Wu et al., 2006). It has also been reported that adenine is preferentially incorporated opposite 8-nitroguanine during DNA synthesis mediated by DNA polymerase η and κ, leading to G → T transversion (Suzuki et al., 2005). Therefore, 8-nitroguanine is a potentially mutagenic DNA lesion, which may contribute to inflammation-related carcinogenesis. In the $ONOO^-$-treated *supF* shuttle vector plasmid, which was then replicated in *Escherichia coli*, the majority of mutations occurred at G:C base pairs, predominantly involving G → T transversions (Juedes & Wogan, 1996; M.Y. Kim et al., 2005). Indeed, this type of mutation occurred *in vivo* in the *ras* gene (Bos, 1988) and the *p53* tumor suppressor gene in lung and liver cancer (Hsu et al., 1991; Takahashi et al., 1989). G → T transversions were most prominently detected in the omentum of asbestos-exposed rats (Unfried et al., 2002). These findings imply that DNA damage mediated by inflammatory reactions may participate in carcinogenesis via activation of protooncogenes and inactivation of tumor suppressor genes.

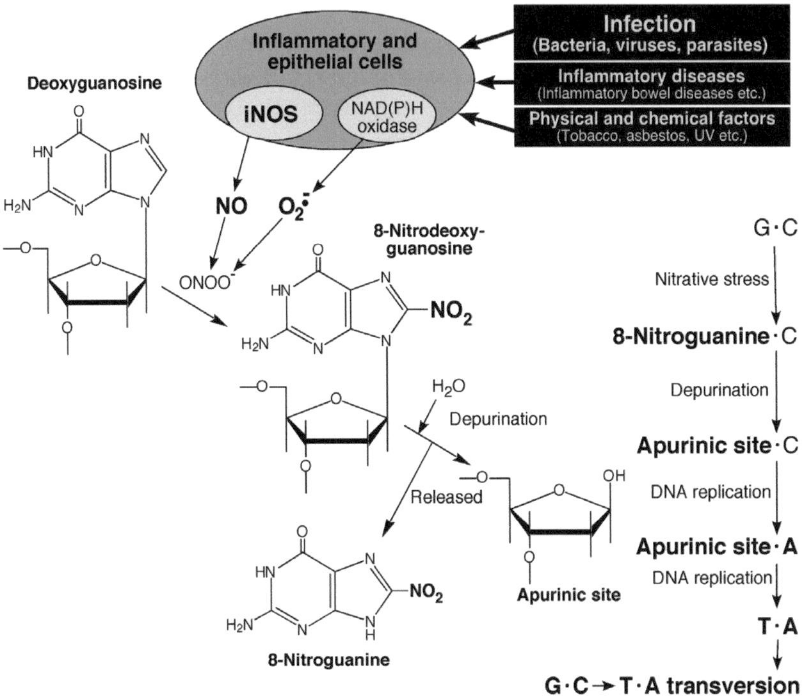

Fig. 1. Proposed mechanism of 8-nitroguanine formation and mutation under inflammatory conditions.

4. Nitrative DNA damage during cervical carcinogenesis

4.1 DNA damage in cervical tissues of CIN patients

To clarify the role of inflammation-mediated DNA damage in cervical carcinogenesis, we performed immunofluorescence staining to examine the formation of 8-nitroguanine and 8-oxodG in biopsy specimens obtained from CIN patients. To detect 8-nitroguanine, we produced a specific antibody and used for experiments (Hiraku & Kawanishi, 2009; Pinlaor et al., 2004a). We compared the fluorescent intensity of these DNA lesions in cervical tissues of patients with different stages of CIN caused by high-risk HPV and condyloma acuminatum, benign cervical warts caused by low-risk HPV. In biopsy specimens of CIN patients, 8-nitroguanine formation was observed in the nuclei of atypical cells (Figure 2), and 8-oxodG showed a similar staining pattern to 8-nitroguanine. Their staining intensity tended to increase with CIN grades. Statistical analysis revealed that the immunoreactivity of 8-nitroguanine in cervical epithelium was significantly increased in the order of condyloma acuminatum < CIN1 < CIN2-3, while there was no significant difference in 8-oxodG formation (Table 2). iNOS expression was also observed in the cytoplasm of both cervical epithelial cells and infiltrating stromal inflammatory cells in CIN patients. 8-Nitroguanine formation was observed in the majority of iNOS-positive epithelial cells. On the other hand, no or weak 8-nitroguanine formation occurred in cervical tissues from patients with condyloma acuminatum. These results raise the possibility that 8-nitroguanine can be used a potential biomarker to evaluate the risk of cervical carcinogenesis.

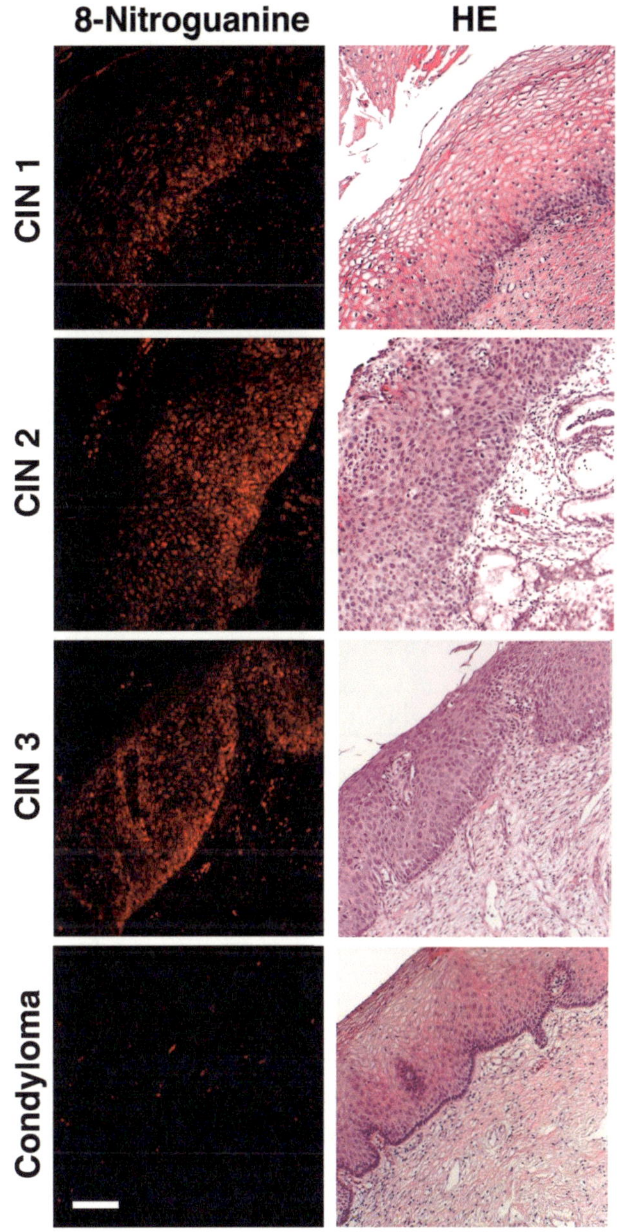

Fig. 2. 8-Nitroguanine formation and histopathological changes in cervical biopsy specimens. 8-Nitroguanine formation was assessed by immunofluorescence staining, and histopathological changes were examined by hematoxylin and eosin (HE) stain. Paraffin sections were incubated with the primary antibody (rabbit polyclonal anti-8-nitroguanine antibody) and then with the secondary antibody (Alexa 594-labeled goat anti-rabbit IgG antibody). 8-Nitroguanine formation was observed in the nuclei of atypical epithelial cells. In the patients with condyloma acuminatum, no or weak 8-nitroguanine formation occurred. Scale bar = 50 μm.

Biomarkers	Immunoreactivity Grading*	Number of cases		
		Condyloma (n = 5)	CIN1 (n = 9)	CIN2-3 (n = 16)
8-Nitroguanine	-	4	4	2
	+	1	2	7
	++	0	3	4
	+++	0	0	3
P	Kruskal-Wallis**		0.024#	
	Scheffe	Condyloma vs CIN1	0.396	
		Condyloma vs CIN2-3	0.030#	
		CIN1 vs CIN2-3	0.359	
8-oxodG	-	4	4	7
	+	1	4	3
	++	0	1	3
	+++	0	0	3
P	Kruskal-Wallis		0.232	
p16	-	1	1	2
	+	3	6	5
	++	1	1	8
	+++	0	1	1
P	Kruskal-Wallis		0.332	

*The immunoreactivity for each specimen was scored as follows: (-) no or few cells were positive, (+) >25% of the cells were positive, (++) >50% of the cells were moderately positive, and (+++) >75% of the cells were strongly positive.
**The statistical difference in immunoreactivities was analyzed by Kruskal-Wallis test, and if there was a statistical significance, Scheffe's multiple comparison was performed. #$P < 0.05$.

Table 2. Difference in immunoreactivies of DNA lesions and p16 in cervical epithelial cells of biopsy specimens obtained from patients with CIN and condyloma acuminatum

The formation of nitrative DNA lesion in relation to cervical carcinogenesis has been supported by a recent study. NO exposure induced DNA damage and increased mutation rates in HPV-positive human cervical epithelial cell lines established from CIN patients (Wei et al., 2009). In addition, NO exposure increased the expression of E6 and E7 genes, resulting in decreased p53 and RB protein levels in these cells (Wei et al., 2009), although precise molecular mechanism has not been understood. These findings raise the possibility that NO serves as a molecular cofactor with HPV infection, and resulting DNA damage and the expression of viral oncoproteins cooperatively contribute to HPV-mediated cervical carcinogenesis. Therefore, modification of local NO concentration in cervical tissues and related molecular events may constitute a strategy to prevent HPV-related cancer.

4.2 Comparison of 8-nitroguanine formation and p16 expression in CIN patients

There are several reports showing that the cyclin-dependent kinase inhibitor p16 is overexpressed in cervical neoplasia (Gupta et al., 2010; Klaes et al., 2001; Sano et al., 1998; von Knebel Doeberitz, 2002; J. L. Wang et al., 2004), and proposed as a potential biomarker of cervical carcinogenesis. The expression of p16 was significantly higher in CIN and squamous cell cancer than in normal or inflammation of the cervix, and p16-positive patients had significantly shorter interval for disease progression from initial biopsy to CIN 3 or invasive cancer than p16-negative patients (J. L. Wang et al., 2004). E7 oncoprotein binds to RB, leading to the release of the transcription factor E2F from the RB/E2F complex (von Knebel Doeberitz, 2002). E2F accumulation leads to the expression of p16-related transcript, although the molecular mechanism remains to be clarified (Khleif et al., 1996).

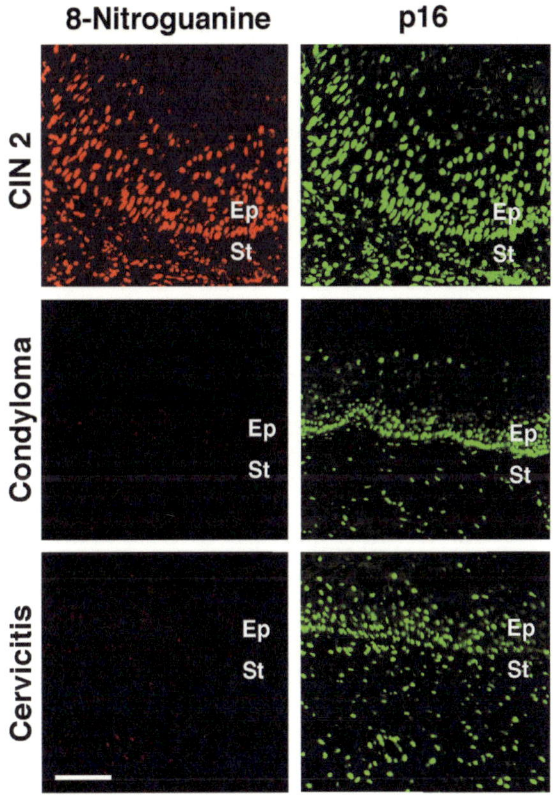

Fig. 3. 8-Nitroguanine formation and p16 expression in cervical biopsy specimens. 8-Nitroguanine formation and p16 expression were assessed by immunofluorescence staining. Paraffin sections were incubated with the primary antibodies (rabbit polyclonal anti-8-nitroguanine and mouse monoclonal anti-p16 antibodies), and then with the secondary antibodies (Alexa 594-labeled goat anti-rabbit IgG and Alexa 488-labeled goat anti-mouse IgG antibodies). Strong p16 expression (green) was observed in cervical epithelial cells of CIN2 patients and showed a similar pattern to 8-nitroguanine formation (red). In patients with condyloma acuminatum and cervicitis (HPV-16-positive), p16 expression was observed in the basal layer but no or weak 8-nitroguanine formation was detected. Ep, epithelium. St, stroma. Scale bar = 50 μm.

We performed immunohistochemistry to compare 8-nitroguanine formation and p16 expression in cervical biopsy specimens of HPV-infected patients. Strong p16 expression was observed in cervical epithelial cells of CIN patients and showed a similar pattern to 8-nitroguanine (Figure 3). However, in cervical tissues of patients with condyloma acuminatum and HPV-positive cervicitis, p16 expression was observed in the basal layer, whereas no or weak 8-nitroguanine formation was detected. Statistical analysis revealed that no significant difference in p16 expression was observed among condyloma and CIN groups, whereas there was significant difference in 8-nitroguanine formation as described above (Table 2). These results suggest that p16 is simply a marker to reflect HPV infection, and that 8-nitroguanine is more suitable marker to discriminate high-risk and low-risk cervical lesions.

5. Role of nitrative DNA damage in inflammation-related carcinogenesis

5.1 8-Nitroguanine formation in inflammation-related carcinogenesis

In addition to cervical cancer, we have investigated 8-nitroguanine formation in tissues of patients and animal models of a wide variety of inflammation-related cancer and cancer-prone diseases by immunohistochemical analysis. We first demonstrated that this DNA lesion was formed at the site of carcinogenesis induced by bacterial, viral, and parasitic infections (Hiraku, 2010; Kawanishi & Hiraku, 2006; Kawanishi et al., 2006). The studies on 8-nitroguanine formation in relation to inflammation-related carcinogenesis are summarized in Table 3.

Infectious diseases			
Cause	Site of DNA damage	Species	References
Helicobacter pyroli	Gastric epithelium	Human	(Ma et al., 2004)
Human papillomavirus (HPV)	Cervical epithelium	Human	(Hiraku et al., 2007)
Hepatitis C virus	Hepatocyte	Human	(Horiike et al., 2005)
Epstein-Barr virus (EBV)	Nasopharyngeal epithelium and tumor tissue	Human	(Ma et al., 2008)
Liver fluke (*Opisthorchis viverrini*)	Bile duct epithelium	Hamster	(Pinlaor et al., 2004a) (Pinlaor et al., 2004b) (Pinlaor et al., 2006)
	Tumor tissue	Human	(Pinlaor et al., 2005)
Inflammatory diseases and conditions			
Cause	Site of DNA damage	Species	References
Inflammatory bowel disease	Colon epithelium	Mouse	(Ding et al., 2005)
Oral licken planus	Oral epithelium	Human	(Chaiyarit et al., 2005)
Oral leukoplakia	Oral epithelium	Human	(Ma et al., 2006)
Soft tissue tumor (Malignant histiocytoma)	Tumor tissue	Human	(Hoki et al., 2007a) (Hoki et al., 2007b)
Asbestos	Bronchial epithelium	Mouse	(Hiraku et al., 2010)

Table 3. 8-Nitroguanine formation in humans and animals in relation to inflammation-related carcinogenesis

We found that 8-nitroguanine was formed in epithelial cells of intrahepatic bile duct using an animal model infected with the liver fluke *Opisthorchis viverrini*, endemic in northeastern Thailand (Pinlaor et al., 2004a; Pinlaor et al., 2004b; Pinlaor et al., 2003). Administration of the antiparasitic drug praziquantel and the antioxidant curcumin significantly reduced oxidative and nitrative DNA damage (Pinlaor et al., 2006; Prakobwong et al., 2011). We have also demonstrated that 8-nitroguanine was formed in the gastric gland epithelial cells from gastritis patients with *Helicobacter pylori* infection (Ma et al., 2004), in the hepatocytes of patients with chronic hepatitis C (Horiike et al., 2005) and in the nasopharyngeal epithelial cells and tumor tissues of patients infected with Epstein-Barr virus (EBV) (Ma et al., 2008). These results suggest that 8-nitroguanine is a promising biomarker providing an assessment of the risk of inflammation-mediated carcinogenesis at the precancerous stage. Moreover, in EBV-infected patients, the staining intensity of 8-nirtroguanine was significantly stronger in nasopharyngeal cancer cells than in epithelial cells of chronic nasopharyngitis patients, suggesting that 8-nitroguanine accumulates during the development of chronic inflammation to cancer (Ma et al., 2008). In addition, 8-nitroguanine formation was observed under inflammatory conditions independent of infection. This DNA lesion was seen in colon epithelial cells of a mouse model of inflammatory bowel disease (Ding et al., 2005), in oral epithelial cells of patients with oral premalignant lesions (Chaiyarit et al., 2005; Ma et al., 2006) and in bronchial epithelial cells of asbestos-exposed mice (Hiraku et al., 2010).

Several studies have raised a possibility that DNA damage is involved in tumor progression. In patients with inhrahepatic cholongiocarcinoma, oxidative and nitrative DNA damage in tumor and adjacent tissues was associated with tumor invasion (Pinlaor et al., 2005) 8-Nitroguanine staining was observed in tumor tissues of patients with malignant fibrous histiocytoma, a soft tissue tumor, which is proposed to be accompanied with inflammatory responses. The statistical analysis using the Kaplan-Meier method revealed that strong 8-nitroguanine formation was significantly associated with a poor prognosis of the patients (Hoki et al., 2007a). These findings indicate that this DNA lesion contributes to not only tumor initiation but also tumor progression and poor prognosis of cancer patients.

5.2 Mechanism of inflammation-related carcinogenesis and the role of DNA damage

On the basis of our previous studies, possible mechanism of inflammation-related carcinogenesis and tumor development via DNA damage is shown in Figure 4. Various infectious agents, including bacteria, viruses and parasites, inflammatory diseases and environmental factors can induce inflammatory responses and the production of ROS and RNS from inflammatory and epithelial cells. A wide variety of inflammatory cytokines mediate the activation of transcription factors, including NF-κB and STATs. NF-κB regulates the expression of a wide variety of inflammation-related molecules including iNOS (Karin, 2006; Kundu & Surh, 2008) and participates in multiple steps of carcinogenesis (Karin, 2006; Pikarsky et al., 2004). RNS can induce the activation of NF-κB under certain circumstances (Janssen-Heininger et al., 2000). Therefore, reciprocal and positive regulation between RNS and NF-κB may lead to persistent inflammatory reactions and nitrative DNA damage, contributing to carcinogenesis.

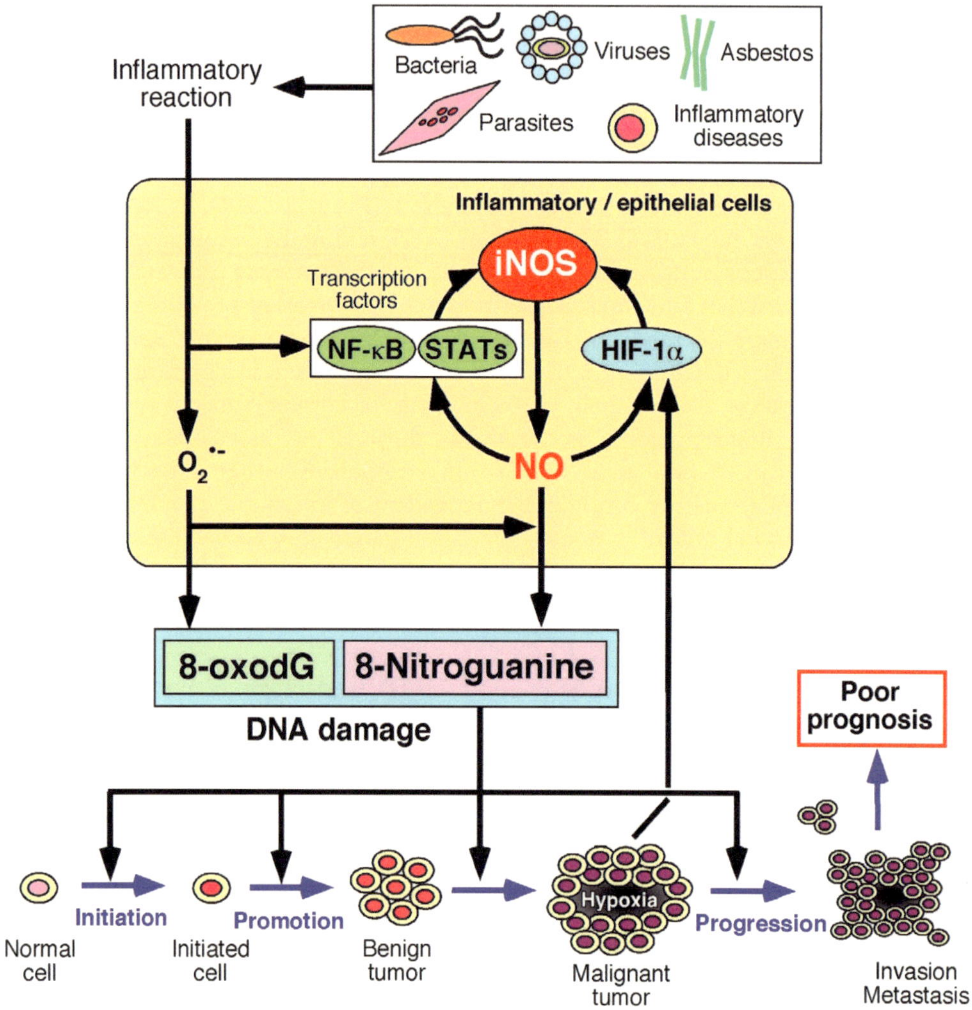

Fig. 4. Possible mechanism of inflammation-related carcinogenesis and tumor progression via 8-nitroguanine formation.

STAT1 and STAT3 are known to mediate the expression of iNOS (Lo et al., 2005; Tedeschi et al., 2003). STAT3 interacts with EGFR in the nucleus to form a complex, which mediates transcriptional activation of iNOS (Lo et al., 2005). Actually, phosphorylated STAT3 (active form) and EGFR were strongly expressed and colocalized in the nucleus of cancer cells of nasopharyngeal cancer patients (Ma et al., 2008). A recent study has demonstrated that excess $ONOO^-$ mediates the activation of JAK/STAT signalling pathway in experimental animals (H. Wang et al., 2009). These findings imply that a positive loop between STATs and iNOS may exist.

Hypoxia-inducible factor (HIF)-1α is an oxygen-sensing transcription factor, which is upregulated in a hypoxic environment during tumor growth. HIF-1α mediates the transcription of various genes, including iNOS and VEGF (Harris, 2002). An increase in iNOS-catalyzed NO production induces the accumulation and activation of HIF-1α (Mateo et al., 2003; Thomas et al., 2004). HIF-1α and 8-nitroguanine were colocalized and associated with poor prognosis of cancer patients (Hoki et al., 2007b). Therefore, reciprocal activation of HIF-1α and iNOS may lead to persistent DNA damage in tumor tissues, contributing to poor prognosis of cancer patients. A recent study has demonstrated that IκB kinase (IKK)-β, involved in NF-κB activation, is required for HIF-1α protein accumulation under hypoxia in cultured cells and animals (Rius et al., 2008), whereas NF-κB bas been reported to be regulated under hypoxia in an HIF-1α-dependent manner (Walmsley et al., 2005). Thus, HIF-1α and NF-κB may positively regulate each other and participate in tumor progression.

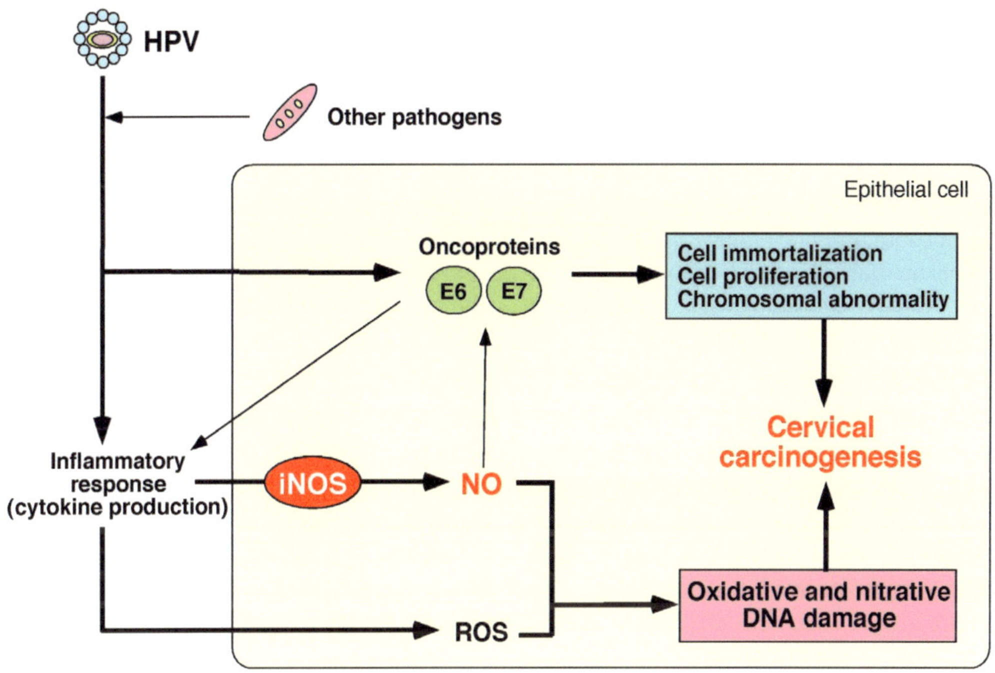

Fig. 5. Possible mechanism of HPV-induced cervical carcinogenesis mediated by chronic inflammation.

Collectively, molecular events mediated by various pathogens converge to nitrative stress, and resulting DNA damage contributes to the accumulation of genetic alterations in tissues throughout the carcinogenic process. In particular, 8-nitroguanine formation may participate in inflammation-related carcinogenesis as a common mechanism, regardless of etiology. Therefore, 8-nitroguanine could be used as a potential biomarker to evaluate the cancer risk and predict the prognosis of cancer patients. In addition, certain pathogens possess unique molecules mediating abnormal cell proliferation and survival, such as E6 and E7 proteins of HPV as described below. Therefore, 8-nitroguanine formation may contribute to carcinogenesis in cooperation with pathogen-specific molecular events.

A recent study has demonstrated that 8-nitro-cGMP, formed by the reaction of RNS with cGMP, regulates the redox-sensor signaling proteins, via *S*-guanylation of cysteine sulphydrils, and mediates an adaptive response against oxidative and nitrative stress (Sawa et al., 2007). *S*-Nitrosylated proteins, formed via reaction of thiols with NO or its reactive metabolites, possess cytoprotective properties (Ishima et al., 2007). In inflammation-related carcinogenesis, nitrated or nitrosylated molecules may participate in protection of initiated cells bearing genetic alterations due to oxidative and nitrative DNA damage, and contribute to tumor development.

5.3 Mechanism of HPV-mediated cervical carcinogenesis via inflammatory reactions

A possible mechanism of HPV-induced cervical carcinogenesis involving inflammatory reactions is shown in Figure 5. We have demonstrated that inflammation-mediated DNA lesions were formed in cervical tissues of CIN patients (Hiraku et al., 2007). To date, no evidence suggesting that HPV infection alone induces inflammatory states has been provided. Therefore, it is speculated that inflammatory reactions are derived from HPV infection and co-infection with other pathogens, although the precise mechanism remains to be clarified. DNA damage mediated by inflammatory reactions would play a substantial role in tumor initiation and also the following steps of carcinogenesis. In addition, HPV oncoproteins E6 and E7 mediate cell immortalization, dysregulation of cell proliferation and chromosomal abnormalities by interacting with numerous target proteins. The molecular events mediated by these oncoproteins may promote the proliferation and transformation of cells initiated by oxidative and nitrative DNA damage, and contribute to tumor promotion and progression.

In addition, several studies have demonstrated that HPV oncoproteins mediate inflammatory responses. The expression of E6 and E7 oncoproteins derived from highly carcinogenic HPV-16 enhanced the release of IL-1α from cultures of normal cervical keratinocytes, and E7 proteins that strongly bound to RB protein (high risk types HPV-16 and HPV-18) induced more IL-1α release than those that bound poorly (low-risk type HPV-6) (Iglesias et al., 1998). A recent study has shown that E7 expression increased the promotor activity of COX-2 and the downstream molecule IL-32 in HPV-positive cervical cancer cell lines (Lee et al., 2011). IL-32 induces the expression of various inflammatory cytokines, including IL-1β, IL-6, TNF-α and chemokines (S.H. Kim et al., 2005). IL-32 expression was detected in cervical tissues of patients with squamous cell carcinoma and increased with the tumor stage (Lee et al., 2011). Therefore, these HPV oncoproteins may participate in inflammatory responses in cervical tissues and contribute to carcinogenesis. In addition, a recent study has shown that NO treatment mediates the expression of E6 and E7 in cultured cells (Wei et al., 2009). A COX-2-selective inhibitor suppressed the expression of E7 in cultured cervical cancer cells (Lee et al., 2011). Inflammatory reactions may reciprocally mediate the expression of HPV oncoproteins, resulting in the persistence of inflammation-related DNA damage and dysregulated cell proliferation, contributing to tumor progression.

6. Conclusion and future perspective

Chronic infection and inflammation are known to contribute to a substantial part of environmental carcinogenesis. Cervical cancer is the second most common cancer among women, and HPV infection is involved in almost all cases. Recent epidemiological studies revealed that chronic inflammation participates in cervical carcinogenesis. Under inflammatory conditions, reactive oxygen and nitrogen species are generated, and resulting DNA damage may play an important role in carcinogenesis. We performed immunohistochemical analysis and demonstrated that 8-nitroguanine, a mutagenic DNA lesion formed during inflammation, was formed in cervical epithelial cells in CIN patients, and its immunoreactivity was significantly increased with CIN grades. The comparison of 8-nitroguanine formation and p16 expression revealed that 8-nitroguanine is more suitable to detect cervical lesions mediated by high-risk types of HPV. Taken together with this and previous studies, it is concluded that 8-nitroguanine can be used as a potential biomarker to evaluate the risk of inflammation-related carcinogenesis, including cervical carcinogenesis. In addition, HPV oncoproteins E6 and E7 are known to mediate cell immortalization, dysregulated cell proliferation and chromosomal instability. Several studies have suggested that these oncoproteins crosstalk with signalling pathways related to inflammatory responses. Therefore, oxidative and nitrative DNA damage mediated by inflammatory reactions and oncoprotein-mediated molecular events may cooperatively contribute to cervical carcinogenesis.

Establishment of methods for quantitative analysis of 8-nitroguanine in biological samples, such as blood and urine, would be useful for evaluation of the risk of inflammation-related carcinogenesis. 8-Nitroguanine formed in DNA is chemically unstable, and is likely to be released from DNA. Thus, this property may hamper the quantitative analysis. An attempt has been made to utilize free 8-nitroguanine in urine for quantitative analysis using high-performance liquid chromatography coupled with electrochemical detection and immunoaffinity purification (Sawa et al., 2006). 8-Nitroguanine has also been measured by liquid chromatography with mass spectrometry and glyoxal derivatization (Ishii et al., 2007).

Moreover, the development of therapeutics targeting inflammation-related molecules may contribute to prevention of cervical carcinogenesis and improvement of prognosis of cancer patients. Animal experiments demonstrated that iNOS inhibitors suppress inflammatory responses and effectively reduce inflammation-related carcinogenesis, although evidence has not yet been provided for their inhibitory effect on cervical carcinogenesis. ONO-1714, an iNOS-specific inhibitor, significantly decreased the degree of cholangitis and reduced the incidence of intrahepatic biliary tumors in bilioenterostomized hamsters (Mishima et al., 2009). Another iNOS inhibitor, 1400W, reduced tumorigenesis in the mammary glands of γ-irradiated mice treated with diethylstilbestrol (Inano & Onoda, 2005). Moreover, administration of the antioxidant curcumin significantly reduced the incidence of liver fluke-induced carcinogenesis via suppression of oxidative and nitrative DNA damage (Prakobwong et al., 2011). To develop a strategy for prevention of HPV-mediated cervical cancer, further studies are needed to clarify the precise molecular mechanisms and the role of chronic inflammation.

7. Acknowledgement

The author is grateful to Dr. Tsutomu Tabata (Mie University Graduate School of Medicine, Japan) and Professor Ning Ma (Suzuka University of Medical Sciences, Japan) for clinical and technical advices, respectively. The author is also grateful to Professor Shosuke Kawanishi (Suzuka University of Medical Sciences), Professor Mariko Murata (Mie

University Graduate School of Medicine) and all collaborators for the encouragement throughout this work. This work was supported by Grants-in-Aid for Scientific Research from the Ministry of Education, Culture, Sports, Science and Technology and the Ministry of Health, Labour and Welfare of Japan.

8. References

Akaike, T., Okamoto, S., Sawa, T., Yoshitake, J., Tamura, F., Ichimori, K., Miyazaki, K., Sasamoto, K. & Maeda, H. (2003). 8-Nitroguanosine formation in viral pneumonia and its implication for pathogenesis. *Proc. Natl. Acad. Sci. USA*, Vol. 100, No. 2, pp. 685-690, ISSN 0027-8424

Balkwill, F. & Mantovani, A. (2001). Inflammation and cancer: back to Virchow? *Lancet*, Vol. 357, No. 9255, pp. 539-545, ISSN 0140-6736

Bos, J.L. (1988). The ras gene family and human carcinogenesis. *Mutat. Res.*, Vol. 195, No. 3, pp. 255-271, ISSN 0027-5107

Bosch, F.X., Lorincz, A., Munoz, N., Meijer, C.J. & Shah, K.V. (2002). The causal relation between human papillomavirus and cervical cancer. *J. Clin. Pathol.*, Vol. 55, No. 4, pp. 244-265, ISSN 0021-9746

Castle, P.E., Hillier, S.L., Rabe, L.K., Hildesheim, A., Herrero, R., Bratti, M.C., Sherman, M.E., Burk, R.D., Rodriguez, A.C., Alfaro, M., Hutchinson, M.L., Morales, J. & Schiffman, M. (2001). An association of cervical inflammation with high-grade cervical neoplasia in women infected with oncogenic human papillomavirus (HPV). *Cancer Epidemiol. Biomarkers Prev.*, Vol. 10, No. 10, pp. 1021-1027, ISSN 1055-9965

Castle, P.E. & Giuliano, A.R. (2003). Chapter 4: Genital tract infections, cervical inflammation, and antioxidant nutrients-assessing their roles as human papillomavirus cofactors. *J. Natl. Cancer Inst. Monogr.*, Vol. 31, pp. 29-34, ISSN 1052-6773

Chaiyarit, P., Ma, N., Hiraku, Y., Pinlaor, S., Yongvanit, P., Jintakanon, D., Murata, M., Oikawa, S. & Kawanishi, S. (2005). Nitrative and oxidative DNA damage in oral lichen planus in relation to human oral carcinogenesis. *Cancer Sci.*, Vol. 96, No. 9, pp. 553-559, ISSN 1347-9032

Chen, Y.C. & Hunter, D.J. (2005). Molecular epidemiology of cancer. *CA Cancer J. Clin.*, Vol. 55, No. 1, pp. 45-54, ISSN 0007-9235

Chun, K.S. & Surh, Y.J. (2004). Signal transduction pathways regulating cyclooxygenase-2 expression: potential molecular targets for chemoprevention. *Biochem. Pharmacol.*, Vol. 68, No. 6, pp. 1089-1100, ISSN 0006-2952

Coussens, L.M. & Werb, Z. (2002). Inflammation and cancer. *Nature*, Vol. 420, No. 6917, pp. 860-867, ISSN 0028-0836

Darnell, G.A., Schroder, W.A., Antalis, T.M., Lambley, E., Major, L., Gardner, J., Birrell, G., Cid-Arregui, A. & Suhrbier, A. (2007). Human papillomavirus E7 requires the protease calpain to degrade the retinoblastoma protein. *J. Biol. Chem.*, Vol. 282, No. 52, pp. 37492-37500, ISSN 0021-9258

David, S.S., O'Shea, V.L. & Kundu, S. (2007). Base-excision repair of oxidative DNA damage. *Nature*, Vol. 447, No. 7147, pp. 941-950, ISSN 0028-0836

Ding, X., Hiraku, Y., Ma, N., Kato, T., Saito, K., Nagahama, M., Semba, R., Kuribayashi, K. & Kawanishi, S. (2005). Inducible nitric oxide synthase-dependent DNA damage in mouse model of inflammatory bowel disease. *Cancer Sci.*, Vol. 96, No. 3, pp. 157-163, ISSN 1347-9032

DiPaolo, J.A., Woodworth, C.D., Popescu, N.C., Notario, V. & Doniger, J. (1989). Induction of human cervical squamous cell carcinoma by sequential transfection with human papillomavirus 16 DNA and viral Harvey ras. *Oncogene*, Vol. 4, No. 4, pp. 395-399, ISSN 0950-9232

Du, M.Q., Carmichael, P.L. & Phillips, D.H. (1994). Induction of activating mutations in the human c-Ha-*ras*-1 proto-oncogene by oxygen free radicals. *Mol. Carcinog.*, Vol. 11, No. 3, pp. 170-175, ISSN 0899-1987

Duensing, S., Lee, L.Y., Duensing, A., Basile, J., Piboonniyom, S., Gonzalez, S., Crum, C.P. & Munger, K. (2000). The human papillomavirus type 16 E6 and E7 oncoproteins cooperate to induce mitotic defects and genomic instability by uncoupling centrosome duplication from the cell division cycle. *Proc. Natl. Acad. Sci. USA*, Vol. 97, No. 18, pp. 10002-10007, ISSN 0027-8424

Duensing, S. & Munger, K. (2004). Mechanisms of genomic instability in human cancer: insights from studies with human papillomavirus oncoproteins. *Int. J. Cancer*, Vol. 109, No. 2, pp. 157-162, ISSN 0020-7136

Erhola, M., Toyokuni, S., Okada, K., Tanaka, T., Hiai, H., Ochi, H., Uchida, K., Osawa, T., Nieminen, M.M., Alho, H. & Kellokumpu-Lehtinen, P. (1997). Biomarker evidence of DNA oxidation in lung cancer patients: association of urinary 8-hydroxy-2'-deoxyguanosine excretion with radiotherapy, chemotherapy, and response to treatment. *FEBS Lett.*, Vol. 409, No. 2, pp. 287-291, ISSN 0014-5793

Gillet, E., Meys, J.F., Verstraelen, H., Bosire, C., De Sutter, P., Temmerman, M. & Broeck, D.V. (2011). Bacterial vaginosis is associated with uterine cervical human papillomavirus infection: a meta-analysis. *BMC Infect. Dis.*, Vol. 11, No. pp. 10, ISSN 1471-2334

Gupta, R., Srinivasan, R., Nijhawan, R. & Suri, V. (2010). Tissue transglutaminase 2 as a biomarker of cervical intraepithelial neoplasia (CIN) and its relationship to p16INK4A and nuclear factor κB expression. *Virchows Arch.*, Vol. 456, No. 1, pp. 45-51, ISSN 0945-6317

Harris, A.L. (2002). Hypoxia-a key regulatory factor in tumour growth. *Nat. Rev. Cancer*, Vol. 2, No. 1, pp. 38-47, ISSN 1474-175X

Hiraku, Y., Tabata, T., Ma, N., Murata, M., Ding, X. & Kawanishi, S. (2007). Nitrative and oxidative DNA damage in cervical intraepithelial neoplasia associated with human papilloma virus infection. *Cancer Sci.*, Vol. 98, No. 7, pp. 964-972, ISSN 1347-9032

Hiraku, Y. & Kawanishi, S. (2009). Immunohistochemical analysis of 8-nitroguanine, a nitrative DNA lesion, in relation to inflammation-associated carcinogenesis. *Methods Mol. Biol.*, Vol. 512, pp. 3-13, ISSN 1064-3745

Hiraku, Y. (2010). Formation of 8-nitroguanine, a nitrative DNA lesion, in inflammation-related carcinogenesis and its significance. *Environ. Health Prev. Med.*, Vol. 15, No. 2, pp. 63-72, ISSN 1342-078X

Hiraku, Y., Kawanishi, S., Ichinose, T. & Murata, M. (2010). The role of iNOS-mediated DNA damage in infection- and asbestos-induced carcinogenesis. *Ann. NY Acad. Sci.*, Vol. 1203, pp. 15-22, ISSN 0077-8923

Hoki, Y., Hiraku, Y., Ma, N., Murata, M., Matsumine, A., Nagahama, M., Shintani, K., Uchida, A. & Kawanishi, S. (2007a). iNOS-dependent DNA damage in patients with malignant fibrous histiocytoma in relation to prognosis. *Cancer Sci.*, Vol. 98, No. 2, pp. 163-168, ISSN 1347-9032

Hoki, Y., Murata, M., Hiraku, Y., Ma, N., Matsumine, A., Uchida, A. & Kawanishi, S. (2007b). 8-Nitroguanine as a potential biomarker for progression of malignant fibrous histiocytoma, a model of inflammation-related cancer. *Oncol. Rep.*, Vol. 18, No. 5, pp. 1165-1169, ISSN 1021-335X

Horiike, S., Kawanishi, S., Kaito, M., Ma, N., Tanaka, H., Fujita, N., Iwasa, M., Kobayashi, Y., Hiraku, Y., Oikawa, S., Murata, M., Wang, J., Semba, R., Watanabe, S. & Adachi, Y. (2005). Accumulation of 8-nitroguanine in the liver of patients with chronic hepatitis C. *J. Hepatol.*, Vol. 43, No. 3, pp. 403-410, ISSN 0168-8278

Hsu, I.C., Metcalf, R.A., Sun, T., Welsh, J.A., Wang, N.J. & Harris, C.C. (1991). Mutational hotspot in the *p53* gene in human hepatocellular carcinomas. *Nature*, Vol. 350, No. 6317, pp. 427-428, ISSN 0028-0836

Huh, K.W., DeMasi, J., Ogawa, H., Nakatani, Y., Howley, P.M. & Munger, K. (2005). Association of the human papillomavirus type 16 E7 oncoprotein with the 600-kDa retinoblastoma protein-associated factor, p600. *Proc. Natl. Acad. Sci. USA*, Vol. 102, No. 32, pp. 11492-11497, ISSN 0027-8424

Hussain, S.P., Hofseth, L.J. & Harris, C.C. (2003). Radical causes of cancer. *Nat. Rev. Cancer*, Vol. 3, No. 4, pp. 276-285, ISSN 1474-175X

Hussain, S.P. & Harris, C.C. (2007). Inflammation and cancer: an ancient link with novel potentials. *Int. J. Cancer*, Vol. 121, No. 11, pp. 2373-2380, ISSN 1097-0215

IARC, (2003). *World Cancer Report*, IARC Press, Lyon

IARC Working Group, (2007). *IARC Monographs on the Evaluation of Carcinogenic Risks to Humans, Vol. 90, Human Papillomaviruses*, IARC Press, Lyon

IARC Working Group, (2011). Human Papillomaviruses, In: *IARC Monographs on the Evaluation of Carcinogenic Risks to Humans, Vol. 100B, A Review of Human Carcinogens, Part B: Biological Agents*, pp. 261-319, IARC Press, Lyon

Iglesias, M., Yen, K., Gaiotti, D., Hildesheim, A., Stoler, M.H. & Woodworth, C.D. (1998). Human papillomavirus type 16 E7 protein sensitizes cervical keratinocytes to apoptosis and release of interleukin-1α. *Oncogene*, Vol. 17, No. 10, pp. 1195-1205, ISSN 0950-9232

Inano, H. & Onoda, M. (2005). Nitric oxide produced by inducible nitric oxide synthase is associated with mammary tumorigenesis in irradiated rats. *Nitric Oxide*, Vol. 12, No. 1, pp. 15-20, ISSN 1089-8603

Inoue, S. & Kawanishi, S. (1995). Oxidative DNA damage induced by simultaneous generation of nitric oxide and superoxide. *FEBS Lett.*, Vol. 371, No. 1, pp. 86-88, ISSN 0014-5793

Ishii, Y., Ogara, A., Okamura, T., Umemura, T., Nishikawa, A., Iwasaki, Y., Ito, R., Saito, K., Hirose, M. & Nakazawa, H. (2007). Development of quantitative analysis of 8-nitroguanine concomitant with 8-hydroxydeoxyguanosine formation by liquid chromatography with mass spectrometry and glyoxal derivatization. *J. Pharm. Biomed. Anal.*, Vol. 43, No. 5, pp. 1737-1743, ISSN 0731-7085

Ishima, Y., Sawa, T., Kragh-Hansen, U., Miyamoto, Y., Matsushita, S., Akaike, T. & Otagiri, M. (2007). *S*-Nitrosylation of human variant albumin liprizzi (R410C) confers potent antibacterial and cytoprotective properties. *J. Pharmacol. Exp. Ther.*, Vol. 320, No. 3, pp. 969-977, ISSN 0022-3565

Janssen-Heininger, Y.M., Poynter, M.E. & Baeuerle, P.A. (2000). Recent advances towards understanding redox mechanisms in the activation of nuclear factor κB. *Free Radic. Biol. Med.*, Vol. 28, No. 9, pp. 1317-1327, ISSN 0891-5849

Juedes, M.J. & Wogan, G.N. (1996). Peroxynitrite-induced mutation spectra of pSP189 following replication in bacteria and in human cells. *Mutat. Res.*, Vol. 349, No. 1, pp. 51-61, ISSN 0027-5107

Karin, M. (2006). Nuclear factor-κB in cancer development and progression. *Nature*, Vol. 441, No. 7092, pp. 431-436, ISSN 1476-4687

Kawanishi, S., Hiraku, Y. & Oikawa, S. (2001). Mechanism of guanine-specific DNA damage by oxidative stress and its role in carcinogenesis and aging. *Mutat. Res.*, Vol. 488, No. 1, pp. 65-76, ISSN 0027-5107

Kawanishi, S. & Hiraku, Y. (2006). Oxidative and nitrative DNA damage as biomarker for carcinogenesis with special reference to inflammation. *Antioxid. Redox Signal.*, Vol. 8, No. 5-6, pp. 1047-1058, ISSN 1523-0864

Kawanishi, S., Hiraku, Y., Pinlaor, S. & Ma, N. (2006). Oxidative and nitrative DNA damage in animals and patients with inflammatory diseases in relation to inflammation-related carcinogenesis. *Biol. Chem.*, Vol. 387, No. 4, pp. 365-372, ISSN 1431-6730

Kemp, T.J., Hildesheim, A., Garcia-Pineres, A., Williams, M.C., Shearer, G.M., Rodriguez, A.C., Schiffman, M., Burk, R., Freer, E., Bonilla, J., Herrero, R. & Pinto, L.A. (2010). Elevated systemic levels of inflammatory cytokines in older women with persistent cervical human papillomavirus infection. *Cancer Epidemiol. Biomarkers Prev.*, Vol. 19, No. 8, pp. 1954-1959, ISSN 1055-9965

Kessis, T.D., Slebos, R.J., Nelson, W.G., Kastan, M.B., Plunkett, B.S., Han, S.M., Lorincz, A.T., Hedrick, L. & Cho, K.R. (1993). Human papillomavirus 16 E6 expression disrupts the p53-mediated cellular response to DNA damage. *Proc. Natl. Acad. Sci. USA*, Vol. 90, No. 9, pp. 3988-3992, ISSN 0027-8424

Khleif, S.N., DeGregori, J., Yee, C.L., Otterson, G.A., Kaye, F.J., Nevins, J.R. & Howley, P.M. (1996). Inhibition of cyclin D-CDK4/CDK6 activity is associated with an E2F-mediated induction of cyclin kinase inhibitor activity. *Proc. Natl. Acad. Sci. USA*, Vol. 93, No. 9, pp. 4350-4354, ISSN 0027-8424

Kim, G.E., Kim, Y.B., Cho, N.H., Chung, H.C., Pyo, H.R., Lee, J.D., Park, T.K., Koom, W.S., Chun, M. & Suh, C.O. (2004). Synchronous coexpression of epidermal growth factor receptor and cyclooxygenase-2 in carcinomas of the uterine cervix: a potential predictor of poor survival. *Clin. Cancer Res.*, Vol. 10, No. 4, pp. 1366-1374, ISSN 1078-0432

Kim, M.Y., Dong, M., Dedon, P.C. & Wogan, G.N. (2005). Effects of peroxynitrite dose and dose rate on DNA damage and mutation in the *supF* shuttle vector. *Chem. Res. Toxicol.*, Vol. 18, No. 1, pp. 76-86, ISSN 0893-228X

Kim, S.H., Han, S.Y., Azam, T., Yoon, D.Y. & Dinarello, C.A. (2005). Interleukin-32: a cytokine and inducer of TNFα. *Immunity*, Vol. 22, No. 1, pp. 131-142, ISSN 1074-7613

Klaes, R., Friedrich, T., Spitkovsky, D., Ridder, R., Rudy, W., Petry, U., Dallenbach-Hellweg, G., Schmidt, D. & von Knebel Doeberitz, M. (2001). Overexpression of p16(INK4A) as a specific marker for dysplastic and neoplastic epithelial cells of the cervix uteri. *Int. J. Cancer*, Vol. 92, No. 2, pp. 276-284, ISSN 0020-7136

Kovacic, M.B., Katki, H.A., Kreimer, A.R. & Sherman, M.E. (2008). Epidemiologic analysis of histologic cervical inflammation: relationship to human papillomavirus infections. *Hum. Pathol.*, Vol. 39, No. 7, pp. 1088-1095, ISSN 0046-8177

Kulkarni, S., Rader, J.S., Zhang, F., Liapis, H., Koki, A.T., Masferrer, J.L., Subbaramaiah, K. & Dannenberg, A.J. (2001). Cyclooxygenase-2 is overexpressed in human cervical cancer. *Clin. Cancer Res.*, Vol. 7, No. 2, pp. 429-434, ISSN 1078-0432

Kundu, J.K. & Surh, Y.J. (2008). Inflammation: gearing the journey to cancer. *Mutat. Res.*, Vol. 659, No. 1-2, pp. 15-30, ISSN 0027-5107

Lee, S., Kim, J.H., Kim, H., Kang, J.W., Kim, S.H., Yang, Y., Kim, J., Park, J., Park, S., Hong, J. & Yoon, D.Y. (2011). Activation of the interleukin-32 pro-inflammatory pathway in response to human papillomavirus infection and over-expression of interleukin-32 controls the expression of the human papillomavirus oncogene. *Immunology*, Vol. 132, No. 3, pp. 410-420, ISSN 0019-2805

Lo, H.W., Hsu, S.C., Ali-Seyed, M., Gunduz, M., Xia, W., Wei, Y., Bartholomeusz, G., Shih, J.Y. & Hung, M.C. (2005). Nuclear interaction of EGFR and STAT3 in the activation of the iNOS/NO pathway. *Cancer Cell*, Vol. 7, No. 6, pp. 575-589, ISSN 1535-6108

Loeb, L.A. & Preston, B.D. (1986). Mutagenesis by apurinic/apyrimidinic sites. *Annu. Rev. Genet.*, Vol. 20, pp. 201-230, ISSN 0066-4197

Ma, N., Adachi, Y., Hiraku, Y., Horiki, N., Horiike, S., Imoto, I., Pinlaor, S., Murata, M., Semba, R. & Kawanishi, S. (2004). Accumulation of 8-nitroguanine in human gastric epithelium induced by *Helicobacter pylori* infection. *Biochem. Biophys. Res. Commun.*, Vol. 319, No. 2, pp. 506-510, ISSN 0006-291X

Ma, N., Tagawa, T., Hiraku, Y., Murata, M., Ding, X. & Kawanishi, S. (2006). 8-Nitroguanine formation in oral leukoplakia, a premalignant lesion. *Nitric Oxide*, Vol. 14, No. 2, pp. 137-143, ISSN 1089-8603

Ma, N., Kawanishi, M., Hiraku, Y., Murata, M., Huang, G.W., Huang, Y., Luo, D.Z., Mo, W.G., Fukui, Y. & Kawanishi, S. (2008). Reactive nitrogen species-dependent DNA damage in EBV-associated nasopharyngeal carcinoma: The relation to STAT3 activation and EGFR expression. *Int. J. Cancer*, Vol. 122, No. 11, pp. 2517-2525, ISSN 1097-0215

Mateo, J., Garcia-Lecea, M., Cadenas, S., Hernandez, C. & Moncada, S. (2003). Regulation of hypoxia-inducible factor-1α by nitric oxide through mitochondria-dependent and -independent pathways. *Biochem. J.*, Vol. 376(Pt 2), pp. 537-544, ISSN 1470-8728

Mishima, T., Tajima, Y., Kuroki, T., Kosaka, T., Adachi, T., Kitasato, A., Tsuneoka, N., Kitajima, T. & Kanematsu, T. (2009). Chemopreventative effect of an inducible nitric oxide synthase inhibitor, ONO-1714, on inflammation-associated biliary carcinogenesis in hamsters. *Carcinogenesis*, Vol. 30, No. 10, pp. 1763-1767, ISSN 0143-3334

Munoz, N., Bosch, F.X., de Sanjose, S., Herrero, R., Castellsague, X., Shah, K.V., Snijders, P.J. & Meijer, C.J. (2003). Epidemiologic classification of human papillomavirus types associated with cervical cancer. *N. Engl. J. Med.*, Vol. 348, No. 6, pp. 518-527, ISSN 1533-4406

Nair, A., Venkatraman, M., Maliekal, T.T., Nair, B. & Karunagaran, D. (2003). NF-κB is constitutively activated in high-grade squamous intraepithelial lesions and squamous cell carcinomas of the human uterine cervix. *Oncogene*, Vol. 22, No. 1, pp. 50-58, ISSN 0950-9232

Nair, J., Gansauge, F., Beger, H., Dolara, P., Winde, G. & Bartsch, H. (2006). Increased etheno-DNA adducts in affected tissues of patients suffering from Crohn's disease, ulcerative colitis, and chronic pancreatitis. *Antioxid. Redox Signal.*, Vol. 8, No. 5-6, pp. 1003-1010, ISSN 1523-0864

Ohshima, H., Tatemichi, M. & Sawa, T. (2003). Chemical basis of inflammation-induced carcinogenesis. *Arch. Biochem. Biophys.*, Vol. 417, No. 1, pp. 3-11, ISSN 0003-9861

Pikarsky, E., Porat, R.M., Stein, I., Abramovitch, R., Amit, S., Kasem, S., Gutkovich-Pyest, E., Urieli-Shoval, S., Galun, E. & Ben-Neriah, Y. (2004). NF-κB functions as a tumour promoter in inflammation-associated cancer. *Nature*, Vol. 431, No. 7007, pp. 461-466, ISSN 1476-4687

Pinlaor, S., Yongvanit, P., Hiraku, Y., Ma, N., Semba, R., Oikawa, S., Murata, M., Sripa, B., Sithithaworn, P. & Kawanishi, S. (2003). 8-Nitroguanine formation in the liver of hamsters infected with *Opisthorchis viverrini*. *Biochem. Biophys. Res. Commun.*, Vol. 309, No. 3, pp. 567-571, ISSN 0006-291X

Pinlaor, S., Hiraku, Y., Ma, N., Yongvanit, P., Semba, R., Oikawa, S., Murata, M., Sripa, B., Sithithaworn, P. & Kawanishi, S. (2004a). Mechanism of NO-mediated oxidative and nitrative DNA damage in hamsters infected with *Opisthorchis viverrini*: a model of inflammation-mediated carcinogenesis. *Nitric Oxide*, Vol. 11, No. 2, pp. 175-183, ISSN 1089-8603

Pinlaor, S., Ma, N., Hiraku, Y., Yongvanit, P., Semba, R., Oikawa, S., Murata, M., Sripa, B., Sithithaworn, P. & Kawanishi, S. (2004b). Repeated infection with *Opisthorchis viverrini* induces accumulation of 8-nitroguanine and 8-oxo-7,8-dihydro-2'-deoxyguanine in the bile duct of hamsters via inducible nitric oxide synthase. *Carcinogenesis*, Vol. 25, No. 8, pp. 1535-1542, ISSN 0143-3334

Pinlaor, S., Sripa, B., Ma, N., Hiraku, Y., Yongvanit, P., Wongkham, S., Pairojkul, C., Bhudhisawasdi, V., Oikawa, S., Murata, M., Semba, R. & Kawanishi, S. (2005). Nitrative and oxidative DNA damage in intrahepatic cholangiocarcinoma patients in relation to tumor invasion. *World J. Gastroenterol.*, Vol. 11, No. 30, pp. 4644-4649, ISSN 1007-9327

Pinlaor, S., Hiraku, Y., Yongvanit, P., Tada-Oikawa, S., Ma, N., Pinlaor, P., Sithithaworn, P., Sripa, B., Murata, M., Oikawa, S. & Kawanishi, S. (2006). iNOS-dependent DNA damage via NF-κB expression in hamsters infected with *Opisthorchis viverrini* and its suppression by the antihelminthic drug praziquantel. *Int. J. Cancer*, Vol. 119, No. 5, pp. 1067-1072, ISSN 0020-7136

Prakobwong, S., Khoontawad, J., Yongvanit, P., Pairojkul, C., Hiraku, Y., Sithithaworn, P., Pinlaor, P., Aggarwal, B.B. & Pinlaor, S. (2011). Curcumin decreases cholangiocarcinogenesis in hamsters by suppressing inflammation-mediated molecular events related to multistep carcinogenesis. *Int. J. Cancer*, Vol. 129, No. 1, pp. 88-100, ISSN 0020-7136

Rius, J., Guma, M., Schachtrup, C., Akassoglou, K., Zinkernagel, A.S., Nizet, V., Johnson, R.S., Haddad, G.G. & Karin, M. (2008). NF-κB links innate immunity to the hypoxic response through transcriptional regulation of HIF-1α. *Nature*, Vol. 453, No. 7196, pp. 807-811, ISSN 1476-4687

Roeters, A.M., Boon, M.E., van Haaften, M., Vernooij, F., Bontekoe, T.R. & Heintz, A.P. (2010). Inflammatory events as detected in cervical smears and squamous intraepithelial lesions. *Diagn. Cytopathol.*, Vol. 38, No. 2, pp. 85-93, ISSN 1097-0339

Romano, G., Sgambato, A., Mancini, R., Capelli, G., Giovagnoli, M.R., Flamini, G., Boninsegna, A., Vecchione, A. & Cittadini, A. (2000). 8-Hydroxy-2'-deoxyguanosine in cervical cells: correlation with grade of dysplasia and human papillomavirus infection. *Carcinogenesis*, Vol. 21, No. 6, pp. 1143-1147, ISSN 0143-3334

Sano, T., Oyama, T., Kashiwabara, K., Fukuda, T. & Nakajima, T. (1998). Expression status of p16 protein is associated with human papillomavirus oncogenic potential in cervical and genital lesions. *Am. J. Pathol.*, Vol. 153, No. 6, pp. 1741-1748, ISSN 0002-9440

Sawa, T., Tatemichi, M., Akaike, T., Barbin, A. & Ohshima, H. (2006). Analysis of urinary 8-nitroguanine, a marker of nitrative nucleic acid damage, by high-performance liquid chromatography-electrochemical detection coupled with immunoaffinity purification: Association with cigarette smoking. *Free Radic. Biol. Med.*, Vol. 40, No. 4, pp. 711-720, ISSN 0891-5849

Sawa, T., Zaki, M.H., Okamoto, T., Akuta, T., Tokutomi, Y., Kim-Mitsuyama, S., Ihara, H., Kobayashi, A., Yamamoto, M., Fujii, S., Arimoto, H. & Akaike, T. (2007). Protein *S*-guanylation by the biological signal 8-nitroguanosine 3',5'-cyclic monophosphate. *Nat. Chem. Biol.*, Vol. 3, No. 11, pp. 727-735, ISSN 1552-4450

Schroer, N., Pahne, J., Walch, B., Wickenhauser, C. & Smola, S. (2011). Molecular pathobiology of human cervical high-grade lesions: paracrine STAT3 activation in tumor-instructed myeloid cells drives local MMP-9 expression. *Cancer Res.*, Vol. 71, No. 1, pp. 87-97, ISSN 0008-5472

Shibutani, S., Takeshita, M. & Grollman, A.P. (1991). Insertion of specific bases during DNA synthesis past the oxidation-damaged base 8-oxodG. *Nature*, Vol. 349, No. 6308, pp. 431-434, ISSN 0028-0836

Sisk, E.A. & Robertson, E.S. (2002). Clinical implications of human papillomavirus infection. *Front. Biosci.*, Vol. 7, pp. e77-84, ISSN 1093-4715

Smith, J.S., Herrero, R., Bosetti, C., Munoz, N., Bosch, F.X., Eluf-Neto, J., Castellsague, X., Meijer, C.J., Van den Brule, A.J., Franceschi, S. & Ashley, R. (2002a). Herpes simplex virus-2 as a human papillomavirus cofactor in the etiology of invasive cervical cancer. *J. Natl. Cancer Inst.*, Vol. 94, No. 21, pp. 1604-1613, ISSN 0027-8874

Smith, J.S., Munoz, N., Herrero, R., Eluf-Neto, J., Ngelangel, C., Franceschi, S., Bosch, F.X., Walboomers, J.M. & Peeling, R.W. (2002b). Evidence for *Chlamydia trachomatis* as a human papillomavirus cofactor in the etiology of invasive cervical cancer in Brazil and the Philippines. *J. Infect. Dis.*, Vol. 185, No. 3, pp. 324-331, ISSN 0022-1899

Song, S., Gulliver, G.A. & Lambert, P.F. (1998). Human papillomavirus type 16 *E6* and *E7* oncogenes abrogate radiation-induced DNA damage responses in vivo through p53-dependent and p53-independent pathways. *Proc. Natl. Acad. Sci. USA*, Vol. 95, No. 5, pp. 2290-2295, ISSN 0027-8424

Suzuki, N., Yasui, M., Geacintov, N.E., Shafirovich, V. & Shibutani, S. (2005). Miscoding events during DNA synthesis past the nitration-damaged base 8-nitroguanine. *Biochemistry*, Vol. 44, No. 25, pp. 9238-9245, ISSN 0006-2960

Tagesson, C., Kallberg, M., Klintenberg, C. & Starkhammar, H. (1995). Determination of urinary 8-hydroxydeoxyguanosine by automated coupled-column high performance liquid chromatography: a powerful technique for assaying in vivo oxidative DNA damage in cancer patients. *Eur. J. Cancer*, Vol. 31A, No. 6, pp. 934-940, ISSN 0959-8049

Takahashi, T., Nau, M.M., Chiba, I., Birrer, M.J., Rosenberg, R.K., Vinocour, M., Levitt, M., Pass, H., Gazdar, A.F. & Minna, J.D. (1989). p53: a frequent target for genetic abnormalities in lung cancer. *Science*, Vol. 246, No. 4929, pp. 491-494, ISSN 0036-8075

Tazawa, H., Okada, F., Kobayashi, T., Tada, M., Mori, Y., Une, Y., Sendo, F., Kobayashi, M. & Hosokawa, M. (2003). Infiltration of neutrophils is required for acquisition of metastatic phenotype of benign murine fibrosarcoma cells: implication of inflammation-associated carcinogenesis and tumor progression. *Am. J. Pathol.*, Vol. 163, No. 6, pp. 2221-2232, ISSN 0002-9440

Tedeschi, E., Menegazzi, M., Margotto, D., Suzuki, H., Forstermann, U. & Kleinert, H. (2003). Anti-inflammatory actions of St. John's wort: inhibition of human inducible nitric-oxide synthase expression by down-regulating signal transducer and activator of transcription-1α (STAT-1α) activation. *J. Pharmacol. Exp. Ther.*, Vol. 307, No. 1, pp. 254-261, ISSN 0022-3565

Thanan, R., Murata, M., Pinlaor, S., Sithithaworn, P., Khuntikeo, N., Tangkanakul, W., Hiraku, Y., Oikawa, S., Yongvanit, P. & Kawanishi, S. (2008). Urinary 8-oxo-7,8-dihydro-2'-deoxyguanosine in patients with parasite infection and effect of antiparasitic drug in relation to cholangiocarcinogenesis. *Cancer Epidemiol. Biomarkers Prev.*, Vol. 17, No. 3, pp. 518-524, ISSN 1055-9965

Thomas, D.D., Espey, M.G., Ridnour, L.A., Hofseth, L.J., Mancardi, D., Harris, C.C. & Wink, D.A. (2004). Hypoxic inducible factor 1α, extracellular signal-regulated kinase, and p53 are regulated by distinct threshold concentrations of nitric oxide. *Proc. Natl. Acad. Sci. USA*, Vol. 101, No. 24, pp. 8894-8899, ISSN 0027-8424

Tindle, R.W. (2002). Immune evasion in human papillomavirus-associated cervical cancer. *Nat. Rev. Cancer*, Vol. 2, No. 1, pp. 59-65, ISSN 1474-175X

Unfried, K., Schurkes, C. & Abel, J. (2002). Distinct spectrum of mutations induced by crocidolite asbestos: clue for 8-hydroxydeoxyguanosine-dependent mutagenesis *in vivo*. *Cancer Res.*, Vol. 62, No. 1, pp. 99-104, ISSN 0008-5472

von Knebel Doeberitz, M. (2002). New markers for cervical dysplasia to visualise the genomic chaos created by aberrant oncogenic papillomavirus infections. *Eur. J. Cancer*, Vol. 38, No. 17, pp. 2229-2242, ISSN 0959-8049

Walmsley, S.R., Print, C., Farahi, N., Peyssonnaux, C., Johnson, R.S., Cramer, T., Sobolewski, A., Condliffe, A.M., Cowburn, A.S., Johnson, N. & Chilvers, E.R. (2005). Hypoxia-induced neutrophil survival is mediated by HIF-1α-dependent NF-κB activity. *J. Exp. Med.*, Vol. 201, No. 1, pp. 105-115, ISSN 0022-1007

Wang, H., Li, Y., Liu, H., Liu, S., Liu, Q., Wang, X.M., Shi, Y. & Duan, H. (2009). Peroxynitrite mediates glomerular lesion of diabetic rat via JAK/STAT signaling pathway. *J. Endocrinol. Invest.*, Vol. 32, No. 10, pp. 844-851, ISSN 0391-4097

Wang, J.L., Zheng, B.Y., Li, X.D., Angstrom, T., Lindstrom, M.S. & Wallin, K.L. (2004). Predictive significance of the alterations of p16INK4A, p14ARF, p53, and proliferating cell nuclear antigen expression in the progression of cervical cancer. *Clin. Cancer Res.*, Vol. 10, No. 7, pp. 2407-2414, ISSN 1078-0432

Warner, T.D. & Mitchell, J.A. (2004). Cyclooxygenases: new forms, new inhibitors, and lessons from the clinic. *FASEB J.*, Vol. 18, No. 7, pp. 790-804, ISSN 1530-6860

Wei, L., Gravitt, P.E., Song, H., Maldonado, A.M. & Ozbun, M.A. (2009). Nitric oxide induces early viral transcription coincident with increased DNA damage and mutation rates in human papillomavirus-infected cells. *Cancer Res.*, Vol. 69, No. 11, pp. 4878-4884, ISSN 0008-5472

Williams, C.S., Tsujii, M., Reese, J., Dey, S.K. & DuBois, R.N. (2000). Host cyclooxygenase-2 modulates carcinoma growth. *J. Clin. Invest.*, Vol. 105, No. 11, pp. 1589-1594, ISSN 0021-9738

Wiseman, H. & Halliwell, B. (1996). Damage to DNA by reactive oxygen and nitrogen species: role in inflammatory disease and progression to cancer. *Biochem. J.*, Vol. 313 (Pt 1), pp. 17-29, ISSN 0264-6021

Wu, X., Takenaka, K., Sonoda, E., Hochegger, H., Kawanishi, S., Kawamoto, T., Takeda, S. & Yamazoe, M. (2006). Critical roles for polymerase ζ in cellular tolerance to nitric oxide-induced DNA damage. *Cancer Res.*, Vol. 66, No. 2, pp. 748-754, ISSN 0008-5472

Xu, M., Luo, W., Elzi, D.J., Grandori, C. & Galloway, D.A. (2008). NFX1 interacts with mSin3A/histone deacetylase to repress hTERT transcription in keratinocytes. *Mol. Cell Biol.*, Vol. 28, No. 15, pp. 4819-4828, ISSN 0270-7306

Yermilov, V., Rubio, J., Becchi, M., Friesen, M.D., Pignatelli, B. & Ohshima, H. (1995a). Formation of 8-nitroguanine by the reaction of guanine with peroxynitrite *in vitro*. *Carcinogenesis*, Vol. 16, No. 9, pp. 2045-2050, ISSN 0143-3334

Yermilov, V., Rubio, J. & Ohshima, H. (1995b). Formation of 8-nitroguanine in DNA treated with peroxynitrite in vitro and its rapid removal from DNA by depurination. *FEBS Lett.*, Vol. 376, No. 3, pp. 207-210, ISSN 0014-5793

Yugawa, T. & Kiyono, T. (2009). Molecular mechanisms of cervical carcinogenesis by high-risk human papillomaviruses: novel functions of E6 and E7 oncoproteins. *Rev. Med. Virol.*, Vol. 19, No. 2, pp. 97-113, ISSN 1052-9276

16

HPVTyper: A Software Application for Automatic HPV Typing via PCR-RFLP Gel Electrophoresis

Christos Maramis, Dimitrios Karagiannis and Anastasios Delopoulos
Dept. Electrical & Computer Engineering, Aristotle University of Thessaloniki
Greece

1. Introduction

The human papillomavirus (HPV) has been proved to be a many-sided virus. Up to date, over 200 types of HPV have been reported, while ongoing research studies constantly discover new types of the virus. Recently, certain HPV types have been associated with the development of several cancer types (Parkin, 2006), including anal, vaginal, penile, oral, and pharyngeal cancer.

The cervical cancer is currently the most prominent case of association between HPV and cancer. The persistent infection of the anogenital tract by a group of HPV types has been proved to be the main causal factor of cervical cancer (Bosch et al., 2002; Walboomers et al., 1999). This group of cervical cancer related types currently includes 30 to 40 types. However, not all the types in the group induce the same risk for the development of cervical cancer. In fact, virologists have classified the aforementioned types with respect to their oncogenic activity as low-risk, high-risk, and potentially high-risk (Muñoz et al., 2003), while other HPV types remain unclassified.

Focusing on the case of cervical cancer, the statistics are overwhelming: With 500.000 cases diagnosed every year (Greenblatt, 2005), it is the second leading cause of cancer related deaths after breast cancer for women between 20 and 39 years old (Landis et al., 1999) and one of the leading cancer types affecting women worldwide (Moore, 2006). When the above facts are combined with the variability of oncogenic activity among HPV types, the need for specifying not only whether a patient has been infected by HPV but also the exact infecting types becomes evident. The task of identifying the specific HPV type(s) that have infected a patient based on their genotypic characteristics is called *HPV genotyping* or – more simply – *HPV typing*.

In the domain of cervical cancer, HPV typing provides valuable and sometimes critical information to the practitioner of a female patient with respect to her risk for developing cervical cancer. However, it should be noted that as soon as the relation of HPV with other cancer types becomes fully understood, it is highly probable that HPV typing will acquire similar importance in those cancer domains as well. Moreover, HPV typing is also performed for epidemiological purposes, i.e., to determine the frequency and type distribution of the virus in various populations.

The need for HPV typing has given birth to a variety of molecular biology methods and associated assays/kits for carrying out this task. The main objectives that are important when comparing these diagnostic tools are (i) the diagnosis accuracy, (ii) the diagnosis cost, and (iii) the automation level of the diagnostic procedure. Although many solutions are currently available – they will be briefly described in the following section – none stands out when compared to its counterparts. In this chapter, we will present a novel diagnostic tool for HPV typing that attempts to optimize all the aforementioned objectives. This tool is HPVTyper, a freely-available software application that processes images resulting from the PCR-RFLP examination of tissue samples (see Section 2.1) and automatically infers the HPV type(s) that have infected the samples. The novel HPV typing methodology that is employed by HPVTyper has been introduced and extensively validated in a series of recent publications.

2. HPV typing methods

As we have already mentioned, owing to the significance of the task, plenty of molecular diagnostic methods for HPV typing have emerged during the last decades. The majority of them is based on detecting type-specific DNA in an investigated tissue sample (DNA testing methods). The most prominent DNA testing methods are outlined in Section 2.1. The method that is employed by HPVTyper is described separately in Section 2.2.

2.1 Methods overview

Four categories of HPV typing methods are presented in this section. For each category, we provide a short description of the corresponding generic method and comment on its advantages/drawbacks with respect to the other categories.

PCR-based assays. The methods of this category employ the polymerase chain reaction (PCR) to amplify a specific part of the viral DNA. Typing is achieved through the use of type-specific pairs of primers that bound the DNA region to be amplified. Gel electrophoresis of the PCR products is employed to visualize the typing results. The PCR-based methods have been among the first HPV typing methods to be employed and, consequently, many applications of them have been reported (Fontaine et al., 2007; Husnjak et al., 2000; Karlsen et al., 1996; Walboomers et al., 1999).

The main drawback of these methods is the need of a different pair of primers for each type that is considered in the typing process, which, of course, increases the cost of the diagnosis. Moreover, in the case of newly-discovered types appropriate sets of primers have to be designed *de novo*.

Hybridization assays. These methods are based on the hybridization of oligonucleotide probes, where each probe is associated with a specific type of the virus. There are several variants of the hybridization method, namely dot blot (Greer Jr et al., 1990), reverse line blot (Kleter et al., 1999; van den Brule et al., 2002), enzyme immunoassay (Jacobs et al., 1997), etc. These methods employ PCR with general primers in their first stages and their results can be read directly from the assay.

The hybridization methods are less laborious than the PCR-based ones, since they do not require the application of multiple PCRs. However, the previously discussed drawback of the PCR-based methods applies here as well: A different oligonucleotide must be produced – and possibly designed – for each HPV type that needs to be identified.

DNA microarrays. This category of methods shares its conception principle with the hybridization assays (i.e., typing is performed through type-specific oligonucleotide probes) but additionally employs the microarray technology. More specifically, the oligonucleotide probes are "printed" on a two-dimensional array structure and the outcome is usually digitized with the help of a microarray scanner.

The DNA microarray assays have been proved to be very popular during the last decade (Gheit et al., 2006; Hwang et al., 2003; Kim et al., 2003; Klaassen et al., 2004) owing to their accuracy and ease of use. However, being mostly industrial products, the set of HPV types that can be typed by a particular microarray is hardwired into the assay and the expansion to new types necessitates redesigning the assay. Moreover, their consumable nature imposes an additional component to their diagnosis cost.

DNA sequencing. This method discriminates among the HPV types by discovering the exact nucleotide sequence of a small region in the viral DNA. This is the golden standard of virus typing in terms of accuracy since it is able to reveal the viral DNA information to its fullest extent. Since the establishment of the method, several DNA sequencing techniques have been applied on the task of HPV typing (Barzon et al., 2011; Gharizadeh et al., 2001; 2005; Vernon et al., 2000).

The early DNA sequencing techniques have been characterized by low throughput (leading to expensive typing examinations) and could be easily confused in the case of multiple infections. However, the recent introduction of massively parallel sequencing assays (next-generation sequencing) has shown promise to minimize the examination cost and revolutionize DNA sequencing as an HPV typing method (Jordan, 2010; Liu, 2008).

2.2 PCR-RFLP gel electrophoresis

The method of interest for this chapter, i.e., the method that is employed by HPVTyper, is called *PCR-RFLP gel electrophoresis*. The standard protocol for performing HPV typing via the aforementioned method is described in detail in the present section. The protocol involves a series of operations that process the examined tissue sample by means of several established molecular biology techniques and a final step that requires the expertise of a molecular biologist. The involved steps are outlined in Fig. 1(a).

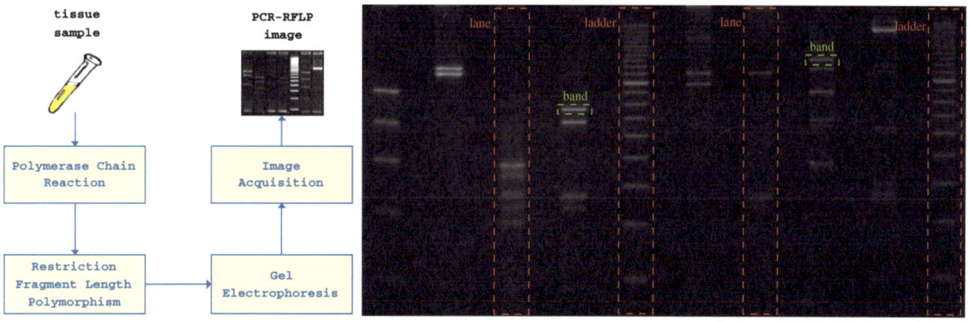

(a) (b)

Fig. 1. HPV typing via PCR-RFLP gel electrophoresis. (a) The steps involved in the standard HPV typing protocol. (b) The outcome of a typical PCR-RFLP gel electrophoresis examination; samples of lanes, bands and ladders are enclosed in rectangles.

First, an organic sample is collected from the tissue of interest and the contained DNA is isolated. Then, the PCR (Tagu & Moussard, 2006, Ch. 24) amplifies a highly preserved region of the hypothesized[1] viral DNA with the help of a general-purpose primer set. After that, a restriction enzyme cleaves the amplified HPV DNA at sites that are characterized by a specific nucleotide sequence (restriction sites). This procedure, which is called restriction fragment length polymorphism (RFLP) analysis (Tagu & Moussard, 2006, Ch. 50), produces for each HPV genotype a set of DNA fragments that is known *a priori*; the RFLP analysis is the cornerstone of the discussed method.

Let us elaborate on this. If we assume that the amplified DNA sequence of an HPV genotype of interest is known, then we can predict the sites that will be cleaved by a specific restriction enzyme and, thus, we can infer the set of DNA fragments that are produced after digestion by this restriction enzyme. This set of DNA fragments or *fragment length pattern* (FLP) serves as the signature of this particular HPV genotype and is the means for successfully carrying out the HPV typing.

Following the RFLP analysis, a solution of the digested PCR product is being injected into an individual well at the front end of a gel matrix. Then, in the presence of an electric field, the negatively-charged DNA fragments are forced to move with different mobilities (i.e., drift velocities) towards the anode in the direction opposite to that of the electric field. During the gel electrophoresis (Tagu & Moussard, 2006, Ch. 5), the large molecules remain close to the well, while the more agile smaller molecules cover a much larger distance. This way, one *lane* starting from each well is formed; each lane contains concentrations of DNA of the same length that are shaped as *bands* perpendicular to the electric field direction. One or more among the wells of a gel matrix are reserved to include *DNA ladders*, i.e., DNA molecules of known lengths. These reference ladders assist the biologists in estimating the unknown length of the DNA that forms the bands of the other lanes during the last step of the protocol.

After the electrophoresis is completed, the viral DNA molecules are stained by soaking the gel in a solution of a certain fluorescent dye. For this purpose one can employ either the highly mutagenic yet still common ethidium bromide or, preferably, some other less hazardous fluorescent substance (SYBR Safe, DAPI, etc). Then, an appropriate light source (usually ultra violet or blue) is used momentarily to excite the dye, which fluoresces to make the viral DNA visible. At that moment, a digitized image of the gel matrix is acquired (see Fig.1(b) for an example).

In the final step, the acquired image is analyzed by a molecular biologist in order to reach a typing decision. This analysis includes two stages. First, the biologist estimates the DNA fragment lengths corresponding to the bands that are observed on a lane of interest; this is achieved by interpolating the bands of the image's ladder(s). Then, the biologist "manually" compares the set of estimated fragment lengths from the investigated lane with the FLPs of all the considered HPV genotypes in order to decide which genotype or combination of genotypes has produced the observed band pattern.

From the previous description, one can realize that HPV typing via PCR-RFLP gel electrophoresis suffers from several shortcomings. First of all, it falls short with respect to the other methods in terms of accuracy, since it does not employ type-specific probes or primers. Moreover, it might require a considerable amount of intellectual effort by the molecular biologist to come to a typing conclusion, while typing by the other methods is

[1] We use the word *hypothesized* because the sample can be HPV-free.

essentially straightforward. Finally, the typing procedure becomes even more complicated and error-prone in cases of multiple infections.

Despite the aforementioned shortcomings, PCR-RFLP gel electrophoresis has been used extensively over the past two decades as a method for HPV typing (Lungu et al., 1992; Nobre et al., 2008; Santiago et al., 2006) and remains today the method of choice for a significant percentage of molecular biology laboratories worldwide. This is because the method also demonstrates a series of noteworthy advantages over its counterparts. It does not require the use of overspecialized devices, expensive consumables and type-specific agents. This way it is relatively inexpensive and can be carried out in every moderately equipped molecular biology laboratory. Moreover, owing to its lack of attachment to type-specific entities, the method can easily be exploited for identifying new HPV types, possibly without even the need to repeat the *in vitro* examination of the sample.

3. The employed HPV typing methodology

HPVTyper builds upon a novel HPV typing methodology (Maramis et al., 2010; 2011), which tackles the main shortcomings of typing via the PCR-RFLP method. This methodology is capable of producing very accurate typing decisions – even in complex cases of multiple infections – in an entirely automatic manner. The methodology's performance has been extensively evaluated through a series of experiments (Maramis et al., 2011) on a well-sized set of real HPV data [2].

The discussed methodology is founded on a novel observation model that describes formally the mechanism by which a set of molecular biology parameters (e.g., the concentrations of several HPV genotypes) generates the observed outcome of a PCR-RFLP gel electrophoresis examination (i.e., an image similar to the one depicted in Fig. 1(b)). The observation model is presented in Section 3.1.

Once the observation model has been established, we proceed with describing the employed methodology. This involves three phases, which are outlined in Fig. 2. In the first phase, the acquired image is preprocessed (Section 3.2). This is a necessary condition for the successful exploitation of the observation model. Then, based on the observation model, accurate information regarding the viral DNA fragments that have resulted from the RFLP analysis is automatically extracted (Section 3.3). The extracted fragment information is fed to a novel HPV typing algorithm (Section 3.4) that identifies – entirely automatically – those HPV genotype(s) that are most probable to have infected the examined sample.

3.1 Observation model

The introduced observation model consists of a set of formulas which associate the visual outcome of a PCR-RFLP gel electrophoresis examination with the underlying parameters of the HPV genotype(s) that have infected the examined sample. In other words, it describes with quantitative terms the mechanism by which the image of such an examination is generated from the infecting HPV genotypes.

In order to present the observation model, let us imagine the following situation: The sample that we are examining has been infected by type T of HPV. After the application of PCR, the

[2] The employed dataset can be accessed via the internet at `http://olympus.ee.auth.gr/~chmaramis/virusTyping`.

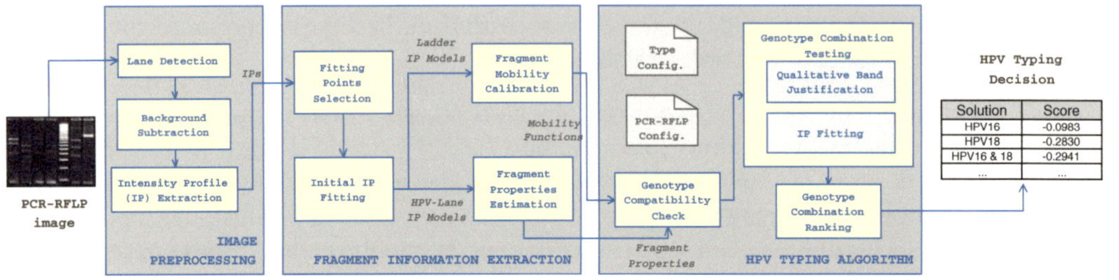

Fig. 2. Outline of the employed HPV typing methodology. The main operations are presented as blocks and the operation sequence is indicated by arrows.

concentration of T in the PCR product is c_T. The digestion of the amplified DNA sequence of T by the employed restriction enzyme yields K DNA fragments, whose lengths in base pairs (bp) are contained in the FLP $\boldsymbol{l} = [l_1, l_2, \ldots, l_K]$. At the end of gel electrophoresis, the digested DNA fragments have formed K bands on the sample's lane – this might look like Fig. 3(a) assuming that $K = 4$.

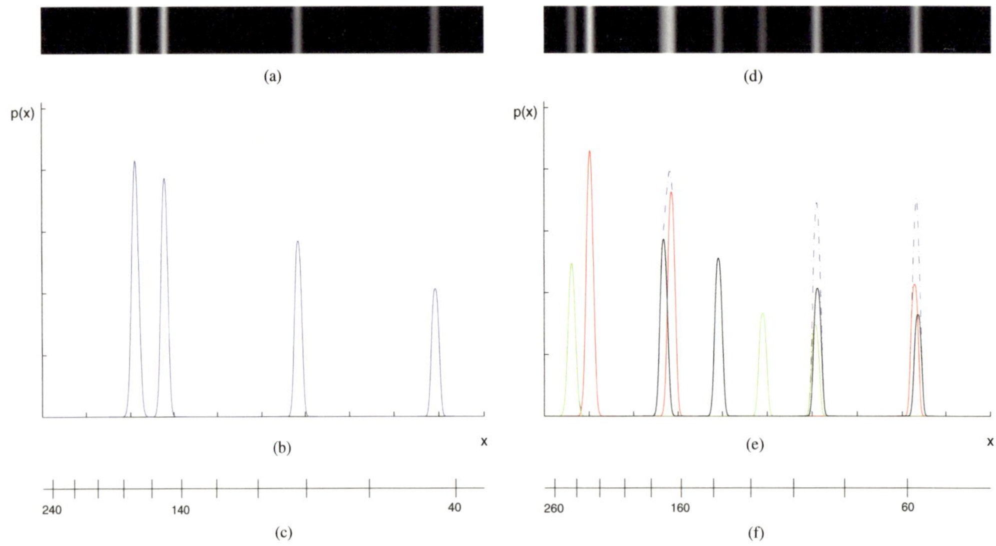

Fig. 3. Illustration of the employed observation model via two examples. (a) Lane image with 4 bands. This corresponds to a sample infected by HPV 53 (GenBank ID X7448) after amplification by MY09/11 (primers) and digestion by HpyCH4V (restriction enzyme). (b) The intensity profile that is extracted from the above lane. The depicted peaks correspond to fragment lengths 171, 151, 83, and 44 bp (left to right). (c) The 20-bp marker that depicts the position-length relation for the above image/profile. (d) Lane image involving triple HPV infection. This corresponds to a sample infected by HPV 30, 62, and 72 (GenBank IDs X74474, AY395706, and X94164) after amplification by MY09/11 and digestion by HpyCH4V. (e) The intensity profile that is extracted from the above lane (blue/dash-dotted line). The contributions of the three infecting types are also displayed with various colors/grayscale levels. (f) The 20-bp marker that depicts the position-length relation for the above image/profile.

Due to the one-dimensional nature of the involved electrophoresis procedure, the information that is conveyed by a lane image lies exclusively in the electrophoresis direction (the X axis in Fig. 3(b)). This means that any two horizontal slices of the lane image are practically replicas of each other. Thus, instead of dealing with the entire lane image, we might as well take a single horizontal slice of it. The resulting one-dimensional intensity curve is called *intensity profile* and is depicted in Fig. 3(b). The intensity profile consists of K bell-shaped peaks, whose centers on axis X are aligned with the positions of the band middles in the lane image.

For a given gel electrophoresis configuration (i.e., fixed gel viscosity, electrophoresis voltage, etc.) the distance that has been covered at the end of the experiment by a certain DNA fragment, and consequently its position, x, on axis X depends only on the length, l, of the fragment. In the described observation model this position-length relation is provided by the following *fragment mobility function*:

$$x = d(l; \boldsymbol{\pi}) = \pi_1 + \pi_2 \log(\pi_3 + \pi_4 l + l^2), \tag{1}$$

where the vector $\boldsymbol{\pi} = [\pi_1, \pi_2, \pi_3, \pi_4]$ aggregates the parameters of the fragment mobility function.

If we assume that $\boldsymbol{\pi}$ is known and recall that the ith peak in the intensity profile of Fig. 3(b) is formed by DNA fragments of length l_i, we conclude that the observed peak centers, $x_1, x_2, \ldots, x_K$, are given by the expression

$$x_i = d(l_i; \boldsymbol{\pi}) \quad i = 1, 2, \ldots, K. \tag{2}$$

Moreover, it has been observed that, during gel electrophoresis, a moving population consisting of DNA fragments of some length tends to constantly lose some of its members, i.e., its concentration attenuates continuously as the population moves. This phenomenon is taken into account by the described observation model by means of the residual function

$$r(x) = \phi x + 1 \quad x \in [0, E]. \tag{3}$$

This function expresses the percentage of DNA fragments that have not abandoned the moving population when its mean position is x.

In our example we have assumed that the concentration of the PCR product of T is c_T. The PCR product is digested to form K DNA fragment populations that correspond to lengths $l_1, l_2, \ldots, l_K$ and are concentrated in the lane's well before the beginning of the electrophoresis. Thus, the concentrations of these populations at the well will also be:

$$\underbrace{c_T, c_T, \ldots, c_T}_{K} .$$

However, due to the aforementioned concentration attenuation, at the end of the electrophoresis, the fragment populations that form the peaks of the intensity profile in Fig. 3(b) will have the following reduced concentrations:

$$\underbrace{r(x_1)c_T, r(x_2)c_T, \ldots, r(x_K)c_T}_{K} .$$

The image intensity that is produced by a DNA molecule is determined by the number of fluorescent molecules that are bound to it. Since this number is proportional to the fragment length, the employed observation model computes the contribution of each of the aforementioned K fragment populations to the intensity of the profile as follows:

$$\underbrace{f \cdot l_1 r(x_1) c_T, f \cdot l_2 r(x_2) c_T, \ldots, f \cdot l_K r(x_K) c_T}_{K},$$

where f denotes the contribution of a single-bp DNA fragment to the profile intensity.

Regarding the peak shape, it has been proved (Maramis & Delopoulos, 2010b) that any intensity profile peak corresponding to fragments of length l_0 can be accurately modeled by the integrated Weibull function,

$$w(x;\beta,\gamma,x_0) = \frac{\gamma}{2\gamma^{1/\gamma}\beta\Gamma(1/\gamma)} \exp\Big(-\frac{1}{\gamma}\big|\frac{x-x_0}{\beta}\big|^{\gamma}\Big), \tag{4}$$

where (i) $\Gamma(\cdot)$ is the complete gamma function, (ii) the parameters β and γ determine the peak shape, and (iii) x_0 is the mean distance covered by the fragments of length l_0, i.e., $x_0 = d(l_0;\boldsymbol{\pi})$.

Finally, the described observation model superimposes K integrated Weibull functions to model the entire intensity profile of the investigated lane as follows:

$$i(x) = f \cdot c_T \sum_{i=1}^{K} l_i \cdot r(x_i) \cdot w\big(x;\beta_i,\gamma_i,x_i)\big), \tag{5}$$

where $i(\cdot)$ denotes the intensity profile model. In order to derive (5) we have taken into account the previously computed contributions of the DNA fragment populations to the profile intensity.

3.2 Image preprocessing

The first phase of the employed HPV typing methodology deals with the preprocessing of the acquired PCR-RFLP image in order to extract the intensity profiles of all the depicted lanes. The processing operations of this phase presume that the image at hand passes certain quality checks (see Fig. 1(b) for a positive example):

1. The image depicts the lane areas exclusively.
2. The bands appear bright on darker background.
3. The vertical axis of the image identifies with the electrophoresis axis.

Assuming that the image at hand passes these checks – as we will see in Section 4, this might require the application of a few manually-guided image processing operations – the employed methodology detects the boundaries of the lanes that are depicted. Then, with the help of the inter-lane regions it models the background intensity of the image as a polynomial of the image coordinates. Next, it removes the background intensity from the lane areas to keep only the intensity component of the acquired image that is induced by the viral material. All these operations are performed automatically and have been documented in detail elsewhere (Maramis & Delopoulos, 2010a).

This produces a set of background-corrected lane images like the one depicted in Fig. 3(a). The extraction of the intensity profile, $p(\cdot)$, of each lane image concludes this phase. However, due to the presence of noise in the image, instead of taking a single slice of the lane image we aggregate the intensity information along the axis that is perpendicular to electrophoresis (let this be denoted by Y). Thus, if $I(\cdot)$ is the background-corrected image of a lane and D is the image size along axis X, the intensity profile of the lane is given by the expression:

$$p(x) = \underset{y}{\text{median}}\{I(x,y)\} \quad x = 1,2,\ldots,D\,. \tag{6}$$

3.3 Fragment information extraction

The objective of this phase is to estimate certain properties of the DNA fragments that are contained in the lane of a sample. More specifically, we refer to an *initial* estimation of the fragment lengths and concentrations that are associated with the molecule populations on the lane. For this purpose, the employed methodology makes use of the previously extracted intensity profiles and the observation model of Section 3.1. The steps of this phase are described in the following sections.

3.3.1 Peak area detection

This step has not been described in the introductory papers of the employed methodology (Maramis et al., 2010; 2011). It is applied on every intensity profile that has been extracted in Section 3.2 and its objective is to determine (i) the number and *approximate* positions of the peaks in the intensity profile, and (ii) the set of datapoints that constitute the body of each peak. The latter information is utilized by all the subsequent steps of the methodology that involve curve fitting (Sections 3.3.2 and 3.4.2).

First, the rolling disk technique (Mikhailyuk & Razzhivin, 2003) is applied to eliminate from the profile any possible background intensity residuals. The disk radius (parameter θ_1) controls the sensitivity of the aforementioned technique to intensity variations in the profile. After that, the intensity profile is smoothed (θ_2 denotes the order of the smoothing filter) and the watershed algorithm (Vincent & Soille, 1991) detects the local maxima (i.e., peaks) of the intensity profile curve. In order to eliminate possible false peaks (i.e., peaks that do not correspond to real HPV-related bands), a thresholding procedure is employed to rule out peaks lower than a certain multiple (parameter $\theta_3 \geqslant 1$) of the median value of the intensity profile. Next, the watershed algorithm is applied for the second time to detect the pair of the profile's local minima that are adjacent to both sides of each profile peak. Each pair of local minima defines a sequence of profile points which includes the corresponding peak. The central part of this sequence ("representing" the peak's body) will be employed for fitting purposes in the rest of the typing process. The parameter θ_4 specifies the percentage of profile points that are selected for fitting. The selected profile points from all the peaks are aggregated into the set, $\boldsymbol{X}_{\mathrm{F}}$, of the profile's fitting points.

The parameters θ_1 to θ_4 are going to be revisited in the description of HPVTyper in Section 4.

3.3.2 Initial intensity profile fitting

In this step, a simplified model originating from the observation model is employed for each intensity profile that has been extracted – this applies to both the image's ladders and

HPV-related lanes. This model deliberately ignores the – unknown at this point – correlation of the intensity profile peaks through the FLPs of the infecting HPV types. For a lane with K peaks the simplified intensity profile model, $p_m(\cdot)$, is given by the formula

$$p_m(x;\boldsymbol{\rho}) = \sum_{i=1}^{K} A_i \cdot \exp\Big(-\frac{1}{\gamma_i}|\frac{x-x_i}{\beta_i}|^{\gamma_i}\Big) \quad x = 1,2,\ldots,D\,, \tag{7}$$

where $\boldsymbol{\rho} = [A_1, \beta_1, \gamma_1, x_1, \ldots, A_K, \beta_K, \gamma_K, x_K]$.

The above model is fitted to the extracted intensity profile using the least squares optimization criterion. Formally, this involves finding the parameter vector $\boldsymbol{\rho}_{\text{opt}}$ that satisfies the following equation:

$$\boldsymbol{\rho}_{\text{opt}} = \arg\min_{\boldsymbol{\rho}} \sum_{x \in \boldsymbol{X}_{\text{F}}} \big(p(x) - p_m(x;\boldsymbol{\rho})\big)^2\,. \tag{8}$$

This optimization procedure is called *initial intensity profile fitting* and is carried out once for each lane of the examined image by means of an established optimization algorithm.

3.3.3 Fragment mobility calibration

This step applies only to the ladders of the image and aims to calibrate the fragment mobility function, $d(\cdot)$, of the observation model. In other words, it attempts to calculate the parameter vector $\boldsymbol{\pi}$ (see Section 3.1) that optimally describes the position-length relation of the DNA fragments in the image at hand. Although ideally this relation should be a constant characteristic of the image, the presence of noise and the approximate nature of the fragment mobility function justify the use of all the available ladders to estimate as accurately as possible the position-length relation for various regions of the image.

Focusing on a ladder that includes K peaks, the positions of the peak centers in the intensity profile have been estimated in the previous step; let these be denoted by x_i^* for $i = 1,2,\ldots,K$. Moreover, the ladder specifications provide the molecular lengths that correspond to the aforementioned peaks; let these be expressed as l_i^* for $i = 1,2,\ldots,K$. Then, the optimal parameter vector $\boldsymbol{\pi}_{\text{opt}}$ is given by the expression

$$\boldsymbol{\pi}_{\text{opt}} = \arg\min_{\boldsymbol{\pi}} \sum_{i=1}^{K} \big(x_i^* - d(l_i^*;\boldsymbol{\pi})\big)^2\,. \tag{9}$$

The described *fragment mobility calibration* is performed for each ladder of the image by means of an established optimization algorithm.

3.3.4 Fragment properties estimation

The fragment lengths and concentrations that correspond to the observed populations of HPV DNA molecules (i.e., the observed intensity profile peaks) of each lane are estimated in this step. This applies only to the HPV-related lanes of the experiment. For this purpose, each HPV-related lane is associated with a ladder (possibly the one lying closer to the lane on the gel matrix), which lends the lane its optimized fragment mobility function (Section 3.3.3).

Since the peak positions, x_i, of a profile have been estimated during the initial intensity profile fitting, the fragment lengths, l_i, that are associated with the peaks can be calculated by the inverse of the calibrated fragment mobility function as follows:

$$l_i = d^{(-1)}(x_i; \boldsymbol{\pi}_{\text{opt}}) \quad i = 1, 2, \ldots, K, \tag{10}$$

where the parameter vector $\boldsymbol{\pi}_{\text{opt}}$ optimizes the fragment mobility function of the employed ladder and we have assumed that the intensity profile includes K peaks.

Equations (5) and (7) are combined to produce the following formula that estimates the fragment concentrations:

$$c_i' = \frac{2\gamma_i^{1/\gamma_i}\beta_i\Gamma(1/\gamma_i)}{l_i\gamma_i} \cdot A_i \quad i = 1, 2, \ldots, K. \tag{11}$$

It is worth mentioning that c_i' denotes the *apparent concentration* of the ith fragment population on the lane, i.e., the concentration that is calculated if we assume that the parameter f in (5) is equal to 1. This assumption does not harm the employed methodology, since we are only interested in the relative concentrations of the observed fragment populations – this will become clear in Section 3.4. For the calculation of the various c_i', the β_i and γ_i values that have been optimized by (8) and the l_i values that have been estimated by (10) are employed.

3.4 HPV typing algorithm

In this phase the actual typing decisions are made. The *HPV typing algorithm* is charged with the task of deciding which HPV types or combinations of them are able to explain the observed intensity profile peaks of a lane both qualitatively and quantitatively – by means of the observation model. First, all the considered genotypes are checked with respect to their compatibility with the observed peaks (Section 3.4.1) and those that are found incompatible are rejected. Then, each possible combination of compatible genotypes is treated as a hypothesis that is tested for its ability to produce the intensity profile (Section 3.4.2). Finally, the combinations of compatible genotypes are ranked (Section 3.4.3) by a certain score that combines their results in the previous test with the combination's prior probability.

3.4.1 Genotype compatibility check

Let us assume that the intensity profile of the investigated lane has K peaks lying at positions $\boldsymbol{x} = [x_1, x_2, \ldots, x_K]$ and we want to check the compatibility of genotype T with aforementioned profile. If $\boldsymbol{l} = [l_1, l_2, \ldots, l_N]$ denotes the FLP of T, then we define the function $a(\cdot) : [1, \ldots, N] \to [1, \ldots, K]$ that assigns the FLP components to the profile peaks such that: $a(i) = j$ denotes that the ith component of $\boldsymbol{l}$ *resides* at the jth peak.

Among all possible assignments, we select $a^*(\cdot)$ that minimizes:

$$C_{T,a(\cdot)} = \frac{1}{N}\sum_{i=1}^{N}\left(d(l_i; \boldsymbol{\pi}_{\text{opt}}) - x_{a(i)}\right)^2. \tag{12}$$

Depending on the gel electrophoresis and imaging parameters, the DNA fragments of lengths l_{i_1} and l_{i_2} ($l_{i_1} \neq l_{i_2}$) that correspond to the FLP components with indices $i_1 \neq i_2$ can be perceived as contributing to the same observed peak. However, in the selection of $a^*(\cdot)$ we permit assignment coincidence for components i_1 and i_2 (i.e., $a(i_1) = a(i_2)$) only if the expected positions of fragments i_1 and i_2 are close enough to each other, i.e.,

$$|d(l_{i_1};\boldsymbol{\pi}_{\text{opt}}) - d(l_{i_2};\boldsymbol{\pi}_{\text{opt}})| \leqslant \theta_5 . \tag{13}$$

The parameter θ_5 is called *coincidence threshold* and, given a parameter vector $\boldsymbol{\pi}_{\text{opt}}$, determines whether two diverse fragment lengths can be assigned to the same peak or not.

The *compatibility degree* of genotype T is defined as $C_T = C_{T,a^*(\cdot)}$ and has to not exceed the *compatibility threshold* θ_6 should the genotype be considered compatible with the intensity profile (i.e., $C_T \leqslant \theta_6$).

3.4.2 Genotype combination testing

In the combination testing procedure, the phenomenon of *partial digestion* is taken into account. Up to this point, the term FLP has been used to denote the pattern of fragment lengths that results from the digestion of *all* the restriction sites in the amplified DNA molecule (*full digestion*). In this sense, if the amplified molecule of an HPV genotype T contains $N-1$ restriction sites, then the genotype's FLP will be $\boldsymbol{l} = [l_1, l_2, \ldots, l_N]$. However, sometimes restriction enzymes fail to digest the amplified DNA at one or more of the above sites; in these cases FLPs corresponding to partial digestion coexist with the FLP resulting from full digestion. For instance, $\boldsymbol{l}' = [l_1 + l_2, l_3 \ldots, l_N]$ is the result of the enzyme's failure at the first restriction site. To avoid confusion, for the rest of this chapter the terms *main FLP* (mFLP) and *partial digestion FLP* (pdFLP) are employed for full and partial digestion respectively.

For a combination of compatible genotypes $\boldsymbol{t} = \{T_1, \ldots, T_M\}$, $\boldsymbol{l}^k = [l_1^k, \ldots, l_{N_k}^k]$ is employed to denote the mFLP of T_k, with N_k being the number of fragments in $\boldsymbol{l}^k$. With respect to the assignment $a_k^*(\cdot)$ of T_k we adopt the optimal assignment that was selected for this genotype during the compatibility check. Then, the operations that are described in the following paragraphs are performed on combination $\boldsymbol{t}$.

Qualitative peak justification

First, the genotype combination is tested for its ability to qualitatively justify *all* the observed peaks of the profile, with or without the help of a number of pdFLPs that result from the participating HPV genotypes. Only the pdFLPs that result from up to a certain number of cleavage failures (parameter θ_7) are considered. These pdFLPs are combined to form a set of *subhypotheses* so that each subhypothesis includes all the mFLPs of $\boldsymbol{t}$ and a specific subset of the possible pdFLPs. A subhypothesis is accepted at this step if it satisfies the following *qualitative peak justification* criterion:

$$\forall j = 1, \ldots, K \quad \exists k, i \text{ such that } a_k^*(i) = j, \tag{14}$$

where the assignments of the involved pdFLPs (i.e., $a_k^*(\cdot)$ for $k > M$) are also considered; these are selected in the same manner as the mFLP assignments (see Section 3.4.1). Among the subhypotheses that satisfy the above criterion, we select the one that includes the fewest pdFLPs and this is propagated to the following step. If no subhypothesis satisfies the criterion, combination $\boldsymbol{t}$ is rejected.

Intensity profile fitting

In this step, the most crucial of the typing algorithm, the investigated genotype combination hypothesis attempts to explain the intensity profile data as the superposition of contributions from the involved FLPs. In this task, each genotype combination is "represented" by its optimally performing subhypothesis from the previous step.

Let us assume that the selected subhypothesis of the investigated combination $\boldsymbol{t}$ consists of Q FLPs (M mFLPs and $Q - M$ pdFLPs). Based on (5) of the observation model, the individual contribution of the qth FLP $\boldsymbol{l}^q = [l_1^q, \ldots, l_{N_q}^q]$ to the observed intensity profile is given by the equation:

$$i_q(x; c'_q, \boldsymbol{\theta}_q, \phi) = c'_q \sum_{i=1}^{N_q} l_i^q \cdot r(x_i^q) \cdot w(x; \beta_i^q, \gamma_i^q, x_i^q) \quad x = 1, 2, \ldots, D, \tag{15}$$

where ϕ is the attenuation factor in (3), c'_q is the apparent concentration of the FLP and $\boldsymbol{\theta}_q = [\beta_1^q, \gamma_1^q, x_1^q, \ldots, \beta_{N_q}^q, \gamma_{N_q}^q, x_{N_q}^q]$.

The intensity profile model of the investigated genotype combination $\boldsymbol{t}$ results from aggregating the contributions of the participating FLPs as follows:

$$\overline{p}_m(x; \overline{\boldsymbol{\rho}}) = \sum_{q=1}^{Q} i_q(x; c'_q, \boldsymbol{\theta}_q, \phi) \quad x = 1, 2, \ldots, D, \tag{16}$$

where $\overline{\boldsymbol{\rho}} = [c'_1, \boldsymbol{\theta}_1, \ldots, c'_Q, \boldsymbol{\theta}_Q, \phi]$. The latter vector plays in the present task the same role with the parameter vector $\boldsymbol{\rho}$ of the simplified intensity profile model of (7). The optimal intensity profile model of $\boldsymbol{t}$ results from the following expression:

$$\overline{\boldsymbol{\rho}}_{opt} = \arg\min_{\overline{\boldsymbol{\rho}}} \sum_{x \in \boldsymbol{X}_\mathrm{F}} \left(p(x) - \overline{p}_m(x; \overline{\boldsymbol{\rho}})\right)^2. \tag{17}$$

In the minimization of (17) the following constraint applies: The concentration of a pdFLP is not allowed to exceed a percentage (parameter $\theta_8 < 1$) of the concentration of the corresponding mFLP. The calculation of $\overline{\boldsymbol{\rho}}_\mathrm{opt}$ in (17) under the aforementioned constraint is undertaken by an established optimization algorithm. The initialization of the optimization procedure is performed with the help of the estimates that have been obtained for the fragment properties from the initial intensity profile fitting (Section 3.3.2).

3.4.3 Genotype combination ranking

The score that is employed for ranking the tested combinations of compatible genotypes takes into account both the fitting results of the previous step (Section 3.4.2) and the prior probability of the combination.

Focusing on genotype combination $\boldsymbol{t}$, if $\overline{\boldsymbol{\rho}}_\mathrm{opt}^{\boldsymbol{t}}$ is the optimized parameter vector of the combination's profile model and $\|\boldsymbol{X}_\mathrm{F}\|$ is the number of employed fitting points, the mean squared fitting error of $\boldsymbol{t}$ is defined by the expression

$$J(\boldsymbol{t}) = \frac{1}{\|\boldsymbol{X}_\mathrm{F}\|} \sum_{x \in \boldsymbol{X}_\mathrm{F}} \left(p(x) - \overline{p}_m(x; \overline{\boldsymbol{\rho}}_\mathrm{opt}^{\boldsymbol{t}})\right)^2. \tag{18}$$

Moreover, if J_0 is the mean squared error obtained from the initial fitting of the investigated profile (Section 3.3.2), i.e.,

$$J_0 = \frac{1}{\|\boldsymbol{X}_\mathrm{F}\|} \sum_{x \in \boldsymbol{X}_\mathrm{F}} \left(p(x) - p_m(x; \boldsymbol{\rho}_\mathrm{opt})\right)^2, \tag{19}$$

$P_0(\boldsymbol{t})$ is the joint prior probability of the HPV types from which the genotypes in $\boldsymbol{t}$ stem, and K is the number of peaks in the profile, then, the score of $\boldsymbol{t}$ is given by the formula

$$R(\boldsymbol{t}) = -2K\frac{J(\boldsymbol{t})}{J_0} + \theta_9 \cdot \ln\left(P_0(\boldsymbol{t})\right). \tag{20}$$

The parameter θ_9, which is called *prior weight*, is employed to adjust the significance of the prior probability in the ranking process. Its value is positive and defaults to 1.

As one can anticipate from (20), the score only takes negative values, and a genotype combination whose score is close to 0 denotes a better solution than an combination with lower score. The *eligibility threshold* θ_{10} is employed to discriminate between the tested genotype combinations that are considered to be solutions to the problem (i.e., $R(\boldsymbol{t}) \geqslant \theta_{10}$) and those that are not.

4. Description of HPVTyper

HPVTyper is a novel software application for analyzing images that have resulted from the PCR-RFLP examination with the intention of performing accurate and automatic HPV typing. This is achieved by employing the typing methodology that has been presented in Section 3. The application consists of an *engine module* that undertakes all the computations which are involved in the typing methodology (e.g., the initial intensity profile fitting of Section 3.3.2) and a *user interface module* that allows the user to interact graphically with the application. The classic client-server architecture has been employed for implementing the communication between the engine and the user interface.

HPVTyper has been designed upon the following principle: The application automates as many of the involved operations as possible while, at the same, it allows the user to intervene essentially at any stage of the typing procedure. This principle is implemented by means of an abundant set of parameters – the already defined parameters θ_1 to θ_{10} are among them. Each parameter possesses a predetermined default value which is used in the involved operations, unless the user wishes to change/adjust it via the graphical user interface.

All the functionalities of the application are made available through four windows, which are described in detail in the following sections.

4.1 Image Processing Window

The main window of HPVTyper is called *Image Processing Window*. This window is presented to the user when HPVTyper initiates and it is mainly concerned with loading the PCR-RFLP images to be analyzed, performing all the required image preprocessing operations on them (Section 3.2), and introducing the depicted lanes. The layout of the Image Processing Window is illustrated in the screenshot of Fig. 4.

As it can be observed in Fig 4, most of the window area is covered by a pane that displays the currently loaded PCR-RFLP image along with a marker indicating positions on the gel

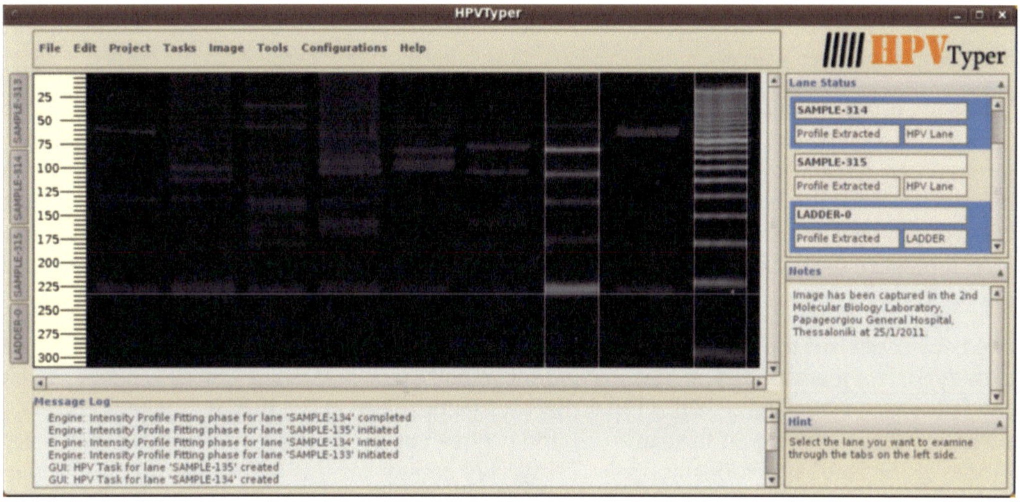

Fig. 4. Screenshot of the Image Processing Window.

electrophoresis axis (the vertical axis of the image). This is the *image workspace pane* and it can also display certain intermediate image preprocessing results (e.g., the lane boundaries). Below this pane, there is the *message log pane* which displays messages from either the engine module or the user interface module regarding the progress of the HPV typing procedure. With respect to the engine messages, these are the means of the application for notifying the user about changes in the status of computationally expensive operations that are queued in the engine module (e.g., the initiation/termination of the genotype combination testing phase for a particular lane.).

On the right side of the window there is a column that includes three more panes. The first from the top is the *lane status pane*, which allows the user to provide a name for each lane of the active image and to classify it as either HPV-related or ladder. Moreover, it informs the user about the processing status of each lane (e.g., "Boundaries Detected", "Profile Extracted"). When the user selects a lane from the current pane, its position on the loaded image is highlighted as illustrated in Fig. 4. The *notes pane* is located in the middle of the column and allows the user to write down their notes on the present HPV typing assignment in free-text format. The notes are saved and reloaded each time the user opens the same HPV typing project – the concept of HPV typing project will be defined later in the present section. Finally, the *hint pane* contains helpful suggestions of the application to the user regarding the subsequent steps of the typing procedure.

In addition to the aforementioned panes, the Image Processing Window includes a series of menus (ordered in a row on the top of the window) that expose most of the HPVTyper's functionalities to the user.

The most simple functional usage scenario of the main window of HPVTyper is summarized in the following paragraphs. All the described operations are triggered by means of the menu that emerges when right-clicking on the image, unless specified otherwise. First, a PCR-RFLP gel electrophoresis image is loaded to the application through the *File menu*. This action creates an *HPV typing project* dedicated to the typing of the lanes that are included in the image. A number of processing operations can be applied on the image so as to ensure that it passes the quality checks of Section 3.2; these operations include cropping the image, rotating it, and inverting its grayscale levels.

When the image is ready, the user triggers the automatic lane detection operation. Once this operation is completed, the detected lane boundaries are overlaid on the image. At this point, the user can revise/adjust the boundaries of some or all the lanes by moving the displayed boundaries with the help of the mouse. When satisfied with the lane boundaries, the user triggers the background subtraction operation. This is performed automatically and, after its completion, the background-corrected image replaces the original in the image workspace pane.

Next, the user visits the lane status pane in order to provide names for the lanes of interest and classify each of them as HPV-related [3] or ladder. When a lane is selected – by left-clicking on its cell in the lane status pane – HPVTyper displays its position on the image (image workspace pane). By right-clicking on the same cell, the user can ask HPVTyper to extract the intensity profile of the lane. When this happens, HPVTyper creates for this lane either an *HPV typing task*, in case of an HPV-related lane, or a *mobility calibration task*, in case of a ladder. The created task is tied to the selected lane and is uniquely identifiable within the active HPV typing project.

4.2 Profile Processing Window

All the operations that are necessary for carrying out an HPV typing or mobility calibration task are performed in the *Profile Processing Window*. This includes mainly the operations described in Sections 3.3 and 3.4. Each of the HPV typing or mobility calibration tasks that have been created in the main window maintains its own Profile Processing Window. Upon the creation of such a task, a button that activates the corresponding Profile Processing Window is added in a column on the left end of the Image Processing Window.

The layout of the Profile Processing Window that corresponds to an HPV-related lane is illustrated in the screenshot of Fig. 5. This includes three panes. Most of the window area is covered by the *profile workspace pane*, which is designed to undertake the fragment information extraction operations described in Section 3.3. On the other hand, the panes in the right column, namely the *compatibility check pane* (top) and the *combination testing pane* (bottom), are meant to carry out the operations corresponding to the HPV typing algorithm (see Section 3.4).

In the profile workspace pane, the horizontal axis identifies with the electrophoresis axis. The pane displays four vertically aligned items, which are (starting from the bottom):

1. The image of the ladder that has been associated with the lane under investigation.
2. The virtual marker that has resulted from the calibration of the aforementioned ladder. This marker specifies the relation between positions and fragment lengths (in bp).
3. The background-corrected image of the investigated lane.
4. The intensity profile that has been extracted from the aforementioned lane.

At the bottom of the profile workspace pane, the user can adjust the values of parameters θ_1 to θ_4 (see Section 3.3.1) and also change the ladder that is associated with the investigated lane.

[3] In the application the term *HPV lane* is employed to denote those lanes that need to be typed.

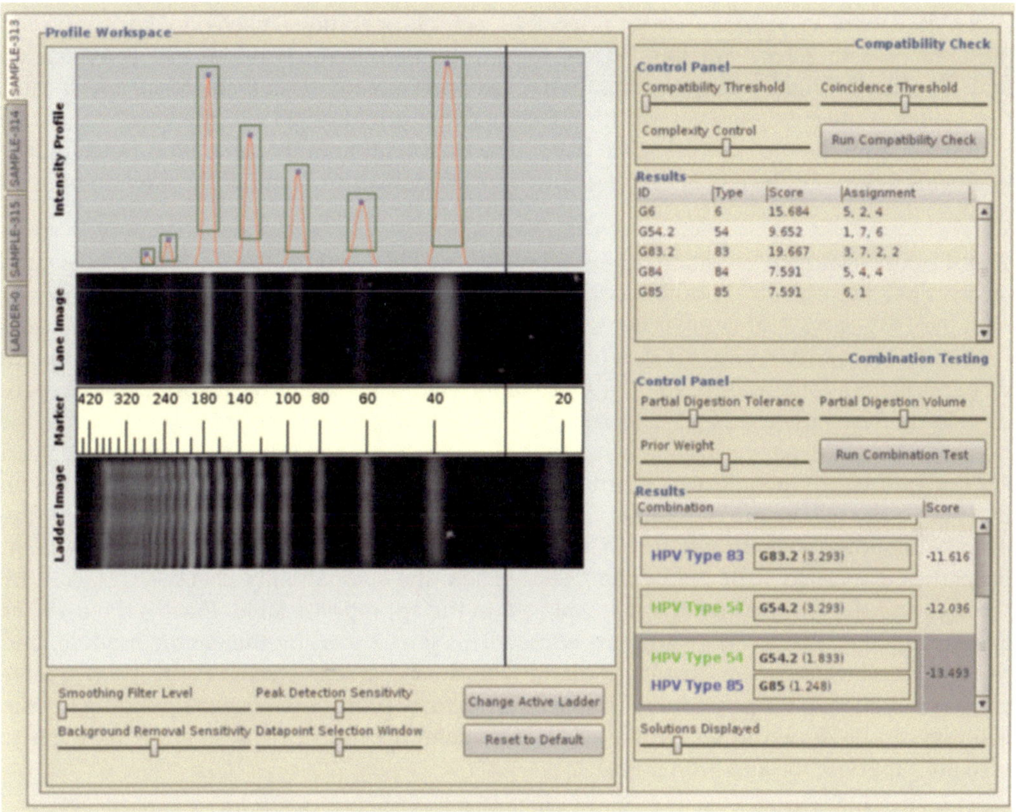

Fig. 5. Screenshot of the Profile Processing Window.

The compatibility check pane, which deals with the procedure described in Section 3.4.1, is divided into two parts. The upper part is employed to control the compatibility check procedure (parameters θ_5 and θ_6) and determine the maximum number of compatible genotypes that can be considered by the application (*complexity control* slider). This way, the computational complexity involved in the combination testing phase of the HPV typing algorithm can be controlled by the user. In the lower part, the compatibility check results are presented in a table which includes (i) the genotypes that are found to be compatible with the profile, (ii) the HPV types to which they belong, (iii) the scores that they have achieved in the compatibility check, and (iv) the selected assignment, $a^*(\cdot)$, of each genotype's FLP.

The combination testing pane, which serves the operations described in Sections 3.4.2 and 3.4.3, resembles in terms of design the previous pane: It is divided into an upper part that controls the combination testing and ranking procedure and a lower part that displays the results. In the upper part the values of parameters θ_7 to θ_{10} can be defined. In the lower part, the solutions of the HPV typing algorithm are displayed – sorted by their scores – in a table that includes for each solution (i) its score, (ii) the participating genotypes and associated concentrations that achieve this score, and (iii) the HPV types to which the genotypes belong. A color-coding scheme is employed for the types based on their oncogenic risk (e.g., green denotes low-risk types). The maximum number of solutions that can be displayed is specified with the help of a slider at the bottom of the pane.

When it comes to ladders, only a reduced set of operations needs to be supported (Sections 3.3.1 to 3.3.3). For this reason, the Profile Processing Window that is associated with a ladder is slightly different from what has been already described. More specifically, the compatibility check and combination testing panes are disabled and the lane image item is missing from the profile workspace pane. The fragment mobility calibration functionality is provided through the corresponding option in the right-click menu of the aforementioned pane.

The shortest sequence of actions that completes an HPV typing task is briefly presented below. First, the user has to calibrate the mobility function from the ladder that is associated with the HPV-related lane under investigation. This procedure is performed on the ladder's Profile Processing Window. At this point, all the operations described in Section 3.3.1 can be performed automatically by HPVTyper via the right-click menu of the profile workspace pane and afterwards modified manually by the user in a context-aware manner. Once the calibration is achieved, the user switches to the Profile Processing Window of the investigated HPV-related lane. Operations similar to those performed for the ladder can be attempted on this profile as well, before requesting HPVTyper to execute the initial intensity profile fitting process. Following the profile fitting, the application automatically estimates the fragment properties associated with the profile peaks. Then, the compatibility check is triggered by the user and the obtained results are displayed in the appropriate table. Finally, the user has to initiate the combination testing procedure. This is executed by the engine module, and the computed solutions are displayed along with their characteristics in the respective table upon completion of the procedure. The optimal intensity profile model corresponding to each solution can be drawn in the profile workspace pane upon user request, allowing them to visually supervise the end fitting results.

4.3 Configuration Editors

By the term *Configuration Editors* we refer to two distinct windows that are employed for editing the information required for making the HPV typing decisions. These windows, namely the *PCR-RFLP Configuration Editor* and the *Type Configuration Editor*, are meant to be used rarely, e.g., whenever new scientific discoveries need to be taken into account in the typing process. They can both be accessed through the *Configurations menu* of the main window and are described in the following sections.

4.3.1 PCR-RFLP Configuration Editor

Since various combinations of primers and restriction enzymes can be employed for a PCR-RFLP examination and also various HPV genotypes may be considered in an HPV typing task, the knowledge of the above parameters – the *PCR-RFLP configuration* – is necessary when one attempts to perform HPV typing on an acquired PCR-RFLP image. The present window allows the user to insert information regarding the above configuration into HPVTyper. The application can store many different PCR-RFLP configurations and the user is responsible for assigning the appropriate one to each HPV typing task through the *Tasks menu* of the application's main window.

The layout of the PCR-RFLP Configuration Editor is illustrated in the screenshot of Fig. 6 and its usage is straightforward. In the upper part of the window, the user can switch between the stored configurations, keep configuration-related notes, and define the associated PCR primers and restriction enzyme(s). In the lower part of the window, the application displays in a tabular form (i) the HPV genotypes that are considered in the present configuration (user-defined names are employed), (ii) their GenBank accession ID, (iii) the HPV types to which they belong, (iv) the length of their amplicon, and (v) their fragment length pattern. On the right side of this table, there is a form for editing the genotype-specific information.

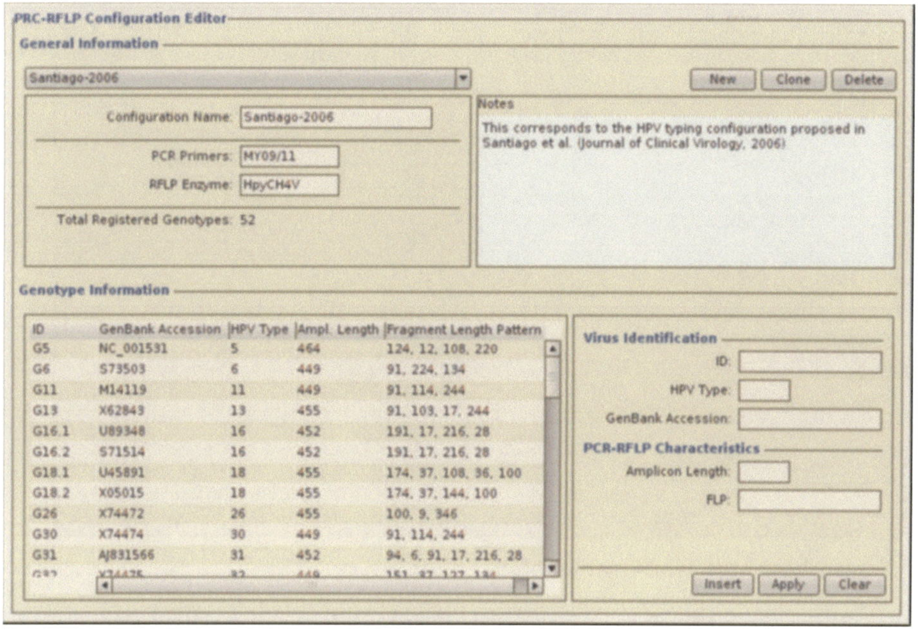

Fig. 6. Screenshot of the PCR-RFLP Configuration Editor.

4.3.2 Type Configuration Editor

The HPV types demonstrate significant variations in their prevalence in different populations and tissue types. Since the typing methodology that is employed by HPVTyper explicitly uses the prior probabilities of the various HPV types to make its typing decisions, it is reasonable to allow multiple sets of prior probabilities to be included in the application. This way, the appropriate set of prior probabilities that best suits an examined tissue sample by geographic and/or anatomic criteria can be employed.

The present window allows the user to edit an existing set of prior probabilities or insert a new set. In addition, it provides the user with the opportunity to define the oncogenic risk of each HPV type; this information is used in the color-coded representation of the types in the Profile Processing Window.

The design of the present window resembles that of the PCR-RFLP Configuration Editor and all the provided functionalities are straightforward. The layout of the Type Configuration Editor is illustrated in the screenshot of Fig. 7.

5. Important features of HPVTyper

As it may have become clear from the presentation of the employed methodology but also from the description of the application itself, HPVTyper demonstrates several noticeable

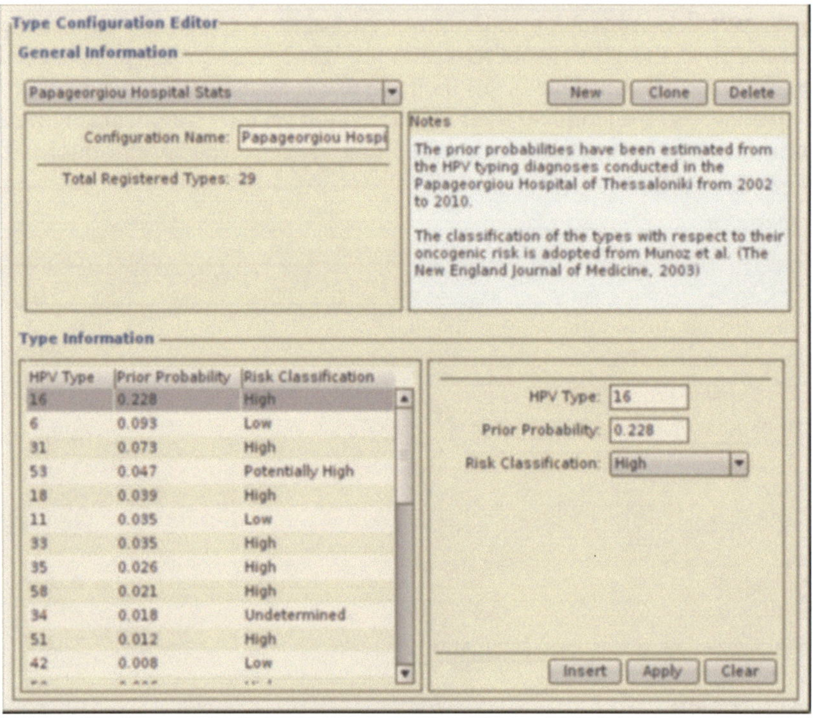

Fig. 7. Screenshot of the Type Configuration Editor.

features. When combined, these features establish HPVTyper as a noteworthy HPV typing approach that is significantly differentiated from its counterparts. The most important of the application's features are outlined in this section.

Accurate typing decisions. The typing methodology that has been presented in Section 3 has been adequately evaluated with respect to its accuracy, yielding very satisfactory results (Maramis et al., 2011). Since HPVTyper employs this methodology, the typing decisions that are made with the help of the application are very accurate. This is true for cases of single HPV infection and – more importantly – for complex cases involving multiple infections. In fact, the aforementioned methodology is the only established way to resolve the latter cases when attempting HPV typing via PCR-RFLP gel electrophoresis.

Automatic typing procedure. HPV typing with HPVTyper can be performed completely automatically. This applies to the entire typing procedure (Sections 3.2 to 3.4) but its importance focuses on the automatic application of the HPV typing algorithm (Section 3.4), since such a feature has been missing from all the previous typing algorithms. In the case of HPVTyper, this feature derives from the computerized nature of the employed methodology along with the use of default values for the set of involved parameters (e.g., parameters θ_1 to θ_{10}) and significantly eases the typing process for the user.

Supervised typing procedure. Although HPVTyper provides the possibility of automatic typing, at the same time, it allows the user to supervise the entire typing procedure. This includes presenting intermediate results to the user (the outcome of initial intensity profile fitting, the outcome of type compatibility check, etc.) and also allowing them to adjust a wide range of parameters that can influence the typing result (e.g., parameters θ_1 to θ_{10}).

This way, the user has full control on the typing procedure and is able to verify themselves step-by-step the correctness of the application's results.

Free availability. Since HPVTyper can be obtained for free, each molecular biology laboratory that possesses the required equipment for performing HPV typing via PCR-RFLP gel electrophoresis can benefit from the presented HPV typing method without any additional cost. In these laboratories the conventional manual method for HPV typing via PCR-RFLP could be replaced with minimum effort by HPVTyper in order to update the employed HPV typing procedure.

Adaptability to emerging discoveries. Scientific research regarding HPV and its connection to cervical cancer is very active. For this reason, it is possible to see in the future new types and genotypes of the virus being discovered, new restriction enzymes and primers being employed for HPV typing, the infection frequency and risk of some HPV types being revised, etc. HPVTyper can easily cope with such scientific discoveries that may emerge by means of its Configuration Editors. The user simply has to edit the information that has become obsolete or add new information through the PCR-RFLP or Type Configuration Editor and the application remains up-to-date. In this sense, HPVTyper is a future-proof HPV typing method.

Expandability to new domains. Although the application has been originally developed as a diagnostic method for the domain of cervical cancer, it can easily find application to every cancer domain in which HPV is involved. Similarly to the previous feature, the information that is related to a new cancer domain can be incorporated in the application with minimum effort by means of the Configuration Editors.

6. Availability

HPVTyper is made freely available to the public through the webpage `http://hippocrates.ee.auth.gr/HPVTyper/` and is subject to the license described therein. The powerful engine module that is installed on the aforementioned server is employed for performing the required computations, while the user interface module is installed to the user's computer by means of the Java Web Start Technology. The use of the aforementioned technology ensures minimum file downloading, automatic updates, and operating system independence at the user's side. A copy of the application's source code can be obtained for free from the above webpage under the same license agreement.

7. Conclusion

In this present chapter, we have introduced HPVTyper, a novel software application for accurate and automatic HPV typing via PCR-RFLP gel electrophoresis. The strength of HPVTyper derives primarily from the underlying HPV typing methodology. This entirely computerized methodology has been justified in parts and as a whole by a series of scientific publications (Maramis & Delopoulos, 2010a;b; Maramis et al., 2010; 2011) and its performance with respect to typing accuracy has been thoroughly evaluated on real HPV typing data (Maramis et al., 2011). By employing this methodology, HPVTyper is able to make accurate typing decisions even for multiply-infected cases in an entirely automatic manner.

The second cornerstone of HPVTyper's strength is its design. The application provides the user with a friendly and straightforward interfacing mechanism to perform all the operations that are involved in the typing process, either as suggested by the application (default parameter values) or according to the user's will (user-adjusted parameter values). Any intermediate results are presented to the user so that they can constantly check the progress of the typing procedure. Owing to the aforementioned design principles, the user has full control over the entire typing process and is able to choose their degree of involvement in the procedure.

The application scope of HPVTyper is impressively wide. By providing tools to easily edit the information that is required for the typing decision, the application can be expanded to include new HPV-related discoveries in the domain of cervical cancer as well as to perform HPV typing in the framework of other cancer domains that are associated with HPV. Finally, it is worth mentioning that the implemented software application could just as well be employed for typing other viruses, should this be required.

A foreseeable future addition to HPVTyper concerns the issue of mutation hotspots in the genome of HPV. When these mutations occur at the restriction sites of the amplified HPV DNA sequence, the resulting FLP of an infecting genotype does not match its expected FLP. Consequently, these mutations constitute a serious threat to the efficacy of the PCR-RFLP typing method in general, no matter whether this is performed manually or by means of HPVTyper.

Fortunately, the powerful decision making mechanism of our application along with the analysis of Section 3.4.2 regarding the phenomenon of partial digestion – already incorporated in the employed methodology – set the ground for future versions of HPVTyper to tackle the aforementioned issue. In fact, these altered mutation-related FLPs are essentially partial digestion FLPs and – just like the latter – they can be foreseen.

With respect to the required modifications on the employed methodology, the compatibility check operation must be updated so as to search for a set of reasonably possible mutation-induced FLPs in addition to the main FLP of an investigated genotype. This flexible compatibility check will allow us to diagnose – with reduced confidence of course (e.g., by adding a penalty to the final score) – infections from HPV types with slightly mutated genomes. However, it should be noted that this approach will induce a significant increase on the computational complexity of the decision making process – an issue that will have to be tackled – and could potentially disturb the accuracy of the employed methodology.

8. References

Barzon, L., Militello, V., Lavezzo, E., Franchin, E., Peta, E., Squarzon, L., Trevisan, M., Pagni, S., Dal Bello, F., Toppo, S. et al. (2011). Human papillomavirus genotyping by 454 next generation sequencing technology, *Journal of Clinical Virology* 52(2): 93–97.

Bosch, F., Lorincz, A., Muñoz, N., Meijer, C. & Shah, K. (2002). The causal relation between human papillomavirus and cervical cancer, *Journal of Clinical Pathology* 55(4): 244–265.

Fontaine, V., Mascaux, C., Weyn, C., Bernis, A., Celio, N., Lefèvre, P., Kaufman, L. & Garbar, C. (2007). Evaluation of combined general primer-mediated PCR sequencing and type-specific PCR strategies for determination of human papillomavirus genotypes in cervical cell specimens, *Journal of Clinical Microbiology* 45(3): 928–934.

Gharizadeh, B., Kalantari, M., Garcia, C., Johansson, B. & Nyrén, P. (2001). Typing of human papillomavirus by pyrosequencing, *Laboratory Investigation* 81(5): 673–679.

Gharizadeh, B., Oggionni, M., Zheng, B., Akom, E., Pourmand, N., Ahmadian, A., Wallin, K. & Nyren, P. (2005). Type-specific multiple sequencing primers: a novel strategy for reliable and rapid genotyping of human papillomaviruses by pyrosequencing technology, *Journal of Molecular Diagnostics* 7(2): 198.

Gheit, T., Landi, S., Gemignani, F., Snijders, P., Vaccarella, S., Franceschi, S., Canzian, F. & Tommasino, M. (2006). Development of a sensitive and specific assay combining multiplex PCR and DNA microarray primer extension to detect high-risk mucosal human papillomavirus types, *Journal of Clinical Microbiology* 44(6): 2025.

Greenblatt, R. (2005). Human papillomaviruses: Diseases, diagnosis, and a possible vaccine, *Clinical Microbiology Newsletter* 27(18): 139–145.

Greer Jr, R., Douglas Jr, J., Breese, P. & Crosby, L. (1990). Evaluation of oral and laryngeal specimens for human papillomavirus (HPV) DNA by dot blot hybridization, *Journal of Oral Pathology & Medicine* 19(1): 35–38.

Husnjak, K., Grce, M., Magdic, L. & Pavelic, K. (2000). Comparison of five different polymerase chain reaction methods for detection of human papillomavirus in cervical cell specimens, *Journal of Virological Methods* 88(2): 125–134.

Hwang, T., Jeong, J., Park, M., Han, H., Choi, H. & Park, T. (2003). Detection and typing of HPV genotypes in various cervical lesions by HPV oligonucleotide microarray, *Gynecologic Oncology* 90(1): 51–56.

Jacobs, M., Snijders, P., Van Den Brule, A., Helmerhorst, T., Meijer, C. & Walboomers, J. (1997). A general primer GP5+/GP6 (+)-mediated PCR-enzyme immunoassay method for rapid detection of 14 high-risk and 6 low-risk human papillomavirus genotypes in cervical scrapings, *Journal of Clinical Microbiology* 35(3): 791.

Jordan, B. (2010). Is there a niche for DNA microarrays in molecular diagnostics?, *Expert Review of Molecular Diagnostics* 10(7): 875–882.

Karlsen, F., Kalantari, M., Jenkins, A., Pettersen, E., Kristensen, G., Holm, R., Johansson, B. & Hagmar, B. (1996). Use of multiple PCR primer sets for optimal detection of human papillomavirus, *Journal of Clinical Microbiology* 34(9): 2095.

Kim, C., Jeong, J., Park, M., Park, T., Park, T., Namkoong, S. & Park, J. (2003). HPV oligonucleotide microarray-based detection of HPV genotypes in cervical neoplastic lesions, *Gynecologic Oncology* 89(2): 210–217.

Klaassen, C., Prinsen, C., De Valk, H., Horrevorts, A., Jeunink, M. & Thunnissen, F. (2004). DNA microarray format for detection and subtyping of human papillomavirus, *Journal of Clinical Microbiology* 42(5): 2152.

Kleter, B., Van Doorn, L., Schrauwen, L., Molijn, A., Sastrowijoto, S., Ter Schegget, J., Lindeman, J., Ter Harmsel, B., Burger, M. & Quint, W. (1999). Development and clinical evaluation of a highly sensitive PCR-reverse hybridization line probe assay for detection and identification of anogenital human papillomavirus, *Journal of Clinical Microbiology* 37(8): 2508.

Landis, S., Murray, T., Bolden, S. & Wingo, P. (1999). Cancer statistics, 1999, *CA: A Cancer Journal for Clinicians* 49(1): 8–31.

Liu, Y. (2008). A technological update of molecular diagnostics for infectious diseases, *Infectious Disorders Drug Targets* 8(3): 183.

Lungu, O., Wright, T. & Silverstein, S. (1992). Typing of human papillomaviruses by polymerase chain reaction amplification with L1 consensus primers and RFLP analysis, *Molecular and Cellular Probes* 6(2): 145–152.

Maramis, C. & Delopoulos, A. (2010a). Efficient quantitative information extraction from PCR-RFLP gel electrophoresis images, *Proc. of 20th International Conference on Pattern Recognition, ICPR 2010*, Istanbul, Turkey, pp. 2564–2567.

Maramis, C. & Delopoulos, A. (2010b). Improved modeling of lane intensity profiles on gel electrophoresis images, *Proc. of XII Mediterranean Conference on Medical and Biological Engineering and Computing, MEDICON 2010*, Porto Karas, Greece, pp. 671–674.

Maramis, C., Delopoulos, A. & Lambropoulos, A. (2010). Analysis of PCR-RFLP gel electrophoresis images for accurate and automated HPV typing, *Proc. of 10th International Conference on Information Technology and Applications in Biomedicine, ITAB 2010*, Corfu, Greece, pp. 1–6.

Maramis, C., Delopoulos, A. & Lambropoulos, A. (2011). A computerized methodology for improved virus typing by PCR-RFLP gel electrophoresis, *IEEE Transactions on Biomedical Engineering* 58(8): 2339–2351.

Mikhailyuk, I. & Razzhivin, A. (2003). Background subtraction in experimental data arrays illustrated by the example of Raman spectra and fluorescent gel electrophoresis patterns, *Instruments and Experimental Techniques* 46(6): 765–769.

Moore, D. (2006). Cervical cancer, *Obstetrics & Gynecology* 107(5): 1152–1161.

Muñoz, N., Bosch, F., de Sanjosé, S., Herrero, R., Castellsagué, X., Shah, K., Snijders, P. & Meijer, C. (2003). Epidemiologic classification of human papillomavirus types associated with cervical cancer, *New England Journal of Medicine* 348(6): 518–527.

Nobre, R., Almeida, L. & Martins, T. (2008). Complete genotyping of mucosal human papillomavirus using a restriction fragment length polymorphism analysis and an original typing algorithm, *Journal of Clinical Virology* 42(1): 13–21.

Parkin, D. (2006). The global health burden of infection-associated cancers in the year 2002, *International journal of cancer* 118(12): 3030–3044.

Santiago, E., Camacho, L., Junquera, M. & Vázquez, F. (2006). Full HPV typing by a single restriction enzyme, *Journal of Clinical Virology* 37(1): 38–46.

Tagu, D. & Moussard, C. (2006). *Techniques for Molecular Biology*, Science Pub Inc.

van den Brule, A., Pol, R., Fransen-Daalmeijer, N., Schouls, L., Meijer, C. & Snijders, P. (2002). GP5+/6+ PCR followed by reverse line blot analysis enables rapid and high-throughput identification of human papillomavirus genotypes, *Journal of Clinical Microbiology* 40(3): 779.

Vernon, S., Unger, E. & Williams, D. (2000). Comparison of human papillomavirus detection and typing by cycle sequencing, line blotting, and hybrid capture, *Journal of Clinical Microbiology* 38(2): 651.

Vincent, L. & Soille, P. (1991). Watersheds in digital spaces: an efficient algorithm based onimmersion simulations, *IEEE Transactions on Pattern Analysis and Machine Intelligence* 13(6): 583–598.

Walboomers, J., Jacobs, M., Manos, M., Bosch, F., Kummer, J., Shah, K., Snijders, P., Peto, J., Meijer, C. & Muñoz, N. (1999). Human papillomavirus is a necessary cause of invasive cervical cancer worldwide, *Journal of Pathology* 189(1): 12–19.